R.Golkow, M.D.

Mammography

Mammography

by W. Hoeffken
and M. Lanyi

Technique · Diagnosis
Differential Diagnosis
Results

with contributions by
H. Gajewski and
K.-J. Lennartz

Translated by L. G. Rigler
and R. D. Arndt
assisted by P. Spiegler

516 Illustrations
(32 in color)

1977
W. B. Saunders Company Philadelphia · London · Toronto
Georg Thieme Publishers Stuttgart

Authors:

Professor Dr. med. WALTHER HOEFFKEN
Chefarzt des Strahleninstituts der Allgemeinen Ortskrankenkasse Köln
Machabäerstraße 19—27, D-5000 Köln, FRG

Dr. med. MARTON LANYI
Facharzt für Röntgenologie und Strahlenheilkunde
Kaiserstraße 17—19, D-527 Gummersbach, FRG

Contributors:

Dr. HEINZ GAJEWSKI
Sophienstraße 83, D-8520 Erlangen, FRG

Professor Dr. med. KARL-JOSEF LENNARTZ
Pathologisches Institut der Universität Köln
Josef-Stelzmann-Straße 9, D-5000 Köln-Lindenthal, FRG

Translators:

Professor LEO G. RIGLER, M.D.
Dept. of Radiological Sciences
University of California
Los Angeles, California 90024
United States of America

Asst. Professor ROLF D. ARNDT, M.D.,
Dept. of Radiological Sciences
University of California
Los Angeles, California 90024
United States of America

Asst. Professor PETER SPIEGLER, Ph. D.,
Dept. of Radiological Sciences (Medical Physics)
University of California
Los Angeles, California 90024
United States of America

Preface

Roentgen examination of the breast has achieved increasing importance in recent years and it should become routine to perform an annual breast examination on all women in the cancer age. This method can no longer be the monopoly of a few specialists; it should be an established procedure in general radiology.

With the advent of molybdenum x-ray tubes the technical problems have been essentially solved. The accuracy of current mammographic diagnosis adequately reflects the present state of medical knowledge.

The roentgen characteristics of pathological processes in the breast are reproducible and are the same whether the mammogram is performed on x-ray film or with the use of xeroradiography. Nonetheless, many xeromammograms have been added to the important chapters for this American edition. It also reflects recent findings, as well as containing some improved illustrations and some new ones. The American edition has thus been brought up to date. We hope it will take its place beside the standard American works on mammography. Now it behooves physicians to correctly understand and interpret the phenomena seen in the roentgenogram. It is the purpose of this book to serve their needs. The best way to gain knowledge in this special method of diagnosis is through the comparison of pathologico-anatomical data with the roentgen findings. This is the fundamental way to formulate a roentgen differential diagnosis.

For this reason, the book is systemically divided into sections dealing with the pathology, clinical findings and radiology of individual breast diseases followed by a section dealing solely with the roentgen differential diagnosis of calcifications and of rounded, stellate, and diffuse densities within the breast.

Special chapters are devoted to the physical and technical aspects of mammography, ductography, technique of puncture and aspiration, cytology, clinical examination of the breast and pneumocystography. Other methods of diagnosis including thermography, ultrasound, and diaphanoscopy (transillumination) are dealt with in the supplement.

It is our hope that this book may shorten the arduous path of gathering personal experience, reduce the incidence of having to learn from one's own errors and allow a high degree of diagnostic acumen to be attained rapidly, in order to make mammography what it should have become long ago: the best method for early detection of breast carcinoma.

WALTHER HOEFFKEN
MARTON LANYI

Cologne and Gummersbach
Spring 1976

Acknowledgments

This book could only be realized through close and intensive cooperation with others. We owe a special debt of thanks to our collaborators Dr. phil. H. Gajewski, Erlangen, Prof. Dr. med. K.-J. Lennartz, Institute of Pathology of Cologne University, and Frau Dr. med. Ch. Merkl, Cytologic Laboratory at Cologne-Rodenkirchen.

Photographic reproduction presented a particular problem. It was necessary to prepare the illustrations by photographic enhancement techniques in order display adequately the significant findings in the final reproductions in the book. We are grateful to our collaborator E. Storch-Rödel for her assistance in this respect.

The first-named author recalls with gratitude his collaboration with Prof. C. Kaufmann, whose wealth of clinical experience helped pave his way into the field of mammography at the University Women's Clinic in Cologne in the late 1950's. Similarly, the second-named author would like to record a debt of gratitude to his sometime chief, the late Prof. P. Deak, for introducing him to mammography and for valuable help during early years at the Budapest Medical Training Institute.

Our thanks are due also to John N. Wolfe for many useful suggestions in regard to xeromammography. It is our great pleasure to have worked with him.

We cordially thank all the others who have assisted us in the preparation and publication of this book:

Dr. E. Albring, Dr. F. Baldus, Dr. F. D. Bückmann, Frau L. Buttenbaum, Priv.-Doz. Dr. P. Citoler, Frau G. Effenberger, Fräulein K. Ferber, Prof. Dr. R. Fischer, Prof. Dr. A. Gregl, Dr. phil. nat. K. Heuss, Dr. J. R. Hüppe, W. Irmer, Dr. H. Jacobs, Ch. Jung, Frau I. Lange, Frau Dr. C. Lendvai-Viragh, R. Mathias, Dr. V. Menges, Dr. R. Michel, Dr. H. Neuhaus, A. E. Noverraz, Dr. M. Rado, Dr. C. Sievert, Dr. K. H. Schlensker, Prof. Dr. W. Schulze, Dr. H. Zwicker.

For their generosity in the production of the book we thank Georg Thieme Publishers. Dr. med. h. c. G. Hauff realized many of the authors' wishes regardless of cost considerations. The supervision of production work lay in the experienced hands of Mr. J. Zimnik.

Finally, we owe a special debt of thanks to Professor Leo G. Rigler, M. D. and his collaborators, Assistant Professors Rolf D. Arndt, M. D. and Peter Spiegler, Ph. D. They have produced a masterly translation for the American edition.

Walther Hoeffken
Marton Lanyi

Introduction to the American Edition

When this volume on breast diseases was brought to my attention I was impressed by the importance of making it readily available to physicians in the United States. A remarkable correlation of the clinical findings, the pathology and the roentgen diagnosis of breast diseases has been achieved by the authors. In addition there is a splendid delineation of the roentgen signs of diseases of the breast and illustrations of extraordinary quality. All of these factors impelled Dr. ARNDT and me to undertake the somewhat arduous task of translation and editing. The result has been most gratifying. The increasing use of mammography in this country should make this volume extremely valuable, not only to those who are doing this as a special procedure but to all physicians interested in the early diagnosis of carcinoma of the breast. I am proud to commend it to the American reader.

LEO G. RIGLER, M. D.

Los Angeles

Contents

Historical Review

The first report concerning roentgen examination of diseases of the breast was made by SALOMON from the Surgical University of Berlin in 1913, not to introduce a new method of clinical diagnosis of diseases of the breast but rather to report on carcinoma and the spread of tumor. SALOMON studied roentgenograms of surgical specimens of breast tumors following mastectomy and recorded the roentgen signs of carcinoma. On reading this first publication on mammography one is astounded by how much SALOMON knew at that time, how much was later forgotten and how little has since been added to that body of knowledge to arrive at the current state of mammography.

Mammography did not achieve any clinical significance with SALOMON's publication because as is often the case with new discoveries, interest is determined on the one side by technical feasibility and on the other by practical need. In 1913 both appeared to be insufficient. The situation in the second half of the 19th Century may be illustrated with quotations from surgeons of that time which bear witness to the hopelessness and resignation regarding breast carcinoma. In England, PAGET (1853) wrote: "We have never observed the failure of recurrence over a seven-year period — our decision in individual cases for or against removal of a carcinomatous breast was never based on the hope of curing the disease."

The French physician VELPEAU (1856) was also not optimistic: "The surgical removal of a carcinoma is in general simple . . . however, . . . the disease always recurs after surgery. In fact, the course of the disease is accelerated by surgery and the fatal end occurs sooner."

In America, AGNEW (1883) was only able to express hope for the future: "I do not doubt that cancer will one day be curable, but I do not believe that this will be procured through the surgeon's scalpel."

A new epoch of breast surgery, however, began with HALSTEAD (1898). In fact, during this time breast surgery attained an enthusiastic high point. With radical mastectomy and axillary lymph node resection HALSTEAD suddenly achieved a 41% four-year survival rate with only a 10% rate of local recurrence. In comparison BILLROTH (1880) reported a 4.7% three-year survival rate and an 82% rate of local recurrence without radical mastectomy. Following HALSTEAD's early reports the new wave of enthusiasm for breast surgery using his technique soon dwindled as further evaluations were made. But optimism returned with the work of STEINTHAL (1905) who brought a new impetus to this method of treatment by defining surgical indications, particularly for radical mastectomy according to STEINTHAL's stages I and II. Everyone was now more satisfied with the results of breast surgery and the dictum went out that every palpable nodule must be removed surgically and examined histologically. There was little interest in further diagnostic methods. This explains why over the next 20 years only one publication on roentgen examination of the breast is to be found. This was by KLEINSCHMIDT and appeared in a medical textbook on malignant tumors by ZWEIFEL and PAYR (1927). In this book KLEINSCHMIDT showed the first roentgenogram of a living breast. Surgeons on the other hand were occupied with extending the radical operation by including removal of the infra- and supraclavicular as well as the mammary lymph nodes. However, as the statistics from these more extensive procedures began to accumulate it became evident that such radical surgery had not altered the survival rates of patients with breast carcinoma. At this time Phase II of mammography began. Over the next 30 years many publications on mammography appeared, particularly in South America by DOMINGUEZ (1929, 1930), BARALDI (1935) and GOYANES et al (1931) and at about the same time in the United States of America with WARREN (1930), RIES (1930), SEABOLD (1931), LOCKWOOD and STEWART (1932). In Germany VOGEL (1932) became interested in the radiological demonstration of breast tumors. He reported cases of carcinoma, sarcoma and chronic cystic mastitis and noted among his observations a case of fibrocystic disease associated with a walnut-sized carcinoma.

A surgeon, Dr. PAYR of Leipzig, was particularly interested in mammography as a diagnostic tool. As a result, during this 30-year period, the next significant publication, by FINSTERBUSCH and GROSS (1934), on the calcification of milk ducts of the breast, came from PAYR's clinic. After this period there was little written on mammography in Germany; however, interest in this method of diagnosis was developing at a rapid rate in the United States. Much is owed to LEBORGNE, a student of DOMINGUEZ, who carried on investigations comparing pathological and mammographical anatomy. LEBORGNE (1953) was also the first to define the various calcifications in the breast; he also became particularly interested in the microcalcifications associated with breast carcinoma. He published very impressive photographs comparing microcalcification in comedocarcinoma as seen in the roentgenogram, the surgical specimen and in the histological preparation. He was the first to differentiate between multiple grouped microcalcifications of carcinoma, singular small calcific deposits and large homogeneous calcification of fibroadenomas as well as describing calcifications in the arteries

of the breast and walls of cysts. GERSHON-COHEN of Philadelphia, in collaboration with the pathologist INGLEBY (1960), refined roentgen signs and pathological-anatomical findings in disease of the breast. GERSHON-COHEN had been working on mammography since 1947. Similar investigations were also published by REIMANN and SEABOLD (1933). Thereafter very little new knowledge was acquired. Everything was attempted: the demonstration of the lactiferous ducts, originally by RIES (1930) using Lipiodol, and later by LEBORGNE (1944) with water-soluble contrast material; pneumomammography (BARALDI, 1935) performed by injecting air into the retromammary space; and stereoscopic examination by FRAY and WARREN (1932). In France LEDOUX-LEBARD and coworkers (1933), ESPAILLAT (1933), and GROS and SIGRIST (1951) had been involved with mammography since its beginning and continued to spawn European interest. In Holland, VON RONNEN (1956) reported on mammography in the Academic Press.

In Germany, however, mammography had in essence been forgotten since the work of KLEINSCHMIDT, VOGEL, FINSTERBUSCH and GROSS. It was not until 1957 that interest in mammography, after extensive research and refinement in the United States, returned to France and thereafter to Germany. In 1956 BECKER and RUNGE of Heidelberg sent their coworkers WERNER and BUTTENBERG to Strasbourg to learn this method of diagnosis from GROS. GROS had already achieved a high degree of technical and diagnostic success in mammography and his method was thereafter introduced in the Heidelberg University Clinic in the winter of 1956—57. KUEBLER (1955) and REINHARDT (1953) had already set the stage in Germany for this development. BUTTENBERG and WERNER published their monograph on mammography, including technique, a roentgenographic atlas and a statistical analysis, in 1962.

From 1930 to 1960 the second phase of mammography, a solid understanding of its diagnostic possibilities and the correlation of roentgen signs with pathological-anatomical data was completed. However, it was limited to only a few centers where interested specialists were accumulating experience and success with this method of diagnosis.

Mammography had not yet achieved any international recognition as a significant diagnostic tool. There did not appear to be any special clinical need for an additional diagnostic method in the examination of the female breast. It was hoped that the combination of surgery and radiotherapy was the answer to improving therapeutic results in carcinoma of the breast. The technique of mammography was refined but no major improvement on the basic principle was made. Phase III of mammography began with a search toward improving the radiographic technique in order to refine diagnostic detail. In America it was particularly EGAN who introduced new techniques to achieve the finest contrast and detail in mammography. DOBRETSBERGER in Austria developed the isodensity method designed to equalize the marked differences in x-ray density inherent in breast radiography. This consisted of placing the breast in a plastic container filled with alcohol prior to the x-ray exposure. Others, in order to circumvent such a cumbersome technique, experimented with various absorption devices such as plastic, foam rubber, etc. in order to achieve better contrast. However, it was soon learned that each additional absorption device led to an increase in exposure factors which resulted in radiographs of poor quality. Eventually intensive efforts were made to improve low kilovoltage techniques. The construction of special tubes with small apertures, the lowering of kilovoltage to 28—20 kilovolts and the use of industrial instead of the usual roentgen film brought a significant improvement in the quality of breast radiography.

The next significant step forward was again achieved by GROS. It was he who introduced the use of the characteristic radiation of molybdenum for mammography. With the construction of molybdenum tubes the last step in technical improvement has been made and thus mammography has attained its current status of widespread clinical application.

During these years a general effort was made to improve therapy for breast cancer. The statistics show that over the years no real improvement in survival rates had occurred. The search for better surgical techniques had led to no result. Mc-WHIRTER (1964) demonstrated that there was no difference in the 5-year survival rate between radical mastectomy and simple mastectomy followed by radiation of the anatomical regions of lymph drainage. Preoperative radiation, although offering some hope originally, had also failed to improve statistics and radiation therapy was again reserved primarily for postoperative treatment.

Supervoltage technique with ultrahard x-ray beams provided a significant improvement in delivery of tumor dose to local lymph nodes and simultaneously diminished damage to the skin and skeletal structures of the thorax. The ice, however, had not yet been broken and most surgical clinicians, pathologists and, in fact, physicians in general were skeptical about the application of mammography as an accurate method of diagnosis.

The removal of this skepticism in Germany has been our endeavor since we began mammography at the University Clinic for Women in Cologne in 1958 and gradually we have convinced clinicians of the value of this method. In collaboration with KAUFMANN, pathologists have also been convinced of the good correlation between mammography and histological findings. Together with HAMPERL we have made efforts to advance mammography to such a degree that it enable us to detect the clinically occult carcinoma early and even to find the preinvasive state of carcinoma in situ. We have been fortunate in achieving such early detection followed by histological diagnosis and appropriate therapy in an increasing number of cases.

Increasing interest in mammography in Germany followed the European symposium on mammography held in Strasbourg in 1966. At this meeting many radiologists were made aware of this method of diagnosis. Interest in mammography was aroused among clinicians through the German gynecological congress held in Hamburg in 1970 and the German surgical congress in Munich in 1971. With these events the second requirement was met for the expansion of mammography: the recognition of the need for a new diagnostic method in the early diagnosis of carcinoma of the breast.

The technical improvements have been achieved, and diagnostic acumen will increase rapidly as experience is gained and more radiologists are trained in this specialty. We hope that the resulting expansion of mammography will some day allow mass application of this diagnostic method. Currently there are great organizational problems in this regard; however, the significance of mammography as a noninvasive diagnostic method for the detection of early breast carcinoma should be recognized.

1*

Basic Physical Aspects of Mammographic Technique

by H. GAJEWSKI

The photographic quality of breast roentgenograms must be assessed in terms of their diagnostic value; that is, in their ability to demonstrate early and unusual lesions. It is conceivable, as unfortunately happens again and again in the evaluation of mammography, that cost considerations may exert such influence that the production of an image of coarse structures is accepted as a proper technique.

Technical Exposure Problems

The difficulties in formulating exposure techniques in radiography of the breast are due to:

> The properties of the objects to be recorded; the larger requirements for radiographic contrast and image sharpness;
> unusual positioning and projection requirements of the object to be examined.

The Object

The breast, its shape, its size, and its tissue composition *vary considerably from one individual to another*. Its conical shape is responsible for the larger differences in thickness between the base and the periphery. The roentgenograms must, therefore, image *a wide range of thicknesses*. The various tissues such as connective tissue, glands, fatty tissue, and skin produce *little subject contrast*. Other structures (for example, arteries, veins and lactiferous ducts) and small but important pathological details (for example, microcalcifications and radiating offshoots of denser tissue) most of which are as small as 0.1 mm, will absorb very little radiation.

Contrast and Image Sharpness Requirements

The exposure techniques must be selected in such a manner that small differences in attenuation between adjacent tissues are recorded with the *highest possible radiographic contrast*. Additionally a wide range of x-ray intensities (*radiation contrast*) transmitted by the thinnest and thickest portions of the subject must by the thinnest and thickest portions of the subject must also be portrayed.

Furthermore the exposure technique must be formulated to yield the *sharpest possible image of the smallest structures* that make up the breast.

Position and Projection Requirements

The position of the breast and the direction of the x-ray beam must be chosen to yield an isolated image, i.e., an image free of overlapping structures provided the anatomical conditions allow this. To fulfill this requirement, the relationship between object, x-ray beam and image recorder should be as close as possible to the *tangential exposure* condition illustrated in fig. 1.1. This is valid for the various projections (see technique formulation p. 34). Properly constructed mammographic cones will meet this condition by their shape and rigid attachment to the x-ray tube housing. The diagnostically important lateral projection of the nipple is met by proper positioning of the breast.

Solution to the Exposure Problem

The solution to the previously described exposure problems, requires an optimum compromise among the various factors that control image contrast and image sharpness. In essence one must consider:

1) The spectral distribution of the x-radiation before and after passage through the object;
2) the geometric requirements of projection and the properties of the image recorder.

One must further observe various *additional requirements* (for example tube rating, film speed and sensitivity) and important practical considerations (for example patient load, radiation dose). Four of the technical solutions that have been used and will be discussed in detail are:

1) the soft radiation technique;
2) the isodensity technique;
3) xerox mammography;
4) photofluorography.

One of these methods, the soft radiation technique has won the widest acceptance because it achieves the most favorable compromise between the many, sometimes contradictory requirements, and produces the most favorable technique for diagnosis.

Soft Radiation Technique

Radiation Quality

The dependence of the attenuation coefficient as a function of tube potential for various tissues is depicted in fig. 1.2. From it, it is evident that large attenuation differences, that is the large contrast between fatty tissue and soft tissue, which is desired, can be achieved in the 20 to 40 kVp range. This general statement on radiation quality or respectively on the radiation spectrum best suited for mammography, must be refined by additional specification of the target material and the total filtration. Further consideration must be given to the changes in spectral distribution as the beam goes through the object and the spectral sensitivity of the image receiver. One

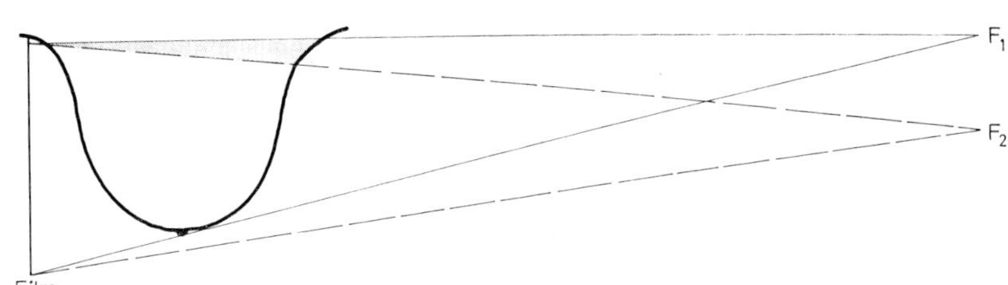

Fig. 1.1 Projection requirements for lateral medial mammographic exposures (outline tracing of x-ray beam). The object is fully imaged when the normal ray of the beam is tangent to the chest wall (focal spot in position F1). This is achieved by an off-axis spot in position F1). This is achieved by an asymmetrical cone or by tilting the x-ray tube. When the central ray is perpendicular to the film (corresponding to focal spot in position Γ2), the grey shaded areas of the breast will no be visualized.

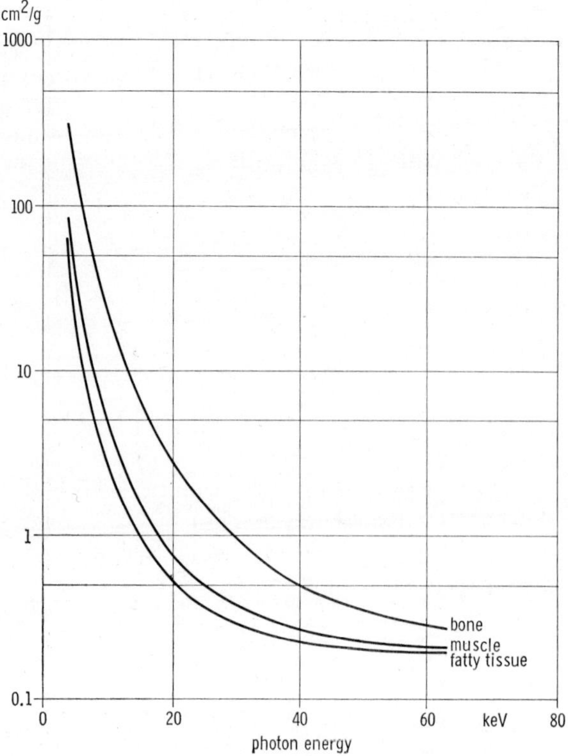

Fig. **1**.2 Mass attenuation for bone, muscle and fatty tissue as a function of photon energy. (see also Table 1.1 and 1.2). Monochromatic radiation. Narrow beam geometry. (From: H. Gajewski, K. H. Reiss: Radiologe 14 (1974) 438—446)

must also not forget that scattered radiation, produced by the object, reduces the contrast, and that the x-ray tube output is limited by rating charts. The radiation dose to the patient must also be considered.

An experimental study aimed at obtaining the optimal spectral distribution of the primary radiation best suited for mammography is too time consuming. It is easier to tackle the problem through numerical calculations. This is now feasible because it is possible to measure quantitatively the spectral energy distribution of the diagnostic x-ray beam with high resolution, and to utilize high speed computers which in a very short time perform calculations that take into account total filtration, variation in object thickness, and spectral sensitivity of x-ray film. Such investigations have been performed by N. Mika and K. H. Reiss (1968).

The Energy Spectrum of X-rays

The radiation emanating from an x-ray tube consists of a continuous *bremsstrahlung* spectrum (brakage radiation) with a cut-off at the photon energy corresponding to the maximum tube potential, and the line spectrum of the target's characteristic radiation. In x-ray tubes with

Table 1.1

Mass attenuation coefficient $\frac{\mu}{\rho}$ (in cm²/g) for a few important elements as a function of photon energy (in keV).

Energy (keV)	Hydrogen $\left(\frac{\mu}{\rho}\right)$ total	Carbon	Nitrogen	Oxygen	Aluminum	Phosphorus	Sulphur	Calcium
5.0	0.471	19.4	30.5	45.2	184.0	280.0	344.0	636.0
6.0	0.430	10.8	17.5	26.2	111.0	168.0	208.0	385.0
8.0	0.399	4.36	7.27	11.2	50.0	76.0	93.9	174.0
CuK$_\alpha$ 8.1	0.398	4.19	7.00	10.79	48.26	73.42	90.74	168.19
10.0	0.388	2.21	3.69	5.72	26.3	40.8	50.9	95.0
15.0	0.376	0.742	1.15	1.74	7.97	12.4	15.6	30.1
20.0	0.369	0.419	0.585	0.817	3.41	5.29	6.63	13.1
AgK$_\alpha$ 22.0	0.366	0.360	0.484	0.656	2.58	3.99	4.99	9.92
I^{125} 27.5	0.359	0.272	0.332	0.419	1.37	2.07	2.59	5.18
30.0	0.357	0.250	0.296	0.363	1.09	1.63	2.03	4.03
40.0	0.346	0.205	0.225	0.252	0.545	0.772	0.945	1.77
50.0	0.335	0.186	0.196	0.210	0.355	0.472	0.562	0.989
WK$_\alpha$ 58.5	0.327	0.176	0.182	0.191	0.279	0.354	0.411	0.679
60.0	0.326	0.175	0.181	0.189	0.270	0.340	0.393	0.642

tungsten targets, the *characteristic radiation* does not play an important role in the 20 to 40 kVp potential range which is best suited for the soft radiation techniques in mammography. For tungsten the K-characteristic radiation is excited at 69.3 kV and appears with appreciable intensity at 80—90 kV. The L-characteristic radiation of tungsten is absorbed by the glass wall. Fig. **1**.3 illustrates the energy spectrum from a tungsten target x-ray tube at a constant tube potential of 25 kV.

If it is also desirable to use characteristic radiation in making the roentgenogram, a target material with an atomic number between 40 and 45 must be used. For technical reason, molybdenum, the atomic number of which is 42 and the Kα-characteristic radiation has an energy of 17.5 keV, is the most important of such elements. GROS (1966) first pointed out the many advantages of this element as a target material for mammography.

Fig. **1**.4 illustrates a molybdenum target x-ray spectrum filtered with 0.5 mm of beryllium at 35 kV constant potential (solid line). A comparison with the dashed curve shows that the spectrum can be favorably manipulated by added molybdenum filtration. The low energy photons, which are predominantly absorbed in the object, as well as the higher energy photons which

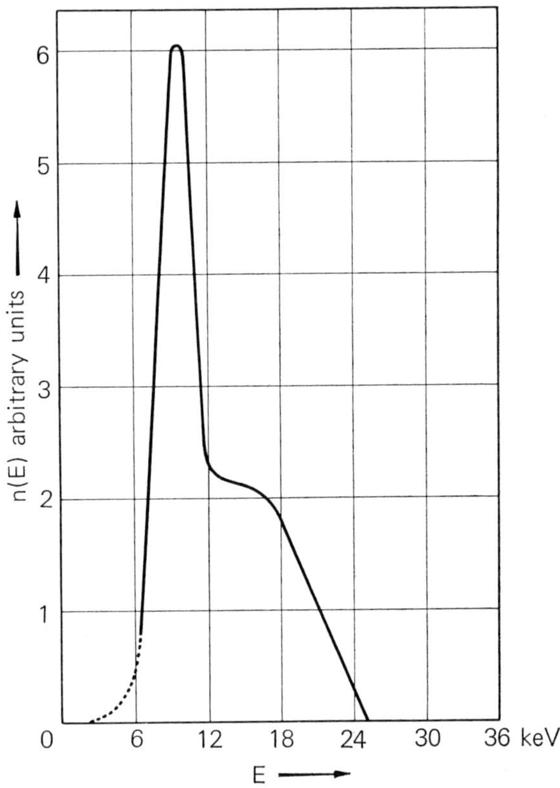

Fig **1**.3 X-ray spectrum from a tungsten target tube with a 0.5 mm beryllium window. Tube potential 25 kV constant potential (Mika and Reiss).
E photon energy
n(E) number of photons with energy E

Table 1.2

Calculated mass attenuation coefficients $\frac{\mu}{\rho}$ (in cm²/g) for various tissues and phantom materials as a function of photon energy (in keV).

Energy (keV)	Fatty tissue $\left(\frac{\mu}{\rho}\right)$ total	Striated muscle	Plexiglass	Polyethylene	Water	Hydroxylapatite
5.0	25.0	40.5	26.1	16.7	40.2	324.2
6.0	14.2	23.5	14.9	9.31	23.4	194.7
8.0	5.96	10.7	6.22	3.79	10.0	88.1
8.1	5.74	10.30	5.99	3.64	9.63	85.1
10.0	3.05	5.21	3.18	1.95	5.12	47.8
15.0	1.00	1.55	1.03	0.689	1.59	15.02
20.0	0.533	0.748	0.542	0.412	0.769	6.54
22.0	0.450	0.612	0.455	0.361	0.626	4.97
27.5	0.326	0.415	0.327	0.284	0.414	2.62
30.0	0.296	0.366	0.295	0.265	0.363	2.06
40.0	0.235	0.263	0.231	0.225	0.263	0.954
50.0	0.210	0.223	0.205	0.207	0.224	0.569
58.5	0.197	0.205	0.193	0.197	0.206	0.417
60.0	0.196	0.203	0.192	0.196	0.204	0.398

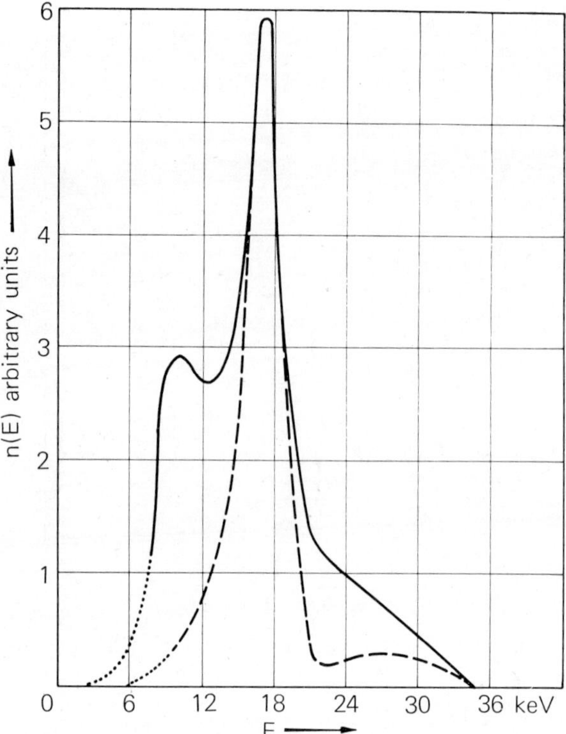

Fig. **1**.4   X-ray spectrum from a molybdenum target tube. Tube potential 35 kV constant potential (Mika and Reiss).
——— 0.5 mm Be window
...... 0.5 mm Be window + 0.04 mm added Mo filtration.
E photon energy
n(E) number of photons with energy E

produce deterioration in the contrast, are preferentially removed, in contrast to the useful middle energy photons to which also belong the molybdenum $K\alpha$-characteristic radiation. This selective effect of the molybdenum filter results from the discontinuous change in the attenuation coefficient at the K-edge of molybdenum. Fig. 1.5 illustrates the transmission as a function of energy for a 0.04 mm thick Mo filter which was also used to obtain the spectrum in fig. 1.4. It easily clarifies the effect of selective filtration. The object alters the impinging primary spectrum qualitatively as well as quantitatively. Fig. 1.6 shows that for a 4 cm thick water phantom, the lower energy photons are more readily attenuated than the higher energy photons which lead to hardening of the primary radiation spectrum. It also shows that only a small fraction of all photons penetrates the object. KYSER (1971) has also measured spectral distributions with regard to the suitability of target materials.

Image Contrast

The changes brought about in the primary spectra of the x-ray beam by the object and their relation to image contrast, are difficult to demonstrate because of the wide ranges in organ size and tissue composition from one subject to another. GAJEWSKI and HEILMAN (1971) have therefore performed experiments with a breast phantom to precisely assess the effect of target material (tungsten, molybdenum), tube filtration and tube potential on image contrast. Their results are:

1) For rotating anode with tungsten target, image contrast is improved by reducing the inherent filtration (replace glass wall by a beryllium window plus 0.03 mm added molybdenum to make a total equivalent of 0.5 mm Al). The improvement in contrast is achieved at the expense of a higher mAs value and a higher skin dose.

2) In the tube potential range of 24—27 kVp, and for a maximum object thickness of 4.5 cm, images with better or equal contrast can be achieved with a rotating-tungsten target anode, if the same filtration (0.5 mm Be + 0.03 mm Mo) as for the rotating molybdenum target anode is used. An advantage of the tungsten radiation is the low mAs value (shorter exposure time respectively); a disadvantage is the higher skin dose.

3) When using a *molybdenum target tube, contrast diminishes more slowly with increasing tube potential* than with a tungsten target tube. This advantage of the rotating molybdenum target anode with beryllium window and 0.03 mm added molybdenum filtration, makes it possible for thick objects to raise the tube potential and avoid long exposure time (and therefore maintain the same skin dose) without appreciable degradation of image contrast.

Scattered Radiation

The radiation contrast is decreased by the presence of scattered radiation originating from within the object. The fact that the image contrast is improved when making exposures of small

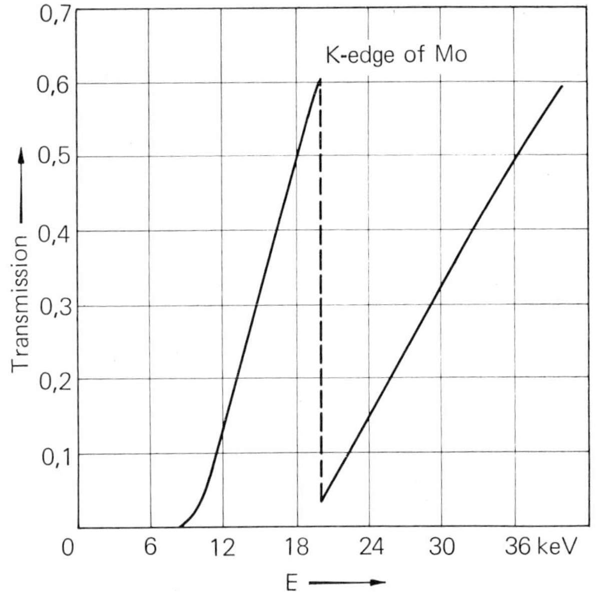

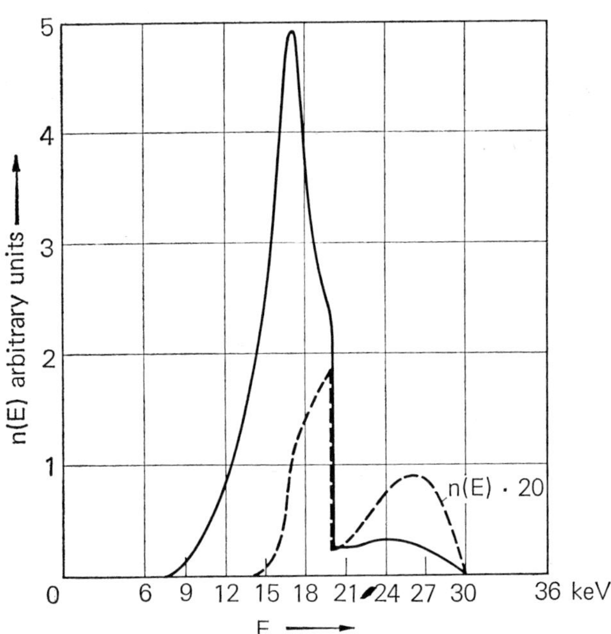

Fig. **1**.5 Transmission fraction for a 0.04 mm Mo filter as a function of photon energy. The transmission fraction rises in the ratio of 1:18.8 at the K-edge of molybdenum.

Fig. **1**.6 Changes in the energy spectrum of a 30 kV molybdenum target x-radiation after transmission through 4 cm of water (after MIKA) which is equivalent to the parenchymal content of an average woman's breast.

E photon energy
n(E) number of photons with energy E
——— 0.05 mm Be filter + 0.03 mm Mo
...... 0.05 mm Be filter + 0.03 mm Mo + 4 cm water (ordinate multiplied by a factor of 20).

areas of the breast with little round cones (i.e. reduction in volume of tissue producing scattered radiation) leads to the conclusion that the ratio of scattered to total radiation is very significant in breast exposures. Phantom measurements made by SEEMANN (1967) and LAVAL-JEANTET et al (1969) yielded values for the *scattered component* which, depending on the experimental condition (thickness of scatterer, tube potential, field size), amounted to 35 to 55% of the total radiation. The degradation in image contrast due to off-focus radiation for rotating anodes is insignificant compared to the larger scattered radiation component (KUHN and GAJEWSKI 1971). The author has performed comparison exposures with and without scattered radiation, by using a breast equivalent phantom. These showed that with practically complete removal of scattered radiation (scanning of exposed object with a narrow lead slit) the image contrast is substantially improved.

However, the use of grids in soft radiation mammography fails for the following reasons:

1) The hardening and the attenuation of the primary radiation in commonly used grids is too high. Special grids for soft radiation mammography should not appreciably attenuate the primary radiation in the tube potential range of 25—35 kVp.

2) Imaging of areas close to the chest wall is made more difficult even when using a special moving grid with a narrow border.

3) The object film distance is increased by the presence of a moving grid, i.e., the image unsharpness is increased.

4) In order to facilitate compression, a stable breast supporting plate, which does not interfere with the moving grid, is necessary. This implies undesirable hardening and attenuation of the primary image producing radiation.

5) The use of grids increases by a factor of 2 the already high mAs and skin dose values.

The opinion (BOHRER 1965, HÜPPE 1970) that compression of the breast reduces scattered radiation is frequently expressed. This effect of compression which is well known for abdomen exposures, is not present in mammary survey

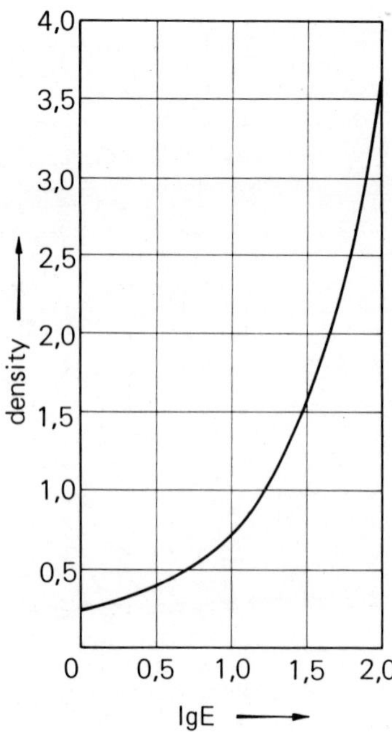

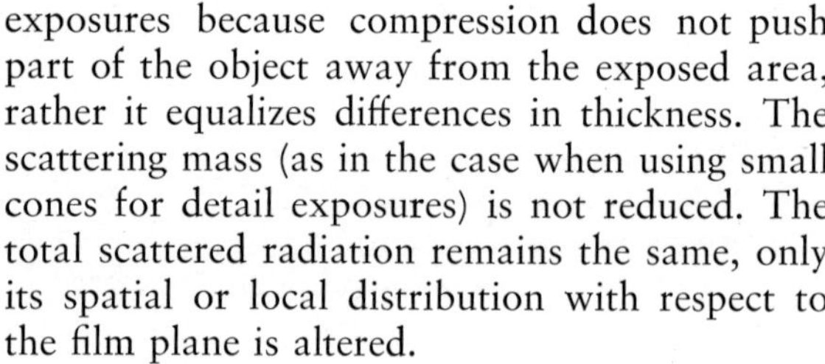

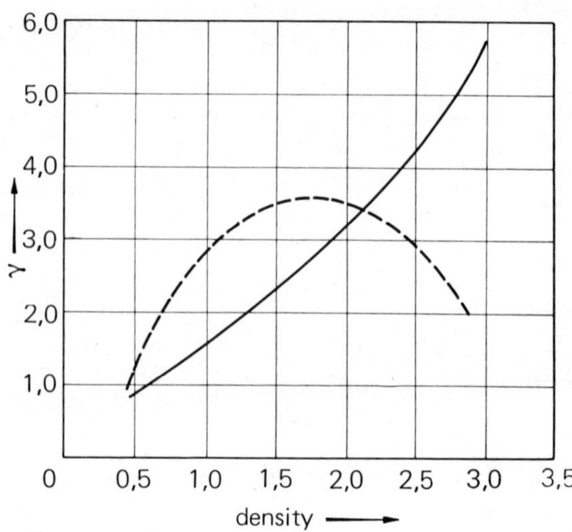

Fig. **1**.7 Left: Characteristic curve for a fine grain, high resolution mammographic film.

Right: Slope of characteristic curve (γ = slope of characteristic curve) as a function of *density*. The broken line curve presents values for a *screen film* combination.

exposures because compression does not push part of the object away from the exposed area, rather it equalizes differences in thickness. The scattering mass (as in the case when using small cones for detail exposures) is not reduced. The total scattered radiation remains the same, only its spatial or local distribution with respect to the film plane is altered.

In the soft radiation techniques, compression of the breast serves three purposes:

1) Reduction in the required exposure time due to lowering of the maximum thickness and the focal spot film distance (only for compression with a compression cone).

2) Equalization of larger differences in thickness.

3) The motionless breast during relatively long exposure times.

Another possibility for recording the large scale of densities of the breast photographically is the *two-film technique*. In this method, two images of the breast are made simultaneously on two films of different speed (speed ratios of 1:2.5 up to 3). The slower film records with good contrast and density the periphery, the faster film the region close to the chest-wall. Two film packages ready for use are available under the trade name Bipackfilm.

A special variation of the two-film technique is the *double film technique* in which two images are simultaneously recorded on a double film.

It consists of a single emulsion film which is perforated in the middle and folded into a double film. The advantages of higher film speed, contrast improvement by superimposition of two images and the possibility of judging the two images separately and thus recognize artifacts more easily is achieved at greater expense in film cost (such as in the two-film technique). The mechanical binding of the two films on the narrow side does not always adequately ensure that the two images will perfectly match when overlaid. A reduced image sharpness of the small details will result.

The image contrast further depends on the properties of the *x-ray film* and its processing. Special mammographic film necessary to attain image sharpness (see following paragraph) have characteristic curves, with increasing gammas (see fig. 1.2). The higher the average density of a mammogram, the higher the radiographic contrast between two neighboring structures with small differences in x-ray attentuation. The average density for properly exposed mammograms should not be less than 2.0.

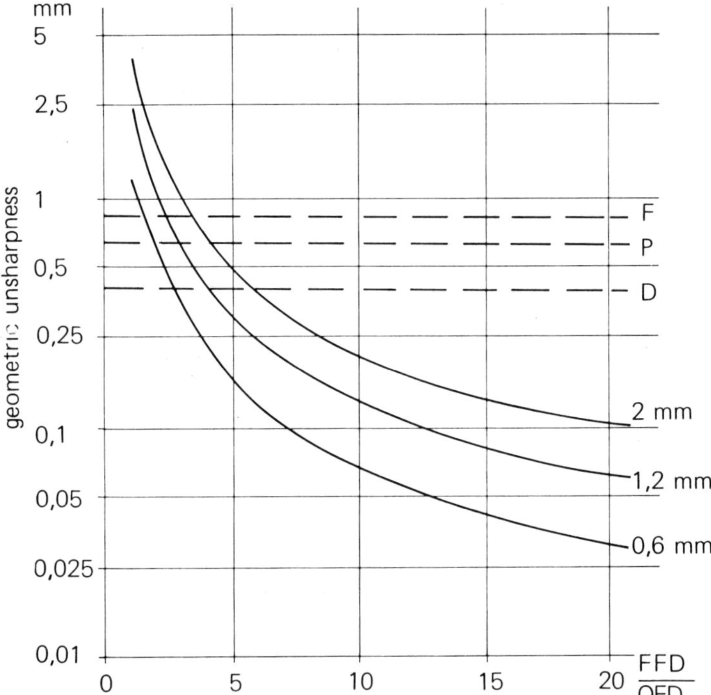

Fig. **1**.8 Geometric unsharpness as a function of the ratio of focus-film distance (FFD) to object film distance (OFD) for three focal spots (2 mm, 1.2 mm and 0.6 mm). The broken lines present values for the screen unsharpness (F fast, P par, D detail); after Stieve and Widenmann (1967).

Examples	FFD	FFD/OFD
grid table	115 cm	4 to 12
spot film device	65 to 80 cm	2 to 6
mammograph	50 cm	5 to 20

Image Sharpness

In soft radiation mammography, image sharpness is controlled by the resolution of the recording system and geometry of the exposure (focal spot size, focal spot film distance). For exposures with intensifying screen, the sharpness is shown by the graph in fig. 1.8. Medical diagnosis requires the imaging of certain structural details (smallest soft tissue septa of 0.1 mm, microcalcification of 0.2 mm). As can be seen in fig. 1.8, this is not possible when using conventional intensifying screens. Also, adequate image sharpness is not achieved with normal nonscreen film, only with special *fine grain x-ray film*. In addition to the specific task, the film should be fast, have a steep gradient or a wide useful range. These, partially contradictory requirements, are resolved into a favorable compromise with *special mammographic film*. This is an industrial x-ray film with high silver content and with an charcteristic curve as illustrated in fig. 1.7. The curve is charcteristic in that the slope and thus the radiographic contrast increases with density (see right side of fig. 1.7). Provided the tube rating charts are not exceeded and provided the radiation dose burden is not excessive, soft radiation mammograms should be exposed to higher densities than conventional roentgeno-

grams, the characteristic curve of which flattens out at higher densities (see broken line in the right portion of fig. 1.7). A basis for the dependence of film speed on photon energy is given by the calculated absorption curve in fig. 1.9. Comparison with the spectral distribution in x-ray energy behind a 4 cm thick water phantom (fig. 1.6) shows that good matching of the spectral distribution of radiation and spectral sensitivity of film is achieved. The slope of the characteristic curve (and thus radiographic contrast) depends on *film processing* (type of developer, replenisher, temperature, development time); thus when unsatisfactory exposures are obtained these factors must also be checked out.

The *use of intensifying screens* — the aim of which is to reduce the skin dose, the energy load to the x-ray tube, and to increase the radiographic contrast — has repeatedly been tried (for example PRICE and BUTTER 1970). A satisfactory radiograph, based on the ability to resolve small calcifications, can be expected, provided only a backscreen is used, there is perfect film screen contact (vacuum cassette), and a fine grain film is the image recorder. Everything else being equal, it is then possible to get an image with half the mAs. Despite the noticeable gain in radiographic contrast, *mammo-*

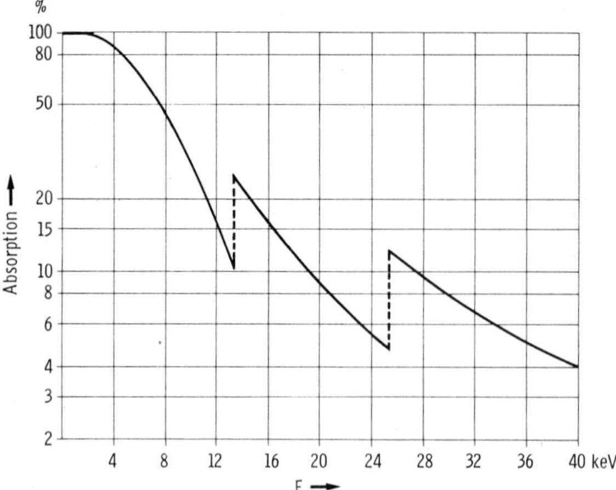

Fig. **1**.9 Absorption (sensitivity) as a function of photon energy for nonscreen x-ray film with a 3.0 mg/cm² AgBr layer (calculated). The rises in absorption correspond to the **K**-edge of bromine ($\approx$ 13.5 keV) and silver (25.5 keV).

graphic exposures with intensifying screens should be rejected for two reasons. First, the manipulation of vacuum cassettes is troublesome and time consuming and second the danger of artifacts by foreign bodies on the surface of the screen (dust and the like) cannot be excluded.*
In soft radiation mammography, the *focal spot size* cannot be chosen on theoretical grounds to achieve optimum image sharpness (geometric unsharpness = inherent unsharpness of the film or equal modulation transfer function of the film and radiation geometry). When using fine grain mammographic film, this would lead to small focal spot sizes which would have a low power rating and this in turn would lead to long exposure time. One may further consider that the choice of focal spot size is also dictated

---

* Since the writing of this paragraph, detail intensifying screens, used with special single emulsion film in a vacuum cassette have been perfected and are now routinely used in many mammographic clinics. The new "low dose" system of DuPont is claimed to show a dose reduction factor of 7 as compared to the Kodak AA film.

** The above discussion is theoretical. In practice, in the U. S. only x-ray tubes with either 0.5 mm, 1.0 mm, or 2.0 mm focal spots are readily available.

*** The presently valid version of DIN 6823 of January 1968 is in the process of revision. In the U. S., the accepted method for the measurement of focal spot sizes is described in the N.B.S. handbook No. 89, also called ICRU report 10f.

by the focus-film distance. For a breast of average thickness and for a focus-film distance of 45 cm, the focal spot — based on equal geometric unsharpness for large object film distance — can be 1.3 to 1.5 times as great as the one used at a focus-film distance of 35 cm. A practical compromise between target rating (duration of exposure time when making exposure with fine grain mammographic film) and focal size (achievable image sharpness) is offered for example by: *target film distance 45 cm, focal spot size 0.6 mm.* If a target film distance different from 45 cm is used, then the focal spot size must be selected according to the following table if it is desired to maintain the same geometrical unsharpness for an object 5 cm above the film.

Table 1.3

Relationship between target film distance (FFD) and focal spot size (F) relative to the same geometric unsharpness of 0.075 mm for an object 5 cm away from the film.

FFD (cm)**	F (mm)**
25	0.3
30	0.38
35	0.45
40	0.53
45	0.6
50	0.68
60	0.83
70	0.98

The focal spot size is generally measured according to the recommendation of the standard sheet DIN 6823.*** The nominal standards are set with reference to the central ray. Discrepancies in the true value of up to 30% of the nominal values are tolerable, since the focal spot size depends on the method of operation (kV, mA). Its measurement in mammographic x-ray tubes should be performed at tube potentials and tube current comparable to the values used in performing mammographic exposures. A detailed analysis of its effect on image sharpness must additionally take into account the line structure of the real focal spot. The effective focal spot size thus varies spatially with respect to the central ray. The geometric unsharpness may vary appreciably over the extent of the image when the magnification remains the same.

Phototiming

In agreement with the experience gained in general radiology, HOEFFKEN, HEUSS and RÖDEL

(1970) have demonstrated that a measurement of the breast's thickness is not a reliable indicator for the proper exposure time. Apart from radiation quality, the important index for the proper timing is the ratio of fatty tissue to parenchyma plus fibrocystically altered tissue. It cannot be accurately estimated even with the help of many years of experience. The proper timing must therefore be obtained by photo-timing based on dose measurements. In contrast to the conditions of radiography with intensifying screens, the radiation detector (ionization chamber or fluorescent screen) must be located behind the film. In mammography, any additional absorber in the path of the useful beam is undesirable. The requirement is, however, easily met since the measurement by the radiation detector is essentially unchanged when the film is placed above the detector.

The detection area which dominates the radiation detector is generally a segment of a circle with a chord lenght of 6.5 cm and an arc height of 3 cm. In most cases, especially for craniocaudal exposures, and for proper correspondence between the dominant and the film holder the detection area lies at the right place for proper phototiming (region of mammary gland close to the chest wall). For mediolateral exposures, one must make sure that the detection area is not too close to the region of the thorax which will yield erroneous dose measurements for phototiming. The following technical means are used to avoid such errors:

1) Use of a transparent film holder which permits visual observation of the detection area with respect to the breast's outline; or
2) a mobile detector that has two dominant areas made visible relative to the radiation field and which are selected by means of a light localizer.

Additionally, both solutions require an alert technologist.

Radiation Dose

The type of examination, the requirements for exposure (such as the focus-skin distance, tube potential, filtration, type of film, etc.) play an important role in the radiation dosimetry of mammography. It is therefore not suprising that the many types of examinations on patients and phantoms have yielded a wide range of skin doses. Our measurements on four commer-

cially manufactured machines (HEUSS and HOEFF-KEN 1972) have shown that the skin dose is always higher with a molybdenum target tube than with a tungsten tube. Large dose variation among the various molybdenum tubes have been found by us as well as by PALMER et al (1971). They are mainly due to differences in filtration. For exposures with soft radiation, the entrance skin dose lies in the range of 2 to 20 R*, which is relatively high, therefore we recommend that every mammographic installation should have available a table which shows the dose per mAs measured at the bottom of the various cones for the usual kVp and tube current values. With a knowledge of the exposure time (which can also be measured for a phototimer when there is a need), it would thus be possible to estimate the skin dose.

Example: For a certain type of mammographic installation, the desired exposure was obtained with 110 mAs at 30 kVp. For a breast of average thickness, the skin dose per mAs for the same target skin distance was measured as 70mR/mAs. The skin dose in the exposure thus amounted to 70×110mR $= 7.7$ R.

In dosimetry measurements, careful attention must be given to ensure that the radiation detector is calibrated for soft radiation. The dose applied in soft radiation mammography is especially important in relation to that which reaches the bone marrow and the gonads. Based on measurements by GILBERTSON et al (1970) the dose at the sternum (2.3% of total active marrow according to ELLIS 1961) has the same magnitude as the dose at the skin entrance. The gonadal dose is less than 1 mR because in a properly constructed mammographic unit, the primary radiation in the direction of the gonads is screened off and the scatter radiation originating in the body has a short range due to its low energy.

In mammography, an optimum *compromise must be achieved between the requirements for a diagnostic image and the acceptable radiation burden.* For small and average breast thickness this compromise is achieved by using an x-ray tube with a molybdenum target, beryllium window and 30 μm added molybdenum filtration and a tube potential of 25 to 30 kVp. For very thick and very dense breasts, a tube potential greater than 30 kVp is necessary in

---

* Based on newer definitions, $1R = 2.58 \times 10^{-4}$ C/kg.

order to avoid excessive skin doses. More than 35 kVp is only necessary for the radiography of the axillary ends of the breast. One danger of the soft radiation technique must be especially emphasized: *Special mammographic tubes with beryllium windows shall under no circumstances be operated without additional filtration.* The primary beam emerging from a beryllium window contains many low energy photons which never contribute to the image formation and are absorbed in the upper skin layer. A high skin dose and a strong skin reaction is unavoidable. Only recently have radiation injuries resulting from inadequate filtration been described in the literature (WRIGHT et al 1971). In clinics specializing in soft radiation mammography, the filter, which represents a favorable compromise between image contrast and radiation burden, is rigidly incorporated in the path of the useful beam. If the mammographic tube is to be used for other purposes, for which, according to radiation safety regulations, the total filtration must be equivalent to 2 mm of aluminum (tube potential greater than 70 kVp), then the equiment must be so designed that, when changing operation mode, the extra filtration can only be removed by activation of interlocks or by making its absence conspicuously noticeable.

Labeling for Identification of the Film

Every mammogram must be marked with the required patient data and must also include the right or left markers and the direction of applied projection. The method of recording patient identification data by means of visible light, which is commonly used in screen film exposures, can lead to practical difficulties when applied to special mammographic film. Its sensitivity relative to the red light of the inscribing units (for example the Filmscriber) is about two orders of magnitude lower than for film screen combinations. To label special mammographic film, one needs a device which is especially designed to adapt to the light filter, the brightness of the lamp, the time of exposure, and the low sensitivity of the film.

It is also possible to label by means of a lead letter marker using x-rays in the same manner as the side of the body and the projection are recorded on the film. In labelling done after the exposure (for example in the darkroom), there is always the danger of erroneously exchanging the films of two patients which can be avoided most safely by marking directly at the time of the exposure. Technical solutions for this method have been achieved.

For the automatic recording of patient data on the film using a light flash Siemens produces a shadow producing data carrier on an index card which can be inscribed with a typewriter.

Viewing the Mammogram

It has already been pointed out that in the interest of good contrast, the mammogram should be exposed to higher densities than normal roentgenograms. It is therefore necessary, when evaluating soft radiation mammograms, to use brighter than normal viewing boxes if it is desired to approach the optimum illumination at which the eye is most sensitive to small variations in brightness (30—60 cd/m²). A viewing box with insufficient illumination leads to underexposure of the mammograms that (especially near the chest wall) are unsatisfactory for good diagnosis.

An *ideal viewing box* for the evaluation of mammograms must have the following properties:

1) The maximum luminous flux should not be less than 6000 cd/m² ($\sim$ 20,000 asb). It must be uniformly diffused over the entire viewing box.*

2) For comparison purpose, it must be possible to view simultaneously four exposures (craniocaudal and lateral exposures from both sides).

3) To avoid blinding the eye, adequate brightness controls and other means of adjustment should be provided.

4) For the viewing of very dark areas, a flashlight, with a halogen lamp and an iris diaphragm should be installed on a mobile stand inside the viewing box or mounted at its side, where it is readily available.

Commercially available viewing boxes do not adequately fulfill these ideal requirements. In practice, the requirements for viewing conditions are not given adequate attention. Because of

---

* In general, the maximum brightness is not shown. In future this number should be required from the manufacturer as a quality index.

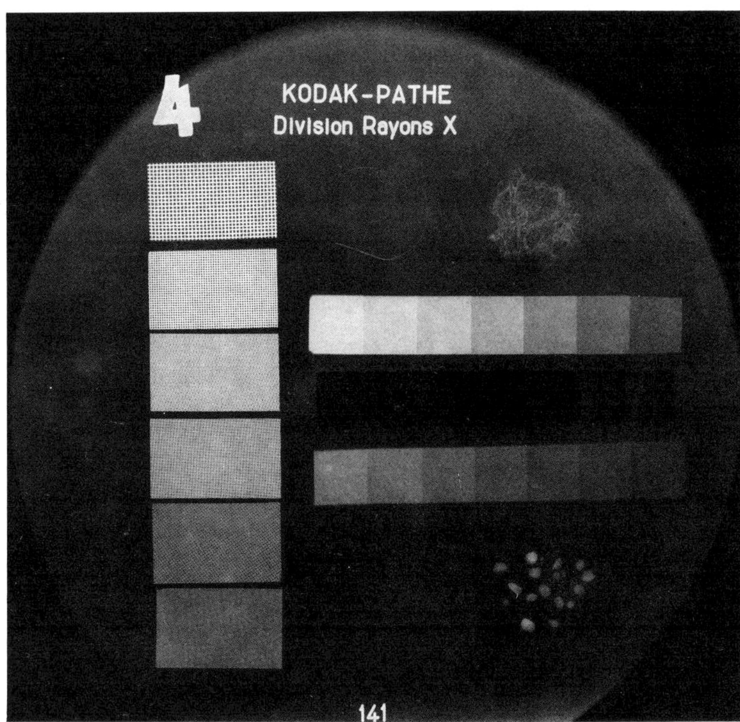

Fig. 1.10   Roentgenogram of the Kodak mammography phantom.

the great need for recognition of detail in mammo-graphy, one should always remind oneself — even more so than when viewing routine roent-genograms — that the total information content can only be extracted under optimum viewing conditions. In this respect, reference is made to the worthwhile monograph by DALICHO (1967). For the recognition of microcalcifications and especially of fine structures, one should have at one's disposition a 2 × magnifying glass of high optical quality with a diameter of 8 cm. To evaluate the size of microcalcifications, magnifiers up to 8 × are even better.

Summary

The *image contrast* (aside from the characteristics of the object) depends on:

1) the target material of the x-ray tube;

2) filtration of primary radiation;

3) kVp and waveform of tube potential;

4) characteristic curve of film and film processing conditions.

The radiographic contrast required to image the breast is achievable with tolerable radiation dose under the following technical considerations:

X-ray tube with a *molybdenum anode, beryllium window and 0.03 mm Mo added filtration;*

kVp between 25—30 (small to medium thick breasts) and 30 to 35 (exceptionally thick or dense breasts);

special non-screen mammographic film with a steep gamma;

average densities greater than 2.0 with strict adherence to prescribed film processing.

The *image sharpness* depends on:
the size of the focal spot;
the magnification factor (ratio FFD:FOD);
the resolving quality of the non-screen film.

A practical and useful compromise between geometry, acceptable focal spot loading and the exposures necessary to achieve the desired densities is accomplished under the following conditions:

1) focal spot size 0.6 mm, 45 cm focus-film distance;

2) for other focus-film distances use the focal spot sizes given in table 1.3 on p. 12;

3) fine grain mammographic film recording without screen.

The Kodak-Pathé mammographic phantom is well suited for quality *control of radiographic contrast and image sharpness.* It consists of a polyester plate in which are embedded contrast

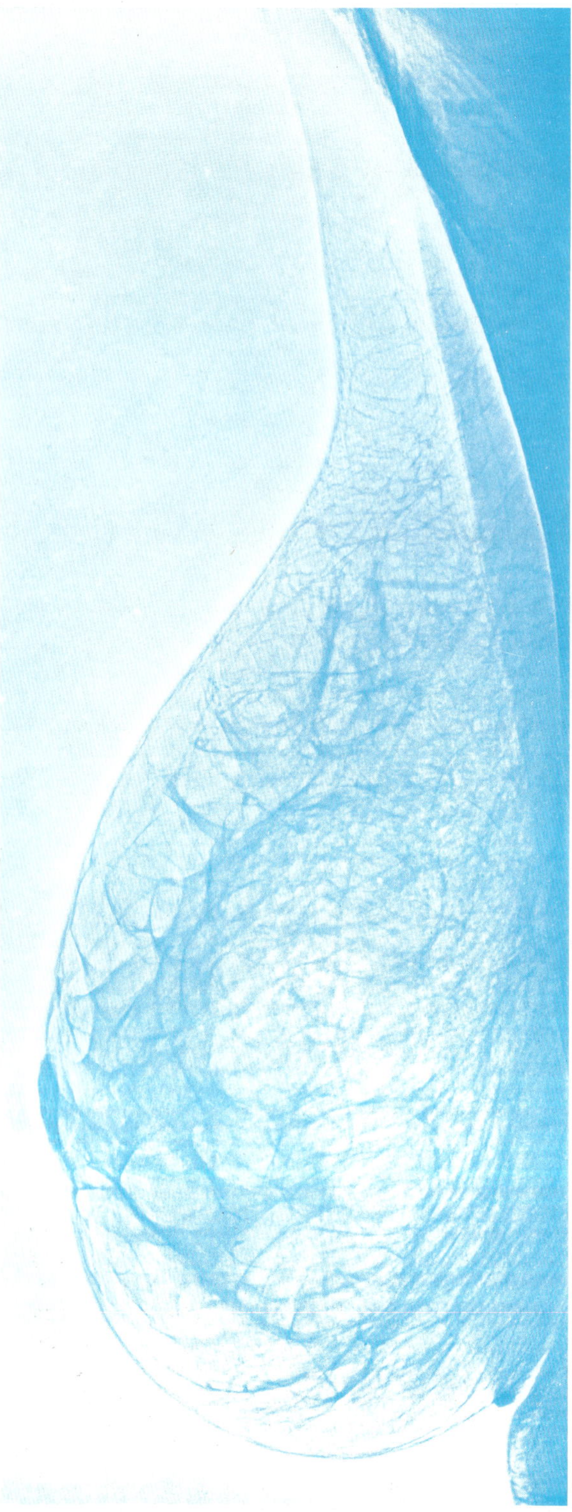

Fig. **1**.11 Xeromammogram.

generating step wedges and various wire meshes (see fig. **1**.10).

Isodensity Technique

The soft radiation isodensity technique has been worked out and described by DOBRETSBERGER (1962, 1965, 1967). It is characterized by the following exposure techniques:

1) Thickness compensation by submerging the breast in a standardized rectangular vessel containing 80% alcohol. For soft radiation it has the same attenuation coefficient and density as the breast.
2) Exposure with a special set-up (see fig. **1**.21). The upper portion of the patients' body as well as the x-ray beam are in a horizontal plane.
3) Reduction of scattered radiation from the alcohol-breast container by means of a moving grid, and beam collimation.
4) Use of screen film in contact with a high detail back screen.
5) Tube potential around 35 kVp.

The advantages are complete imaging of the breast in its natural shape and the ability to exactly reproduce the geometric conditions in the case of retakes for purpose of comparison. Because the organ and alcohol have the same density, the breast floats (even soft and flabby breasts) in the fluid and maintains its natural shape. The isodensity technique produces uniformly graded images with an equally dense background from the region close to the chest wall to the skin at the periphery. The method, however, has not been readily accepted. The reasons for this are its disadvantages. For physical reasons, detail recognition at the periphery is poorer than for conventional soft radiation techniques (HOEFFKEN and GAJEWSKI, 1966). In immersing the breast in alcohol, the thickness of the object to be imaged is increased to that of the fluid container and for similar exposure conditions, it is more difficult to demonstrate small objects embedded in a thick layer than in a thin one. This lack of "image emptiness" in the periphery of the breast also occurs in the proposed modifications of NIEVELSTEIN (1968) and VAN DER PLAATS and NIEVELSTEIN (1967). These investigators used non-screen film to avoid screen unsharpness, a moving grid and a cone to limit scattered radiation and (to adjust for the low sensitivity of the exposure system) higher tube potentials (45 kVp to 55 kVp).

Xeromammography

This electrophotographic process uses a thin layer of amorphic selenium, deposited by evaporation on an electrically conductive plate such as aluminum, to record the image. The selenium layer is charged in the dark by applying an electrical potential of 600 to 800 volts. Because of the high electrical resistance of selenium, the charge remains uniformly distributed over the plate for a long period of time. The selenium layer turns into an electrical conductor when exposed to x-rays in a light tight cassette. The discharge in any area is proportional to the quantity of radiation reaching that area. The remaining charge makes up the latent electrostatic image, which contains the x-ray image. The electrostatic image is made visible by dusting the selenium layer with a fine layer of charged powder (so-called toner) which brings out a fine-grained colored (e.g. blue) image. The dry development procedure (Greek word "xeros" = dry) takes about 10 seconds; for a permanent image, the powder image is transferred electrostatically to paper. Heat treatment is used to melt the thermoplastic dust onto the paper's surface. The entire developing process is performed in the completely automatic Rank-Xerox-System 125, 90 second processer. Cleaning of the plate and reloading for a repeat exposure occurs in the conditioner.

The xerographic image (fig. 1.11) differs in certain respects from the usual x-ray image. Usually a positive xeroradiograph is completed. However, a negative may be obtained by simply activating an appropriate switch on the apparatus. A negative xeroradiograph may have certain advantages in examining dense breast structures. Especially worth noticing is the large image latitude which characterizes xeroradiography and makes it very useful in mammography. The high requirement for resolution is also met. The vivid representation of the long scale of densities is intrinsic in the production of the xerographic image. It is characterized by the so-called "edge enhancement effect". Sharp edges are imaged electrostatically by step potential differences, the amplitude of which is independent of the dose.

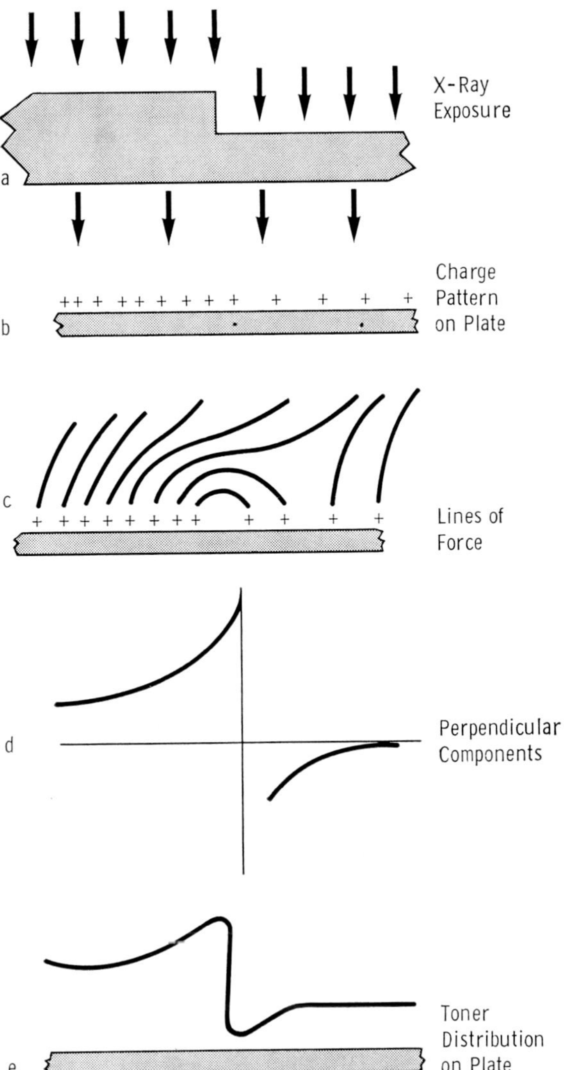

Fig. **1**.12 Edge enhancement in xeroradiographic development. (From: Technical Application Bulletin 1, November 1974, Xerox Corporation.)

Edge enhancement occurs when there is an abrupt change in charge. An edge or boundary is developed in a distinct manner because of the charge step in the latent image. Fringe fields arise because of this charge step and strongly affect toner attraction to the plate. This influence is confined to a narrow region near the edge and results in more toner at the high-charge side of the edge. Consequently, reduced toner reaches the lower charge side of the edge (fig. 1.12). Density increases and then drops significantly. Edge enhancement exaggerates the actual contrast at borders. This helps delineate details of nearly equal x-ray density by accentuating contours.*

---

* From *Technical Application Bulletin* 1, Nov. 1974, Xerox Corporation.

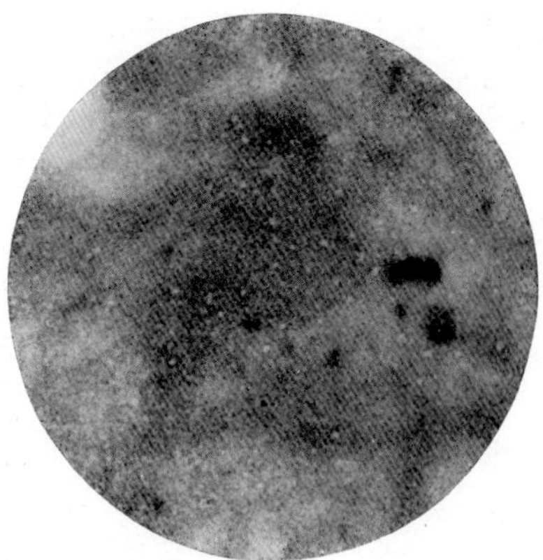

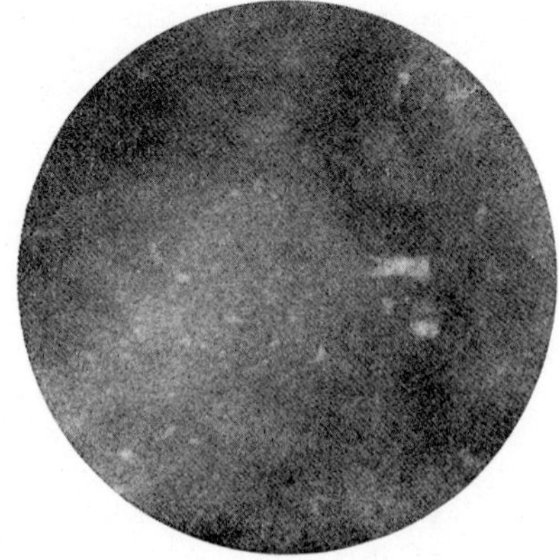

Fig. **1**.13a Xeromammogram, five-fold enlargement. Microcalcifications as a result of the conglomeration of toner powder, have been magnified at the sacrifice of detail. The number of microcalcification is smaller than shown in the conventional mammogram.

Fig. **1**.13b Conventional mammogram, five-fold enlargement. The specific configuration of the microcalcification is easily differentiated. Numerous tiny microcalcifications are visible. Thus appreciation of detail is more advantageous in the conventional film mammograms than on the xeroradiographs.

The dose necessary to produce the image is some 25% less than necessary for nonscreen film exposures. The authors who have used xerography on a large scale (Ruzicka et al 1965, O'Mara et al 1967, Wolfe 1968, 1969, 1972) point out the following advantages:

1) wider image latitude;

2) lower radiation dose since it is possible to work at higher kVp without loss in contrast (about 40 kVp, 400 Mas);

3) simple and fast processing of images without a darkroom.

The evaluation of the xeroradiographic image is probably less difficult than the interpretation of a conventional roentgenogram but a magnifying glass must be used in viewing the xeromammogram.

Artifacts are sometimes disturbing although they are readily recognized. But insufficient illumination can strongly influence the interpretation when using the xerographic system, and enhance the possibility of error in diagnosis. For this reason the xerographic system should make use of an automatic exposure control in order to standardize the image quality, especially when used for routine examination. The recognition of increased density as a result of thickened connective tissue which lies in one plane is more

difficult in the xeroradiograph than in ordinary films, because of the equalization of contrast. The resolution in the xeroradiograph does not match that of industrial film especially with regard to microcalcifications. In the xeroradiographic image, however, fine flecks of microcalcification are magnified due to the conglomeration of the toner powder and they are thus easier to see. At the same time this characteristic destroys their actual configuration (fig. 1.13a). Using fivefold magnification it can be shown that, under identical techniques, industrial film exhibits smaller calcifications than is possible with xeroradiography (fig. 1.13b). The xerographic procedure is superior for imaging large and dense breasts because the system is less sensitive to scattered radiation, so that microcalcifications are more effectively demonstrated. In the conventional roentgenogram, scattered radiation leads to reduced contrast which may impair the possibility of a correct diagnosis (fig. 36.6).

Photofluorography

of the breast the successfull technique of mass chest surveys ,especially since the radiation dose necessary to record the image is lower than the skin dose of soft radiation mammography with fine grain nonscreen film.

The authors who have occupied themselves with photofluorography for serial examinations of the breast (GRAVELLE 1969, NAPPI et al 1966; STRAX and OPPENHEIM 1965 and 1968, TOTI 1969) point out that this procedure is capable of detecting a large number of breast tumors of clinical significance (TOTI 1969). If one recalls, however, that the imaging properties of a photofluorographic system are substantially poorer than those of fine grain nonscreen film, then one could not expect that photofluorography would be a good method for the detection of cases of pathological significance by mass screening. It has therefore not been accepted. LANYI (1970) opposes the application of photofluorographic techniques in mammography.

Technical Equipment Arranged for Mammography

In the previous sections, it has been pointed out that the necessary diagnostic information as well as the photographic quality of the mammogram produce stringent requirements. The technical aids used in general diagnostic radiology are not readily applied to the soft radiation techniques of mammography. Optimum conditions for processing exposure data and for formulating proper projection techniques, especially when applied to examining large groups of patients, as is the case in mass screening, can only be achieved in clinics with special units for mammography. Even in places where mammography is practiced occasionally, a minimum outlay for specialized equipment is unavoidable.

Minimum Equipment Requirements for a Mammographic Installation

The soft x-ray technique requires:

An *x-ray generator* that produces a potential in the range of 25 to 40 kVp. The generators used in general diagnostic radiology are not readily usable since their lowest potential is limited to 35 kVp. The potential range can be lowered, however, by changing certain switching operations. An *x-ray tube assembly* with minimum total filtration. It should have an HVL of 0.5 to 0.8 mm Al. This requirement can only be met with special x-ray tubes that have either a thin glass wall or a beryllium window with additional filtration. Such x-ray tubes are then no longer useful for general purposes (for exam-

ple high kV techniques). Molybdenum is a better target material than tungsten but because of its low energy ratings and poor efficiency in x-ray production, the areas of application of an x-ray tube with molybdenum anode are severely limited. The usual collimator with light localizer cannot be used in breast exposures. It must either be removed or replaced by a system in which the glass backed mirror is replaced by a mirror made of aluminum deposited by evaporation on a thin plastic foil which does not contribute to the filtration.

Special cones are needed which guarantee the proper projection, allow compression of the breast and narrow the useful beams to small regions, necessary to achieve high contrast in the images. The compression plate of such cones should be rigid and contribute as little as possible to the filtration.

A *film holder* which simultaneously acts as a positioning surface for the breast and, if possible, is combined with the detection chamber of the *automatic exposure timer*. The film holder can be rigidly connected with the x-ray tube housing (constrained centering) or detached (free adjustment of the x-ray tube). Figure 1.14 shows the "Mammoset" system which is used for exposures of the sitting or prone patient and which is coupled to a free adjustable x-ray tube. KRÜGER (1972) describes a simple auxiliary tool for the exposure of the patient standing with the upper part of the body leaning forward. It allows exposure of the breast in both directions (patient rotated around 90°) without movement of the x-ray tube, which also represents a minimum use of time. The back of the film holder or of the ionization chamber, respectively, must be shielded to prevent exposures to the ovaries when craniocaudal exposures are made.

Summary

A mammographic installation must meet the following *minimal technical requirements*:

x-ray generator (2, 6 or 12 pulse) with a minimum rating of 1 kW at 30 kVp and variable tube potential between 25 and 35 kVp;

x-ray tube assembly with a total filtration between 0.5 and 0.8 mm Al;

special cones;

holders for the breast and the film that are either mobile or attached to the x-ray tube housing

an automatic exposure timer is recommended.

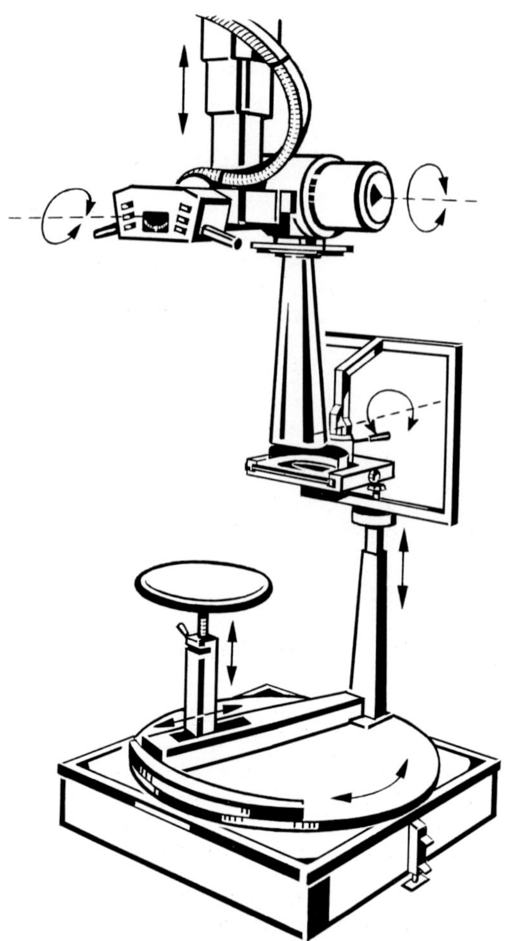

Fig. 1.14 Special mammographic stand "Mammo-set" Kreuzer system (F. W. Hänel, MAVIG, Munich). Vertically adjustable patient swivel stool mounted on a rotating platform. The stool can be rotated, and shifted sideways on the mobile platform. The object-film carrier is also mounted on the platform. The film carrier can be rotated by ± 90° for lateral projections. The stand can also be used for lateral exposures with the patient lying on a table.

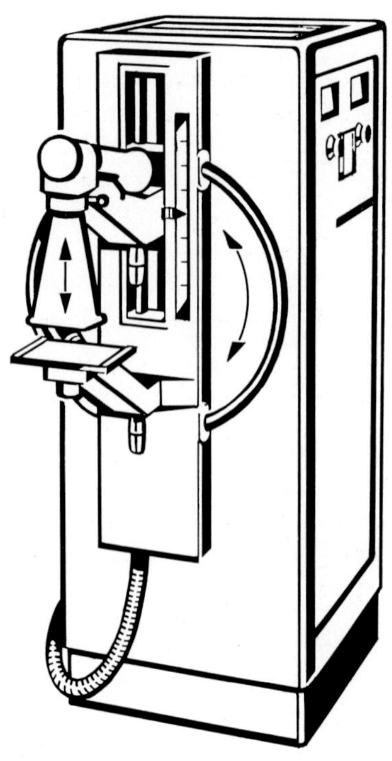

Fig. 1.15 Senograph (Compagnie Générale de Radiologie/Koch & Sterzel). Mammographic unit for exposures with the patient sitting and lying on her side (see fig 3.3). The unit incorporates a high voltage generator with a Greinacher circuitry. X-ray tube with single focal spot, water cooled stationary anode, molybdenum target, beryllium window and 0.03 mm added Mo filtration. Continuous rated power 1.2 kW, focal spot size 0.6 mm; continuously variable kVp selector up to 40 kVp, tube current selector up to 40 mA and timer up to 10 seconds with the possibility of control during a trial exposure (no radiation dose to the patient). Phototimer is optional. The x-ray tube gantry has magnetic brakes and can be rotated ± 180°. It cannot be moved vertically. Compression with interchangeable cones. Focus-film distance is variable (depending on the thickness of the object and compression). In a newer version, the Senograph II, the x-ray tube gantry can be moved vertically. The high voltage generator comes with push button selectors. This unit can also be used to take lateral exposures on patients, lying on their side (mediolateral projection).

Another version, the Senoplex, is a combination of a vertically moving x-ray tube with a positioning table, and a built-in high voltage generator with push button selectors. Special clinical procedures such as galactography and cyst puncture on patients lying on their side (mediolateral) can be performed with ease.

Special Installations for Mammography

With a larger patient load, the time necessary to make mammograms plays an important role. Special units have been developed for serial examination, which, through standardization, and automation of certain techniques, insure optimum contrast and resolution, and through simplicity and ease of use allow a large number of patients to be examined in a short time.

Soft Radiation Technique

The soft radiation technique has been developed mostly in the USA. The craniocaudal exposure was made with the patient sitting, the mediolateral exposure with the patient prone. The change in position necessitated too much time so this procedure was abandoned in serial examination. In clinics specializing in mammography, both projections are made with the patient sitting or standing by means of a *rotating tube gantry*, i.e., a rigid U-shaped arm that can be moved in several directions as well as rotated around its horizontal axis, to which are attached the x-ray tube and object holder centered to each other.

Mammographic units often have a generator, the rating and use of which is especially adapted to their needs. Such installations partly can be combined with coventional generators as well, if mammographic exposures are made occasionally. Rotating anode tubes (sometimes with one grounded electrode) and a molybdenum target have become popular. The grounded electrode type is used at shorter focus film distances and permits compensation for the difference in exposure between the chest and the region of the areola, by exploitation of the heel effect. So far as radiographic contrast is concerned, the molybdenum target tube with beryllium window and added molybdenum filtration is superior to a glass window tube.

All specialized installations for mammography are equipped with *automatic exposure timer*. The detector chamber is located behind the film. *Compression* is achieved at fixed focus-film distance by means of a telescopically adjustable cone or by means of a special device such as a compression plate or cloth. With the adjustable cone there is no need for a compression plate which would only act as a filter and is thus not

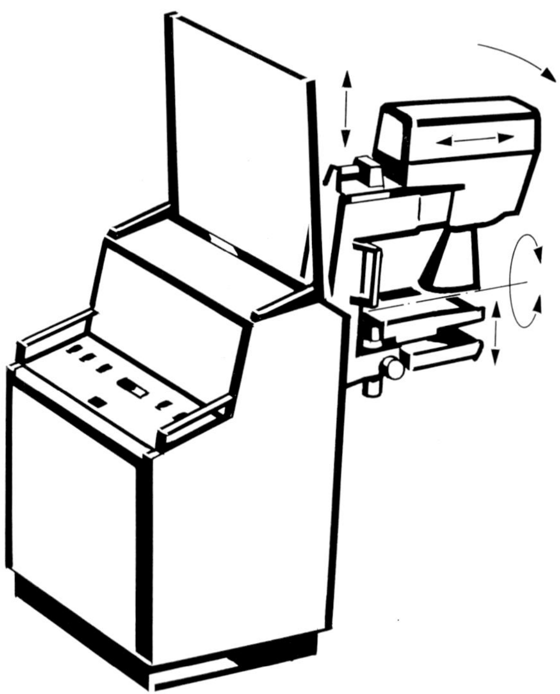

Fig. **1**.16   MMX (General Electric)

Mobile mammographic unit exposures on sitting and lying patients. Built-in high voltage generator (25 to 60 kVp, 200 and 400 mA for both focal spot sizes). Phototimer "Quantamat" is optional.

"GE Maxitron 75" x-ray tube with rotating anode, molybdenum target, beryllium window and two added filters (coordinated with tube potential). Focal spot sizes 1 mm and 2 mm. The x-ray tube gantry can be moved vertically and rotated around its horizontal axis. It can be tilted at an angle of 15° to the chest-wall. Compression by means of a transparent plastic plate. Semicircular cone. The exposure field can be limited, with the help of a light localizer, down to a diameter of 5 cm. Localization is further made easier by diminishing the x-ray intensity in the surroundings of the exposure field. Focus-film distance 58 cm. The operator is protected by a lead-glass barrier.

desirable. The use of a compression cone rigidly coupled to the x-ray tube always brings about an interdependence between focus-film distance and breast thickness.

A *special chair for the patient* makes the positioning easier. When it is movable in two directions, two angles of motion in the x-ray tube gantry are saved (motion parallel and perpendicular to the chest wall).
Radiation protection for the technicians is usually achieved by radiation shields equipped

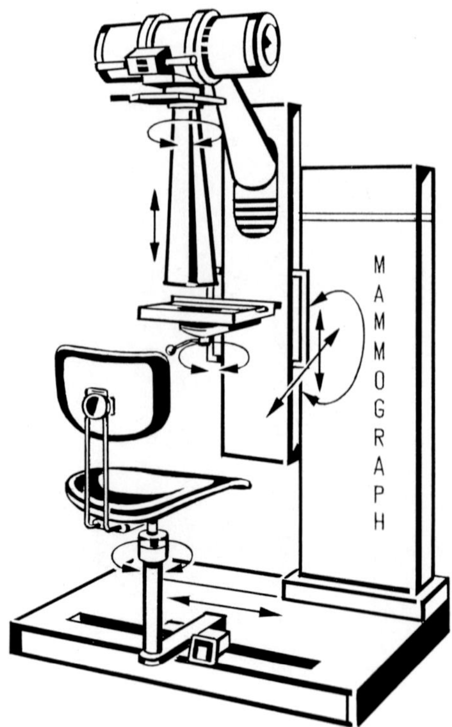

Fig. **1**.17   Mammograph (Fritz Hofmann GmbH, Erlangen). Mammographic unit for exposures of the patient sitting and standing. High voltage generator comes separately (200 to 400 mA at 30 kVp). X-ray tube with rotating anode, molybdenum target, beryllium window and added Mo filtration. Focal spot size 0.6 mm. X-ray tube gantry has magnetic brakes, can be moved vertically and rotated through ± 135º.

Exchangeable compression cones, variable focus-film distance (depends on the breast's thickness and compression; on the average 52 cm); chair can be rotated and moved transversely.

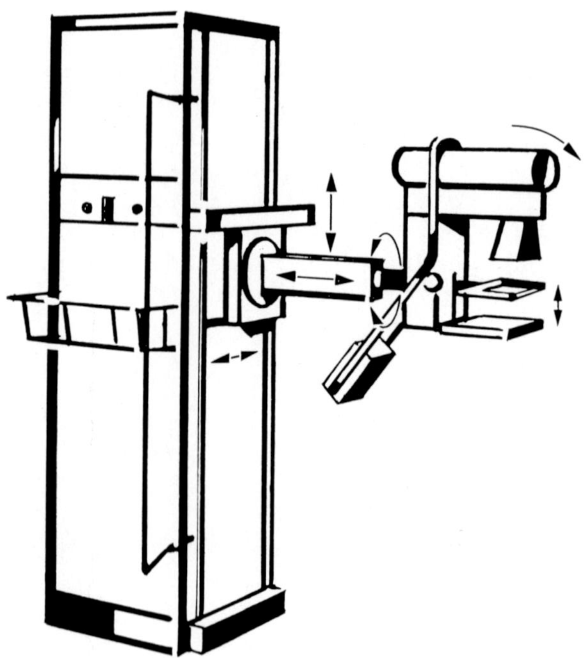

Fig. **1**.18 Diagnostic M. (Philips/C. H. F. Müller). Mammographic unit for exposures of the patient sitting, lying, and standing. Built-in six pulse generator (tube potential is varied in fixed increments from 25 kVp to 50 kVp, maximum tube current 200 mA); automatic exposure timer Amplimat with mobile ionization chamber and the light localizer which shows the extent of the area used for automatic timing. X-ray tube with rotating anode, Mo target, beryllium window and added molybdenum filtration. Single focal spot, 0.6 mm. The x-ray tube gantry can be moved vertically, perpendicularly or parallel to the chest wall. It can also be tilted at an angle of 15° from the chest; electromagnetic brakes. Compression by means of a transparent plastic plate. Focus-film distance 40 cm (for axilla and spotfilm radiographs with small format 45 to 50 cm also possible). Exposures initiated by operator behind a transparent radiation shield.

with observation windows. Figs. 1.14 through 1.20 show sketches of various mammographic installations and their most important characteristics. The legends contain further technical information.

Fluidograph of Dobretsberger

Apart from those installations which usually are not equipped for optimum image quality, only one unit, the Fluidograph of Dobretsberger, is available for the isodensity technique described on page 16. Fig. 1.21 shows the characteristics of this installation.

Mammographic Unit of Odelca

For mammographic photofluorography, a 70 mm Odelca camera with mirror optics is available. It has an input screen of 26 cm × 26 cm. Since the image quality is limited by the resolution characteristics of the fluoroscopic screen, a special fine grain detail screen is used. It naturally requires a higher dose. The following technique factors have been described in the literature: focus-film distance 40 to 65 cm, 20 to 30 kVp, 80 to 150 mAs. Figure 1.22 illustrates a photofluorographic installation for mammography with the Odelca camera.

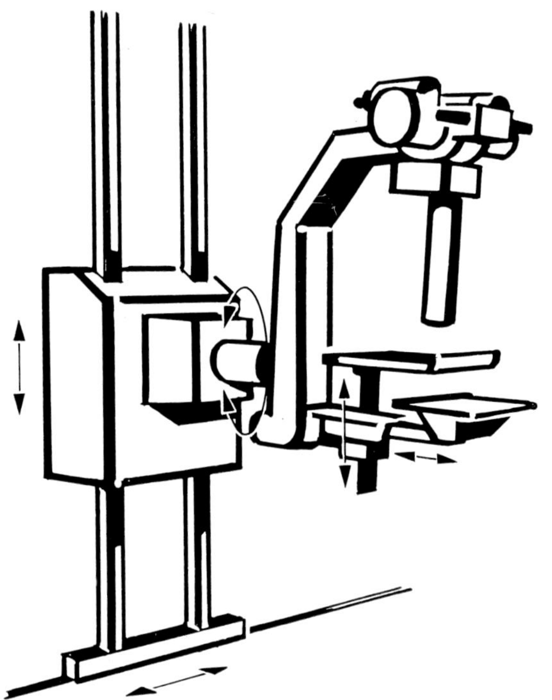

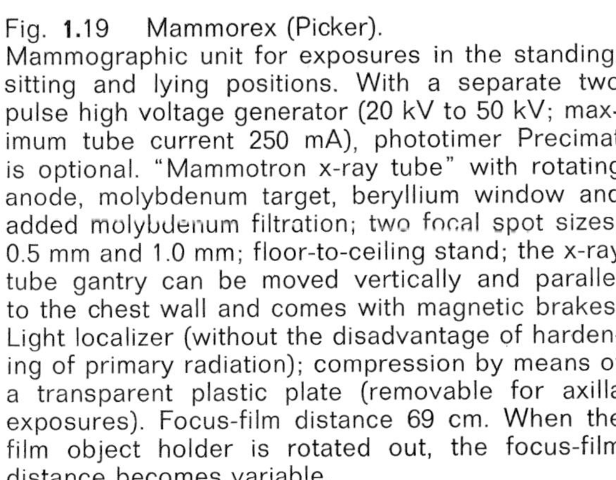

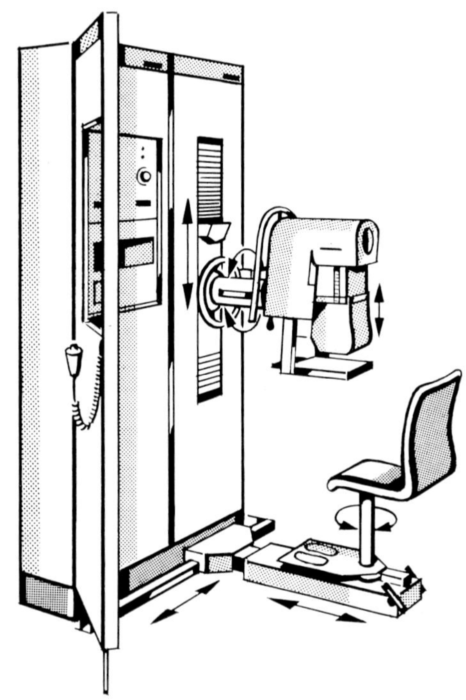

Fig. **1**.19   Mammorex (Picker).
Mammographic unit for exposures in the standing, sitting and lying positions. With a separate two pulse high voltage generator (20 kV to 50 kV; maximum tube current 250 mA), phototimer Precimat is optional. "Mammotron x-ray tube" with rotating anode, molybdenum target, beryllium window and added molybdenum filtration; two focal spot sizes, 0.5 mm and 1.0 mm; floor-to-ceiling stand; the x-ray tube gantry can be moved vertically and parallel to the chest wall and comes with magnetic brakes. Light localizer (without the disadvantage of hardening of primary radiation); compression by means of a transparent plastic plate (removable for axilla exposures). Focus-film distance 69 cm. When the film object holder is rotated out, the focus-film distance becomes variable.

Fig. **1**.20   Mammomat (Siemens AG, Medical technology division). Mammographic unit for exposures in standing, sitting, and prone positions. Six pulse generator (300 mA at 25 kVp; 100 mA at 50 kVp) with push button selectors. Automatic exposure timer "Iontomat 7" (or manual mAs selector); detector built into the film carrier. Visual control of the position of the detector for the lateral exposures. Grounded electrode x-ray tube with rotating anode, molybdenum target, beryllium window and added Mo-filtration. Focal spot size 0.6 mm. The x-ray tube gantry has magnetic brakes, can be moved vertically and rotated through angles of 270°. Transparent compression cone with telescopic motion. Focus-film distance (45 cm). Film change without disturbing the object. Patient data recorded during the exposure. Patient chair can be rotated horizontally and transversely. Swivel-mounted door shield with large lead window.

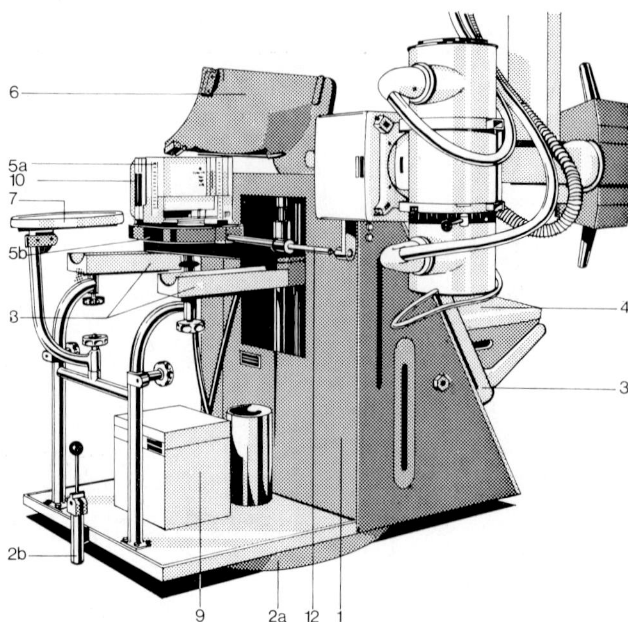

Fig. **1.**21   Fluidograph after Dobretsberger (Siemens Corp., Austria, Medical x-ray division).

1) stand;
2) rotating plate and 2b) stopping mechanism;
3) motor driven patient chair;
4) knee cushion;
5a) "Isodensity" tank and cassette holder;
5b) collecting vessel with central drainage pipe;
6) support for breast not to be exposed;
7) head rest;
8) arm rest;
9) radiation shielded cassette box;
10) moving grid;
11) coupling arm between x-ray tube and collecting vessel 5b, or isodensity tank 5a. Used to center the x-ray beam and the grid.

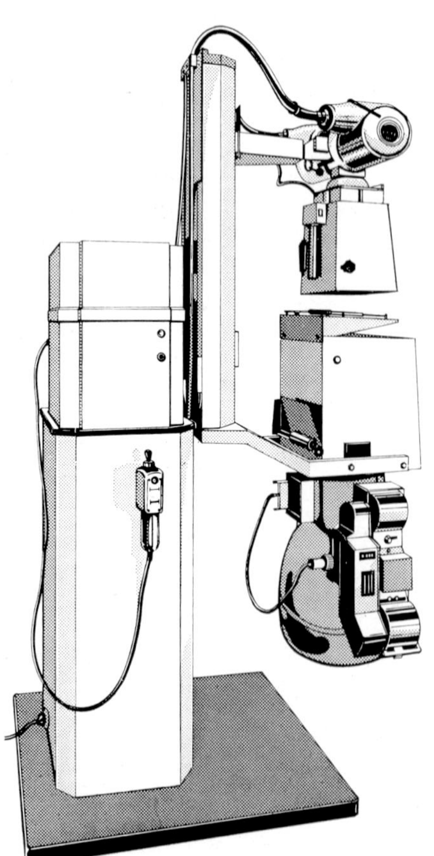

Fig. **1.**22   Odelca 70 mm mammographic unit with special stand for serial photofluorography (N. V. Optical Industries "De Oude Delft" Delft, Netherlands). Set for craniocaudal exposures. Above: x-ray tube with cone. Below: Fluorographic cone with object holder (7 cm above the entrance plane of the cone), Odelca camera, and serial cassette.

Methods of Breast Examination

Chapter 2

Clinical Examination

Only the basic principles of clinical examination of the breast will be discussed. Further details may be sought in the monograph by ZINSER (1972).
The clinical examination of the breast is based on history, inspection and palpation.

History

This provides very important information regarding the breast. Family and gynecological history allow evaluation of the overall risk of breast cancer. One should ask regarding the occurrence of malignant disease in the family and the organ of involvement. The patient's personal history should include any previous malignant diseases, age of menarche, live births and abortions, age of menopause and its cause (physiological, hysterectomy, oophorectomy, castration by radiation therapy). With regard to lactation one should ask about the frequency and length of lactation and the amount of milk produced. The history of puerperal mastitis should be obtained. One should know whether there has been any breast surgery. This will help in interpretation of the mammograms and also provide information about the probability of breast cancer. Further points in the history should include an evaluation of the patient's hormonal state including the use of hormone preparations and knowledge of what

clinical complaints brought the patient in for mammography (pain, trauma, lumps, abnormal secretions or skin changes).

The occurrence of pain immediately preceding menses is probably on the basis of some pathological changes in the breast. Such pain often awakens the patient at night. Breast pain not associated with menses in the pre- or postmenopausal woman is often the earliest sign of carcinoma. The more localized the pain the more it suggests carcinoma. Tingling or the sensation of ants crawling over the breast is suspicious of comedocarcinoma. Pulsating pain generally indicates inflammatory disease.

Hematomas and ecchymoses follow trauma (blunt injury, chronic pressure or vigorous breast examination, etc.). A spontaneous hematoma may be an early symptom of breast carcinoma. In regard to lumps it is important to ascertain whether there has been a recent increase in size. It is also important to understand whether the lump was discovered by the patient or found during a routine physical examination.

Spontaneous lactation in the absence of pregnancy is part of the CHIARI-FROMMEL syndrome (see page 78).

The color of the discharge provides a clue as to its origin (see page 28). Eliciting the history of soiled undergarments (brassiere, nightgown)

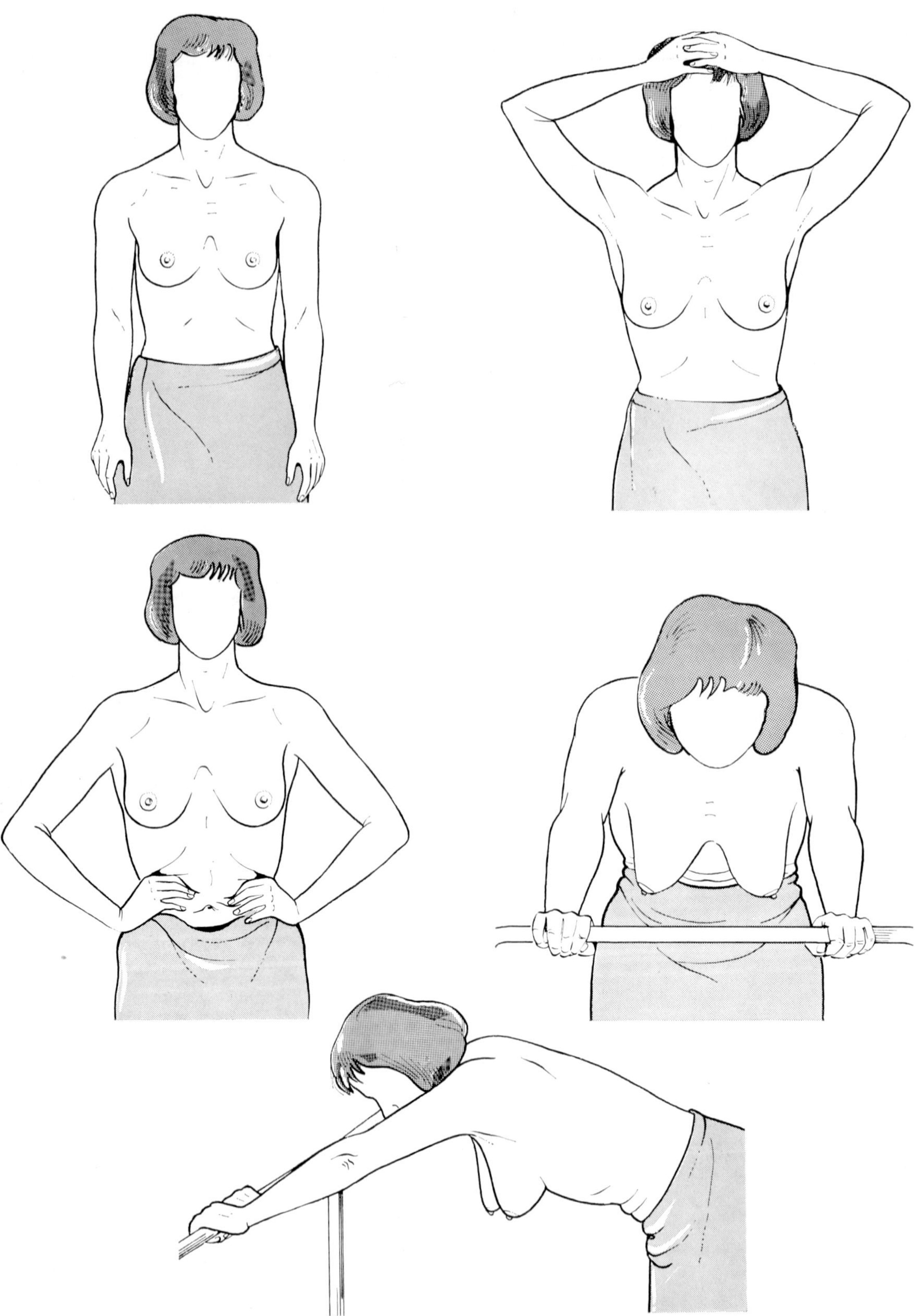

Fig. **2.1**   Positioning of the patient during clinical examination.

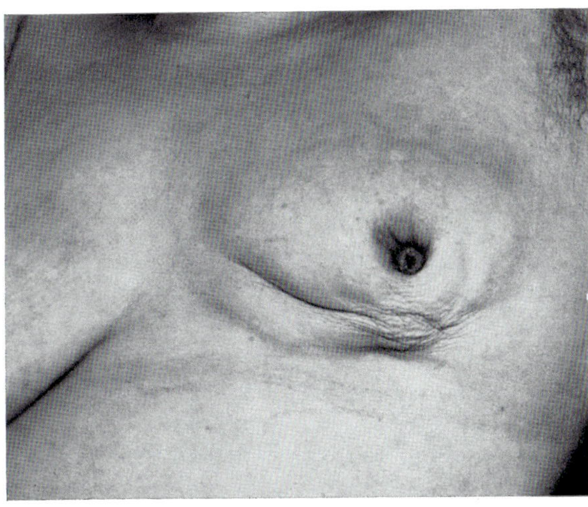

Fig. 2.2   Breast is reduced in size and deformed from scirrhus carcinoma. Nipple retraction. Skin fixation.

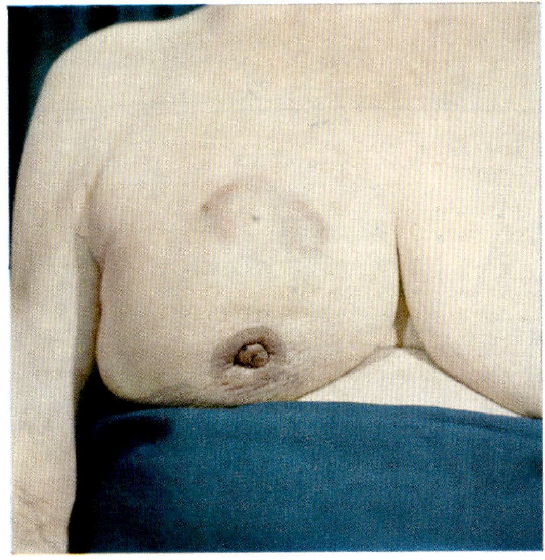

Fig. 2.4   Subcutaneous extension of carcinoma simplex immediately prior to ulceration. Nipple retraction and peau d'orange of the inferior portion of the breast and areola.

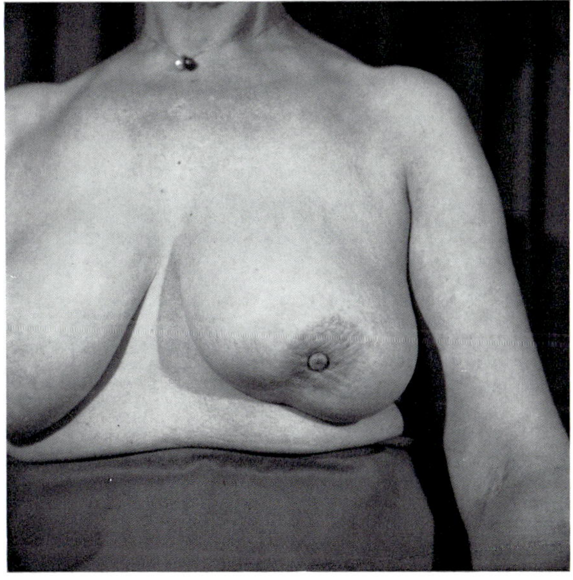

Fig. 2.3   Alteration of the normal curvilinear shape of the breast and nipple retraction secondary to scirrhus carcinoma.

indicates that the patient is not aware of nipple discharge.

One should inquire regarding any previous mammography in order to obtain those films for comparison.

Inspection

Like palpation this part of the examination is performed with the patient standing, supine and bending forward with both breasts suspended from the thorax. During the examination the arms should be placed in the following positions: hanging at the side, raised over the head, and the hands placed on both hips (fig. 2.1). One should note the size and shape of the breasts. A difference in breast size is frequently physiological; however it can also indicate tumor (widespread scirrhus carcinoma: decrease in breast size, fig. 2.2; enlarging tumor: enlargement of the involved breast). In regard to the shape of the breast it is important to note alteration of contour from the usual curvilinear shape (fig. 2.3), localized protruding masses (fig. 2.4), retraction and flattening. These appearances may be very subtle and can all be produced by previous incision or surgery. Alterations of skin color may be caused by inflammatory processes, trauma or by inflammatory carcinoma. One must take careful note of dermatological lesions. Warts for example may cause difficulty in mammographic interpretation. Retention cysts of sebaceous glands, which appear as small yellow nodules, have a tendency toward calcification and may mimic intramammary calcification in the roentgenogram. These must be distinguished on physical examination from skin metastases which are larger reddish nodules (fig. 2.5). Widespread carcinoma produces the so-called "cancer en cuirasse" or may ulcerate.

The so-called "peau d' orange" (orange peel skin) represents skin edema secondary to disturb-

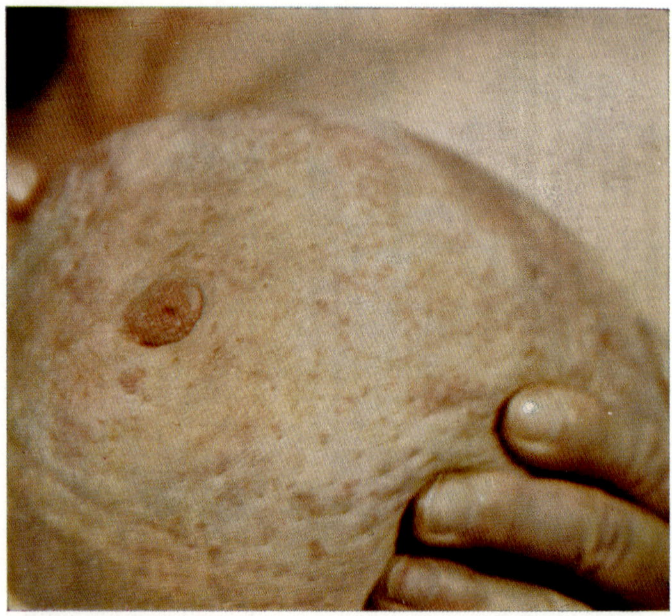

Fig. **2**.5   Skin metastases in diffuse carcinoma. Peau d'orange secondary to carcinoma extending into lymphatics.

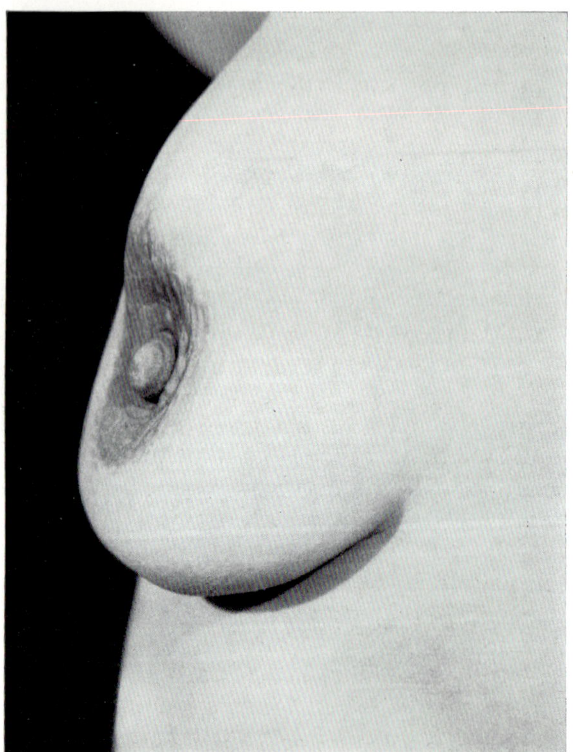

Fig. **2**.6   Nipple retraction from carcinoma.

ed lymph drainage from multiple tumor metastases blocking the lymphatics. Such skin edema may also be caused by right- and left-sided heart failure, cicatricial contraction and the reticuloendothelioses.

Prominent veins may be a sign of malignancy. Most frequently there is dilatation of the veins in the upper half of the breast. This same venous dilatation may be seen with a large fibroadenoma. Symmetrical venous dilatation has no clinical significance. The areola should be examined for signs of retraction, nipple secretion and inflammatory changes. Retraction of the areola does not always indicate carcinoma although this is the most frequent cause (fig. 2.6, 2.2, 2.3, 2.4). Clinical history should allow a differentiation between areolar retraction on a congenital basis, scar formation (fig. 2.7), repeated infections or chronic progressive retraction secondary to plasma cell mastitis (Fig. 2.8). The various degrees of skin retraction, ranging from flattening of the skin surface to fixed inversion, are simply various grades of the same process and do not signify any inference as to pathogenesis.

Spontaneous secretion may be recognized by yellow or brown crusty deposits on the areola even when the patient does not indicate this as her major complaint. Such silent nipple discharge is most frequently seen with fibrocystic disease. In this disorder the discharge has a milky-yellow or green-brown color, is primarily bilateral and originates from numerous ductal openings. Bloody discharge suggests the possibility of ductal carcinoma or papilloma, or of ulceration of a lactiferous duct. In ductal ulcer the secretion most commonly has a brown color. Lactiferous duct ulcer is the result of stasis and inspissation of secretions which exert pressure on the inner wall of the duct, resulting in erosion and ulceration similar to a decubitus ulcer. If the patient has a milky nipple discharge which is persistent, even for several years since the last period of lactation, it may represent the galacturia part of the CHIARI-FROMMEL syndrome.

With any nipple discharge a sample must be taken for cytological examination (this should be done before any galactogram). Inflammatory breast disease results from a sunken nipple, secretory disease and poor hygiene. Inspissated secretions, resembling smegma, may result in frank mastitis. A focus of acute mastitis behind the areola may result in swelling and redness of the nipple (fig. 2.9). Eczematous changes of the nipple (associated with transudation, crust formation, itching, burning, scaling of the epidermis, punctate hemorrhages as may be seen following trauma) may occur not only with eczema but also with PAGET's carcinoma (fig. 2.10). Eczema of the areola can only be distinguished from early PAGET's carcinoma by mammography. Failure of such a lesion to resolve completely after one month of therapy constitutes an absolute indication for further diagnostic workup.

Palpation

In addition to bimanual examination of both breasts, including the inframammary folds (fig. 2.11), palpation of both axillae, the supraclavicular region and an attempt at expression of the secretions from the nipple should be performed. The quality of information obtained is not related to the pressure of the palpating hand.

Ecchymoses and hematomas result in pain for the patient and an inaccurate examination for any subsequent examiner.

The object of palpation is to determine breast disease by noting changes in consistency within the breast. The entire breast must be systematically palpated.

Whichever scheme one chooses to use is unimportant as long as it is a consistent and repeated one. Usually one begins the examination by palpating the presumed normal breast. Any area of localized pain deserves particularly careful examination.

The comparison of palpatory findings in both breasts helps in the determination of the signific-

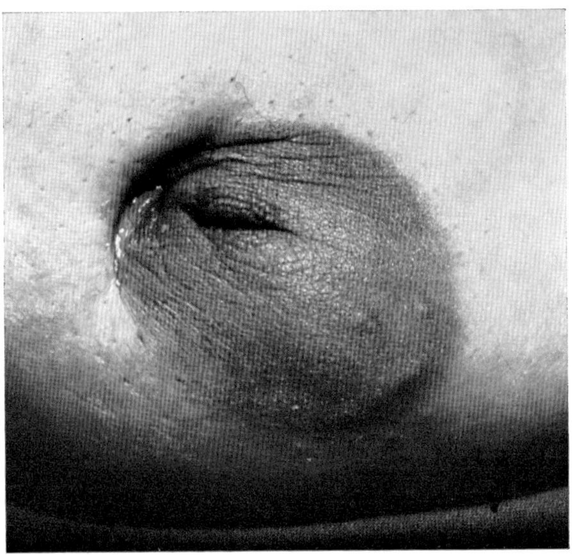

Fig. **2.**7   Nipple retraction secondary to a surgical scar from incision and drainage of breast abscess following mastitis.

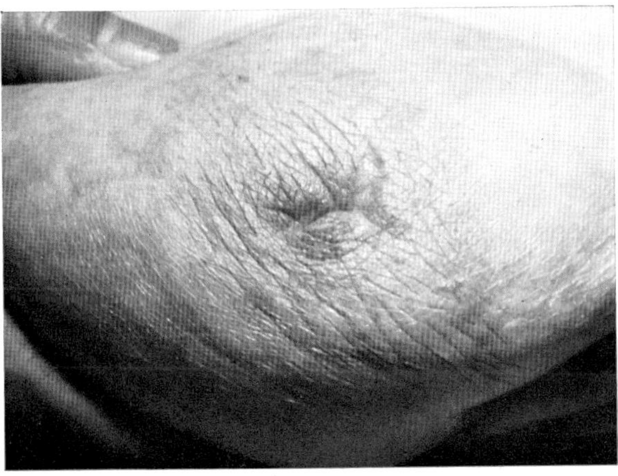

Fig. **2.**8   Retraction of the nipple in plasma cell mastitis.

ance of the difference in consistency found in one breast. If fatty involution is asymmetrical a persistent focus of parenchyma may feel like a lump.

If the palpatory findings are not clear the examination should be repeated in three months. If mammography of both breasts still leaves the diagnosis in doubt biopsy should be performed. In the normal breasts definite differences in consistency are not palpable. The consistency of the breast may be greater laterally than medially insofar as there is a more lateral distribution of parenchymal tissue. A uniform nodularity diffu-

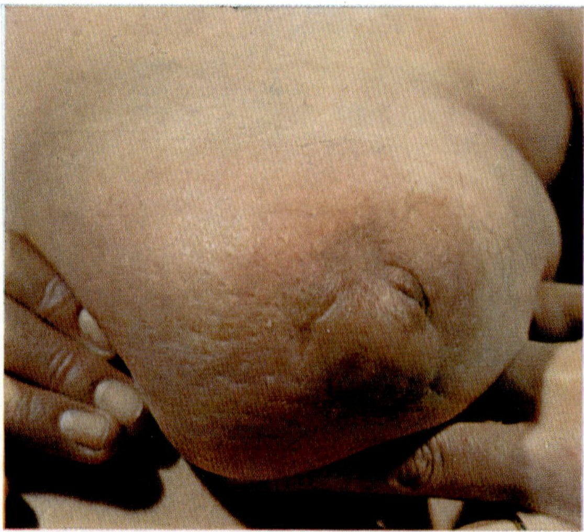

Fig. **2**.9   Erythema and swelling of the nipple in subareolar mastitis. Peau d'orange.

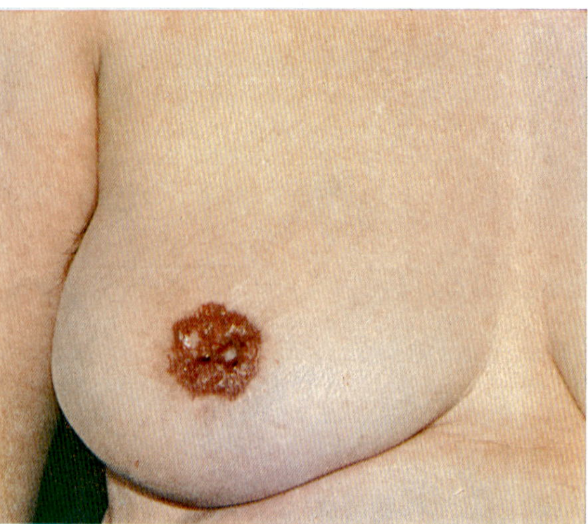

Fig. **2**.10   Eczematous changes of the right nipple in advanced Paget's carcinoma

sely distributed over both breasts suggests fibrocystic disease. In these cases one must palpate with extra care to be able to detect differences in breast consistency. Palpatory findings often give a clue to the underlying pathology. A fibroadenolipoma is frequently soft, a cyst is firm and smooth. Lesions that appear hard to palpation include fibroadenomas, carcinomas, sarcomas, occasionally lipomas, residual parenchyma, scars, focal areas of fibrosis and regions of inflammation. A fluctuant mass suggests abscess. Compression of a premenopausal breast, rich in parenchyma, between the thumb and index finger allows demonstration of a lump. This may be facilitated by bimanual examination.

With any palable lesion one must determine size, consistency, shape, the degree of separation from surrounding tissue, mobility in relation to the skin and underlying tissues, localization and tenderness. The size of a lesion itself gives little information regarding the cause. Changes in size over a period of time, however, may be significant. Young women frequently complain about painful premenstrual breast nodules which may not be demonstrable on x-ray examination. Clinical examination 10 days after menses in such cases is often diagnostic. An obvious difference in the size of a breast mass between palpation and what is visible on the mammogram is an important sign of carcinoma (see page 204).

Sizes of breast lesions should be described in centimeters rather than in terms of their resem-

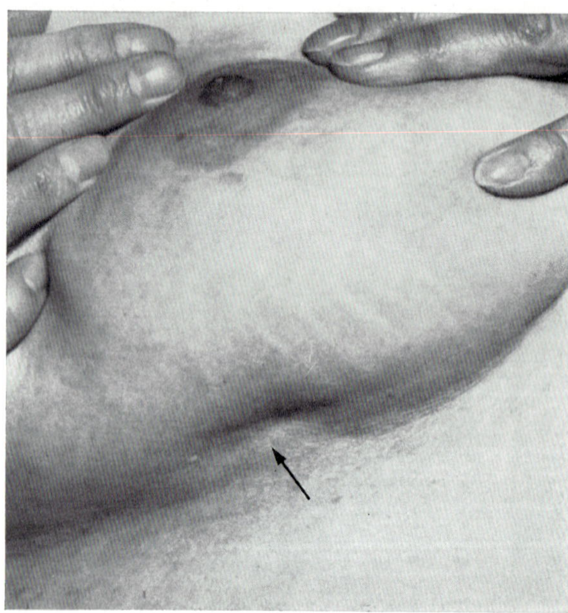

Fig. **2**.11   Skin fixation from a carcinoma near the inframammary fold.

blance to agricultural items such as beans, peas, cherries or nuts. The shape of a breast mass is less likely to provide a clue as to its pathology. It is true that lipomas are frequently oval and cysts or fibroadenomas classically are round and sharply defined from neighboring tissues. However, sharply marginated rounded masses may also be carcinoma, sarcoma, abscess or hematoma.

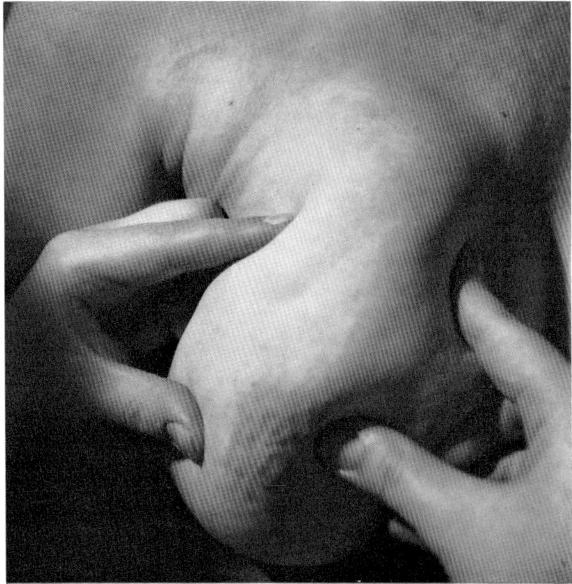

Fig. **2**.12 Flattening of the skin (plateau sign) demonstrated by pressing the skin surfaces together using the thumb and index finger of both hands in order to detect the earliest stages of skin fixation.

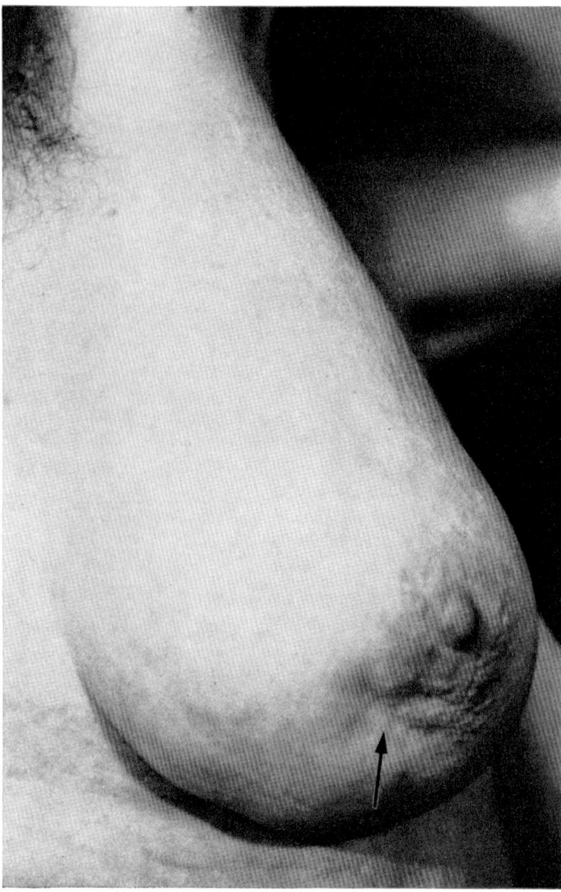

Fig. **2**.14a Circumscribed skin fixation along the inferior aspect of the areola secondary to a foreshortened fibrosed Cooper's ligament.

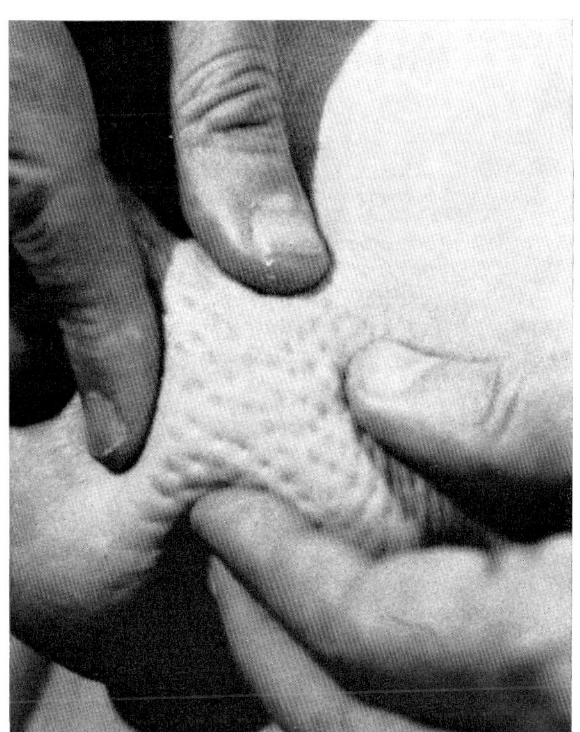

Fig. **2**.13 "Peau d'orange". This phenomenon is demonstrated by compressing the skin using thumb and index finger of both hands.

Smooth margins and sharp demarcation from neighboring tissue suggests a benign process. Poor margination is found with carcinoma, hematoma and inflammatory processes.

It is important to determine clinically whether a lump is freely movable in regard to the overlying skin or the underlying thoracic wall. By attempting to move the lump or the entire breast back and forth across the thoracic wall one can determine fixation by an infiltrative process. In order to determine whether a mass is fixed to the overlying skin various maneuvers are helpful (fig. **2**.1): elevation of both arms over the head, placing both hands on the hips and flexing the pectoralis muscles, and having the patient lean forward in order to suspend both breasts from the chest.

By compressing the skin with thumb and index finger of both hands one may frequently elicit a

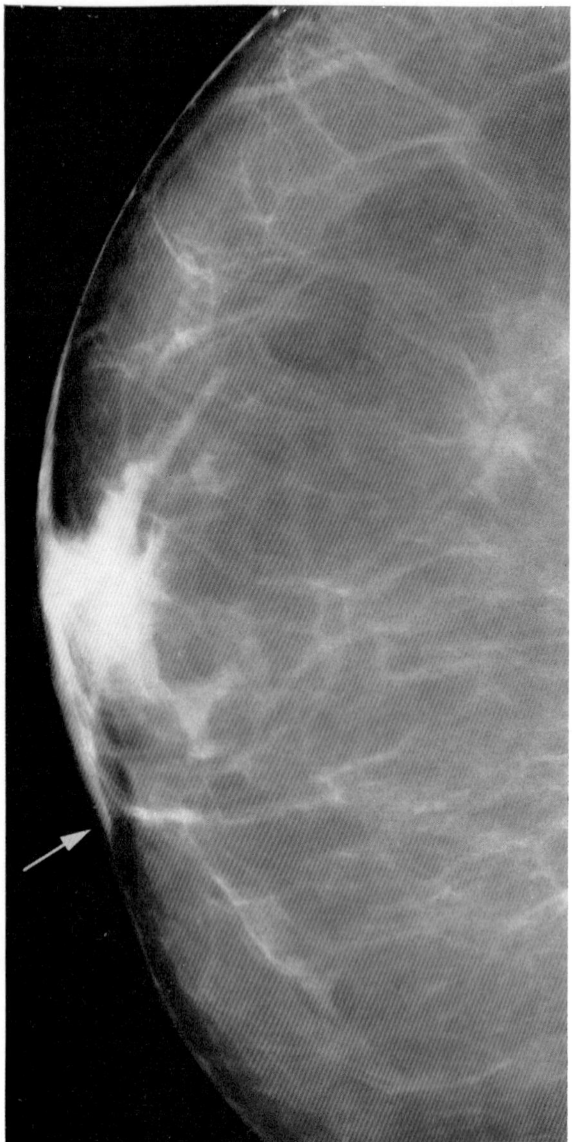

Fig. **2**.14b   The corresponding mammogram verifies the skin retraction to be the result of a scar. No evidence of carcinoma.

plateau formation of the overlying skin (fig. 2.12) or demonstrate "orange peeling" of the skin (fig. 2.13). The multiple punctate skin retractions demonstrated by this maneuver may indicate an underlying carcinoma or fat necrosis as a result of trauma, foreshortened COOPER's ligaments or a small area of local fibrosis (fig. 2.14a and 2.14b). With this compression maneuver one is better able to evaluate disease processes in the inframammary fold, an area which is frequently difficult to evaluate (fig. 2.11). It is

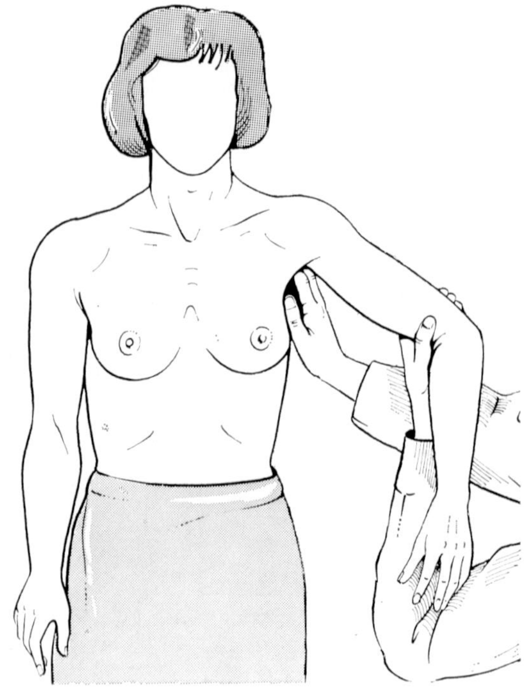

Fig. **2**.15   Palpation of the axilla.

important to localize a mass during palpation and to correlate this with the mammographic findings. This becomes particularly important when a process localized by palpation cannot be found in the mammogram.

Easily palpated lipomas for example are frequently not demonstrable in the x-ray film and only with careful search can one visualize the fibrous capsule of such a mass with any degree of frequency. Likewise one may see an occult carcinoma adjacent to an easily palable cyst. The patient's complaint of localized breast pain may indicate carcinoma, even in the absence of palpatory evidence. It is not true that breast pain rules out carcinoma.

In order to facilitate examination of the left axilla the patient places her left hand on the anterior aspect of the examiner's left forearm and the axilla is then examined with the right hand (fig. 2.15). This position is reversed for palpation of the right axilla. It is important that the pectoralis musculature not be flexed during this portion of the examination. One must remember that soft axillary lymph nodes 5 to 6 mm. in diameter may be found following nail bed inflammatory processes of the finger (McNAIR & DUDLEY, 1960, in 37% of their cases).

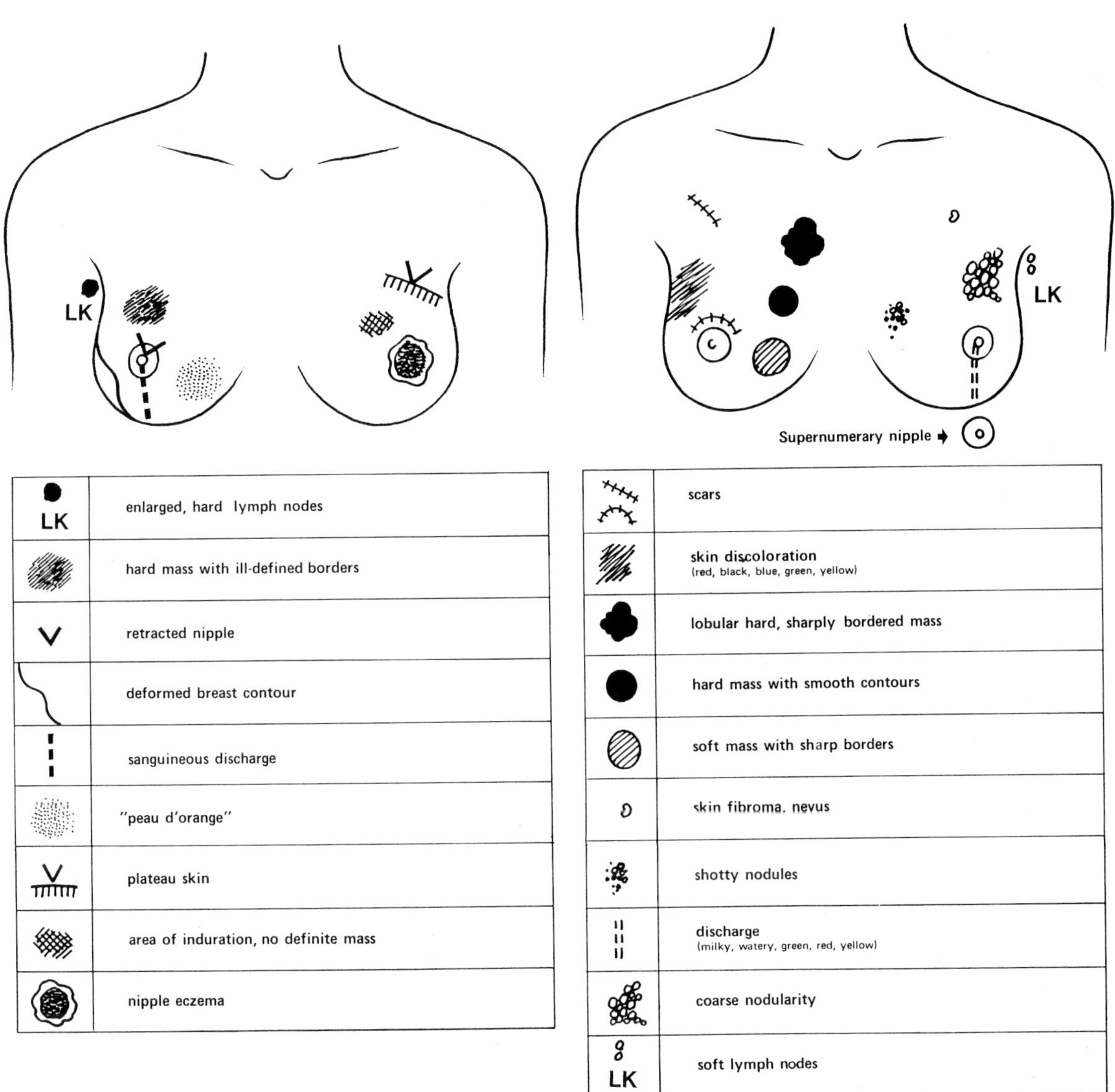

Fig. 2.16 Symbols for clinical findings.

Metastatic lymph nodes are as a rule harder and larger.

Next, the supraclavicular lymph nodes should be examined and a search made for metastatic changes although involvement of these nodes is a late finding.

With each breast examination one should attempt to express secretions from the nipple. The breast is placed in the palm of the examiner's hand while pressure is placed on the dorsal aspect of the breast with the other hand in a motion extending from the wall of the thorax towards the areola. If discharge is obtained a smear should be performed and sent for histological evaluation (page 44).

The use of symbols has been helpful when trying to document the findings at physical examination and these are described in fig. 2.16.

Chapter 3

Mammographic Technique

Positioning

Correct positioning is of the greatest importance because this determines whether the entire breast is included in the roentgenogram. It is particularly important to achieve visualization of the thoracic wall. It is necessary that the roentgenograms be made in standard positions in order to allow accurate comparison and follow-up studies.

Mention should be made of a few problems. Earlier the roentgenogram was performed without compression (so-called "EGAN Technique") but today the examination consists exclusively of compression mammograms. The advantage of compression technique is that it produces a more uniform density, better image quality with easier differentiation between real findings and summation effects.

The craniocaudad projection is exposed while the patient is sitting or standing. The lateral examination should be made with the beam directed in a mediolateral direction. The best technique unqualifiedly is with the patient supine because in this case the breast distributes itself symmetrically onto the film and a portion of the thoracic wall may be included in the roentgenogram. For purposes of technical simplicity, however, the lateral projection is performed with the patient sitting or standing. This requires strong compression of the breast in order to secure it between the x-ray tube and the film. The dependent breast therefore must be pulled forward and elevated by the technician. This may be facilitated by slight tilting of the examining table, approximately 15° towards the outside with subsequent tilting of the upper portion of the patient's body.

Large breasts require several projections to make a composite examination.

Coned-down views with small tube heads (diameter approximately 5 to 6 cm.) are very helpful in questionable lesions. The size of the tube head depends on the size of the area in question. Preceded by accurate localization of the suspicious lesion the area is centered and compressed as much as possible with the tube. Coned-down views in the lateral projection while the patient is sitting can only be performed by pulling the breast forward and upward and then securing it with compression using the tube. Coned-down views in this projection are easier and more reproducible when the patient is supine.

Craniocaudal Projection (Fig. 3.1)

The patient sits on a stool the height of which may be altered and which is both movable and can be locked into position. More recent mammographic units allow examination while the patient is standing. The patient is placed in front of the film holder and the breast laid upon it. The film holder is then set at the correct height which is when the film holder and table elevate the breast slightly so that it compresses itself. The inferior margin of the breast must be exactly

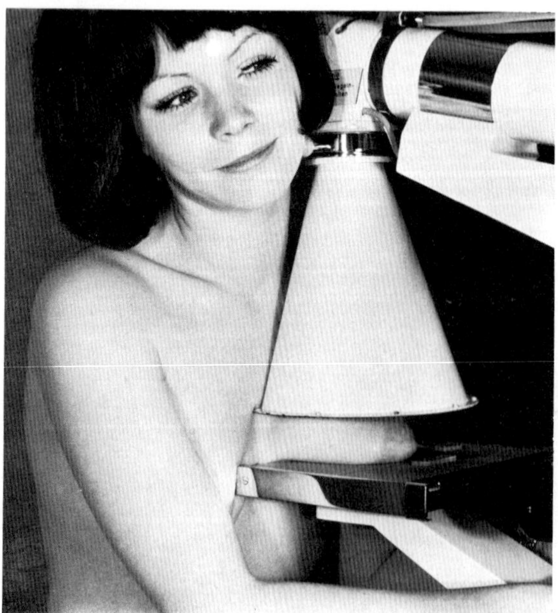

Fig. **3**.1 Positioning for craniocaudad projection.

at the edge of the film and this requires that the patient press the thorax against the film table.

The ipsilateral shoulder must be relaxed and pulled slightly inferiorly and posteriorly in order to allow good projection of the lateral quadrants of the breast on the film. The patient places both hands loosely on the examining table or sometimes grasps hand grips. The head must be turned in the opposite direction. The x-ray tube is pressed against the superior surface of the breast and is adjusted to produce as much compression as is tolerable. One must be careful that the breast is not turned inferiorly nor that skin folds be produced by the compression from the tube. The beam should be centered on the center of the breast not the nipple.

Lateral Projection Sitting or Standing (Mediolateral) (Fig. 3.2)

The roentgen apparatus is adjusted into the lateral position. The patient bends forward slightly, the ipsilateral hand grasps an appropriate hand grip on the unit and the film carrier is pushed as high as possible into the axilla. The shoulder is relaxed. The lateral rib margins must be pressed firmly against the film cassette. The technician elevates the dependent breast into its normal form, pulls the breast slightly forward and compresses it as much as possible between the cassette and the x-ray tube. The nipple should be positioned far laterally towards the film cassette. Demonstration of that part of the breast close to the thoracic walls and ribs is not possible in the lateral examination when performed while the patient is sitting (one cannot achieve the desired amount of breast compression in this

position). This is the main disadvantage of performing the lateral projection with the patient sitting or standing.

Lateral Examination while the Patient is Supine (Mediolateral) (Fig. 3.3)

The patient lies on her side on the examining table. The arm of the side being examined is

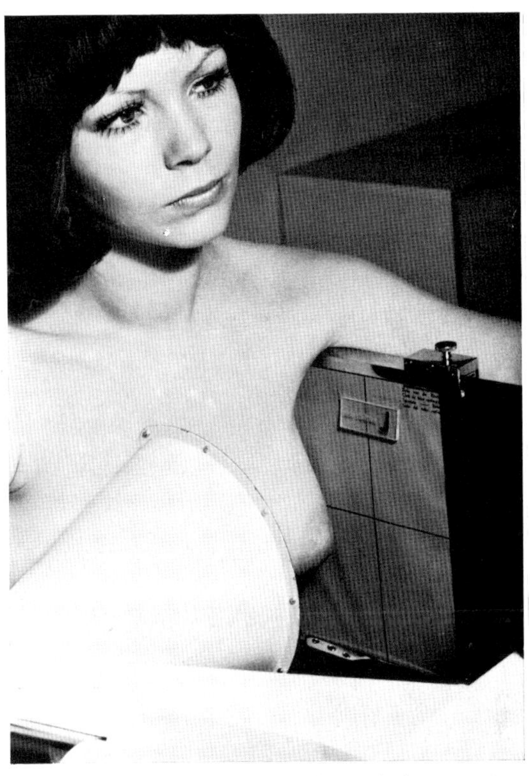

Fig. **3.2** Positioning for the lateral (mediolateral) projection.

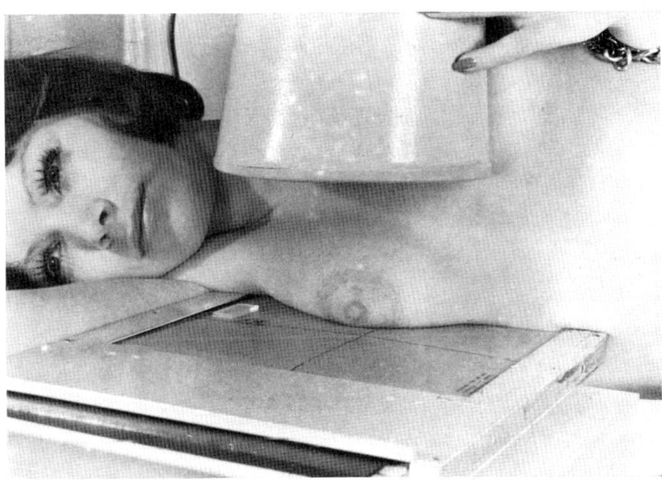

Fig. **3.3** Positioning for the lateral mediolateral projection with the patient supine.

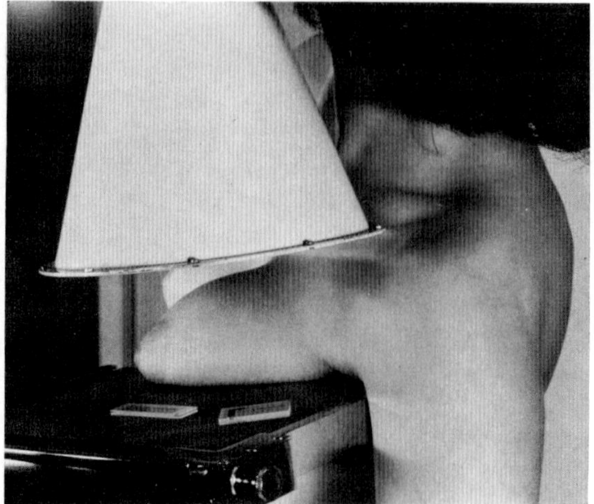

Fig. **3.4** Positioning for the projection of the lateral portion of the breast (so-called "third projection"). (a) Note orientation and arrangement of the breast on the film holder.

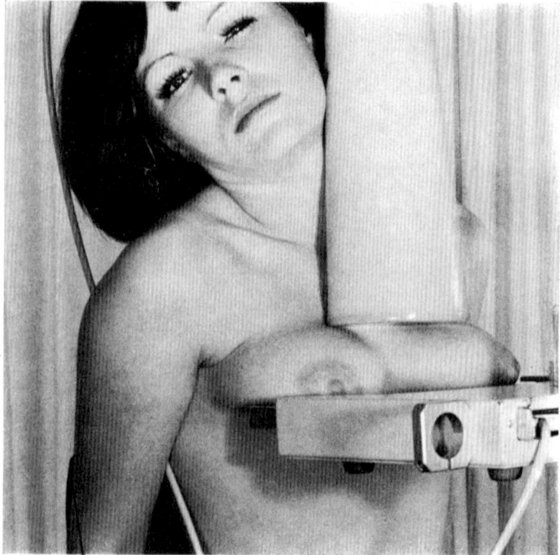

Fig. **3.5** Positioning for the projection of medial portions of both breasts.

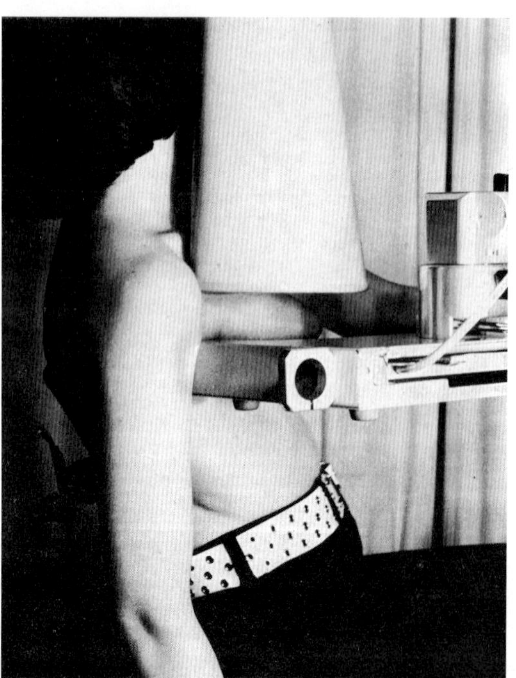

(b) Final position for this projection including compression.

placed as high as possible under the head. The film cassette is placed as far as possible into the axilla underneath the breast. The cassette is elevated by the use of various articles (this is not necessary in a variable film holder) until the breast is elevated and flattened and the nipple is in exact profile. The arm is then moved anteri-

orly until it forms a right angle with the body, the forearm flexed and the hand held in supination under the head (no pillow). The contralateral breast and shoulder are pulled posteriorly and the tube is positioned directly against the sternum. The tube is then used to compress the breast to be examined.

Lateral Portions of the Breast, the So-Called "Third Projection" (Fig. 3.4a, b)

The lateral portion of the breast including the axilla is placed on the film cassette. The patient leans towards the side being examined and the shoulder of the ipsilateral side is pulled far down letting the arm hang. The patient supports herself with the opposite hand by grasping the examination table. The tube head is positioned so that it comes in contact with the head of the humerus and the upper ribs. One must be careful to prevent skin folds from projecting over the breast parenchyma.

This projection is made easier by those units which allow tilting to the side. 10° to 15° of tilt towards the axilla is sufficient.

Examination of Medial Portions of the Breast (Fig. 3.5)

The patient leans forward as far as possible pressing the sternum against the film holder and supports herself by grasping the examination

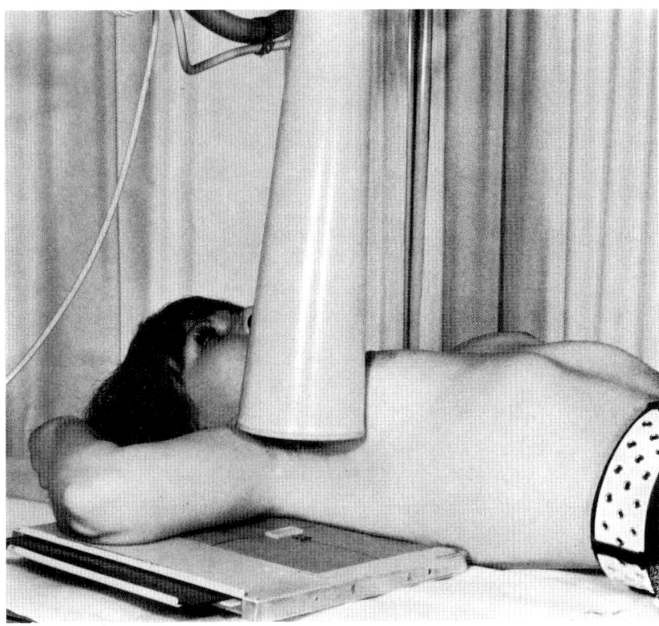

Fig. **3**.6 Positioning for the axillary projection.

table. The medial portions of both breasts are distributed over the film by pulling the breast forward and flattening them. The smallest tube head is used and positioned firmly against the sternum and thereafter compressing the parenchyma and skin from above. It is recommended that Bipac film be used in this projection in order to clearly differentiate the transition of skin and subepidermal tissues as well as the tissue of one breast from that of the other.

Instead of combining the medial portions of both breasts on one film one may choose to project the breasts separately on separate films.

Axillary Projection (Fig. 3. 6.)

The patient is supine. The upper arm is at right angles to the body, the forearm flexed and the hand placed under the head in supination. The film is placed underneath the axilla in such a way that the upper arm and ribs will be included in the projection. The breast is pulled medially and the tube head is positioned against ribs and head of the humerus.

This projection is performed without compression but the kilovoltage must be increased.

Localized examination with compression may be performed; however, this will not permit the inclusion of the entire axilla and soft tissues of the thorax. Furthermore there need not be an increase in kilovoltage.

Localized Projection

To localize a suspicious area in the craniocaudad projection, one draws a line from the nipple perpendicular to the base of the breast and a second line extending from the suspicious area vertically to the first line. The length of the two lines up to the point where they coincide is measured and these measurements are transferred to the breast. The cone-down view is centered on this position (Fig. 53.1a—c).

One proceeds similarly for the lateral projection. There may be differences in localization in the actual breast when measurements from the craniocaudad and lateral projections are transferred but these are due to the differences in the projections and must be taken into consideration. One proceeds in a similar fashion when using the roentgenograms to localize a nonpalpable lesion for biopsy.

Other Projections

Roentgenograms of the suspended breast (KEATS and co-workers 1963) have not proved themselves of value.

The isodensity method of mammography according to DOBRETSBERGER has been described on page 16.

Other methods such as those dealing with interpositioning of materials of varying density

-to achieve equalization of contrast on the film have also not been generally accepted (SEIDEL 1964).

Marking the film

The marking of the films must be uniform. The following method is used internationally:

a) Craniocaudad projection: Demarcated with `craniocaudad` in the middle of the film opposite the nipple; the left breast is indicated with the letter `L` and the right breast with the letter `R`, each respective letter being placed on the lateral side of the breast towards the axilla. Next to the letter indicating the side the word `lateral` is included.

b) Lateral projection: This is indicated with the words `lateral projection`. This demarcation is positioned at the level of the upper portion of the breast. In other cases it may be necessary to add the words `upper` or `lower`. Right and left is demarcated with the letters `R` and `L` and these letters are placed in the upper portion of the film.

c) Demarcation of the axillary, medial and lateral and localized views is undertaken in a similar fashion as those above. Special localized view of smaller fields may not be demarcated with the use of lead markers and must be marked by hand prior to development.

Film*

Cassette films with screens cannot be used because any screen damage or debris or dust particle collections on the screen may lead to the misdiagnosis of microcalcification. Furthermore, even small grain screens do not have sufficient resolution.

Nonscreen film is also not utilized because the resolution is inadequate. Special films used in mammography are constantly being improved. It is desirable that when the film is examined with a magnifying glass (magnification factor of 2 to 3) that one be unable to discern the film grain. This requirement is filled by several brands, for example Gevaert Mammoray T_3, Kodak Definix Medical, DuPont Microtest NDT75.

* See page 12; footnote.

Films must not be bent. Singly packed film must be shaken so that the film within the package moves towards that edge of the package which is positioned against the thoracic wall.

Bipac film (two films of different sensitivity in one package) are particularly suitable for simultaneous delineation of dense central breast parenchyma as well as subcutaneous tissues and skin. A similar effect may be achieved through the use of a "folded film", a single film folded into a double film.

Curvilinear cutting of the film to achieve closer apposition to the thoracic wall (DONOVAN 1964) does not appear to allow better projection of the breast in the craniocaudad view.

Film development

Mammographic films may be developed by hand with the usual developers at 20° centigrade for a period of 5 minutes. Films with lesser sensitivity (for example, Structurix D4) require a development time of 10 minutes.

The film should be sufficiently exposed (no less than an optical density of 2.0) Underexposed mammograms, although they are appealing, do not allow the detection of subtle density differences or adequate evaluation of the skin and subcutaneous tissues on the usual view box. Microcalcifications within dense parenchyma are detectable only on overexposed films. Such heavily exposed films should always be obtained if one is searching for microcalcifications.

Mammographic film with thick emulsion layer and a high silver content can only be developed through a slowly processing developing machine. Films with the characteristics for example of Gevaert Mammoray T_3 require a machine developing time of 10 to 12 minutes at 22° centigrade and a drying temperature of 45° centigrade. Films with the characteristic of Kodak Definix Medical may be developed over a period of 3½ minutes in an automatic developer.

If all the requirements are satisfied then there is no difference in quality between mammograms developed by hand or those developed in an automatic processor. A few special types of films used in mammography may be developed in an automatic processor over a period of 4½ minutes; however, some compromise regarding the size of film grain and contrast must then be accepted.

Chapter 4

Pneumocystography

This examination consists of cyst puncture, aspiration of the contents and subsequent air inflation of the cyst followed by roentgenograms taken at right angles to one another (GROS et al 1954; GROS 1963; HAAGE and FISCHEDICK 1964; HOEFFKEN and HINTZEN 1970).

Indications

This examination is indicated in all smoothly-marginated breast masses having a typically benign appearance and also for clinically palpable nodules which cannot be definitely identified in the roentgenogram because of overlying dense parenchyma.

There are no completely reliable roentgen criteria that can allow definite differentiation between a breast cyst or a fibroadenoma. Differential diagnosis is only possible by aspiration. Occasionally medullary carcinoma or carcinoma simplex is difficult to differentiate from benign cysts or fibroadenomas.

Equipment

(1) Skin disinfectant; (2) sterile towels, gloves and sponges; (3) 14 gauge needle and syringe for local anesthetic (for example, 2% novocaine with epinephrine); (4) cc. syringe for aspiration; (5) specimen container, slides.

Technique

After the usual sterile preparation of the entire area, the breast is palpated with sterile gloves. Sterile technique must be observed at all times during the procedure.

In accordance with the mammograms and palpatory findings one orients one's self as to the exact position of the lump and introduces local anesthesia into the skin and subcutaneous tissue at the proper location. Some feel that local anesthesia is not necessary; however, according to our experience, the procedure can be quite uncomfortable without local anesthesia, partic-ularly if puncture is made in the vicinity of the areola. Additionally local anesthetic containing epinephrine should be used to diminish the risk of hematoma formation.

The breast mass is held firmly between thumb and index finger and a needle is advanced into the mass. A cyst wall can be so firm that it simulates a solid tumor and not infrequently one is surprised to see fluid coming from the needle. The syringe is now connected to the needle and the contents of the cyst are completely aspirated. The patients position may be shifted to facilitate total aspiration.

The emptied cyst is now filled with air, the quantity slightly less than the amount of fluid aspirated. Thereafter roentgenograms are made at right angles to one another. It is recommended that the lateral view be obtained while the patient is sitting in order to document the total removal of the cyst contents. With incomplete aspiration an air-fluid level will be detected (fig. 14.3).

The aspirate is sent for cytological examination (see page 44).

Results and significance

1) The main objective of cyst puncture and pneumocystography is to allow differential diagnosis between a cyst and a solid mass. If it is a solid mass rather than a cyst, cellular material will be aspirated and cytological examination will decide the etiology of the mass. 2) Following complete aspiration of the cyst and subsequent instillation of air 90% of such cysts collapse completely and scar down. Observations have been made histologically of such collapsed and fibrosed cysts following aspiration. Incompletely aspirated cysts may not collapse and become fibrotic; they can recur and may require repeat aspiration later on. In our opinion the instillation of air is particularly important for the desired therapeutic effect of aspiration. Recurrence is more frequent if the aspiration is done without injection of air. Complications

are uncommon. We have experienced one case of mastitis and three hematomas in 250 pneumocystographies (1971).

Operative removal of a solitary cyst is not necessary when the following requirements are fulfilled: (1) The inner wall of the cyst is completely smooth in the pneumocystogram; (2) there are no paracystic masses; (3) cytology of the aspirate is negative; (4) there is complete regression of the cyst within a period of three months following aspiration.

A further advantage of the use of pneumocystography in preference to surgical removal is that even though larger cysts may appear to be solitary at clinical examination, in reality a great number of these are associated with smaller cysts. These can develop into large "solitary cysts" at any time and this may require repeated surgical interventions. The result is a rather difficult management of the patient and also the cosmetic disadvantage of numerous scars.

3) Those cysts which do not fulfill the above-described criteria must be removed surgically. Intracystic malignant changes are very rare. Malignant changes are more inclined to occur in the outer portion of the cyst wall or with an area of mammary dysplasia in the vicinity of the cyst. Particular attention to the region of the cyst must be paid at pneumocystography. It is easier to evaluate these areas following complete emptying of the content of the cyst. Furthermore, it is important at pneumocystography to carefully examine the other portions of the breast roentgenologically as well as by clinical examination in order not to overlook a carcinoma developing completely independent of the cyst under investigation.

4) If puncture reveals that one is dealing with a solid mass rather than a cyst, cellular material should be aspirated from the mass at several sites and smears made for histological examination (see page 48).

Chapter 5

Galactography

The first investigator to demonstrate lactiferous ducts by injecting Lipiodol was E. RIES (1930).

The complications included infection and abscess formation (RIES 1930; ROMANO & MCFETRIDGE 1938).

At one time thorotrast was also used as the contrast agent. However, the danger of inducing malignancy with this material prohibited its use.

LEBORGNE (1944) evolved the technique of galactography using aqueous contrast material. Further reports using this method were made by BJOERN-HANSEN (1965), BJOERN-HANSEN and TALLE (1966), GREGEL and POPPE (1967), and WEISHAAR et al (1970). GROS (1963) coined the term galactography to describe the examination of lactiferous ducts with positive contrast material. SPRATT and DONEGAN (1967) named this technique mastography, and ZUPPINGER (1952) called it glandulography.

Indications

Galactography is an appropriate and useful extension of mammography. It is indicated in all patients with abnormal nipple discharge.

Any nipple discharge is considered pathological when it occurs at a time other than gestation and lactation or persists beyond the normal postpartum lactational period. Unilateral breast secretion whether serous, milky or pastelike, and discolored secretion, green, brown, reddish or frankly bloody are always considered pathological. It is normal, however, to see a clear drop of liquid appearing at the nipple after vigorous attempts at expression. In such a case galactography is difficult because it is only with great patience and frequently with some injury that one is able to cannulate the tiny milk duct. In states of pathological nipple discharge galactography is almost always possible since the ductal opening is larger and more amenable to dilatation and cannulation.

Instrumentation

(1) Sterile gloves; (2) sterile preparation materials (3) dilating sound (lacrimal duct probe, etc.); (4) lacrimal cannula or lymphangiography cannula; (4) water-soluble contrast material (Urografin, Conray, etc.); (6) suitable lighting (surgical lamp); (7) magnifying spectacles are advantageous.

Technique

Galactography should be preceded by a smear and histological examination of the discharge. Galactography may be performed in the sitting or suspine position. In the sitting position the craniocaudal projection and in the supine position the mediolateral view are the most easily obtainable. We prefer to conduct the examination with the patient supine.

After sterile preparation of the nipple an attempt is made to express secretion in order to localize the opening of one of the lactiferous ducts and begin dilatation. Following this, cannulation is performed with a nasolacrimal or lymphangiography cannula attached to a syringe. The cannula should not be inserted deeper than 1 cm. because the lactiferous duct then becomes tortuous and the danger of perforation increases.

Gentle hand injection of contrast material is performed while compressing the papilla in order to improve the seal around the cannula. Care must be exercised that the contrast material does not contain air bubbles since these may be mistakenly interpreted as intracanalicular papillomas.

The concentration of contrast material used during galactography must be much less when xeroradiography rather than film mammography is used. With the xerox technique the recording of a high contrast shadow will result in a halo phenomenon which can obliterate any structures in the immediate vicinity. The toner is concentrated in the region of radiographic contrast material to such an extent that none is available for deposition in the immediate neighboring areas. Important small details (for example microcalcifications which may indicate intraductal or periductal carcinoma) may thus become invisible. Therefore, a 10:1 dilution of the contrast material is recommended whenever ductography is being done with xeromammography (FISCHEDICK and EVERS 1974).

The amount of contrast material varies from 0.2 to 2 ml according to the size of the duct being injected and the extent of the ductal system one is trying to demonstrate. One must rely on pressure sensation during the injection in order to know when enough material has been injected. If the injection pressure is too high extravasation results, secondary to rupture of one of the lactiferous ducts or parenchymal infiltration of the contrast material. A burning sensation felt by the patient suggests extravasation or too much contrast material injected. Slight leakage of contrast material from the mammary duct opening at the end of the injection indicates intra- rather than paraductal injection. In papillomatosis, associated with increased lactiferous secretion there may be dilution of the contrast material. In this case one must frequently use a rather high injection pressure to even introduce contrast material into the ductal system. This problem may in some cases be circumvented by alternately aspirating and injecting the duct and thus achieving a higher concentration of the contrast medium in the system.

Immediately after filling of the lactiferous duct films are made in two projections. One must be careful in positioning the patient for the exposures in order to prevent out-flow of contrast. This is best achieved by having the patient compress the nipple. Mammography during galactographic examination is performed without compression to avoid expressing the contrast material. In most cases the examination is painless. Complications such as inflammation or abscess formation do not occur when water-soluble contrast agents are used and sterile technique is observed. Ductal perforation or extravasation of contrast, secondary to high injection pressure, may cause a tense sensation in the breast or frank pain. However, these generally resolve within 30 to 60 minutes. Breast binding may be helpful in cases of painful irritation of breast parenchyma following the injection. Prophylactic antibiotic therapy is not necessary. However antibiotic treatment is indicated in the event of inflammatory complications following the procedure.

We have had no complications in 178 galactographies (1971).

Significance and Results

In "secretory disease" one finds ductal ectasia and variation in caliber of the lactiferous ducts. In fibrocystic disease one may not uncommonly demonstrate one or several small cysts during galactography.

Papillomas appear as smooth round or wormlike filling defects within the milk ducts. The smooth margins of such filling defects indicate benignancy. Papillomatous carcinoma, in the galactogram, presents as a filling defect with ill-defined margins. However, there is some overlap and a definite differentiation between benign and malignant papillomas is not possible with this procedure. The main purpose of galactography is to demonstrate the location of the lesion rather than to differentiate between its benign or malignant character. Only with this method of diagnosis is it possible to engage upon a localized surgical resection of the lesion. Surgical removal of a diseased lactiferous duct is facilitated by injection of methylene-blue into the duct immediately before surgery.

Carcinoma results in displacement, encasement and irregularity of the contours of the lactiferous ducts within and in the vicinity of the tumor. WEISHAAR et al (1970) have reported their experience with galactography in 75 patients: 11 cases of lactiferous duct ectasia and cysts with or without periductal inflammatory changes or simple fibrocystic disease; 18 cases of intracanalicular papilloma; eight cases of widespread papillomatosis; eight ductal carcinomas. Of interest is that these authors were unable to determine any clinical or abnormal roentgen findings in 16 of their 18 cases of intracanalicular papilloma. Also in their eight cases of papillomatosis there were only three patients who had abnormal clinical or mammographic findings. Of the eight patients with ductal carcinomas only three were demonstrable by mammography or clinical examination, and the remaining five carcinomas would not have been detected without galactography.

A year later this same group of workers reported an additional 11 cases of ductal carcinoma diagnosed exclusively by galactography (RUMMEL et al 1971).
Undoubtedly, papillary ductal carcinoma which grows and spreads in an intraductal fashion cannot be recognized on mammography unless there has been necrosis and subsequent calcification. In these relatively infrequent cases of breast carcinoma an early diagnosis is only possible by recognition of an intraductal filling defect at galactography, followed by injection of methylene-blue into the involved duct to facilitate accurate biopsy.

Chapter 6

Cytology of the Breast

There are three applications of cytology in breast disease diagnosis:

Nipple secretion → exfoliative cytology
Cyst contents → exudative cytology
Solid mass → aspirational cytology

Indications

Breast cytology is indicated in the following cases:

1) breast secretion not associated with lactation;

2) cyst puncture;

3) evaluation of questionable palpatory findings with negative roentgen findings;

4) evaluation of questionable findings;

5) evaluation of diseases in which surgery is contraindicated; for example, the differential diagnosis between mastitis and inflammatory carcinoma or the determination of the tumor type in inoperable carcinoma prior to radiotherapy (GIBSON and SMITH 1957; WEBB 1970).

The significance of breast cytology in the diagnosis of breast diseases is currently under lively discussion. Experts in gynecological cytology are critical of mammary cytology (ZINSER 1972), whereas specialists in mammary cytology rely heavily on this method because of its exceptional reliability and degree of accuracy (FRANZEN and ZAJICEK 1968). In the Radium Institute of the University of Stockholm, all palpable breast changes are punctured and examined histologically. The results and conclusions of their studies are summarized by ZAJICEK (1969) in Table 6.1.

The data obtained in our own patient population are tabulated in Table 6.2.

On the basis of our own experience we are overwhelmingly convinced of the great value of breast cytology. The accuracy rate depends on the one hand on the experience of the cytologist and on the other on the proper removal of the diseased tissue and the correct preparation of the specimen. Unquestionably even with carefully localized aspiration of a breast mass there will be cases where cytological examination will fail to reveal the true diagnosis, particularly in the case of very firm scirrhus carcinomas and in fibroadenomas with very indurated connective tissue components. This is a lesser problem, however, because in these particular cases differential diagnosis on the basis of mammography is relatively easy and fairly reliable.

There are no contraindications to puncture and aspiration. In the event of breast abscess the lesion is punctured and aspirated followed by surgical and antibiotic therapy. No complications of aspiration have been reported. Puncture of cysts and fibroadenomas is harmless. Occasion-

Table 6.1

Cytological findings in 417 cases of histologically verified breast abnormalities from the Radium-Hemmet of Stockholm.

Cytological Findings	Benign 211	Precancerous 16	Carcinoma 190*	Total 417
Benign cells or cellular material	171 (81.0%)	13 (81.3%)	11 (5.8%)	195
Cellular atypia	36 (17.1%)	0	4 (2.1%)	40
Suspicious for carcinoma	4 (1.9%)	2 (12.5%)	24 (12.6%)	30
Carcinoma	0	1 (6.2%)	151 (79.5%)	152

* In one of these cases there was only suspicion of carcinoma.

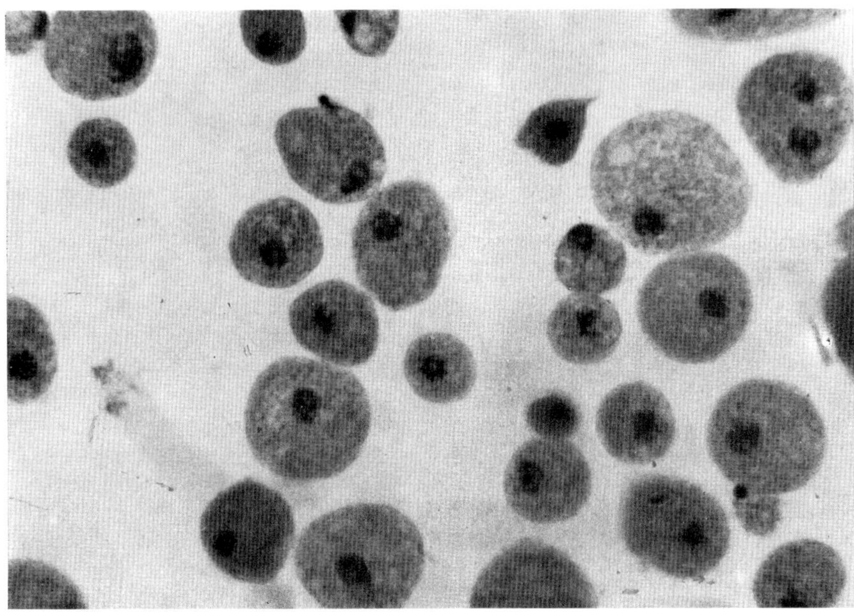

Fig. **6**.1 Breast secretions. Histiocytes, so-called "foam cells".

Table 6.2

Cytological Findings in 894 patients during 1971 (Radiation Institute AOK, Cologne and cytological laboratory of Dr. Merkl, Cologne).

	Total	Acellular or benign	Malig-nant
Breast secretion	497	494	3
Aspiration	397		
a) Cyst	230	228	2
b) Solid masses	167	149	18

ally a hematoma results but this is well and easily tolerated by both the patient and the physician as is any hematoma resulting from an injection or other medical therapy. The occurrence of such hematomas is rare and even though it may make any subsequent excisional biopsy a little more difficult, diagnostic puncture should not be omitted because of this minor complication.

The only real contraindication against puncture would be the risk of hematogenous dissemination of cancer. This problem was studied by ROBBINS et al (1954) as well as BERG and ROBBINS (1962). They compared the survival rate of patients who had puncture of a carcinoma preceding mastectomy with those who did not have the diagnostic puncture preceding mastectomy. There was no difference in 10-year survival rate between the two groups of patients. One may conclude on the basis of these studies that aspirational biopsy is not dangerous even in the case of carcinoma. The implantation of carcinomatous cells in the needle tract is possible and has been observed (Radium Institute); however, the tissue and the needle tract will be removed with mastectomy in the event that carcinoma is diagnosed on the aspirational biopsy.

Techniques of Mammary Cytology

Cytology of Breast Secretion

A. The secretion is uniformly spread onto a slide with another slide or a cover slip.

Technical error: The smear is too thick and therefore fissures occur on drying. If the secretion is thick it is better to divide it among several slides.

B. Fixation:

1) Dry fixation, in other words, drying with air. Advantage: Cytological material does not float away because of dissolving of the fix. Disadvantage: Only suitable for Giemsa stain. Autolysis interferes with Papanicolaou stain.

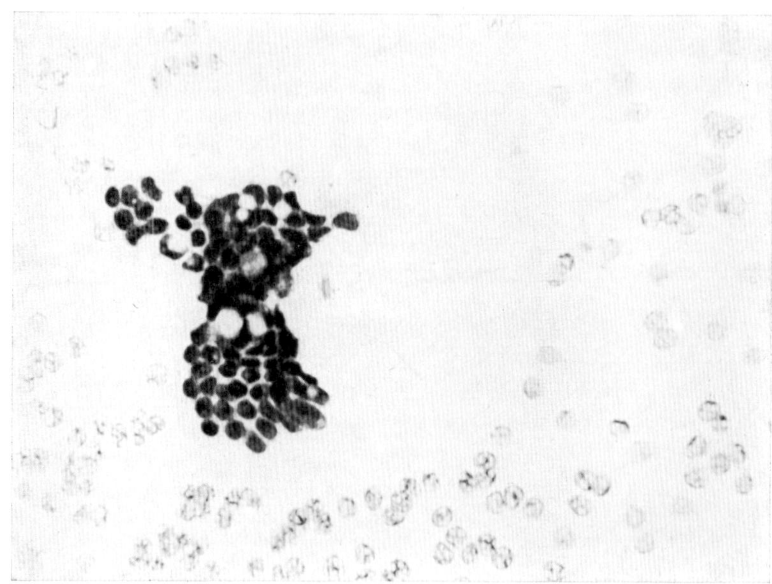

Fig. **6**.2 Ductal epithelial cells in a breast smear. The cells are cohesive and nuclei are small and uniform in size.

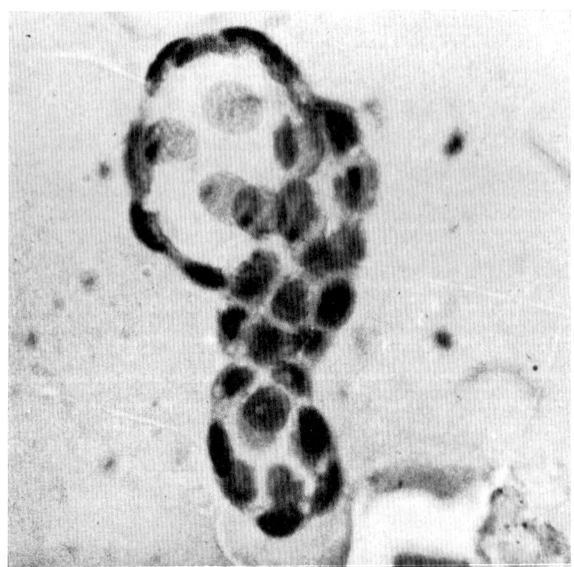

Fig. **6**.3 Breast smear. Intraductal papilloma. Adherent, uniform ductal epithelial cells arranged in a papillary formation.

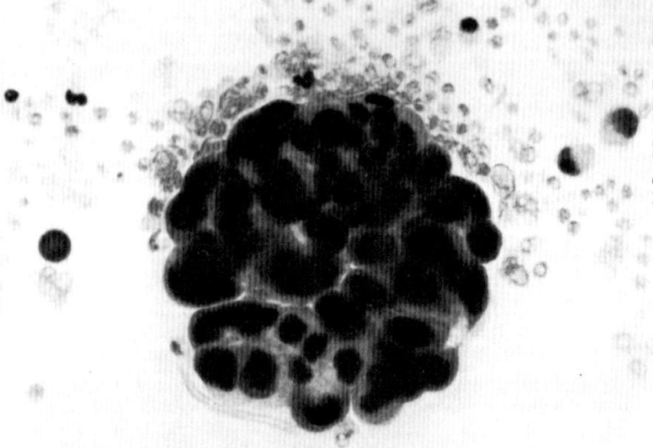

Fig. **6**.4 Breast secretion smear. Intraductal carcinoma. Clump of polymorphic overlapping and non-ordered epithelial cells.

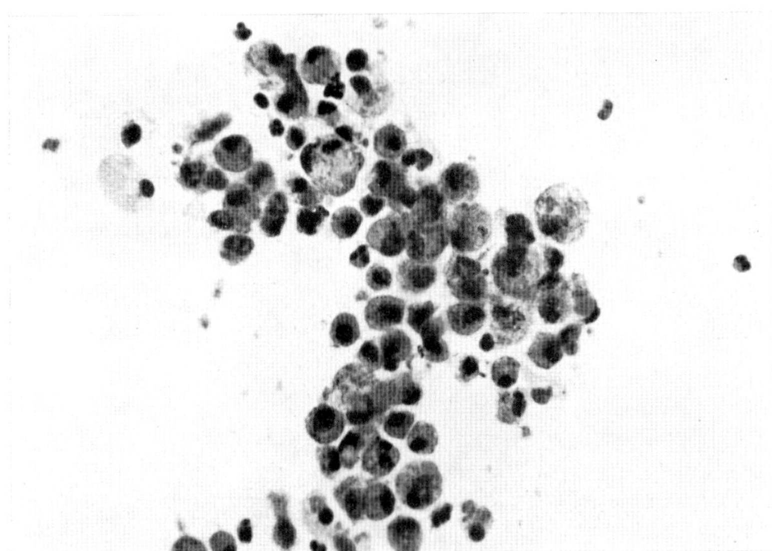

Fig. **6**.5 Cyst aspirate. Histio-cytes.

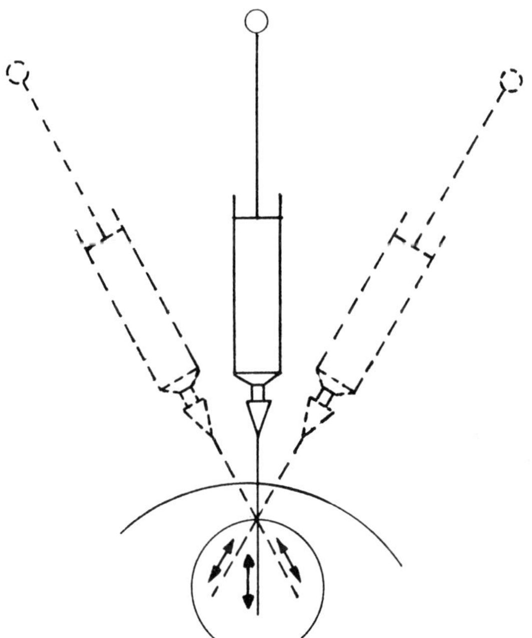

Fig. **6**.6 Technique of aspiration to obtain material for cytological examination from a solid breast mass.

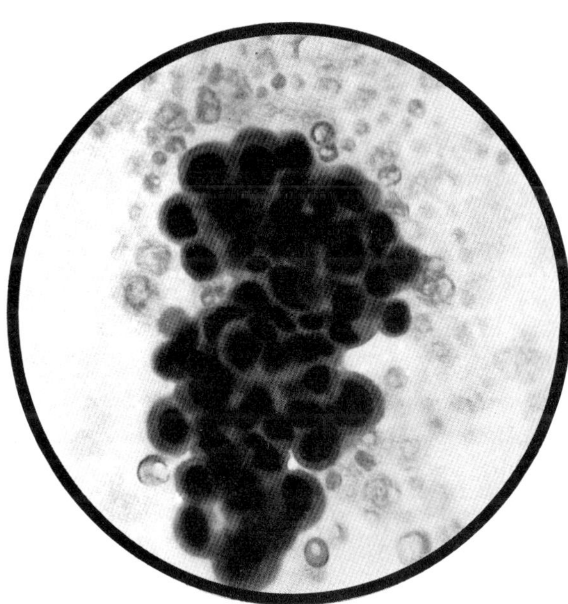

Fig. **6**.7 Aspirate from a breast carcinoma. Poly-morphic, hyperchromatic cancer cells arranged in a papillary formation.

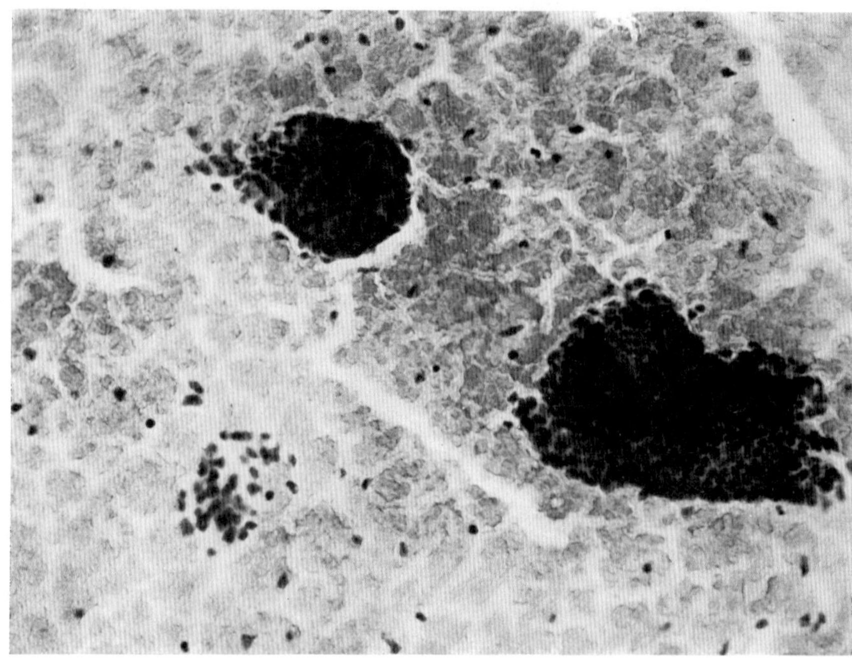

Fig. **6**.8   Aspirate from a fibroadenoma. Small uniform epithelial cells with definite intercellular cohesive pattern. Isolated nuclei are seen in the vicinty.

2) Wet fixation with 80% alcohol, methanol, acetone or alcohol-ether mixture.
Advantage: Easy stainability.
Disadvantage: Cellular material may float away.

3) Fixation spray (for example, Mercko-fix)
Advantage: The most suitable method resulting in good stainability and no loss of cellular material.

C. Stain:
Giemsa and Papanicolaou stains are the most suitable.

Cytology of Cyst Aspirate

The entire cyst contents collected in a clean test tube should be examined as soon as possible. No additives. The solution is centrifuged for 10 minutes at 2,000 revolutions per minute. The sediment is smeared onto several slides some of which are dried in air for Giemsa stain, others fixed in alcohol for Papanicolaou stain.

Aspirational Cytology of Solid Masses

Various biopsy needles may be used.
Following puncture the needle should be directed in several directions within the mass to obtain cells from several portions. The material is immediately spread onto several slides and smeared, using a cover slip (fig. **6**.6).

The material should first be smeared onto one-half of the slide and then with the other side of the cover slip spread evenly onto the other half of the same slide. If the Papanicolaou stain is planned, fixation must be immediate (best done with fixation spray).

Methods of Staining:

1) necrotic material:
Giemsa stain is not suitable, Papanicolaou staining is better.

2) Mucinous material:
Giemsa stain is most suitable. Mucus will not pick up Papanicolaou stain. As a general rule we prefer the Papanicolaou stain. The type of fixation is always indicated at the time of biopsy.

Interpretation of the Histological Materials

Diagnosis of Secretions

The following cells are present within mammary secretions:

Normal:

Histiocytes and degenerated histiocytes, "foam cells" (fig. 6.1);
small cuboidal ductal epithelial cells (fig. 6.2).

Pathological:

Erythrocytes (papilloma? carcinoma?);
leucocytes (mastitis?);
epithelial cells joined together as papillae (fig. 6.3);
tumor cells (fig. 6.4).

In sanguineous breast discharge the epithelial cells may be recognized only with difficulty because of extensive autolytic changes. In the case of a pathological breast secretion and a negative cytological examination repeat smears over a period of several days should be performed.

Diagnosis of Cyst Aspirate

A clear, colorless aspirate generally contains no cells. The following cells may be found in milky, yellow or green as well as brown or darker colored secretions:

Normal:

Mostly degenerated histiocytes (macrophages). Small cuboidal epithelial cells (rare) (fig. 6.5).

Pathological:

Leucocytes in great number; tumor cells (see fig. 30.3c).

Diagnosis of Cellular Material from Puncture of a Solid Mass

It is very difficult to aspirate material from a scirrhus carcinoma. In this case the number of cells in the aspirate may be very sparse, and this is similar to aspiration of a fibroadenoma with connective tissue predominant.

In all other types of tumors numerous cells are easily obtained if the aspirating needle has been correctly placed within the tumor mass (fig. 6.7 and 6.8).

Sanguineous material is difficult to evaluate. In the presence of severe autolytic changes and very few cells, a diagnostic impression should not be given. In such doubtful cases puncture and aspiration should be repeated.

If the aspirate contains mostly normal cells with an occasional atypical epithelial cell there may be a carcinoma in situ. A repeat examination is indicated.

Chapter 7

Arteriography

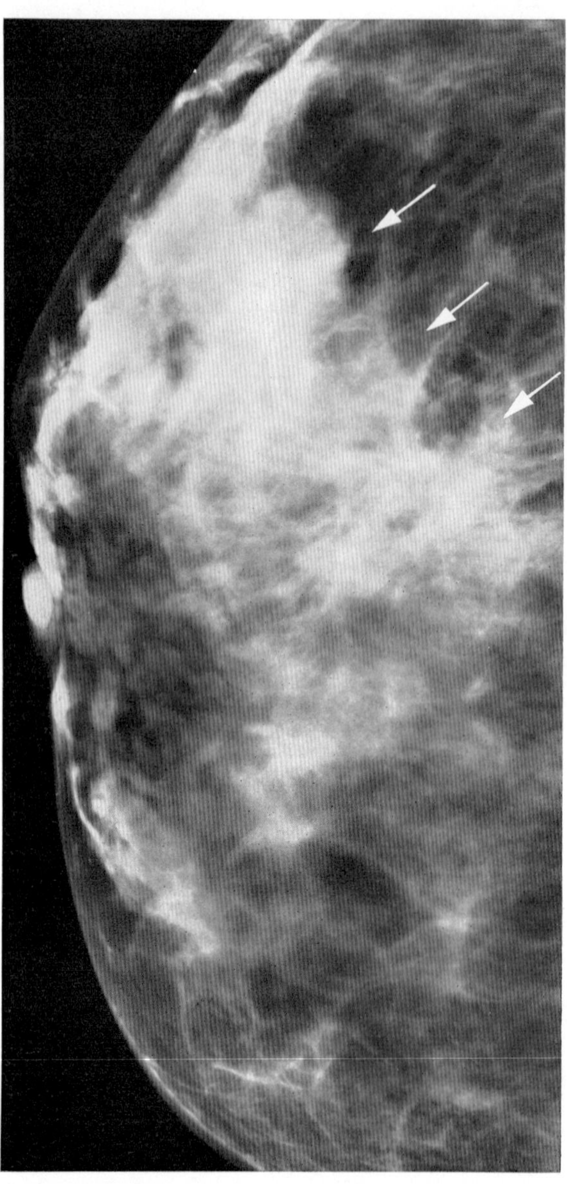

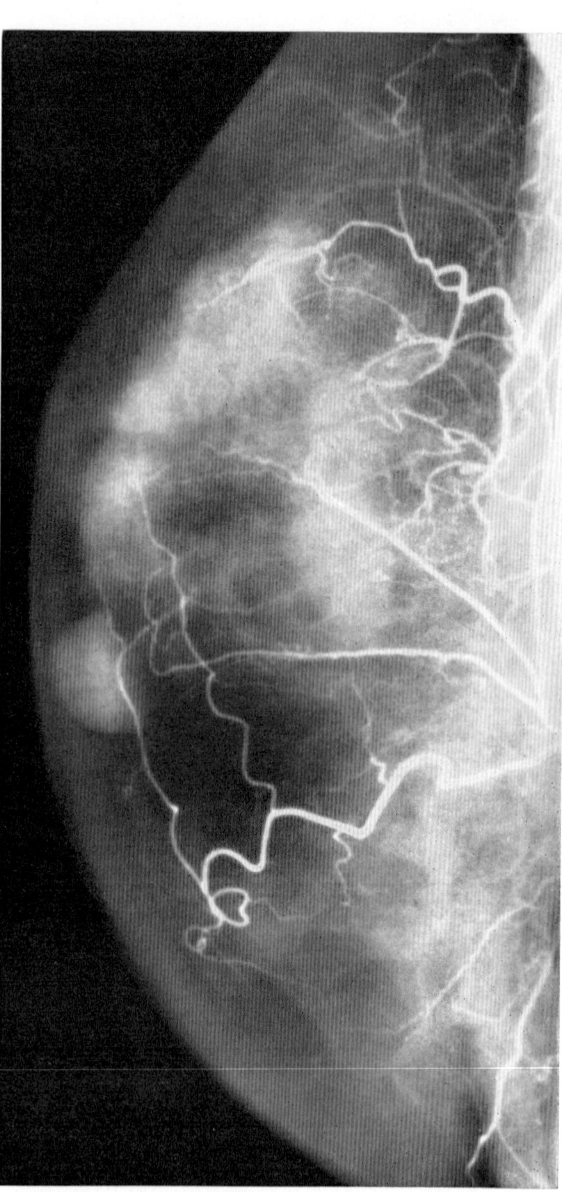

Fig. **7.**1a Mammogram: Abnormal structure in the upper region of the breast parenchyma with radiating borders and connective tissue strands extending into the fatty tissue: Invasive breast carcinoma. Histology: Carcinoma simplex with scirrhus type of extension.

Fig. **7.**2a Mammogram: Rounded mass 3 cm in early arterial phase: Interruption of arteries, narrowing of arteries, cork screw type vessels as well as neovascularity in the periphery of the tumor. Tumor stain not yet visible.

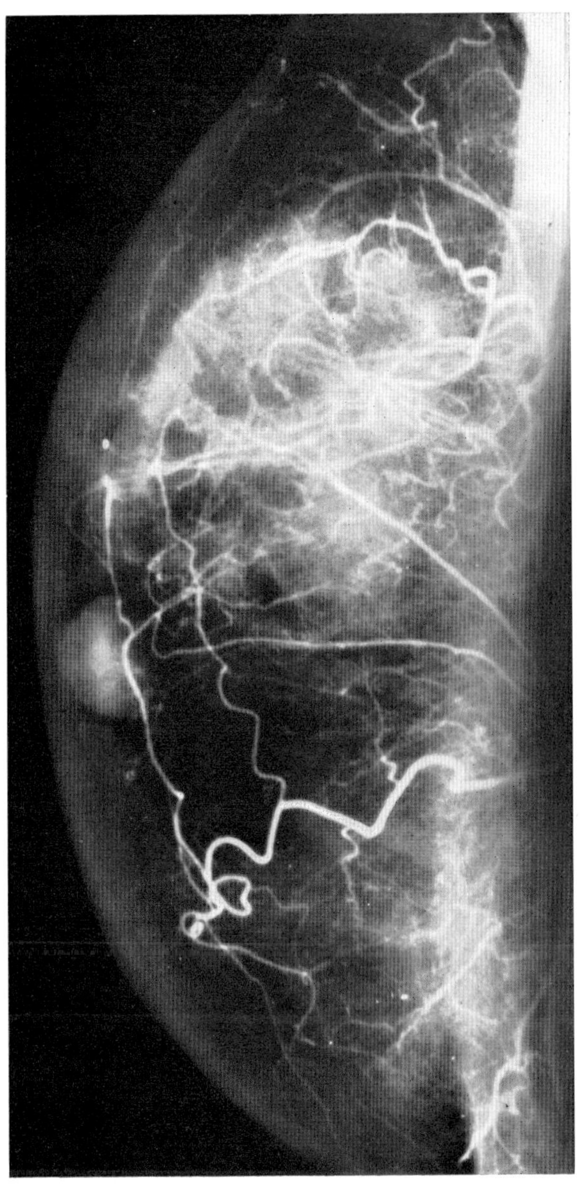

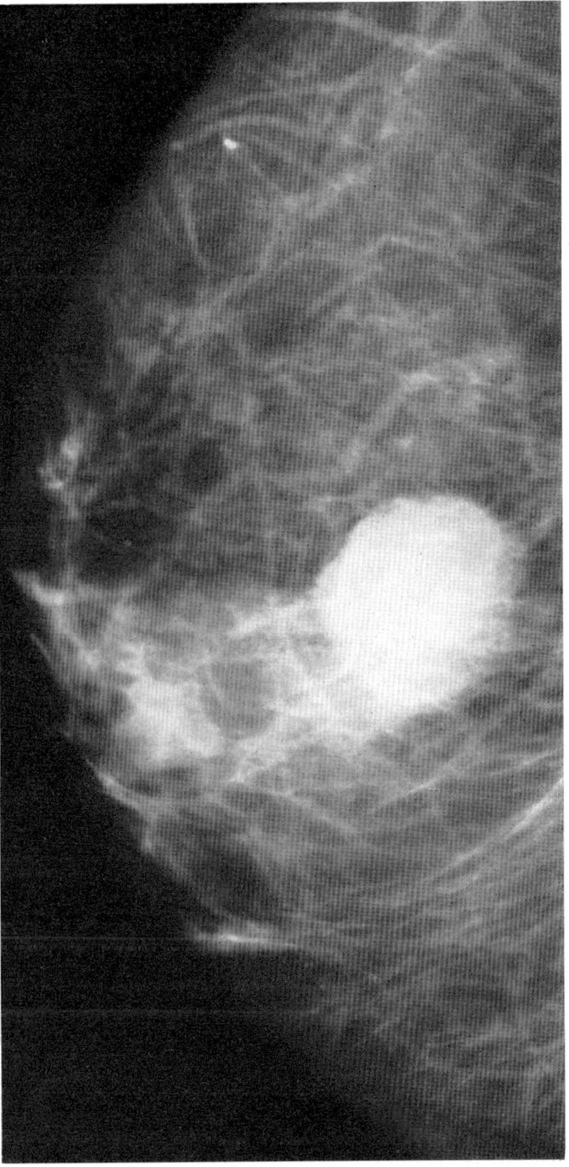

Fig. **7**.1c   Later arterial and capillary phase: Extensive neovascularity in the periphery of the tumor with cork screw vessels. Staining is seen in certain portions of the tumor. The majority of the tumor mass is hypovascular and reveals no staining.

Fig. **7**.2a   Mammogram: Rounded mass 3 cm in diameter with poorly defined slightly lobular margins. Some coarse central calcifications. Radiating extensions from the tumor mass in the direction ol the subareolar region. Carcinoma with early invasive changes. Histology: Adenocarcinoma.

Arteriography of the breast (FELDMANN, et al 1967; FELDMANN 1969; ANACKER et al 1970) permits the demonstration of the arterial vascular supply of the breast, and a differentiation between malignant and benign tumors and hypervascular, pathological lymph nodes.

Indications

Breast arteriography as a tool for the differential diagnosis of diseases of the breast is not in routine usage. This is because arteriography adds little more information for therapeutic purposes than that obtained or obtainable by

4*

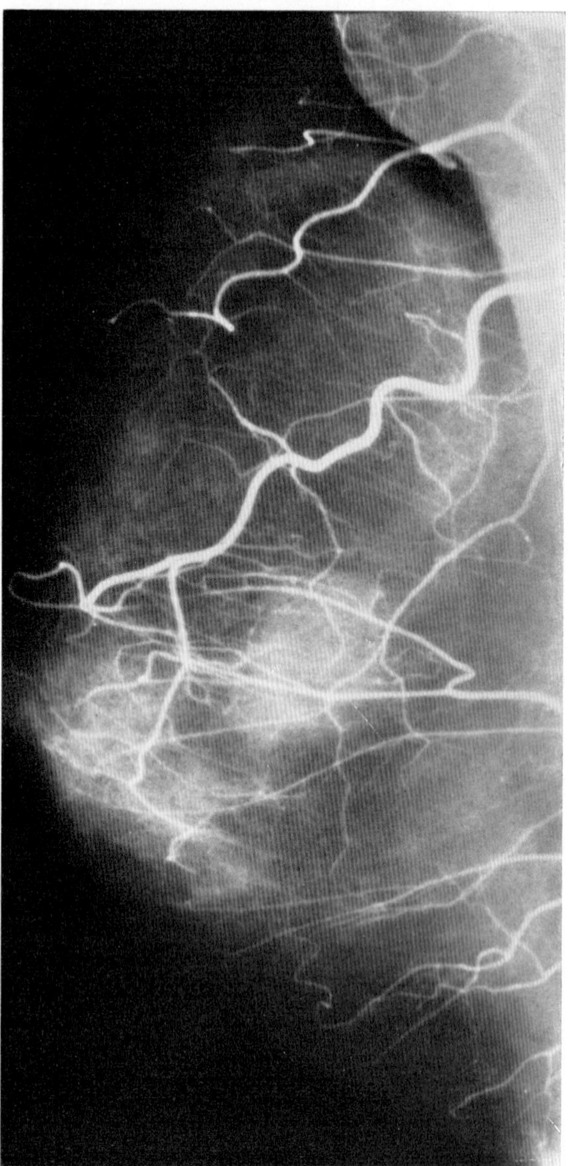

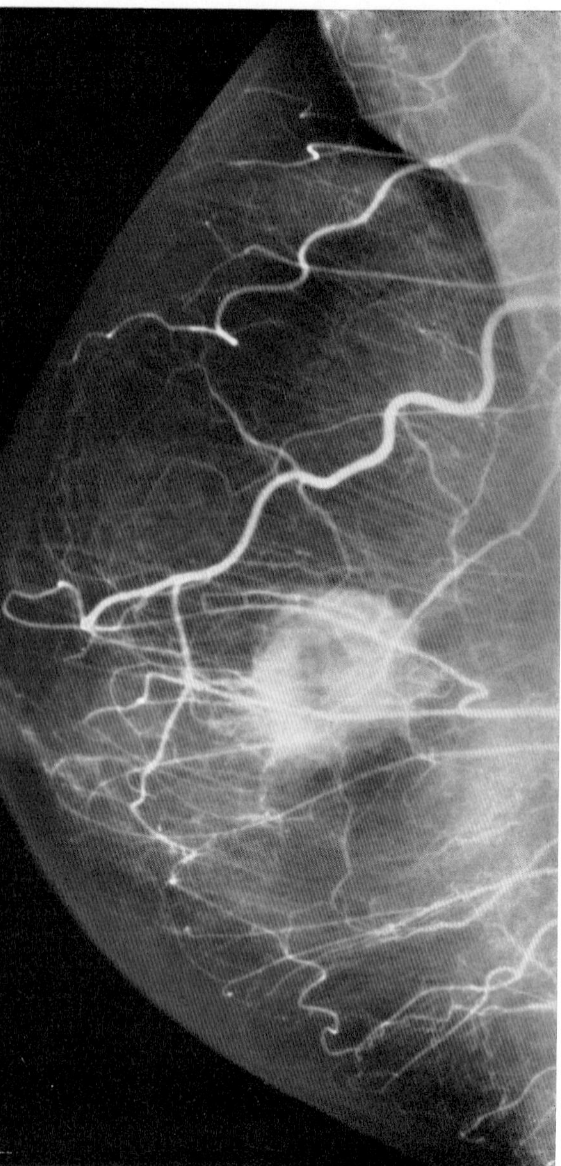

Fig. **7**.2b Early arterial phase of a transfemoral angiogram: No neovascularity or tumor stain.

Fig. **7**.2c Late arterial and capillary phase: Very intensive, almost homogeneous staining of the entire tumor. This represents a highly vascular carcinoma.

clinical and mammographic examination. Although impressive arteriographic demonstrations of breast carcinomas have been achieved and it is possible to differentiate between fibroadenomas and carcinomas, it still does not rule out the need for histological diagnosis. Additionally there is the consideration of certain complications, inherent in any arteriography.

Technique

1) Retrograde arteriography, brachial artery approach on the ipsilateral side (FELDMANN 1969): After puncture of the brachial artery with an 18 gauge needle 35 cc. of Conray-60% are injected mechanically with pressure. Serial roentgenograms are made according to the

following sequence: One film per second for 3 seconds, then one and a half films per second. Total filming time is 10 seconds.

2) Catheter angiography: ANACKER et al (1970) originally used the axillary artery approach but because of technical difficulties and frequent complications abandoned this technique for the transfemoral route. We also prefer the femoral approach to mammary arteriography using the SELDINGER technique (fig. 7.1a—c, 7.2a—c).

It is essentially a nonselective angiogram that is performed when the catheter tip (red ÖDMANN catheter with 4 to 6 side holes) is positioned at the level of the shoulder joint. A semiselective study may be performed using a catheter with primary and secondary curves, end hole only, and positioning it in selected arterial branches going to the breast.

Diagnosis

ANACKER et al indicate the following angiographic signs of mammary carcinoma (these agree with those reported by FELDMANN et al):

In the arterial phase:
> Pathological vessels
>> Corkscrew appearance of vessels
>> Stellate or brush-like distribution of group of vessels
>> Bizarre vascular pattern
>> Hypervascularity
>> Encasement of vessels
> Irregular contours of arteries
> Displacement of arteries
> Stenosis or complete occlusion of arteries

In the capillary phase:
> Tumor blush
> AV shunting
> Rapid circulation rate
> Very slow circulation rate
> Puddling of contrast

In the venous phase:
> Dilated and increased number of veins
> Stenosis of veins

Lymphangiography

Indications

The demonstration of lymphatic drainage of the breast as well as the primary lymph nodes is important in carcinoma of the breast both to identify the location of the lymphatics as well as to determine the presence of metastases to these lymph nodes (KETT et al 1969 and 1970; JACOBS 1972).

However, the tendency to reduce the surgical approach to simple mastectomy followed by radiotherapy has resulted in decreasing interest in lymphangiography of the breast. Therefore breast lymphangiography is not commonly a part of the preoperative diagnostic evaluation of mammary carcinoma.

Two different methods of lymphangiography have been developed.

Direct Lymphangiography

Technique

Intradermally into the areola are injected 0.2 cc of a mixture of 1% methylene-blue and 1% local anesthetic. Within a few minutes the lymph

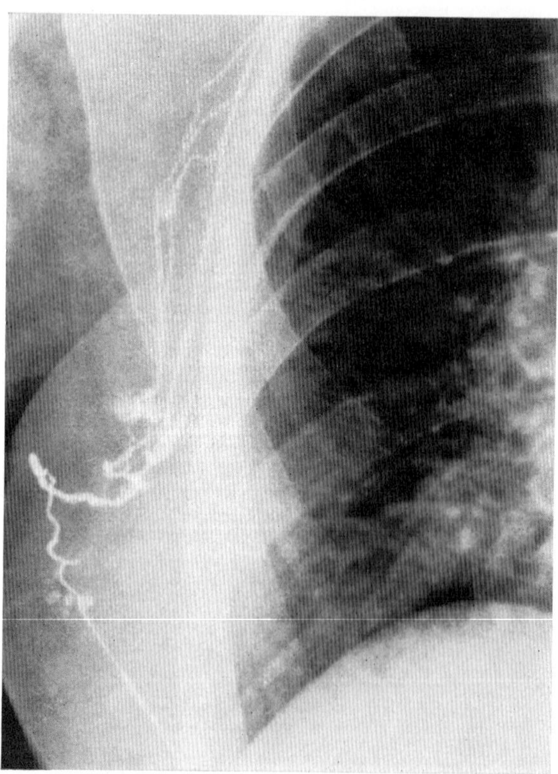

Fig. **8.**1a Injection of a lymphatic, early filling phase; a few pectoral lymph nodes are already demonstrated. (Courtesy of Jacobs, H. Fortschr. Roentgenstr. 116 (1972).

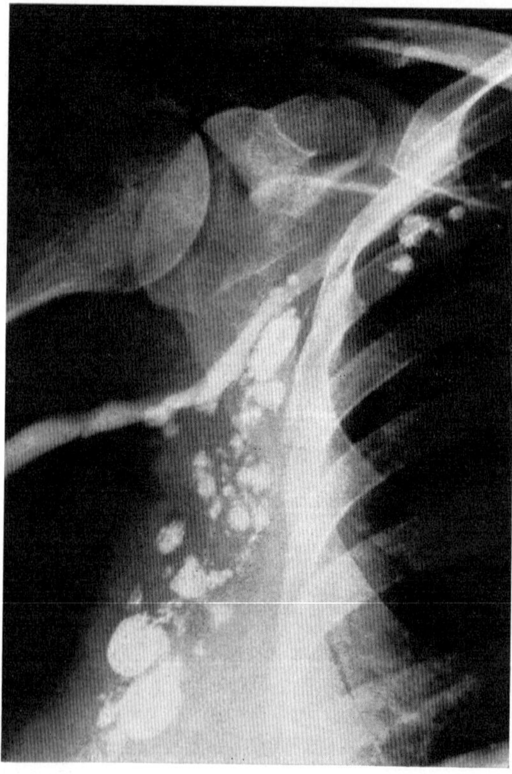

Fig. **8.**1b Normal right-sided lymphangiogram. Simultaneous axillary venography shows topographical relationship.

ducts are recognized by their blue color immediately beneath the skin. A skin incision is made over a visible duct which is dissected and then punctured with a lymphangiographic cannula. The cannula is secured within the lymphatic with a ligature and also to the skin by a second ligature or steristrip. Using a mechanical pressure injector about 2 mm of Lipiodol is instilled over a period of 30 minutes.

Radiographs are obtained in the craniocaudal, mediolateral and oblique projections in order to demonstrate lymphatics, and lymph nodes. An additional axillary view and a parasternal PA projection are obtained.

The same projections are repeated after 24 hours for primary evaluation of the lymph node phase of the study.

Results

The appearance of lymphatics of the breast is typical (fig. 8.1). Nonfilling of lymphatics occurs when there is an obstruction secondary to metastatic destruction of lymph nodes. Under these conditions the contrast material will flow via collaterals or spread out into the connective tissue. Lymph node metastases are recognized as filling defects in the opacified lymph node. KETT et al (1970) have demonstrated lymph node metastases as small as 2 to 3 mm in diameter. Stagnation of contrast material and failure to fill a lymphatic indicate a metastatic block in the afferent lymph node. Noninvolved lymphatics and lymph nodes will opacify in the usual manner. The parasternal lymph node group, according to KETT et al, is only opacified when metastatic spread to this group has occurred.

Indirect Lymphangiography

Occasionally one can obtain opacification of lymphatics during galactography when contrast material has been extravasated into the parenchyma. This type of indirect lymphangiography, however, is accidental and cannot be used as a practical routine approach.

KVASNICKA et al (1961) have described the routine use of indirect lymphangiography with aqueous contrast material. Other authors however have not agreed that this is a useful technique (GILBRIDE 1938; KETT et al 1969; PRIVES 1948).

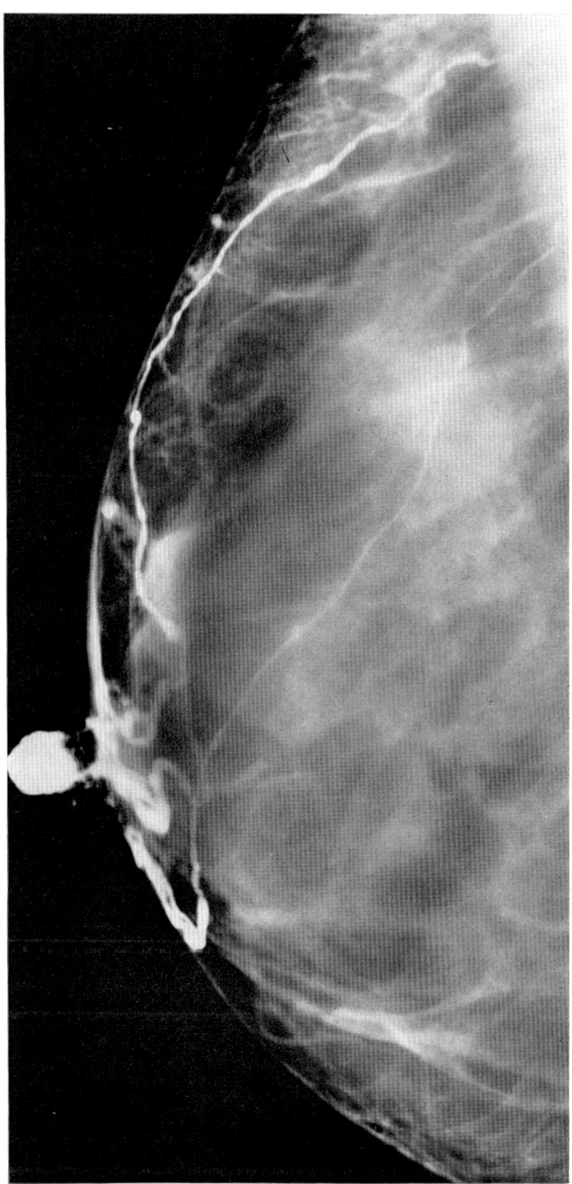

Fig. **8**.2   Indirect lymphangiography.

Technique

This consists of intradermal injection of 1 to 2 cc of aqueous contrast material of 35% concentration into the nipple with a very fine needle under local anesthesia. Consequently the subareolar lymphatic plexus and efferent lymphatics are opacified (fig. 8.2). The opacification of these structures lasts about 15 minutes, and completely disappears after about 30 minutes.

Results

The immediate opacification of the subareolar lymph system with only about 1 to 2 cc of contrast material indicates that most of the intradermal injection must be directly into lymphatic ducts. The direction of lymphatics from the subareolar region determines which lymph ducts are opacified by this method. Any value of this method in determining the presence or absence of lymph node metastases from breast carcinoma has yet to be demonstrated.

The Normal Breast

Chapter 9

Anatomy

The female breast is one of the secondary sex characteristics and its function is the secretion of milk during lactation. It is a differentiated apocrine sweat gland.

Breast Parenchyma

The parenchyma consists of approximately 15 to 20 lobes. The lobes are distributed so that

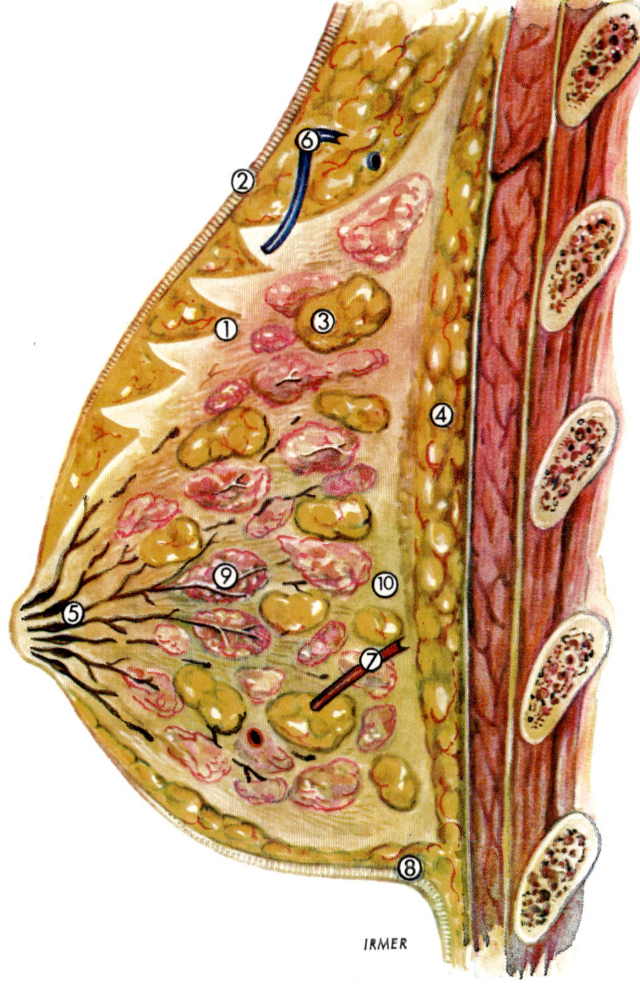

Fig. **9**.1 Structural anatomy of the female breast

(1) Cooper's ligaments
(2) and (8) Skin and subcutaneous tissues with ducts of skin glands
(3) Fat lobule
(4) Retromammary fatty layer
(5) Dilated subareola lactiferous ducts
(6) Vein
(7) Artery
(9) Parenchymal lobe
(10) Connective tissue

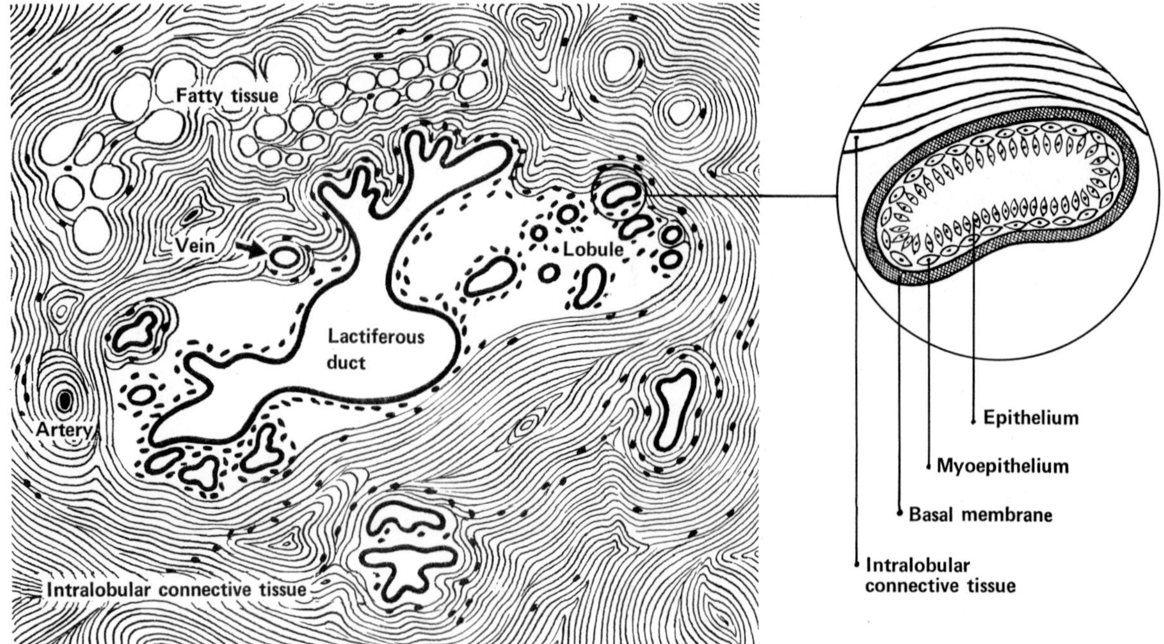

Fig. **9**.2   Schematic drawing of microanatomy of the breast (according to Maximow, A. A., and Bloom, W: A Textbook of Histology. Philadelphia, Saunders, 1945).

(1) Intralobular connective tissue
(2) Artery
(3) Vein
(4) Fatty tissue
(5) Lactiferous duct
(6) Lobule
(7) Epithelium
(8) Myoepithelium
(9) Basal membrane
(10) Intralobular connective tissue

there are more superiorly and laterally than inferiorly and medially. A lobe is divided into numerous lobules which contain the acini. The lobule is the basic structural unit of which the entire breast is composed. At maturity several hundreds of lobules constitute a single breast; however, these involute in size and number with increasing age. Each lobule consists of several acini, ducts and intralobular stroma (fig. 9.2). The stroma is functionally a part of the parenchyma and partakes in hormonal changes. The acini are surrounded by a layer of myoepithelial cells resting upon a basement membrane. These have a contractile function resuting in emptying of the acinar secretion. The excretory ducts of the acini join to form lactiferous ductules draining the lobules, which in turn join to form approximately 15 to 25 lactiferous ducts which empty into the nipple immediately beyond an ampullary dilatation at their most distal aspects (lactiferous sinus) (fig. 9.1). Some of the lactiferous ducts and sinuses may join before their termination so that the number of ductal openings in the nipple may be less than the actual number of lactiferous ducts.

Nipple

The nipple protrudes from the pigmented areola. Numerous crypts are seen at its surface into which the lactiferous ducts open. Normally there is no spontaneous secretion in the mature woman except during gestation and lactation. Ten to 15 small nodular prominences are seen over the areola surrounding the nipple. These are known as the areolar glands or glands of MONTGOMERY, the sebaceous glands and the odoriferous glands. Additional epidermal structures to be found in the areola are sweat glands, epidermal hairs and smooth muscle fibers. The skin of the areola is slightly thicker than that of the breast.

Skin

The skin of the breast (epidermis and dermis) is about 0.5 to 2 mm in thickness. At the base

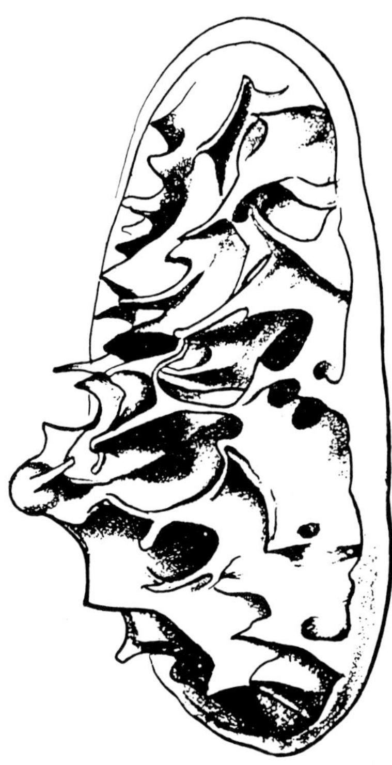

Fig. **9**.3   Drawing of Cooper's ligaments (The Anatomy and Diseases of the Breast, by Sir Astley Cooper, Lea and Blanchard, Philadelphia, 1845).

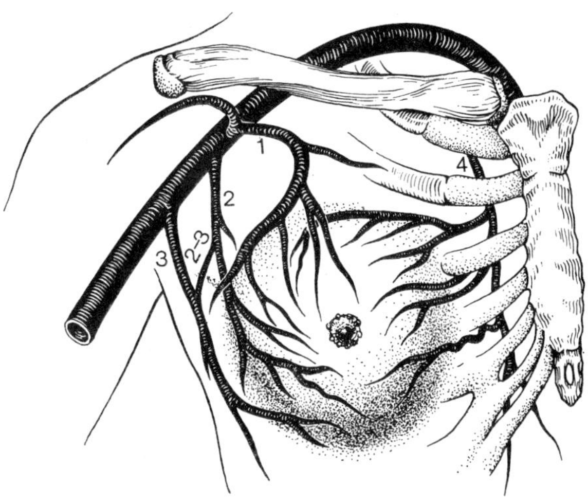

Fig. **9**.4   Arterial supply of the breast
(1) Thoraco-acromial artery;
(2) lateral thoracic artery;
(2, 3) anastomoses between lateral thoracic artery and dorsal thoracic artery;
(3) dorsal thoracic artery;
(4) internal mammary artery.
The medial quadrants of the breast have a further blood supply via branches from the second, third, fourth and fifth intercostal arteries (after Anacker).

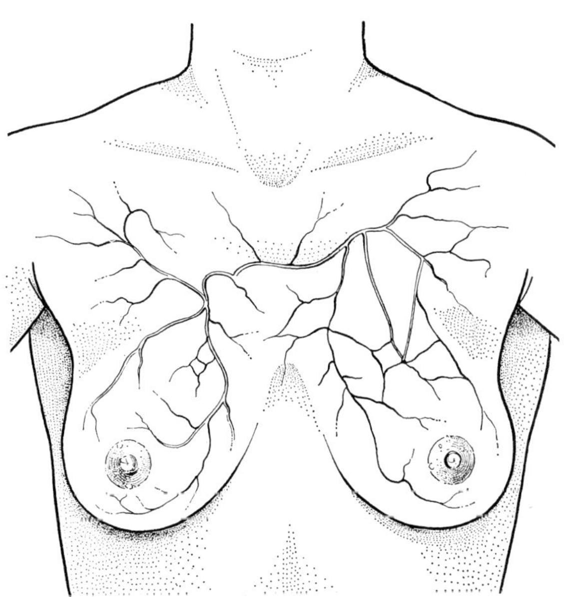

Fig **9**.5a   Transverse distribution of the superficial veins (after Egan).

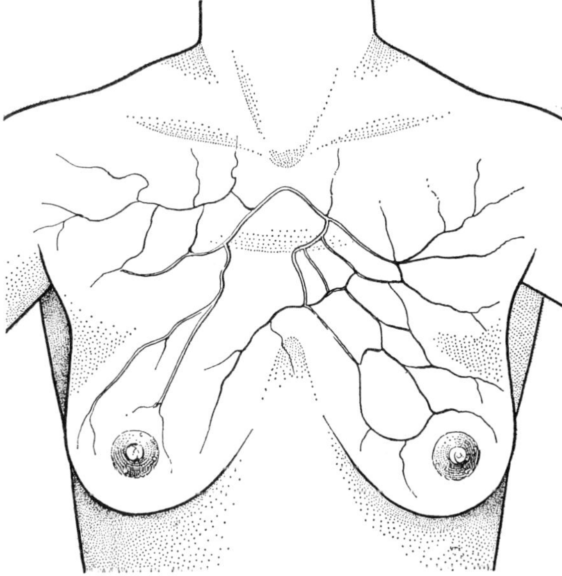

Fig. **9**.5b   Longitudinal distribution of the superficial veins (after Egan).

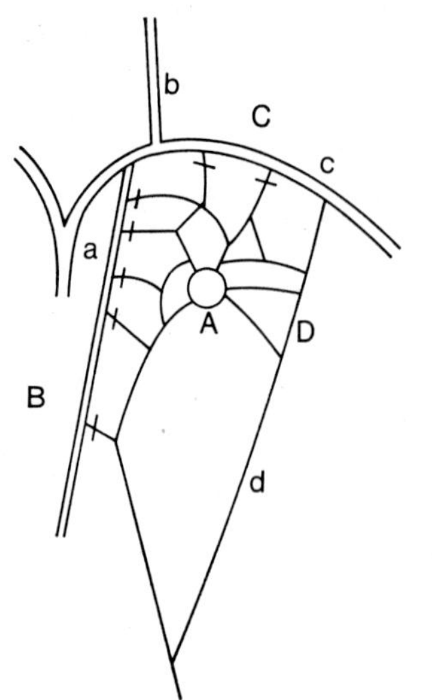

Fig. **9**.6   Venous drainage of the female breast

A = Plexus venosus areolaris;
B = medial flow;
C = cranial flow;
D = lateral flow;
a = internal thoracic vein;
b = jugular vein;
c = subclavian vein;
d = thoraco-epigastric vein.

of the breast this thickness increases. Fine pores formed by sweat glands, sebaceous glands and hair are seen here as elsewhere in the skin.

Stromal Tissue

This provides the shape and consistency of the female breast. Even a fatty breast with little parenchyma may maintain normal shape and tone if the stromal tissue is well developed. The entire breast is enveloped in a duplication of the superficial pectoral fascia. The posterior reflection of this fascia is connected to the pectoral musculature, while the anterior reflection is connected to the skin by thin connective tissue septa. The posterior and anterior fascial planes are connected by curvilinear connective tissue septa known as COOPER's ligaments (1845), which envelop the lobules, and lobes of the breast and are the primary source of support for this organ (fig. 9.3).

Fatty Tissue

The entire breast parenchyma is surrounded by subcutaneous fat. There is also a layer of fat in a retromammary location separating the

breast from the soft tissues of the thorax. Fat is also interspersed in a lobular fashion throughout the entire breast parenchyma.

Arteries

The arterial blood supply of the breast arises medially from the internal mammary arteries and laterally predominantly from branches of the thoracodorsal, lateral thoracic and thoracoacromial arteries. These are branches of the axillary arteries (fig. 9.4).

Veins

Superficial veins of the breast form an irregular netlike pattern in the subcutaneous fatty layers readily visible through the skin by their blue color. Two basic patterns are recognized, one is a predominantly transverse flow in the direction of the sternum and the other a longitudinal flow in the direction of the jugular fossa (MASSOPUST and GARDNER 1950) (fig. 9.5a and b).

The deep veins are distributed in the same course as the arteries. They join behind the areola to form the areolar venous plexus.

Superficial and deep veins anastomose and have the following drainage (fig. 9.6):

The areolar venous plexus drains into the internal mammary vein:

veins may drain medially into the jugular vein;
veins may drain cephalad into the subclavian vein;

veins may drain laterally into the thoracic and epigastric veins.

Veins draining into the internal mammary vein have direct collateral communication with the pulmonary capillary bed allowing hematogenous dissemination of breast carcinoma directly into the lungs (fig. 9.7). There are also collateral branches that connect draining veins of the breast to intercostal veins which in turn provide direct connections with veins of the vertebral plexus and azygos system (fig. 9.8). The azygos venous connections are particularly important in allowing tumor cells to metastasize directly to the vertebral column and pelvis without first passing through the lungs (BATSON 1942; HAAGENSEN 1956).

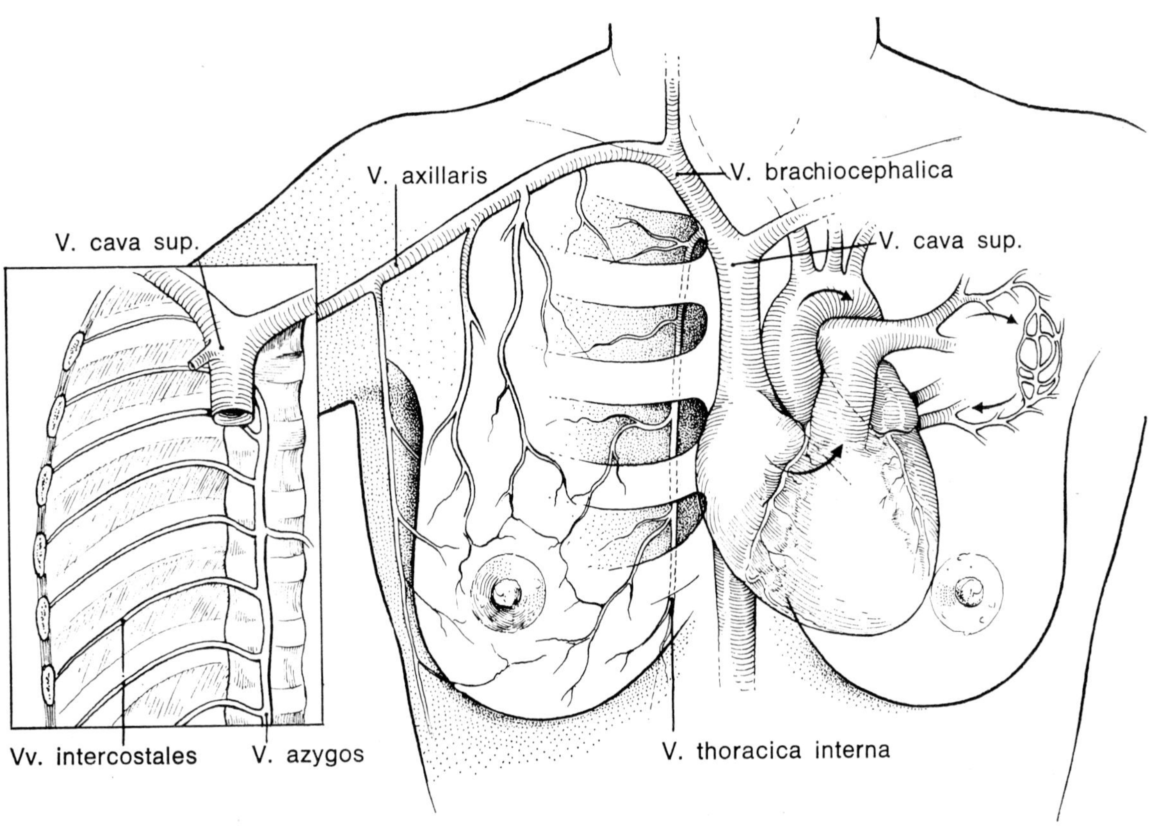

Fig. 9.7 Venous drainage of the female breast and three venous pathways for metastasis of breast carcinoma to the capillary network of the lung (after Haagensen 1971).

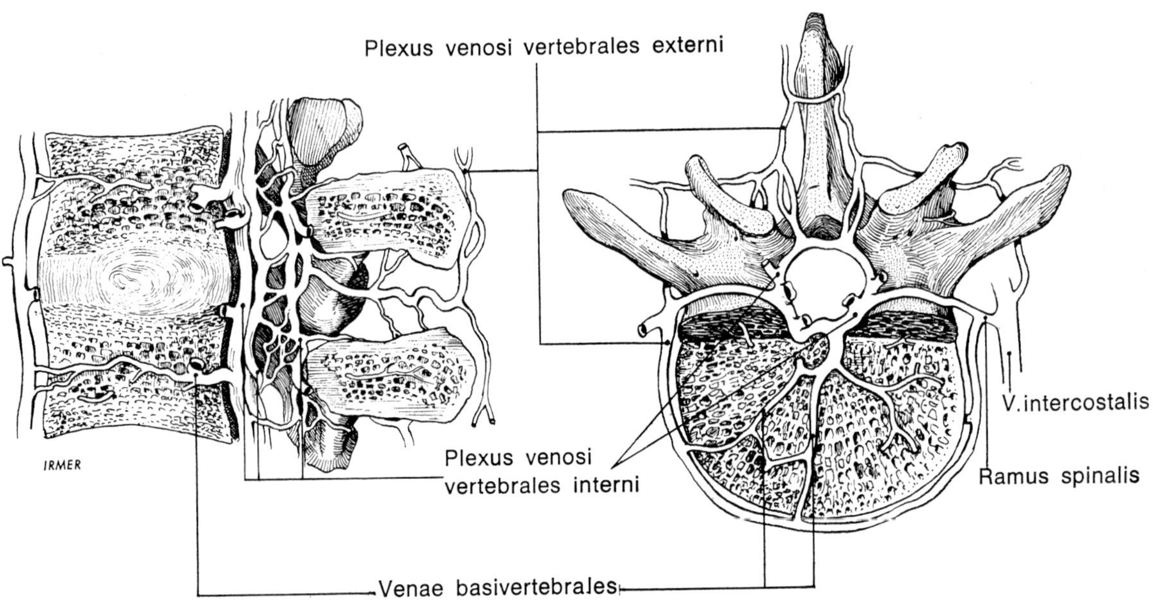

Fig. 9.8 Transverse and sagittal sections of the vertebral body to demonstrate the venous plexus and its connection with intercostal veins. (after Gray's anatomy, 26th edition, by Charles M. Goss, Lea and Febiger, Philadelphia 1954).

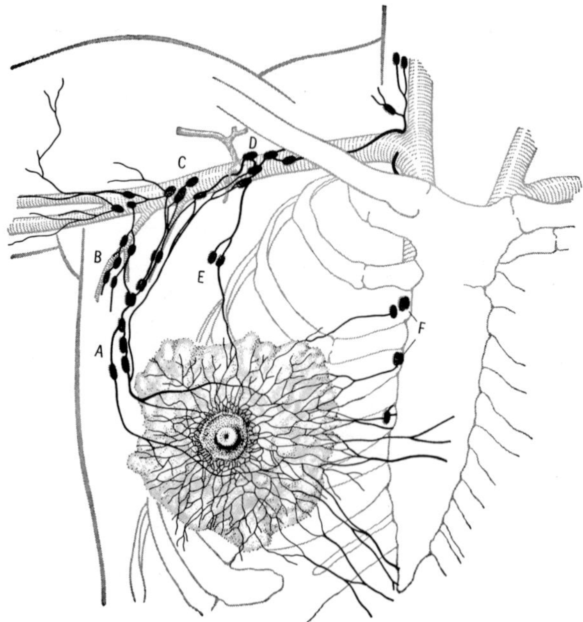

Fig. **9**.9 Lymphatics of the female breast and lymph flow to the axillary and parasternal lymph nodes. Regional lymph nodes.

A) Anterior, pectoral lymph nodes;
B) subscapular lymph nodes;
C) central axillary lymph nodes;
D) subclavicular lymph nodes;
E) interpectoral lymph nodes (Rotter);
F) internal parasternal lymph nodes.
(From Zinser H.-Kl., Mammakarzinom, Thieme, Stuttgart 1972).

Lymphatics

The major lymph drainage of the breast is toward the axilla (fig. 9.9). The first lymph nodes involved in carcinoma of the breast are those occurring along the inferior margin of the pectoralis major (SORGIUS). From these nodes lymph flow is directed towards the central axillary node group and infraclavicular nodes. Flow may also be directed to groups of lymph nodes around the third, fourth and fifth prongs of the serratus anterior muscle as well as towards intercostal and posterior mediastinal node groups. Lymphatic pathways may pierce the pectoralis major to subpectoral lymph nodes (ROTTER 1899) or directly from here to infra and supraclavicular lymph nodes (GROSSMAN's pathway 1896). Medial lymph drainage eventually reaches the parasternal and anterior mediastinal lymph nodes (GEROTA's paramammary pathway, 1896). And lastly there are also lymphatic connections to the opposite breast (cross-mammary-pathway).

Chapter 10

Roentgen Anatomy

The schematic anatomy and roentgen appearance of the mammogram is demonstrated in the examples shown in fig. 10.1 and 10.2a—c.

Breast Parenchyma

The parenchyma absorbs more radiation than does fatty tissue. Consequently the lobules are discernible as densities surrounded by more radiolucent fatty tissue. The number of lobules as visualized in the roentgenogram, is always less than reality because of summation and super-imposition of lobules as they are scattered throughout the breast. The acini are visible only microscopically, not roentgenologically.

Galactography (ductography) may allow demonstration of separate lobules composing a parenchymal lobe (fig. 10.3).

Lactiferous Ducts

The small peripheral lactiferous ducts are not visible in the mammogram; however, they may be demonstrated to their fullest extent including

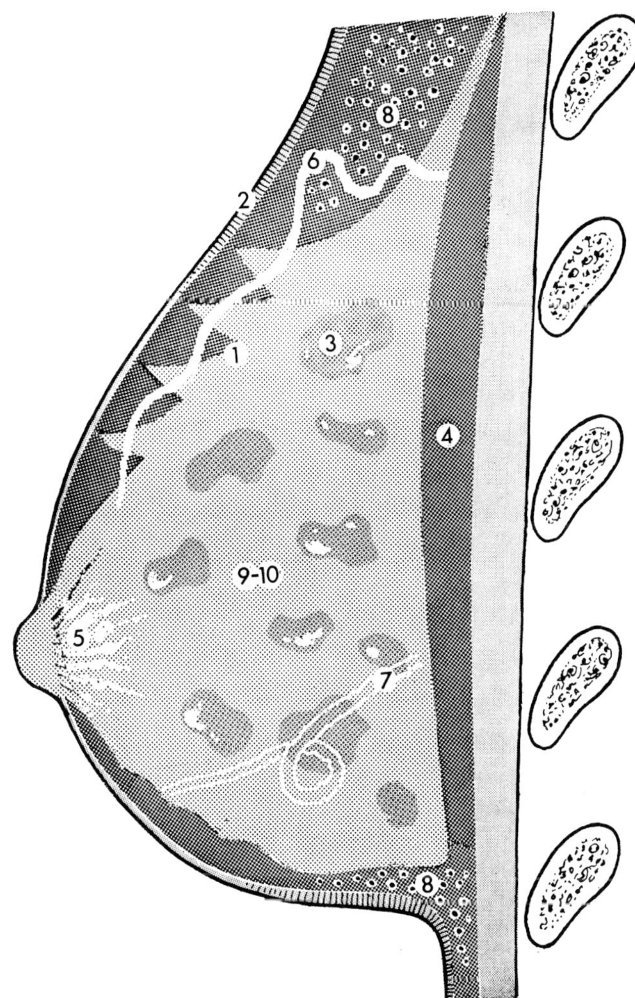

Fig. **10.1** Normal anatomy of the breast in the mammogram (see also Fig. **9**.1).

1) Cooper's ligaments;
2) skin and subcutaneous tissue with ducts from cutaneous glands;
3) fat lobule;
4) retromammary fatty layer;
5) enlarged subareolar lactiferous ducts;
6) vein;
7) calcified artery;
8) skin pores;
9) to 10) breast parenchyma.

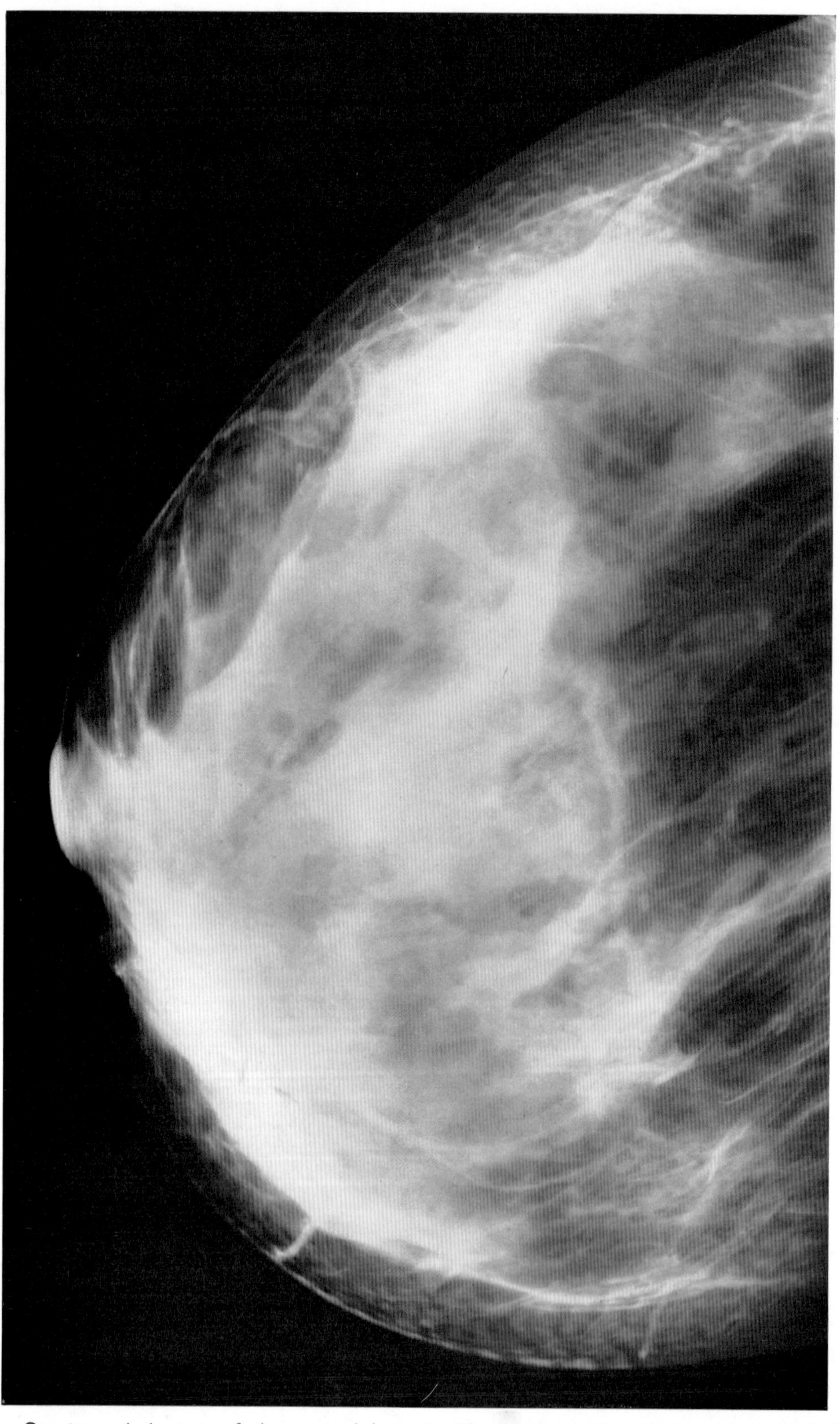

Fig. **10**.2a Craniocaudad view of the normal breast with demonstration of parenchymal lobules, interspersed fatty tissue, supportive connective tissue, skin, subcutaneous tissue and nipple. Veins are of normal caliber. Numerous skin pores are clearly demonstrated.

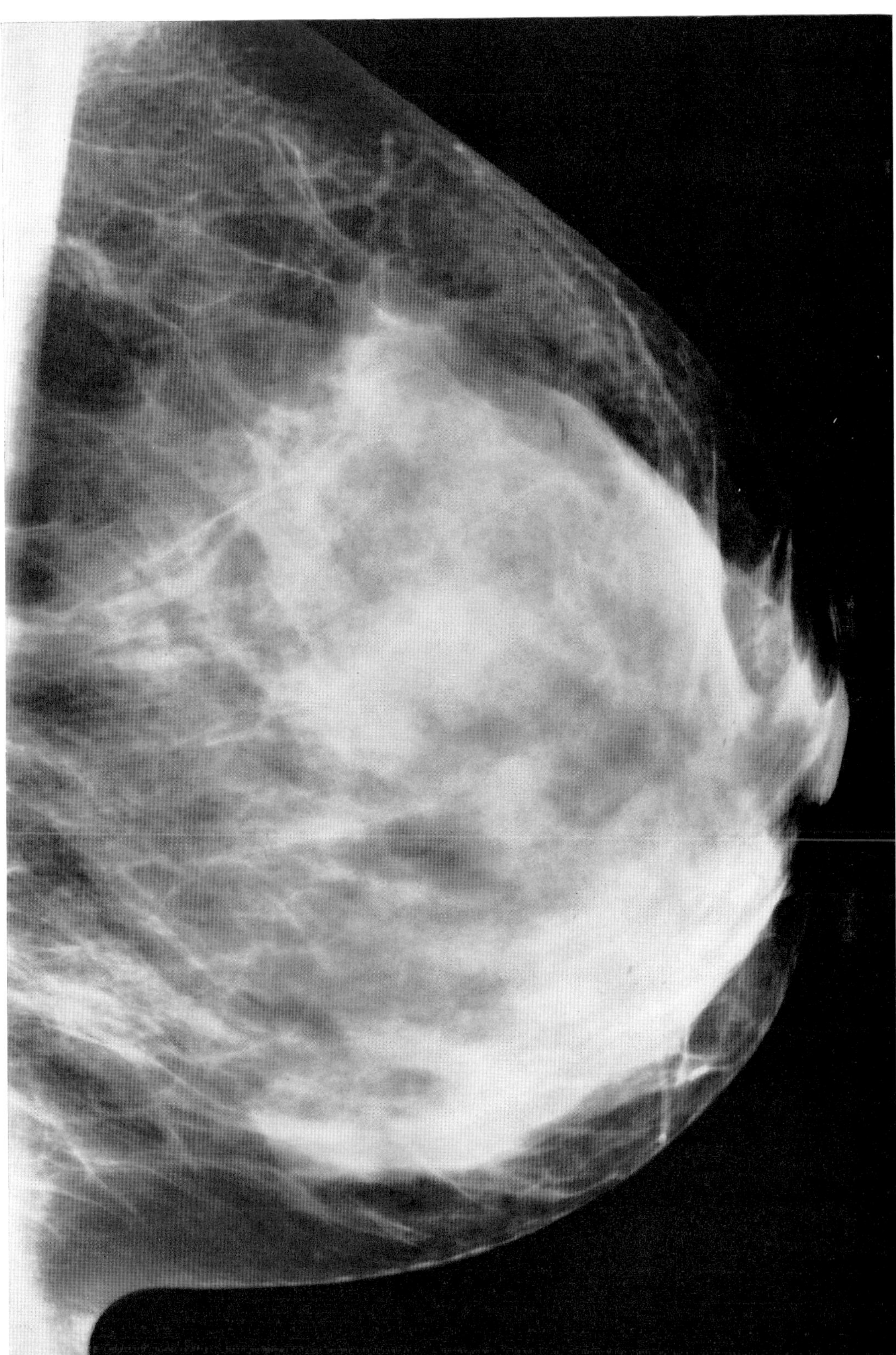

Fig. **10**.2b   Lateral mammogram of the same breast. In addition to the structures seen on Fig. **10**.2a one can see the axillary fold in the upper portion of this film, and Cooper's ligaments are seen beneath the skin.

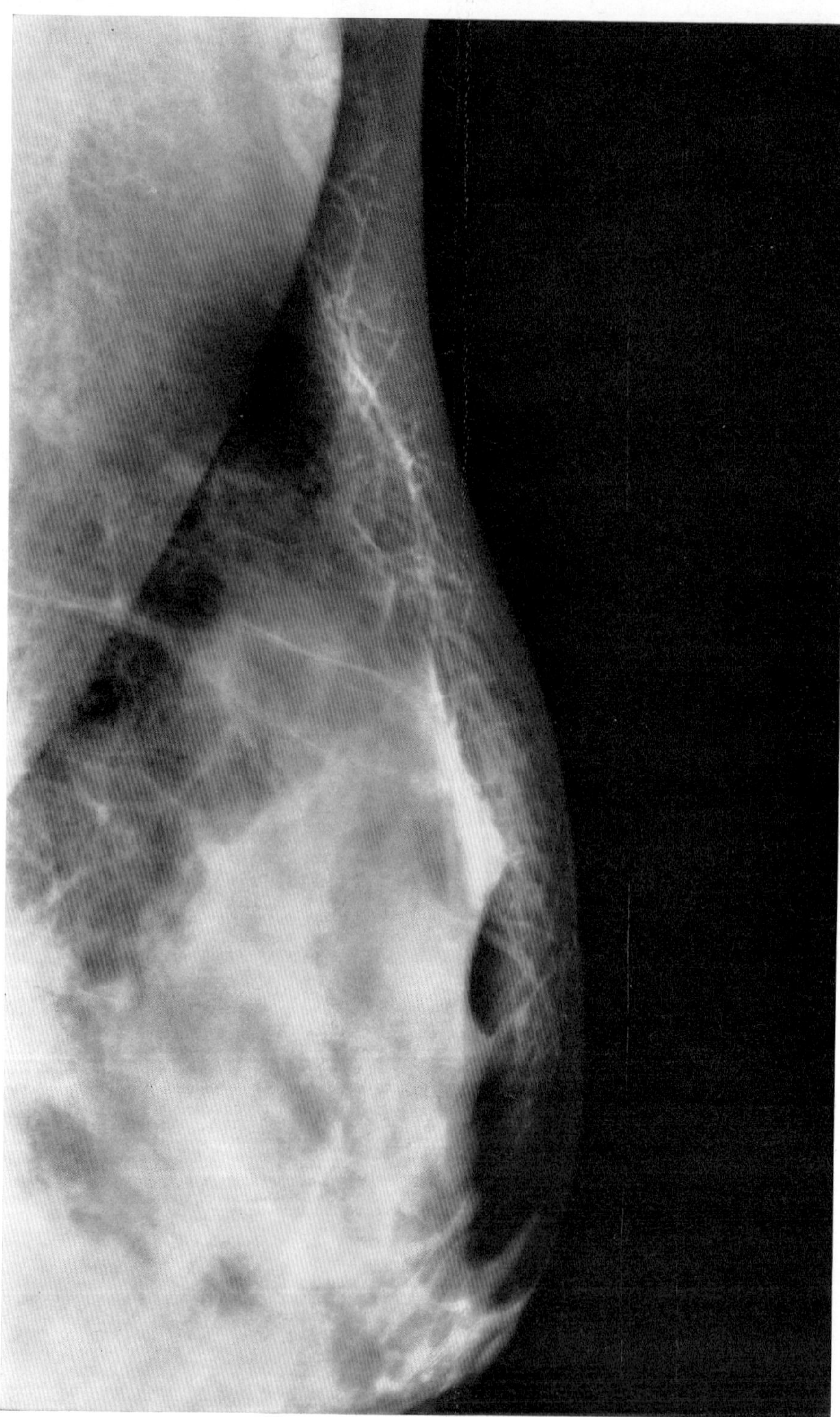

Fig. **10**.2c   So-called third projection with demonstration of the axillary fold and the anterior portion of the axilla.

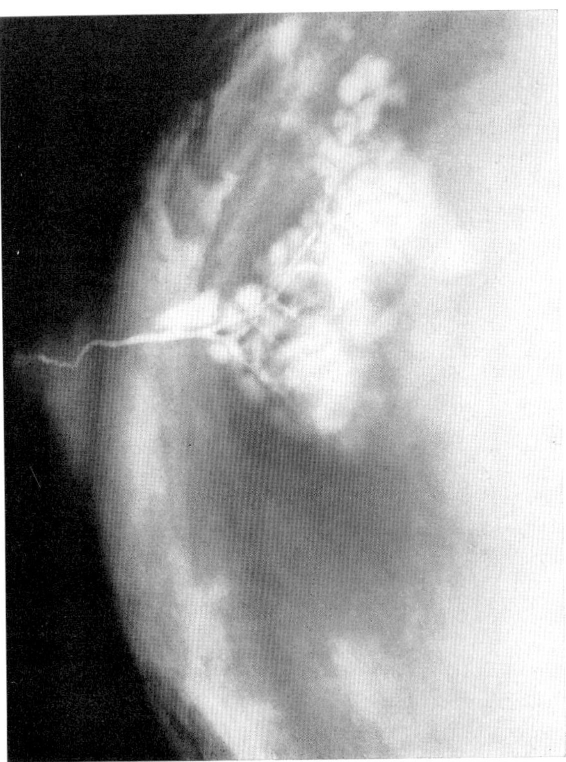

Fig. **10**.3 Ductography. Normal caliber lactiferous ducts with demonstration of numerous lobules which make up a parenchymal lobe.

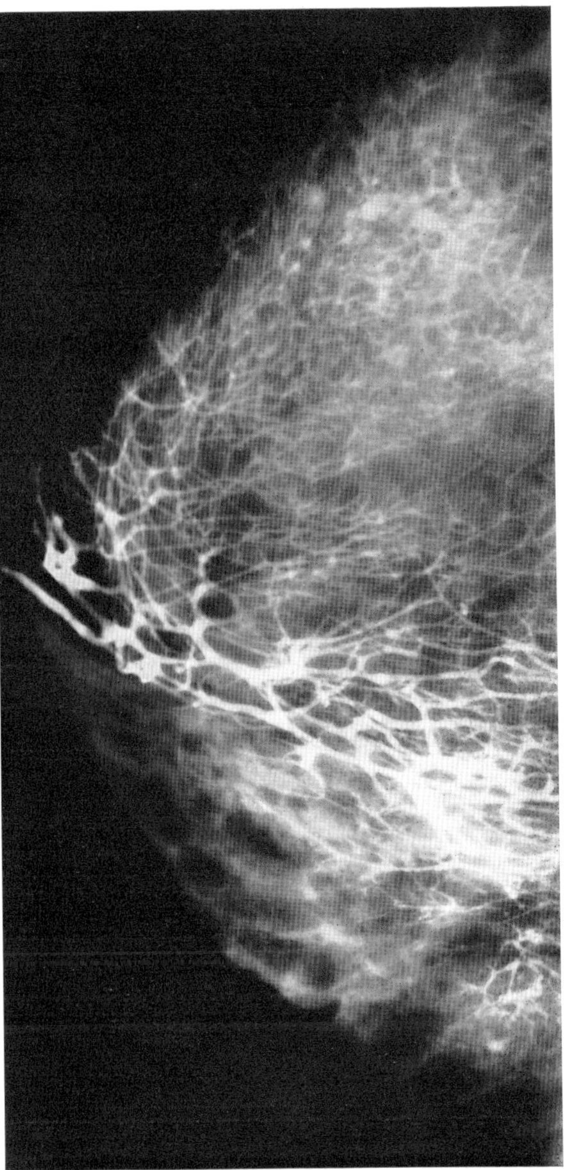

Fig. **10**.4 Ductography demonstrating the widely branching lactiferous duct system. The milk ducts in the lower aspect of the breast are slightly ectatic and of varying caliber.

secondary branches with ductography (fig. **10**.4). However, the retroareolar lactiferous sinuses in the fatty involuted breast of the older woman, may be demonstrated in the mammogram, without the use of contrast injection, as radiating shadows converging on the nipple, each approximately 2 to 3 mm in diameter. They may also appear as a conglomerate density converging on the papilla (fig. **10**.5).

There are various opinions on this matter. LEBORGNE (1953) feels that the milk ducts cannot be differentiated in the mammogram; BACLESSE and WILLEMIN (1967) agree; EGAN (1964) feels that although lactiferous ducts are not recognizable as distinct entities in the mammogram, they may be recognized as separate shadows consisting of a combination of lactiferous ducts and stromal tissue; WOLFE (1967) indicates that ducts less than 1 mm in diameter are not distinguishable. We tend to agree with the view of EGAN and WOLFE (fig. **10**.6a and b).

The Nipple

The nipple may be recognized in profile when the mammogram is examined under a bright light. One can identify the irregular contour of this structure as it projects from the areola. The nipple may be flat, failing to produce a local convexity in profile or may be retracted in which case a rounded lump is seen beneath the center of the areola.

5*

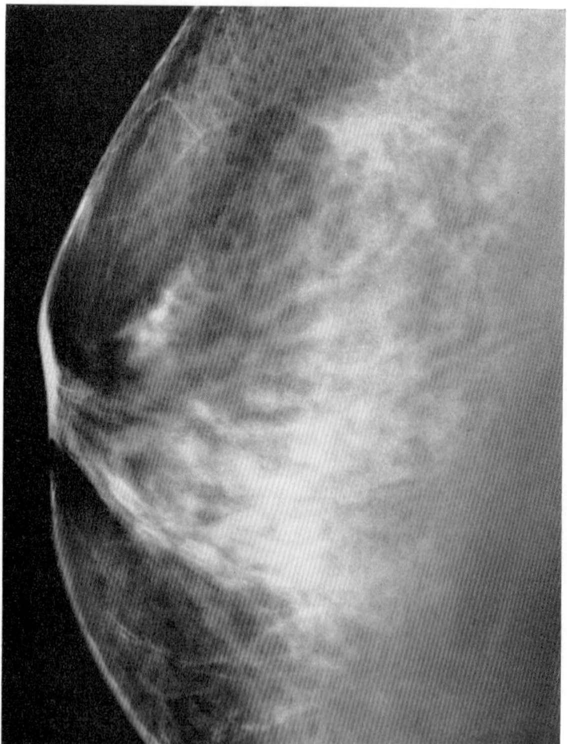

Fig. **10**.5   Illustration of large subareolar lactiferous duct in the plain mammogram with periductal fibrosis and antrophy of breast parenchyma.

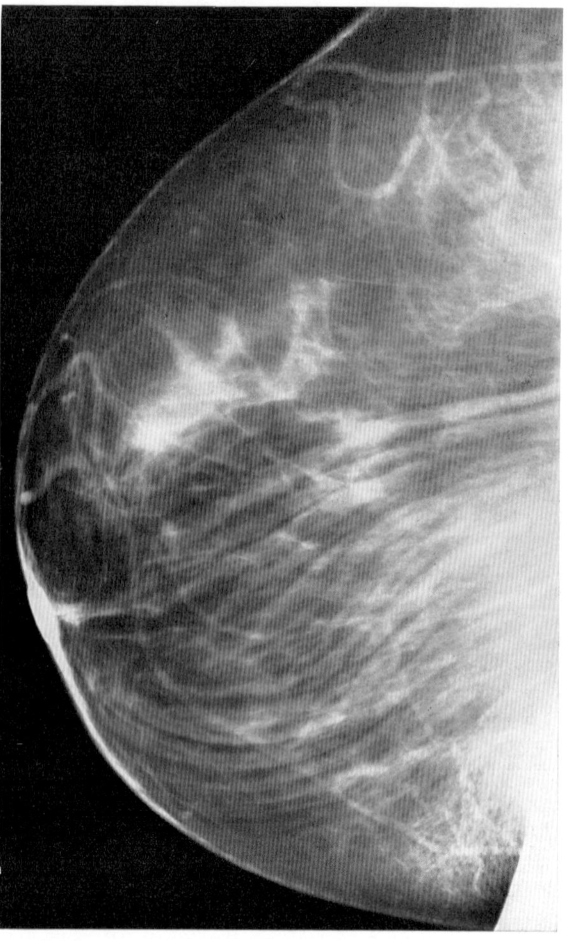

Fig. **10**.7   Skin folds overlying the inferior half of an atrophic breast. Arterial calcifications in the breast.

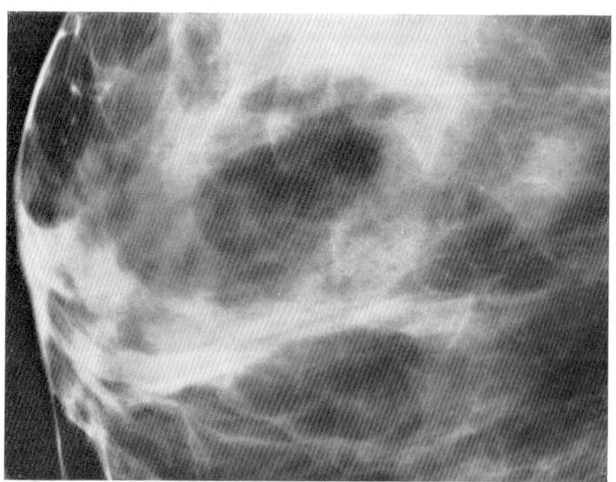

Fig. **10**.6a — Routine mammogram: Periductal fibrosis mimics ductal ectasia.

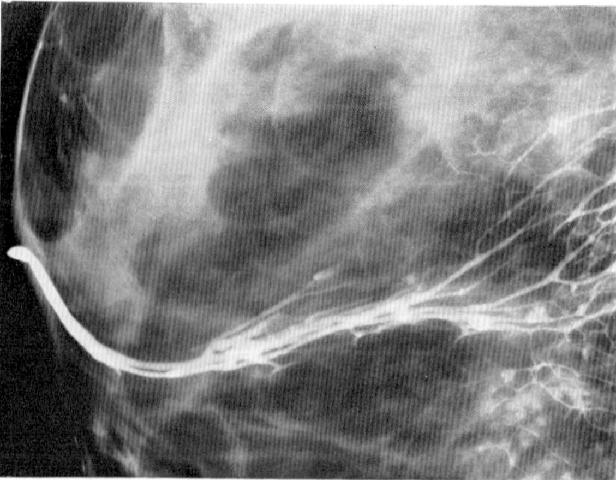

Fig. **10**.6b   Galactography: Lactiferous duct with normal caliber. Small cysts in the periphery.

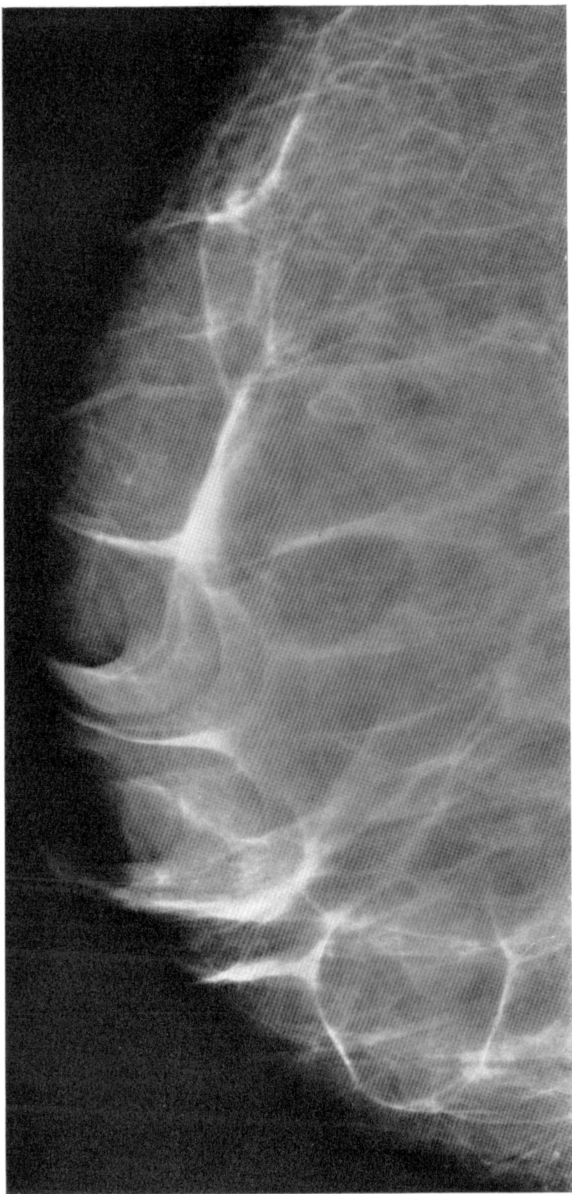

Fig. **10**.8 Cooper's ligaments in the roentgenogram: they extend as curvilinear densities from the parenchymal tissue through the subcutaneous fatty layer to the posterior surface of the skin. They are most numerous and easily defined in the upper half of the breast, less so in the lower portion. It is important not to mistake these for fibrous strands or extensions of scirrhus carcinoma.

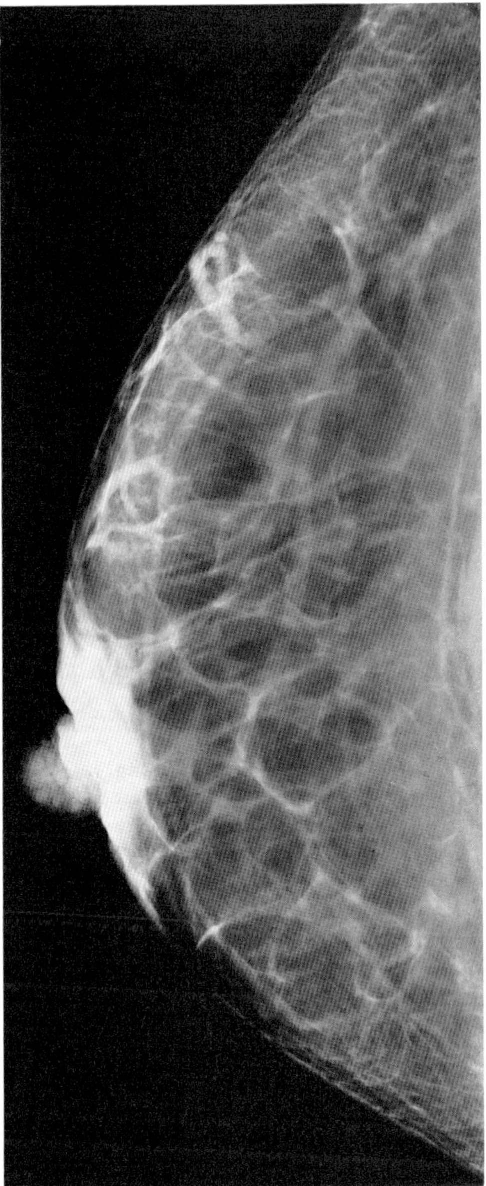

Fig. **10**.9 Involutional breast of the aged with replacement of parenchyma by adipose tissue. The connective tissue structure is maintained. (described as "fibrolipomatosis" by Baclesse-Willemin).

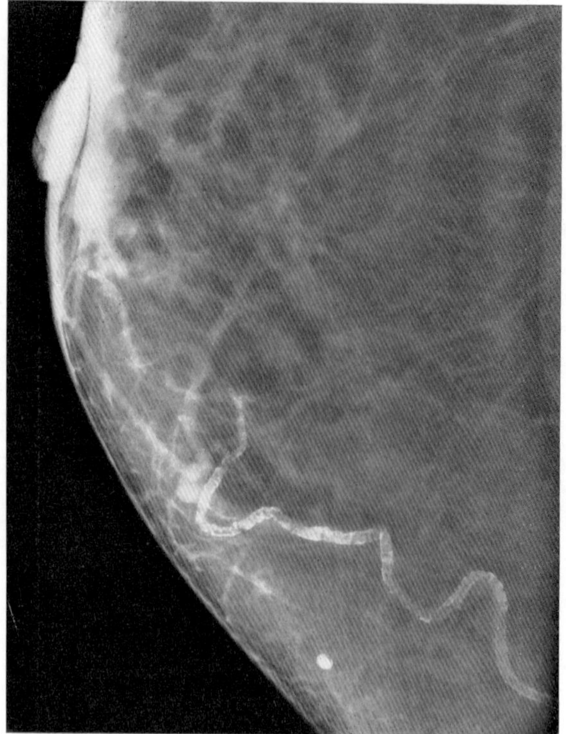

Fig. **10**.10. Calcified arteries in the mammogram. Additionally there is an area of liponecrosis microcystica calcificans.

The thickness of the areola in the mammogram is approximately 2 to 4 mm, slightly thicker than the skin covering the breast.

Epidermis

The overlying skin of the breast may be recognized in a mammogram with suitable lighting and is approximately 0.5 to 2 mm thick. There is normal thickening of the skin in the region of the inframammary fold. The skin may be relatively thicker in an otherwise normal but small breast. EGAN explains that this is the result of a greater orthograde projection of most of the skin because of better film contact obtained with the smaller breast. It seems to us that this explanation might also apply to the observation that the skin appears thicker along the medial, lateral and superior margins of the breast whereas in factit is anatomically actually thicker only along the inferior aspect. Recognition of these factors is important in evaluating pathological skin changes. Pendulous, atrophic breasts may have numerous skin folds which should not be misinterpreted as intramammary pathology (fig. **10.7**). Skin pores,

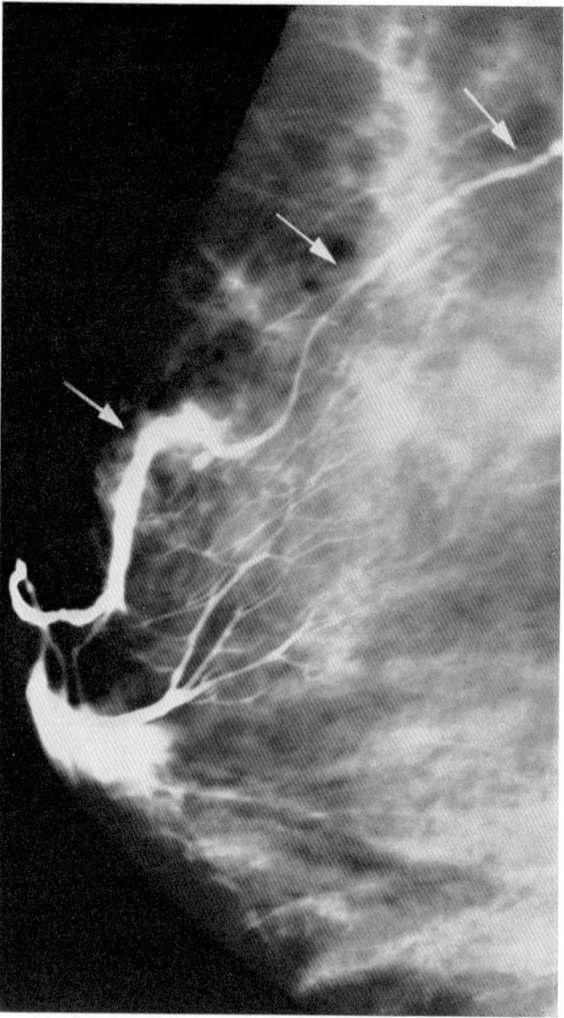

Fig. **10**.11   Demonstration of a lymphatic channel (arrows) following paraductal contrast collection during ductography.

if in orthograde profile, may occasionally be seen in the mammogram as very small irregular pits. In the lateral view, openings of various epidermal glands may be recognized as streaky radiolucencies along the inferior periphery of the breast.

Stromal Tissue

Stromal fibers are recognized in the subcutaneous fatty tissue as hairlike septa extending from the parenchyma to the skin. These are very difficult to see in dense breasts with an abundance of parenchyma or fibrocystic disease. COOPER's ligaments (fig. **10.8**) are easily recognized as curvilinear densities which extend from the parenchyma to the posterior aspect of the overlying epidermis and which provide the main support for the breast. They should not be confused with spicules seen in breast carcinoma. The curvilinear or reticular stromal tissues dominate the mammographic pattern of the fatty atrophic breast (fig. 10.9).

Fatty Tissue

Subcutaneous fat is observed as a lucent zone between the skin and breast parenchyma which is seen along all the margins; the retromammary fatty layer separates the breast mass from the soft tissues of the thorax. The quantity of fatty tissue is not a reliable indication of the functional potential of the breast.

Arteries

These are difficult to identify in the mammogram of a young patient and cannot be differentiated from other structures such as veins. They may, however, occasionally be identified with their more tortuous course, particularly when involved with arteriosclerotic calcification (fig. 10.10). Arterial calcifications are recognized as parallel, circular or interrupted streaks of calcium. Vascular calcification although most commonly found in old age groups, may occur in the middle-aged woman (we have seen vascular calcification in a 22-year-old patient).

The complete demonstration of the larger and smaller arteries of the breast is possible with arteriography. With this mode of diagnosis the entire arterial tree of the breast may be examined with the occasional exception of a few medial or deeper branches originating from the internal mammary artery (see page 50).

Veins

These consist of curvilinear densities measuring 2 to 4 mm in diameter following a long sweeping course in the immediate subcutaneous tissue as well as within the parenchyma, best visualized in the predominantly fatty breasts. The caliber of veins is often much greater in the upper outer quadrant than elsewhere. The venous pattern and caliber are generally symmetrical in both breasts. The difference in the caliber of the veins between one breast and the other normally does not exceed a ratio of 1.5:1. The venous circulation is varible in each individual patient.

Lymphatic Circulation

Lymphatics are not visible in the mammogram. The routine demonstration of the lymphatic circulation of the breast is not currently in use (direct lymphangiography has been reported by KETT et al 1970; indirect lymphangiography has been described by KVASNICKA et al 1971; JACOBS 1972).

Opacification of several lymphatics may occasionally occur during ductography following injection of large amounts of contrast material with extravasation or perforation of lactiferous ducts (fig. 10.11). Lymphatics are then recognized as very small delicate ducts having the appearance of a string of pearls and failing to branch in the periphery. Opacification of lymph ducts in this fashion has heretofore not found any practical or clinical application of significance.

Normal and Abnormal Development, Hormonal Influences

Normal Development

At birth the breast consists of a circumscribed thickening of the skin in the embryonal mammary line overlaying a collection of lactiferous ducts. The newborn already possesses about 15 to 20 lactiferous ducts whose lumen shows only a few protrusions. The breast of the young child is recognizable in the roentgenogram as a small bud of tissue around the nipple.

At puberty these ducts enlarge and proliferate under the influence of estrogen. Usually this is symmetrical; however, it may not be and it is important that during this time the developing but asymmetrical ducts and breast parenchyma not be misinterpreted as a solid nodule, cyst or fibroma (fig. **11.**1a and b). This asymmetry in breast development has no clinical significance and does not indicate that there will be significant breast asymmetry when development is final.

Development of the lactiferous ducts is primarily the result of estrogen influence. The parenchymal acini, on the other hand, grow as a result of cyclical progesterone stimulus. During pregnancy chorionic gonadatropine stimulates final parenchymal growth and secretion.

Abnormal Development

Amastia. Complete absence of one breast is relatively rare.

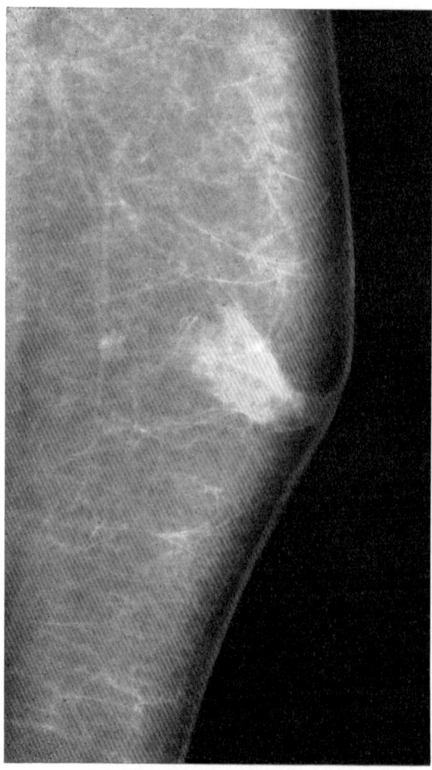
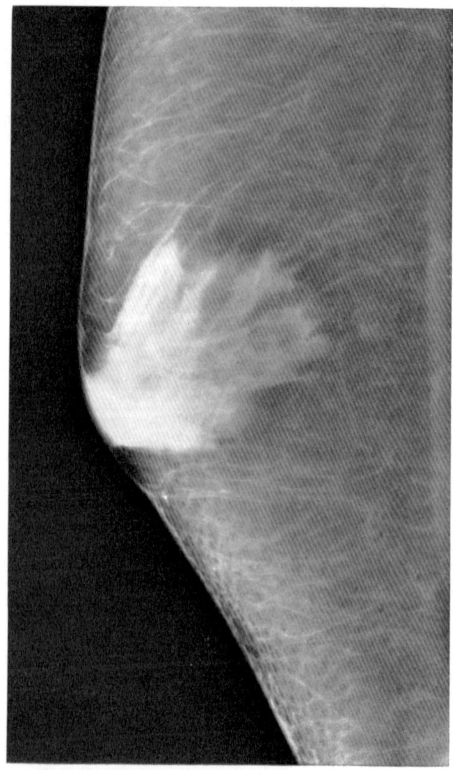

Fig. **11.**1a.b   Asymmetrical development of breast parenchyma prior to puberty in a 9-year-old girl. Clinically insignificant.

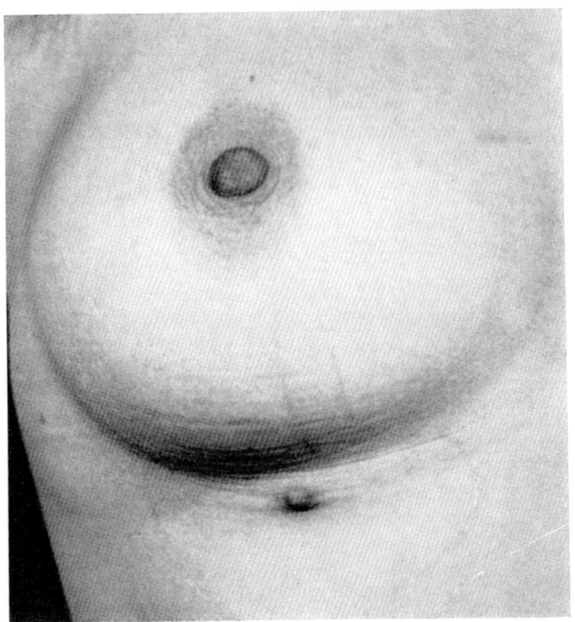

Fig. **11**.2 Supernumerary nipple; development of a second nipple beneath the breast.

Extranumerary Nipples (fig. **11**.2). This consists of the presence of several nipples along the prenatal mammary line without underlying parenchyma. One can determine the presence of absence of an underlying ductal system or a true parenchyma by means of radiography, if indicated.

Polymastia. This indicates an extranumerary nipple in association with underlying parenchyma tissue (fig. **11**.3). A fully or partially developed additional breast may make its appearance during puberty (DeCholnoky 1939).

Acessory Breast Parenchyma (fig. **11**.4). This refers to ectopic foci of breast parenchyma without ductal systems or nipples which are most frequently found in the anterior axillary fold or within the axilla (DeCholnoky 1951). Any breast disease may occur in such ectopic parenchyma.

Mammary Hypertrophy

Hypertrophy of the breast may be unilateral or bilateral, may represent an individual or familial error of development, may be idiopathic but is also occasionally associated with corpus luteum cysts of the ovary (fig. **11**.5). There has been some discussion regarding the relationship of this condition to pituitary growth hormone.

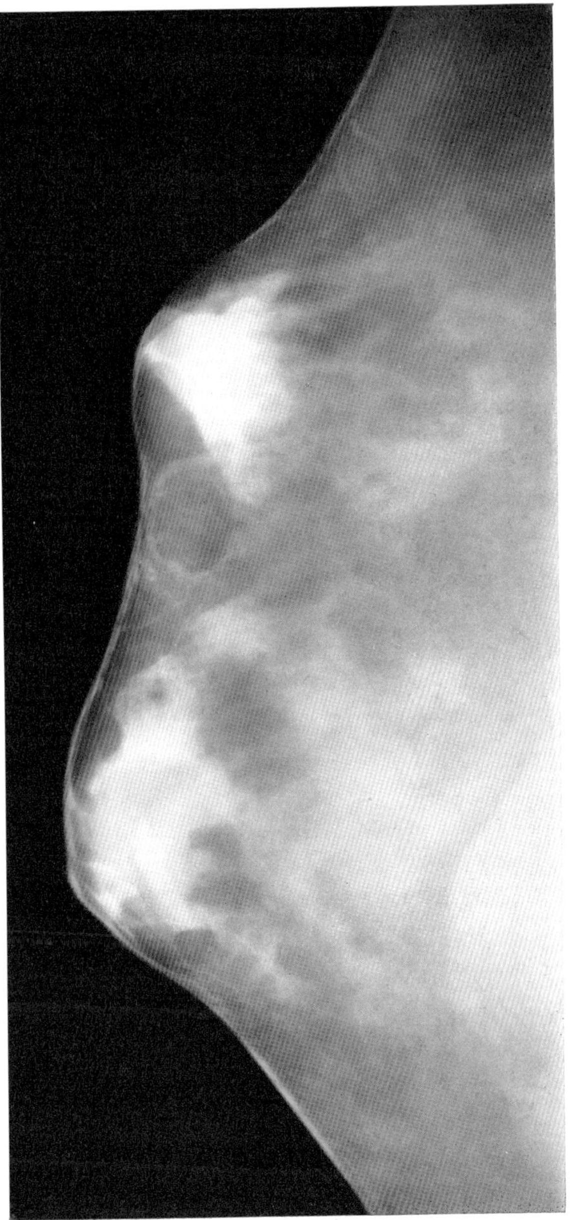

Fig. **11**.3 Supernumerary nipple with associated supernumerary breast parenchyma. Polymastia.

Hormonal Influence

The entire development and growth of the breast from infancy until lactation is under the influence of estrogen and progesterone (fig. **11**.6).

Estrogen, which is produced in the thecal cells of the ovary, in the placenta, in the adrenals, and in the testes of the male, produces the growth of lactiferous ducts.

Progesterone, on the other hand, which is elaborated in the corpus luteum during the

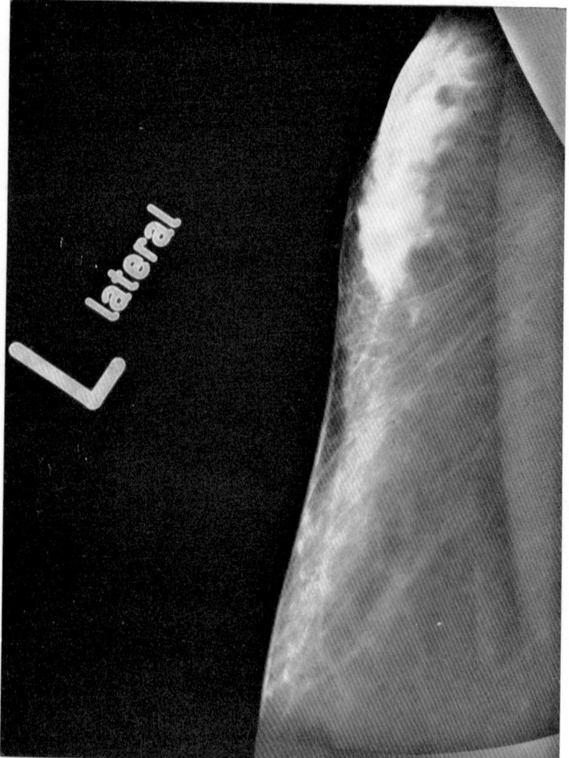

Fig. 11.4 Accessory breast parenchyma underneath the anterior axillary fold.

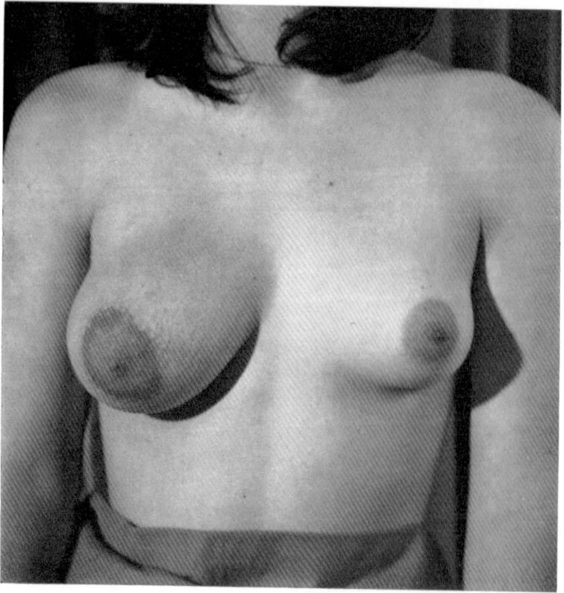

Fig. 11.5 Breast hypertrophy on the right in a 16-year-old girl.

postovulatory phase of the ovarian cycle, and predominant from the placenta approximately after the sixth week of pregnancy, as well as in the adrenals, results in the development of the parenchymal acini.

These two hormones control the primary development of the female breast and are responsible for the physiological changes of the mature breast throughout the menstrual cycle.

An additional hormone that influences the breasts is the lactotrophic hormone, prolactin, produced by the anterior pituitary and secreted by the mother following birth, initiating lactation. Abnormal physiological states result from over or underproduction of any of these hormones or by abnormal cyclical production of the same hormones.

Precocious Breast Development

Accelerated normal breast development during childhood may be a normal variant or indicate precocious puberty. Such precocious breast development may be bilateral or unilateral.

Causes of precocious breast development include adrenal tumors, pituitary tumors, ALBRIGHT's syndrome and granulosa cell tumors of the ovary.

Influence of the Menstrual Cycle on the Breast

Following ovulation there is a generalized enlargement of breast parenchymal tissue secondary to progesterone.

Clinically, this is manifested as increased size and tension within the breast and occasionally pain (mastodynia). This is a normal physiological event and does not always indicate fibrocystic disease. Mammography during the premenstrual phase demonstrates increased size and confluence as well as greater density of the parenchymal tissues, and greater prominence of the venous system (fig. 11.7a and b). As menses appears and estrogen effects predominate there is a generalized involution of parenchyma with lesser density and confluence of these structures.

It is claimed that the recognition of pathological processes with mammograms is better during the postmenstrual state.

The previously described cyclical changes within the breast, however, are more profound clinically than mammographically (MAASEN 1966). Most of the time there is very little definite difference between the pre- and postmenstrual mammogram.

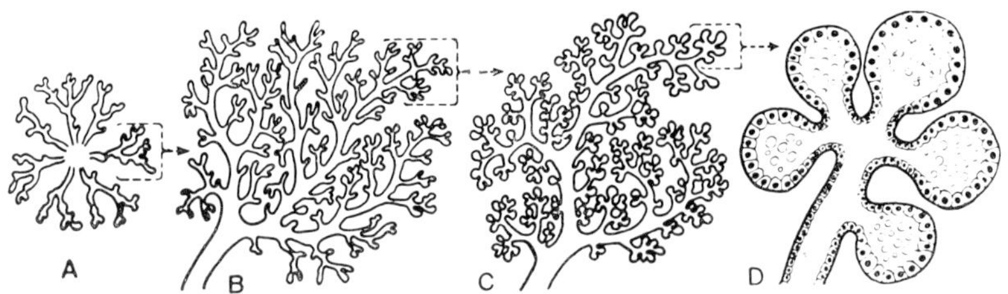

Fig. **11**.6   Schematic demonstrations of parenchymal development in the female breast (after Corner)
A: Immature state. B: Development of the ducal systems in the mature, virgin breast (esrogen effect).
C: Proliferation of ductal system (chorionic estrogen effect) and formation of acini (chorionic progesterone
effect) during pregnancy. D: Milk secretion (prolactin effect).

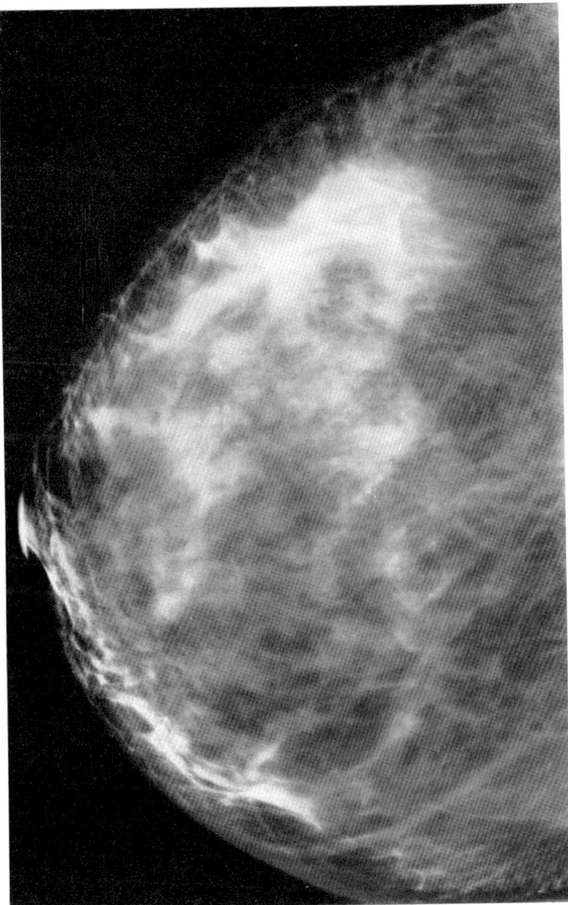

Fig. **11**.7a Premenstrual phase in a 39-year-old
Woman with relatively dense breast parenchyma
particularly in the lateral aspect.

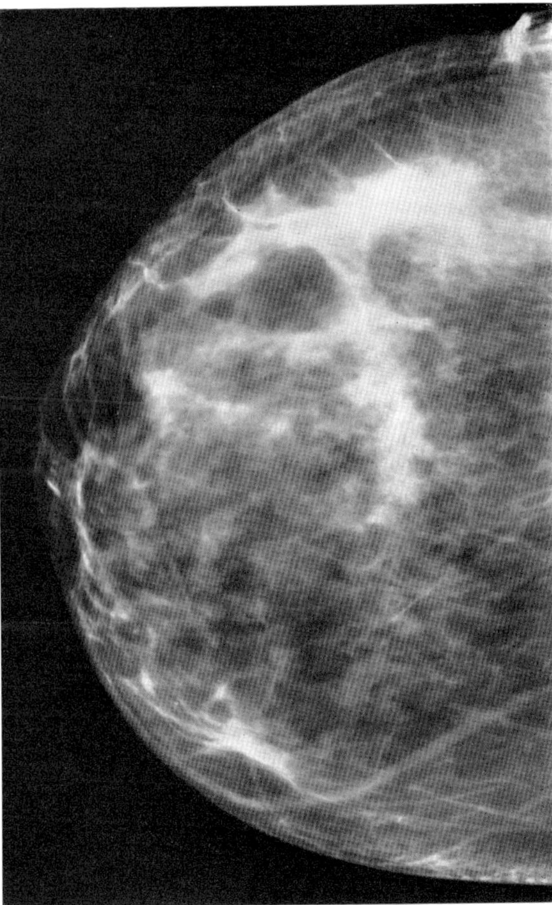

Fig. **11**.7b   The same case in the postmenstrual
phase. The entire breast is somewhat smaller. The
parenchyma Is less dense.

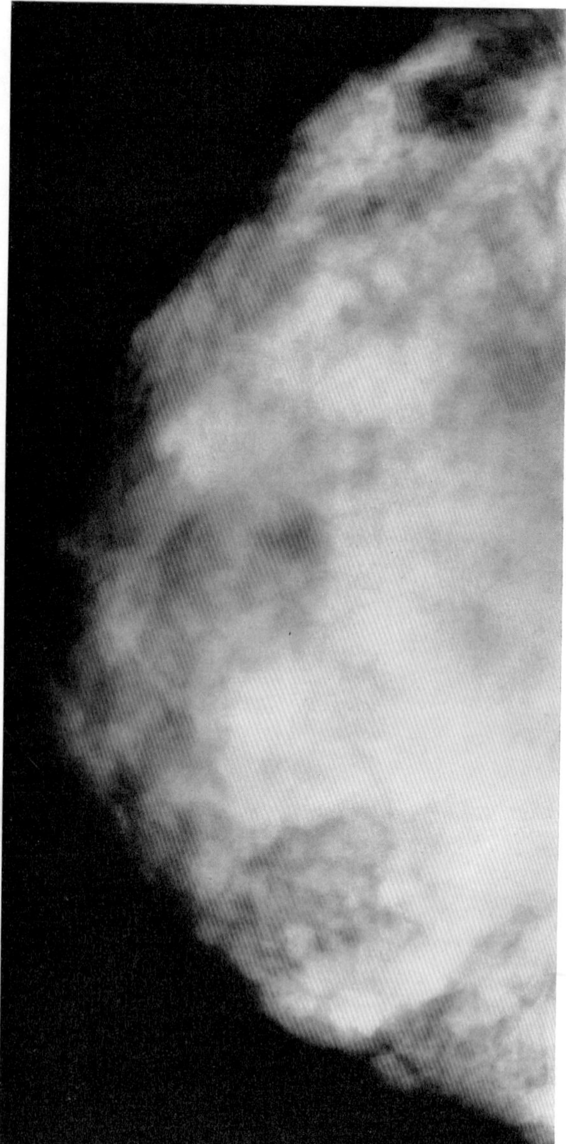

Fig. **11**.8 Lactating breast with increased density and coarsening of the parenchymal strukture. There is confluence of parenchymal lobules filled with milk. The appearance resembles that of pathological adenosis.

Gestational Changes in the Female Breast

During pregnancy there is total maturation and development of the breast parenchyma, under the influence of progesterone.

In the mammogram the density of the parenchyma is increased. The glandular lobules enlarge and the total mass shows a coarser and denser structure. Hyperemia and increased water content of the breast stroma obscure the fatty tissue

which, added to the parenchymal changes, results in an overall dense breast in which it is difficult to recognize individual structures. Sometimes the breast may assume a uniform ground-glass density. It is very difficult during this state to define or recognize pathological processes. In spite of the fact that the changes of pregnancy are rather characteristic in the mammogram, this study is not indicated as proof of pregnancy (FOCHEM and NARICK 1957) because of the obvious desire to avoid additional irradiation and because, other better tests of pregnancy are available.

During lactation milk is secreted from apocrine cells into the lumen of the milk ducts. Eventual filling of the lactiferous ducts results in widening of their caliber. The lactiferous sinuses function as reservoirs of milk. In the mammogram one can recognize the lactation phase as a generalized coarsening, increased density and a tendency towards confluence of the parenchymal lobules (fig. **11**.8) (LOCKWOOD and STEWART 1932; INGELBY et al 1957).

At the conclusion of lactation there is a gradual involution of breast parenchyma which is later followed by a decrease in the caliber of the lactiferous ducts. Ductography (fig. **11**.9a and b) will demonstrate some persistence of widening of the lactiferous ducts even months after the end of lactation particularly if there is some continued mild secretion. There may be tortuosity and varying caliber of the ducts, which become involuted.

The generalized parenchymal involution following the end of lactation results in smaller and more pendulous breasts. Most of the parenchyma is replaced by fatty tissue. Generally some ductal ectasia remains and involution of the lactiferous ducts may be prolonged and remain incomplete. The delicate ductal system demonstrated in ductograms in the prelactational phase is altered to a more coarse and tortuous system following gestation and lactation. Involutional changes also affect the stromal tissue and in the mammogram one notes that the trabeculae of the breast are smaller and less distinct. The degree of involution following lactation is variable. It can be quite extensive with almost total replacement of stromal and parenchymal tissue by fat with only fibrous septa, ducts and vessels remaining. In spite of this, however, the breast retains its ability to redevelop parenchyma and secrete milk during any subsequent pregnancy.

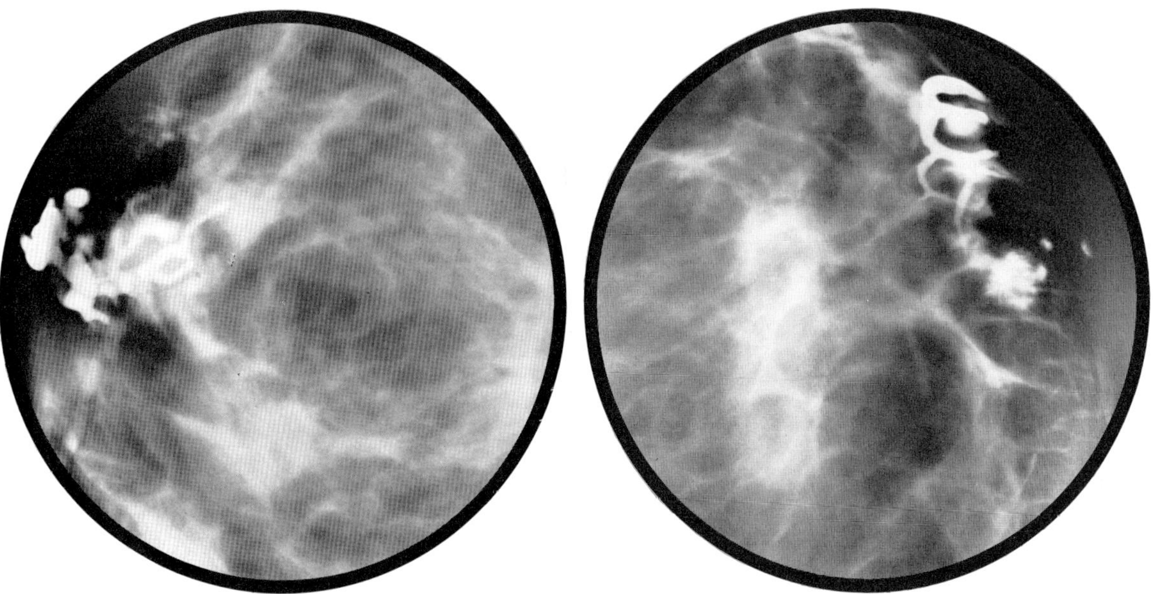

Fig. **11**.9a, b   Chiari-Frommel syndrome in a 31-year-old woman. Ductography: Extensive ductal ectasia bilaterally.

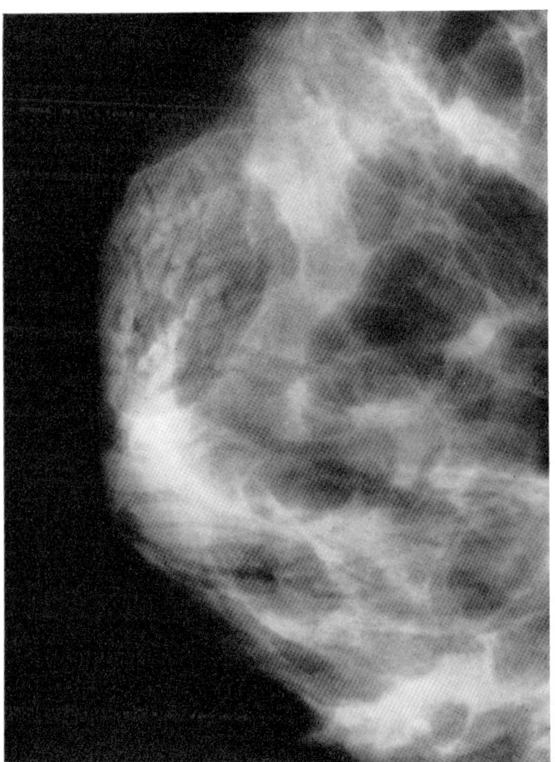

Fig. **11**.10a   Natural contrast produces demonstration of a lactiferous duct by virtue of secretions within the duct containing a high concentration of fat.

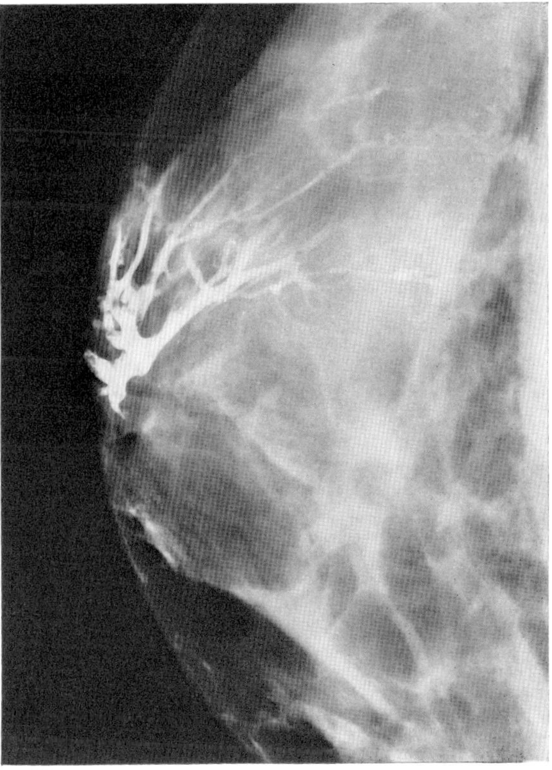

Fig. **11**.10b — Demonstration of several enlarged lactiferous ducts following instillation of contrast material.

Chiari-Frommel Syndrome

In this condition there is prolonged lactation which may persist for month or years after pregnancy. It appears to be related to abnormal secretory and neural ovarian function (LEIBER and OLBRICH 1963). Other components of the syndrome include uterine atrophy, secondary amenorrhea, headaches, back pain and depression. The Chiari-Frommel syndrome is rare and should not be confused with the much more frequent occurrence of persistent serous breast secretions following cessation of lactation. The latter belongs to the spectrum of "secretory disease" and is caused by incomplete or prolonged involution of lactiferous ducts (fig. 11.9a and b). This condition may be verified with ductography. A natural contrast ductogram results whenever there is a high concentration of fat in the ductal contents, resulting from pathological lactation. Because of the low x-ray absorption for fat it serves as a negative contrast material (fig. 11.10a and b).

A variant of the Chiari-Frommel syndrome is the Forbes-Albright syndrome which consists of amenorrhea and galactorrhea associated with acromegaly, without any preceding pregnancy.

Senile Involution of the Breast

This occurs during and after the menopause and is based on atrophy of parenchymal acini. The lactiferous ducts either become small and there may be associated periductal fibrosis or they may enlarge and the lumen becomes filled with inspissated secretion. There is marked proliferation of fat which then becomes the dominant tissue of the breast. Involution of the stromal tissues occurs and the fibrous septa atrophy so that the breast loses its firmness and becomes pendulous. In other cases there may be linear or reticular proliferation of stromal tissue resulting in a firm, well suspended breast even in advanced years. The beginning and the extent of breast involution is variable and dependent upon hormonal influences, nutritional status of the patient and familial background.

Involution of the parenchyma begins inferomedially and progresses superolaterally. The parenchymal tissue in the superolateral aspect of the breast is the longest to persist. Involution may not be symmetrical. Should this process be asymmetrical the breast containing persistent parenchymal tissue may appear to be pathological (fig. 11.11a and b).

Involutional, fatty breasts have been given the name of "empty" breasts in the mammogram. This loose and undesirable term evokes a concept of a nonfunctional status of the organ. This is completely untrue. A predominantly fatty breast with little or no parenchymal substance may be found in young as well as mature patients and simply reflects sparse current development of parenchymal tissue. The so-called "empty" breast changes into a very functional organ with the onset of pregnancy. It is therefore inadvisable to interpret mammograms with words or phrases which imply a certain functional status which may be dependent on the patient's age, history, physical status, and other such factors which may or may not be known: "The Functionally Extinguished Breast", BRASNIKOV (1964); "The Breast Following the Menopause", INGLEBY and GERSHON-COHEN (1960); "The Breast in the Older Woman", BACLESSE and WILLEMIN (1963). STRAX and OPPENHEIM (1960) have therefore pleaded for a more strict mammographic interpretation into three categories as described below:

1) The fibrous type, in which the stromal tissue predominates and the breast demonstrates an overall density in the mammogram surrounded by a narrow small border of subcutaneous fat.
2) The glandular type, in which parenchymal tissue predominates and the mammogram reveals fairly sharply circumscribed parenchymal lobes and lobules through which some fatty tissue is interspersed.
3) The fatty type, in which the predominant tissue is adipose and the mammogram demonstrates a generally radiolucent fatty breast interrupted only by stromal septa, retro-areolar milk ducts and blood vessels.

This type of group differentiation provides a reliable statement regarding the hormonal, functional and age status of the breast. The drawback to this categorization is that it results essentially in a radiographic anatomical description and has very little clinical significance.

Influence of Exogenous Hormones

The response of the breast to exogenous or endogenous estrogen is essentially the same. The effect does not appear to be dose dependent. The estrogen level found in ovulation inhibitors

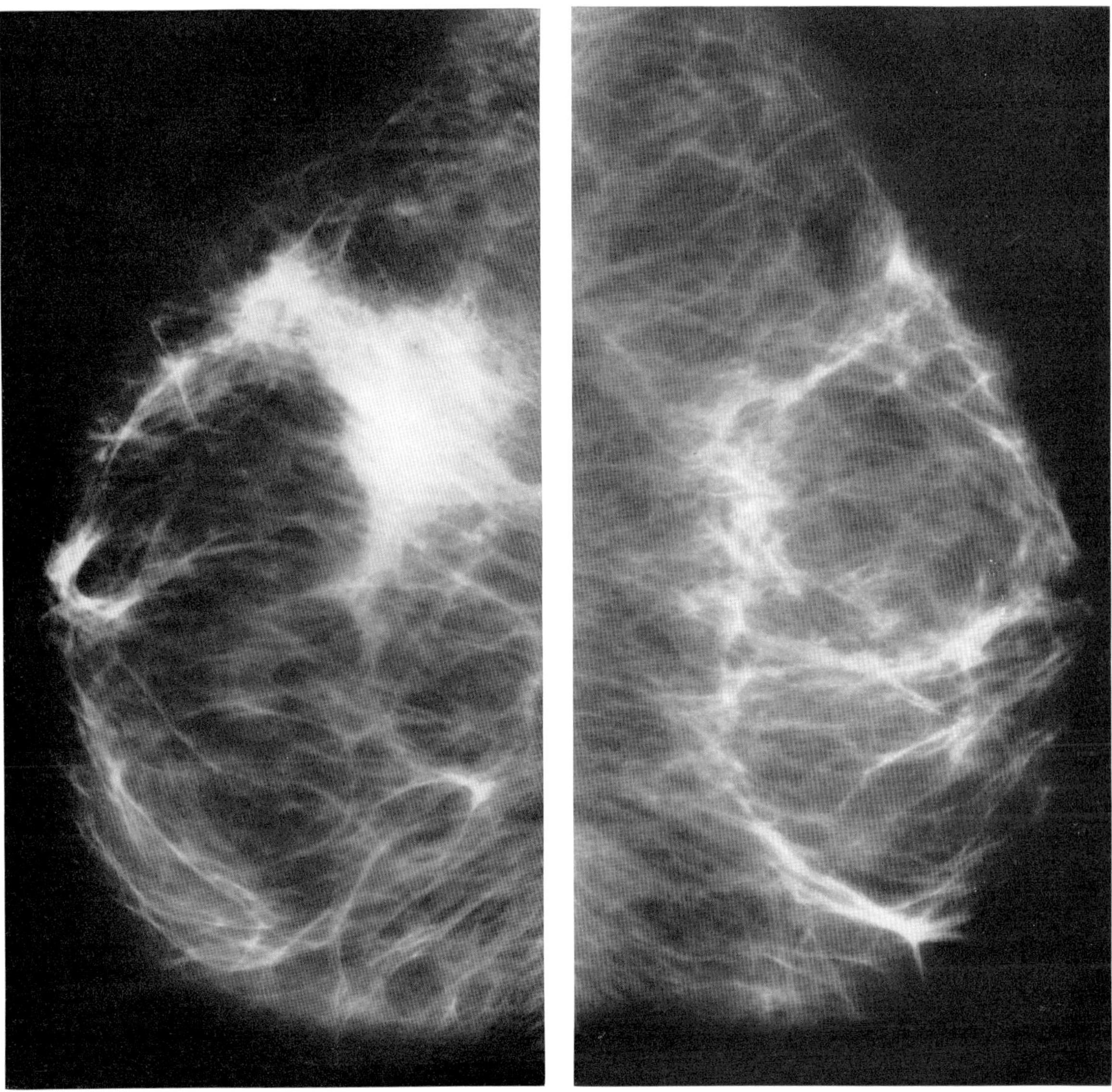

Fig. **11**.11a, b — Asymmetrical parenchymal atrophy with increased residual parenchyma in the left breast, in the lateral projection.

(by virtue of the body's gradually increasing tolerance to higher estrogen levels) manifests itself clinically by transient enlargement of the breasts which return to normal size after the hormonal influence wears off. The histology of the breast reflects the clinical changes. Likewise the roentgen findings change under the influence of hormonal stimulation. If estrogen is administered to the premenopausal woman, mammography seldom will show any changes in the breast parenchyma. The same is true of the postmenopausal mammogram (REINARTZ et al 1970). However, the influence of this hormone is not well evaluated with a single mammographic examination. Follow-up examinations over a period of months and years invariably show regeneration of the parenchyma as a result of the estrogen administration. The effect of exogenous estrogen depends on the patient and varies with each individual, some experiencing obvious changes in breast parenchyma and others none. Gestational preparations may evoke the typical mammographic appearance of chronic fibrocystic disease, including cysts and stromal proliferation. This results from acinar enlargement and from stasis of secretions.

Androgen therapy results in involution of the breast. Marked involution of the parenchyma and fatty proliferation is observed and may produce the roentgen finding of the "empty breast". Again, however, this androgen effect, like all hormonal influences, is individually dependent. In the mammogram it varies from the classical picture of breast involution to essentially no detectable changes (REINARTZ et al 1970).

Chapter 12

The Male Breast

The rudimentary breast fails to develop in the male following birth because of the absence of proper hormonal stimulation.

However, prominence of the nipple and the retro-areolar density may be seen in the male newborn even including actual secretion, and this reflects the effect of maternal hormones. Occasionally similar changes are transiently observed during puberty; however, growth and development of breast parenchyma does not occur in the male. In older men unilateral or bilateral gynecomastia suggests a benign or malignant tumor. The mammogram of the normal male breast reveals predominantly fatty tissue with some rudimentary ductal system behind the nipple (fig. 12.1).

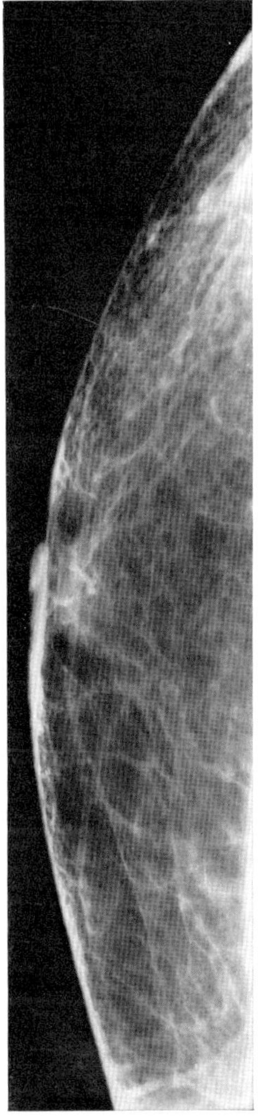

Fig. **12**.1 Male breast. No parenchyma, only fatty tissue. Rudimentary lactiferous ducts are seen in the subareolar region.

Benign Diseases of the Female Breast

Chapter 13

Mammary Dysplasia (Fibrocystic Disease)

Definition and Pathology

Fibrocystic disease is a benign proliferation of the breast stroma. One differentiates a cystic form when the changes are predominantly in the periductal stroma as well as in the ducts and consist of cystic dilatations of varying size (fig. 13.1). In some cases large cysts, in others small cysts predominate. In most cases, cysts of varying sizes are present as seen macroscopically (fig. 13.2). The degree of periductal fibrosis varies as well. In fact periductal fibrosis may be an isolated finding without any evidence of cystic changes (fibrous type of fibrocystic disease). Another form of fibrocystic disease consists of hyperplasia of parenchymal lobules. Proliferation results in adenosis. Of particular interest here is fibrosing or sclerosing adenosis which may mimic carcinoma both histologically and roentgenologically.

Among the forms of fibrocystic disease is the so-called "complicated" proliferative fibrocystic disease which is a papillary epithelial proliferation of ectatic milk ducts. It is recognized that this type of fibrocystic disease predisposes to increased incidence of carcinoma. Varying deformities of the milk ducts are found in fibrocystic disease and these are discussed under ductal ectasia.

Synonyms

Mastitis fibrosa cystica; chronic cystic mastitis; SCHIMMELBUSCH's disease; chronic-cystic masto-pathy; fibroadenomatosis; adenosis; cystic desquamative epithelial hyperplasia; general breast hyperplasia; RECLUS' disease (cystic enlargement of breasts), mazoplasia.

History

SCHIMMELBUSCH was the first to describe the disease that bears his name in 1892; KÖNIG in 1893 reported those changes which he felt were secondary to an inflammatory process and evolved the concept of chronic cystic mastitis.

In the English literature this disease even to the current day is associated with the names of surgeons COOPER (1845) and BRODIE (1846) who reported on these benign changes in the breast over 100 years ago.

In France it was RECLUS (1883) and BRISSAUD (1884) who first reported the disorder in the female breast.

In the Scandinavian literature, SEMB (1928) described this disease as fibroadenomatosis. Many studies, monographs, and publications about this disorder have appeared in the last ten years, authored by well-known clinicians and pathologists. Among these are the following: CHEATLE and CUTLER (1931), HAMPERL (1939), GESCHICKTER (1943), FOOTE and STEWART (1945), HAAGENSEN (1956), INGLEBY and GERSHON-COHEN (1960), CUTLER (1961), BÖHMIG (1964), and KUZMA (1966).

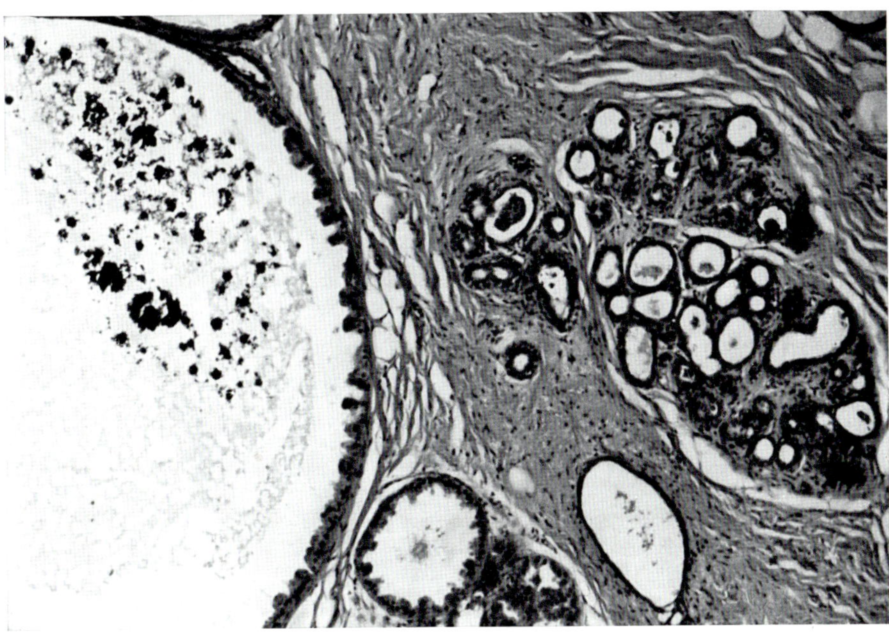

Fig. **13**.1   Cystic dilatation of lactiferous ducts with inspissated secretion, some apocrine metaplasia of the epithelium and nodular proliferation of terminal ductules associated with fibrosis. Cystic fibroadeno-matosis.

Frequency

Fibrocystic disease is such a frequent disorder of the female breast that in its uncomplicated state it is to be recognized almost as an obligatory condition of the breast which from the 20th to the 50th year of life may be present in varying degrees of severity according to whatever its hormonal influence may be.

BORCHARDT and JAFFE (1932) did histological examinations of the breast tissue of over 100 women over age 40 who had no symptoms nor signs of disease. They found that in 93% there were changes consistent with fibrocystic disease.

FRANTZ et al in 1951 reported on a histological study of breasts on 225 female patients who died without signs of breast disease. Macroscopic inspection revealed 19% of the cases had definite cystic changes in the breasts, with cysts ranging in diameter from 1 to 2 mm. These changes were bilateral in half the cases. In a further 34% there were definite changes of fibrocystic disease consisting of intraductal epithelial proliferation, apocrine metaplasia of ductal epithelium and formation of microcysts. In a further 53% of the cases in the absence of clinical symptoms there was histological or macroscopic evidence of fibrocystic disease.

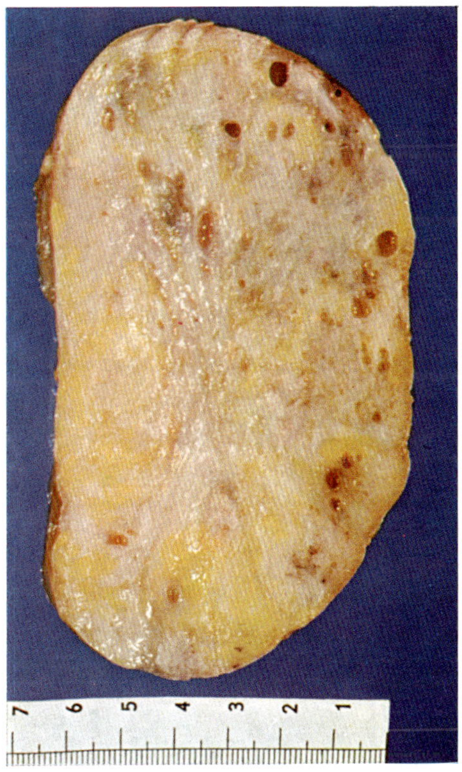

Fig. **13**.2   Specimen photograph: Fibrocystic disease; numerous cysts and fibrotic strands coursing throughout fatty tissue are visible in this section of breast parenchyma.

6*

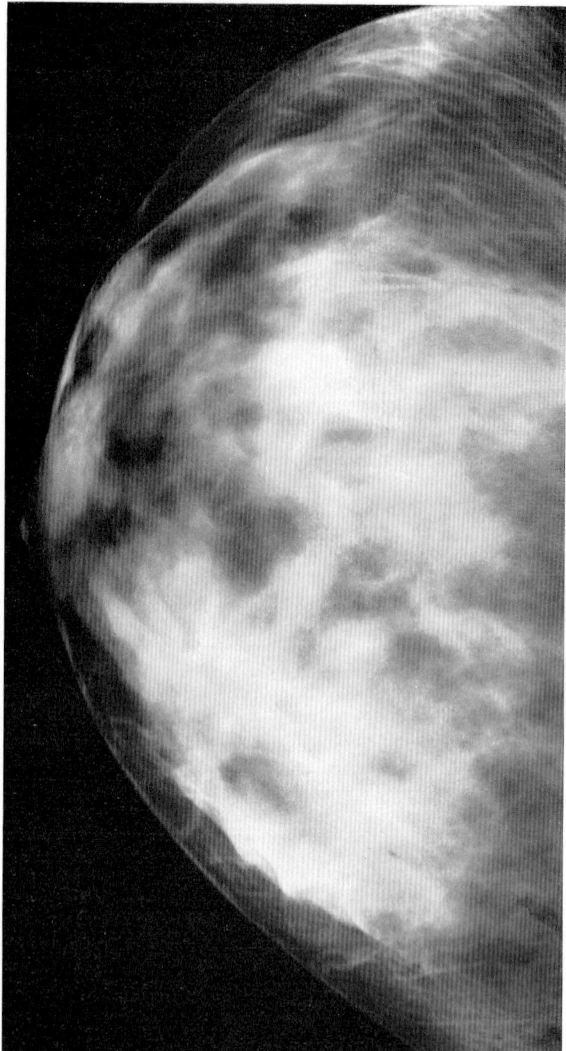

Fig. **13**.3 Extensive mammary dysplasia with coarsening of parenchymal structure.

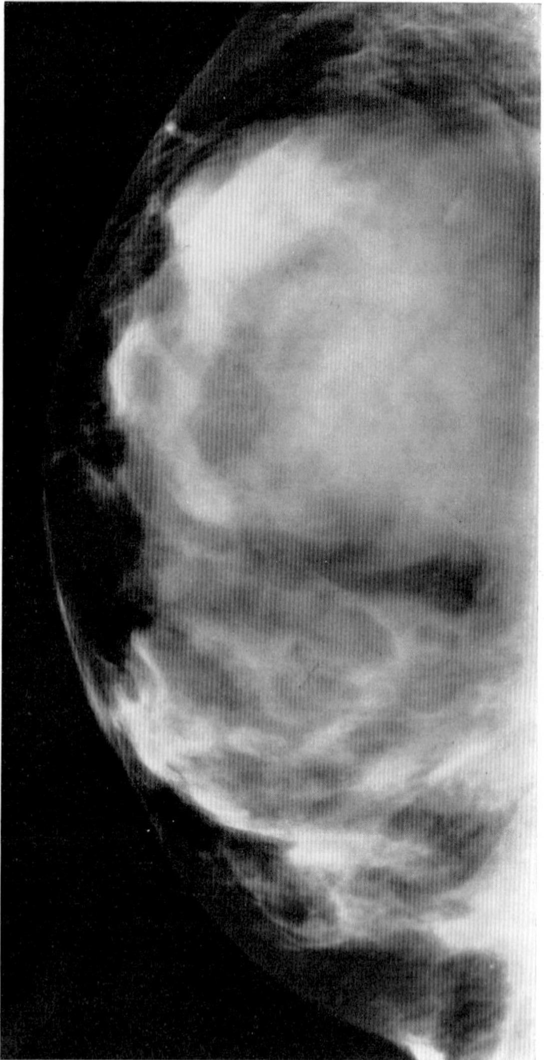

Fig. **13**.4 Circumscribed lobular mass in the upper portion of the breast. Mammary dysplasia.

Numerous other reports on similar investigations which differ little from one another and all indicate the high percentage of patients demonstrating changes in the breast consistent with fibrocystic disease.

It is concluded that fibrocystic disease is only clinically significant when associated with real symptoms or complications.

Clinical Symptoms

Mastodynia or painful sensation of tension within the breast is the least important clinical sign of this disorder. This symptom is most frequently experienced in the first half of the menstrual cycle, abates suddenly with the onset of menses and reappears at the time of ovulation. In the American literature the term used to describe uncomplicated fibrocystic disease is mazoplasia (CHEATLE and CUTLER 1931). This includes a painful breast and palpatory nodules which appear and disappear in the above-described cyclical fashion in relation to the menstrual period. Histologically mazoplasia indicates an overwhelmingly adenomatous stage of fibrocystic disease with ductal ectasia but a few fibrotic changes.

Roentgenology

The changes of fibrocystic disease seen in the mammogram depend on the extent, arrangement,

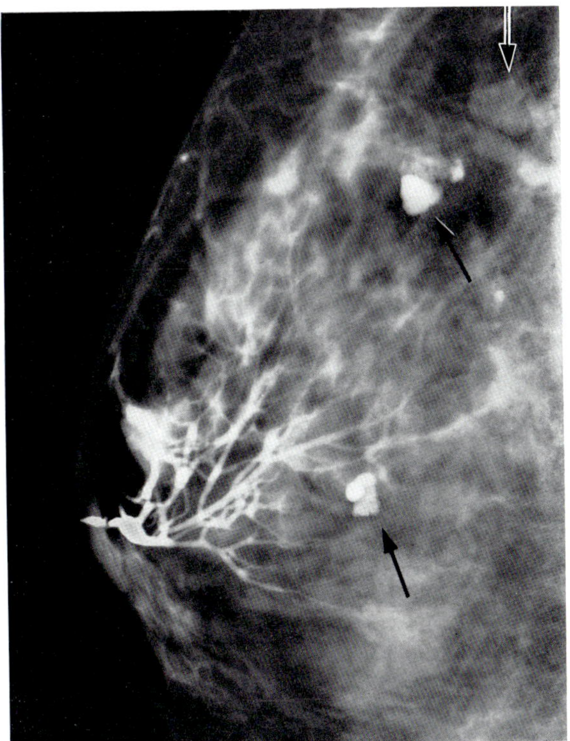

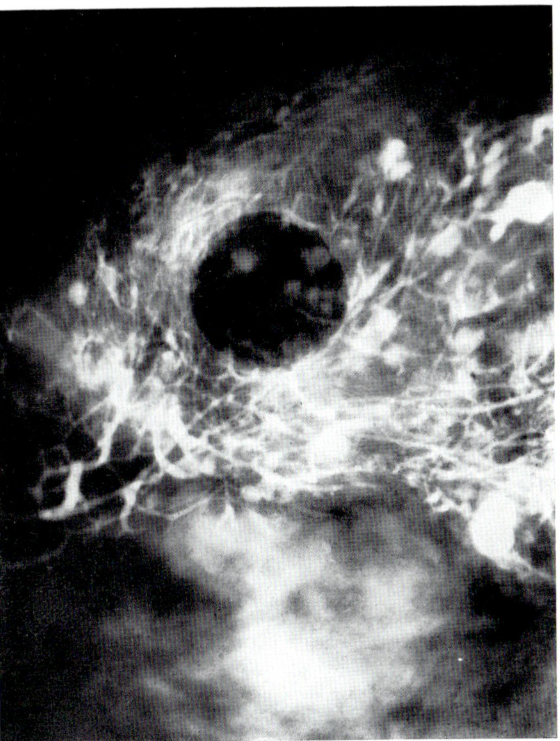

Fig. **13**.5 Ductography performed because of green discolored breast secretion. Cysts approximately 5 mm in size are filled deep within the breast (arrows). In the vicinity of the duct system filled with contrast there are other smaller cysts not filled with contrast (white arrow). Combined ductography and pneumocystography. A smooth contoured large cyst has been aspirated and filled with air. Ductography demonstrates numerous smaller cysts in the vicinity of the large one. Mammary dysplasia with large and small cysts.

Fig. **13**.6 Combined examination (galactography and pneumocystography). A smooth marginated cyst has been aspirated and filled with air. Numerous smaller cysts are demonstrated in the vicinity. Fibrocystic disease with large and small cysts.

and histological type. They consist primarily of fine, coarse, round or lobulated densities and masses scattered in a combination of parenchymal and stromal proliferation. There are linear strands as well.

The mammographic appearance is as variable as the histological one. Only in certain cases are the signs characteristic enough to allow identification of the type of fibrocystic disease in the mammogram. In the majority of cases only the general diagnosis of mammary dysplasia may be made. For example, in principle it is impossible to definitely differentiate between a cyst and a solid fibroadenoma without calcification, unless the cyst is punctured and thereby reduced in size. In the following discussion attempts will be made to separate the various types of fibrocystic disease as they appear in the mammogram,

with the thought in mind that pure forms of this disease are probably never found and that the predominating type is, in fact, a mixture.

Uncomplicated, minimal fibrocystic disease, in the young patient, is demonstrated in the mammogram as a generalized coarsening of the breast structures with varying degrees of increased density. The overall picture is one of multiple nodular densities with irregular and ill-defined borders (fig. 13.3). The diagnosis is simpler in those cases where interspersed fatty tissue allows more accurate demonstration of the coarse. dense parenchymal foci with irregular borders. The diagnosis is most difficult when there is primarily parenchymal dysplasia and the interspersed fat is sparse. In such cases the disorder may be recognized by noting signs of confluence of these coarse, dense nodular structures. If these changes are generalized in a single breast or in fact even bilateral, it is difficult to differentiate hyperplasia from normal parenchyma or from fibrocystic disease. If only focal regions of a breast are involved with such changes the presence of the

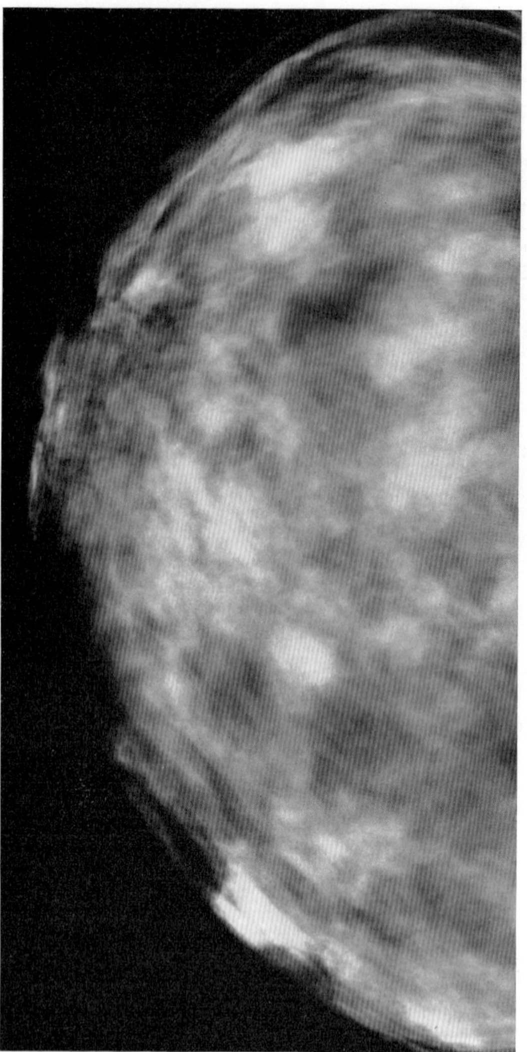

Fig. **13**.7   Mammary dysplasia with coarse parenchyma through which fatty tissue is interspersed.
Small and large, in part confluent, rounded densities are visible which either represent small cysts
or adenomatous changes of parenchymal lobules.

large nodular masses render easier the diagnosis
of the mastopathy (fig. 13.4).

It is essential that the palpatory findings be
correlated with the roentgen findings in order
to come to a correct conclusion. If a dominant
mass is palpated but cannot be discerned in a
dense breast, it assumes important clinical
significance. Further diagnostic steps are then
indicated and dependent primarily on the
palpatory findings. On the other hand it is
equally important if roentgen findings cannot
be correlated with the palpatory examination.
There are numerous cases in which large and

multiple cysts, although easily seen and identified
in the mammogram, cannot be palpated as
readily as fibroadenomas and fibromas. In such
cases the roentgen findings are the primary
indication for further diagnostic measures. It is
incorrect and illogical to assume the view point
that a palpable mass should be biopsied or
removed, but that a mass identified in the mammogram should not be biopsied just because it is not
palpable. Mazoplasia as described in the American literature is recognized in the roentgenogram
primarily as a "coarsening of structure" and
deals with adenosis and microcystic fibrocystic
disease which is definitely related to the menstrual
cycle.

The microcystic type of fibrocystic disease is
impossible to differentiate roentgenographically
from adenomatosis because both conditions
manifest themselves as small grainlike radio-
densities giving no clue as to their actual anatomical origin. Positive contrast ductography, however, does allow differentiation. In microcystic
fibrocystic disease the small cysts projecting off
dilated lactiferous ducts may be filled with
contrast and demonstrated (fig. 13.5 and fig.
13.6). The lactiferous ducts in spite of these
cystic changes may be delicate and uniform but
may also have the typical ectatic changes and
irregular variations in caliber, associated with
- mammary dysplasia.

However, ductography should be performed only
in an abnormally secreting breast and since the
majority of cases of fibrocystic disease is not
associated with nipple discharge, this method of
diagnosis does not find routine application in
this disorder. Fibrocystic disease of a coarser
variety than that described above, including
cysts of 1 to 2 cm in diameter or focal regions of
adenomatosis, presents in the mammogram as a
breast with a generalized coarse and lymph
structural pattern. Cysts need not necessarily
have sharp curvilinear margins since the borders
are often abscured by adjacent adenomatous
tissue, again providing an overall, confluent and
nodular pattern in the roentgenogram. A predominantly coarse adenosis may have a similar
appearance in the mammogram. In such cases
the condition should be designated only as fibrocystic disease of the coarse or nodular type
(fig. **13**.7). The determination of multiple
distinctly rounded shadows ranging from 1
to 2 cm in diameter does not necessarily mean
that one is dealing with numerous cysts (fig.

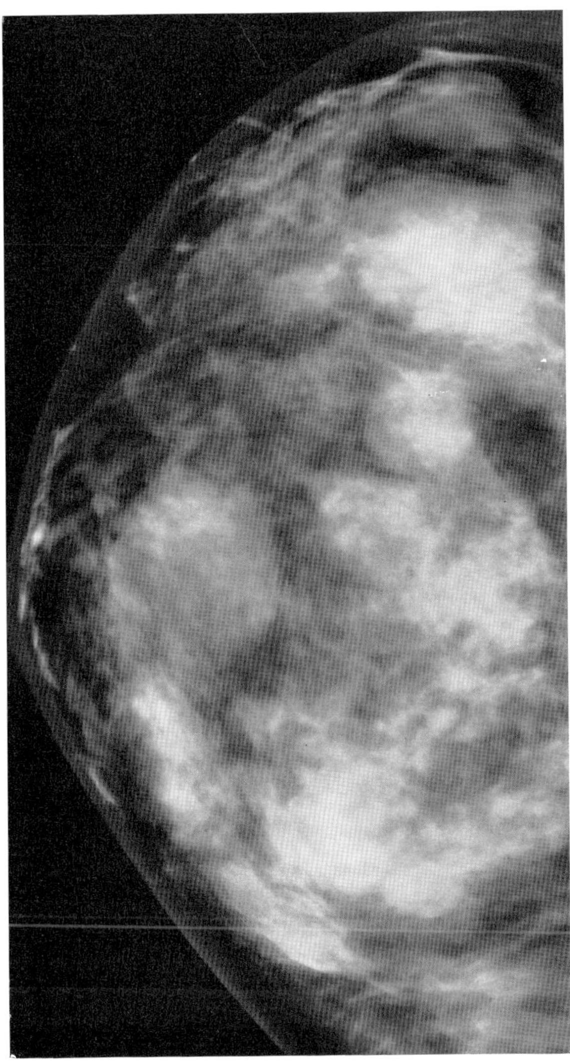

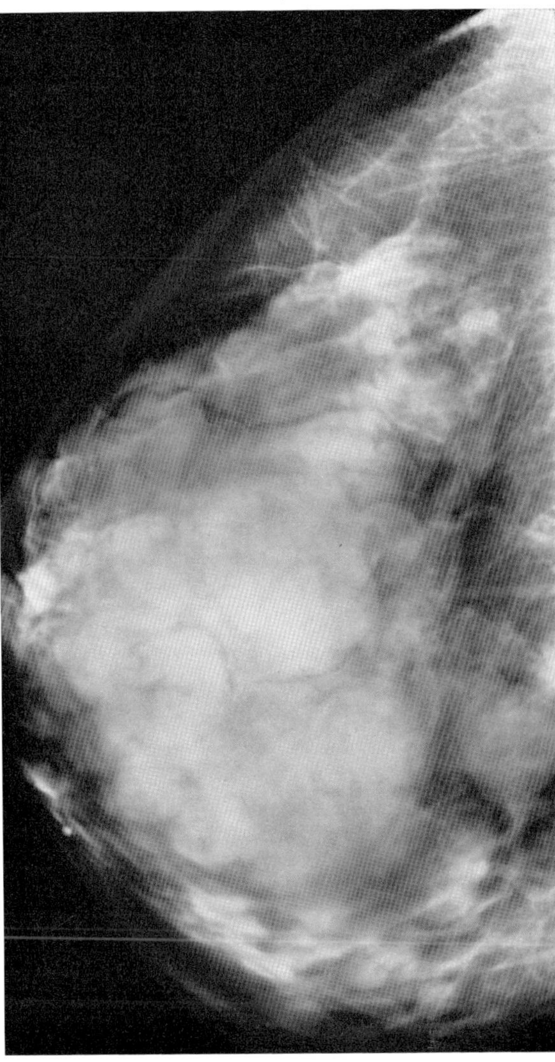

Fig. **13**.8 Mammary dysplasia with large and small cysts. Rounded, smoothly marginated densities ranging from 1 to 2 cm in diameter and separated from one another by interspersed fatty tissue are seen. These could represent fibroadenomas and/or cysts.

Fig. **13**.9 Mammary dysplasia with large cysts; however, any of these rounded densities could be a fibroadenoma. The parenchyma is very coarse and dense and consists of numerous rounded shadows ranging from 1 to 2 cm in diameter and surrounded by a radiolucent zone. The margins of these masses are smooth.

13.8) because a similar appearance may be provided by fibroadenomatous changes (fig. 13.9). If a differential diagnosis is necessary in these cases it can be done only through cyst puncture and instillation of air. It is often astounding that such obvious parenchymal changes, even such as seen in fig. 13.8 and 13.9 may not be palpable as distinct or dominant masses. On occasion the difficult question arises as to whether biopsy should be performed on the basis of mammographic findings alone. Since it is impossible to completely remove every nodule or cyst, in every questionable case one should always biopsy in order to decide whether one is dealing with a solid mass or a fluid-containing cyst and benefit from cytological examination regarding a decision on further therapy. If there are abnormal palpatory findings and a puncture with aspiration of the palpated mass followed by air injection fails to unequivocally demonstrate a cyst whose walls are uniform and smooth, biopsy should then also be performed.

Chapter 14

Fibrocytic Disease with Large Cysts
Solitary Cysts

Definition and Pathology

Large cysts, solitary or multiple, as well as small cysts, are included in the spectrum of fibrocystic disease. Such cysts are the result of enlargement of the lactiferous ducts. The cyst wall consists of a single layer of epithelium and its contents consist of clear, yellow fluid. The staining of this fluid from bleeding results in a gray, brown, or black color. If the fluid is cloudy it indicates a high content of albumin. If there is proliferation or metaplasia of the epithelial layer of the cyst wall, the disease enters the category of "complicated" fibrocystic disease.

A cystic type of mammary dysplasia may be part of the so-called Cowden's syndrome (LLOYD DENNIS). This consists of multiple congenital anomalies (microstomia, tooth anomalies, bird-like facies) as well as hyperkeratotic papillomas of the mucocutaneous junction and thyroid cysts. The breast over the skin is very thin allowing easy visualization of venous patterns and the nipple is hypoplastic.

Clinical Findings

Some cysts are very firm to palpation. If a cyst is discovered following pregnancy and puncture reveals a milky content it probably represents a galactocele. The discovery of bloody fluid within a simple cyst is unusual and should arouse the suspicion of intracystic papilloma. Medullary carcinoma is another possibility. However, aspiration of bloody fluid from a cyst may also be the result of traumatic puncture, if the needle passes through a vein. Not infrequently the patient will insist that the lump in her breast was not palpable a few days ago. In other cases the appearance of the lump will be associated with trauma. Cysts may be palpable as firm or hard nonfluctuant freely movable nodules; thickening (peau d'orange) and retraction of the skin or of the nipple is not associated. Large solitary cysts

containing 10, 15, and 20 cc of fluid are palpable only when completely filled and tense. These are frequently clinically insignificant.

Frequency

The exact statistical frequency of cysts is impossible to determine clinically or pathologically. Only a portion of all cysts are detected by palpation. Histological examination is restricted to biopsy material, and therefore also includes only a portion of the cysts. Additionally, in many cases a cyst may be removed from the breast and not submitted for histological examination because of its benign appearance clinically and at surgery. Furthermose, the definition as to the maximum diameter of a cyst which constitutes small cystic mammary dysplasia or what should be considered large cystic mammary dysplasia has not been determined. The frequency of mammary dysplasia with large cysts described by HAAGENSEN (1971) as 70% multiple cysts and 30% simple cysts, is probably too high, his patient population being a selected one, only those requiring biopsy. Our own series deals with 7,000 patients seen in 1970, including 250 cyst punctures (3.6%). Our patients, however, were also selected insofar as 50% of them were examined for only minimal mastodynia or simply because of concern over breast disease. Furthermore, the figures are not entirely valid, since not all the cysts were punctured, only those which were diagnostically suspicious.

Thus, a cyst is a disease of the breast which occurs in middle-age, most frequently between 30 and 50 years. Younger women and girls are less inclined to have solitary cysts; fibroma or fibroadenoma is more common in such a population. Cysts are rare in postmenopausal women and particularly rare in the elderly. They are more often multiple than solitary (3 to 1). Bilateral occurrence is not uncommon.

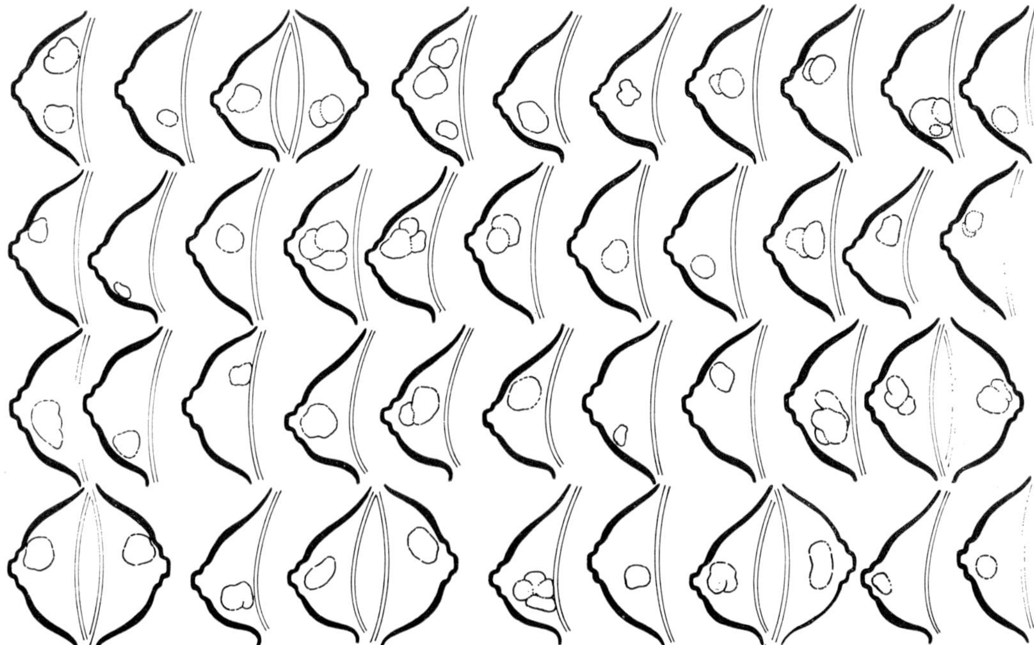

Fig. **14**.1   Drawing of the frequently occurring variations found in solitary, multiple, single or loculated cysts during pneumocystography.

Roentgenology

The shape, size and number of mammary cysts varies (fig. 14.1). Large uncomplicated cysts are seen as round or oval densities in the mammogram. Their contours are smooth and sharp. With progressive enlargement there is compression of surrounding fatty tissue resulting in a radiolucent border. The sharp border of the typical cyst may be obscured by overlying adjacent stromal tissue. A cyst may be loculated.

If so the surface may be slightly lobulated rather than smoothly curvilinear. In such cases it is difficult to differentiate the cyst from a fibroadenoma. On the whole the differentiation between a cyst and a noncalcified fibroadenoma is very difficult if not impossible (GERSHON-COHEN and INGLEBY 1953). This applies to the unicameral round cyst, which, neither through the character of its contour nor the degree of its density can be distinguished from a solid nodule in the roentgenogram. It is to be noted that even a carcinoma may in special cases have a very smooth and sharp contour, very rarely even a radiolucent fatty margin and thus simulate a benign cyst. This is particularly true for carcinoma *solidus simplex* and for medullary carcinoma.

Some authors claim that the position or the direction of the long axis are characteristic. This is not true.

The only certain verification of the nature of the cyst is by puncture and aspiration (fig. **14**.2a and b). If the aspirate is dark, yellow or green then all the fluid should be aspirated and the cyst thereafter filled with air. The amount of air injected should be slightly less than the amount of fluid removed. Pneumocystography, the technique of which has been described in Chapter 4 is then performed with mammograms taken in at least two projections. Uncomplicated cysts will demonstrate a smooth inner contour and the outer margin of the cyst should be smooth as well. If aspiration of the cyst is not complete (fig. **14**.3), a repeat puncture is not necessary if the residual is minimal (see page 39). Using these precautions, if the cytological examination of the cyst contents is negative, surgical removal of the cyst is not necessary. However, it is important to repeat the examination in three to six months in order to determine whether the cyst has recurred (fig. **14**.4a—e). Generally this does not happen as histological studies have shown that there is collapse of the cyst following aspiration and the only residual is a small scar (HAMPERL 1969).

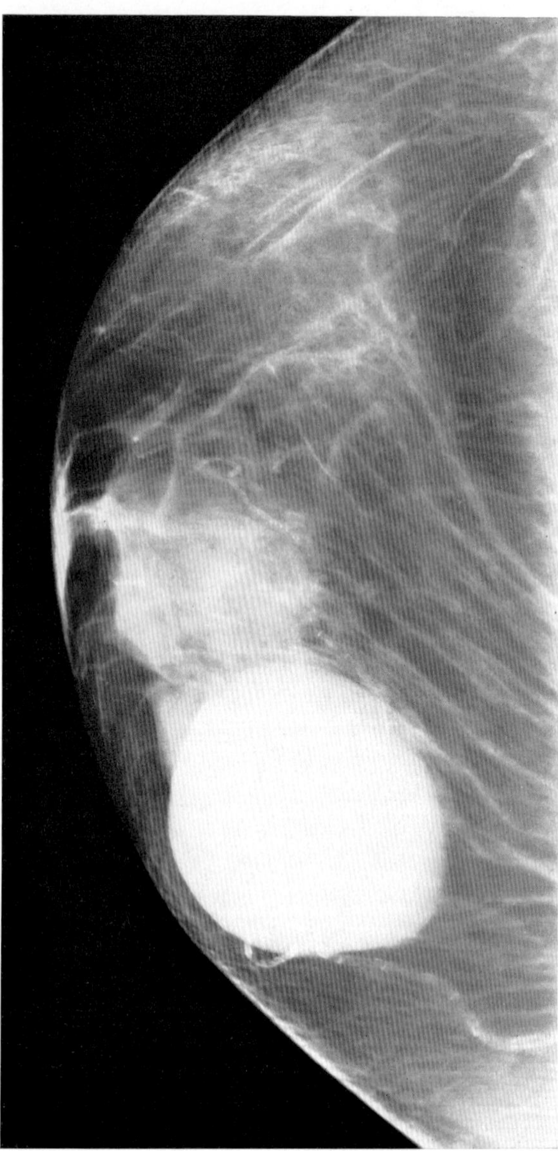

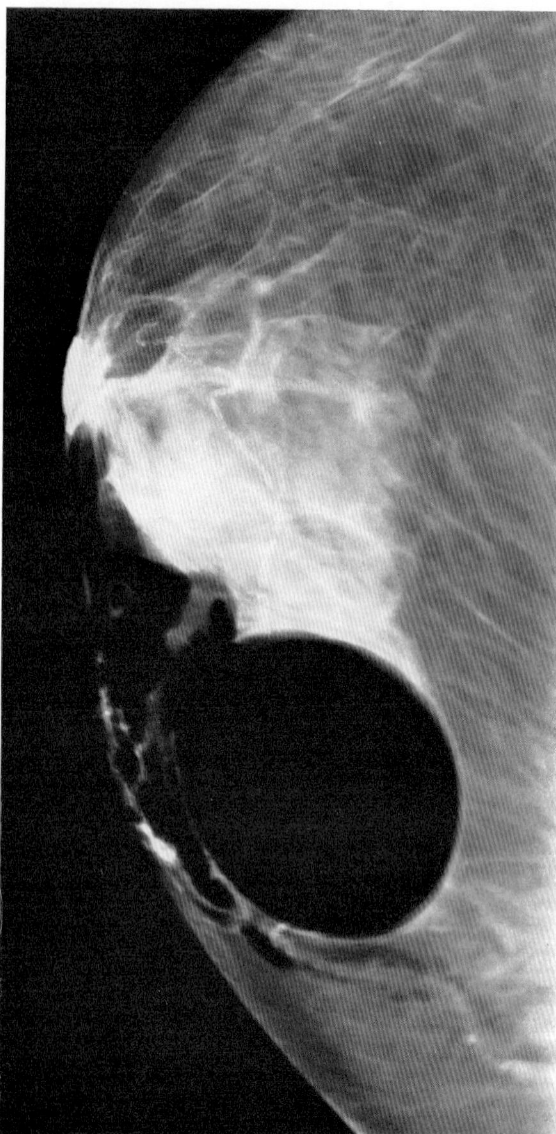

Fig. **14**.2a   Large round mass with smooth contours with diameter of 4.5 cm in an 82-year-old woman (arterial calcifications!). Subareolar fibrosis without areolar skin thickening.

Fig. **14**.2b   After puncture and aspiration of 15 cc of yellow fluid air was instilled revealing a smooth inner controur of the cyst. There is subcutaneous air in the periphery of the cyst.

The collapse and sclerosis of the cyst after pneumocystography is probably the result of the injected air. At any rate, with this technique, success in collapsing a cyst is greater than 95% (HOEFFKEN and HINTZEN 1970). Multiloculated cysts are generally in communication with one another and thus they may be emptied and injected with air by means of a single puncture (fig. 14.5a and b). Such cysts often have lobulated surfaces, mimicking fibroadenoma (fig. 14.6a and b).

In the typical dense breast of mammary dysplasia it is rarely possible to clearly differentiate a single cyst in the mammogram. In these cases it is best to puncture and aspirate any palpable mass. However, it is good practice to do an exploratory puncture of a focus of mammary dysplasia in order to determine whether any large cysts are indeed present (fig. 14.7a and b). This should be

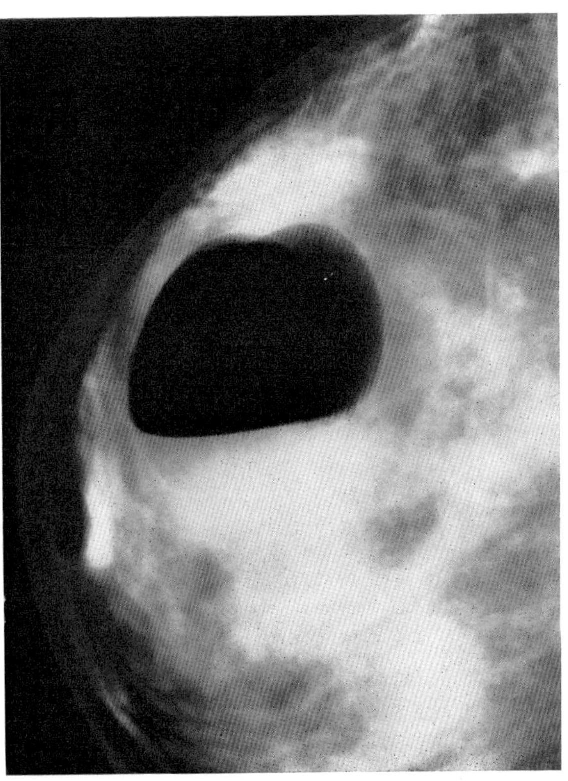

Fig. 14.3 Pneumocystogram with air-fluid level indicating incomplete aspiration of contents (lateral projection, patient sitting).

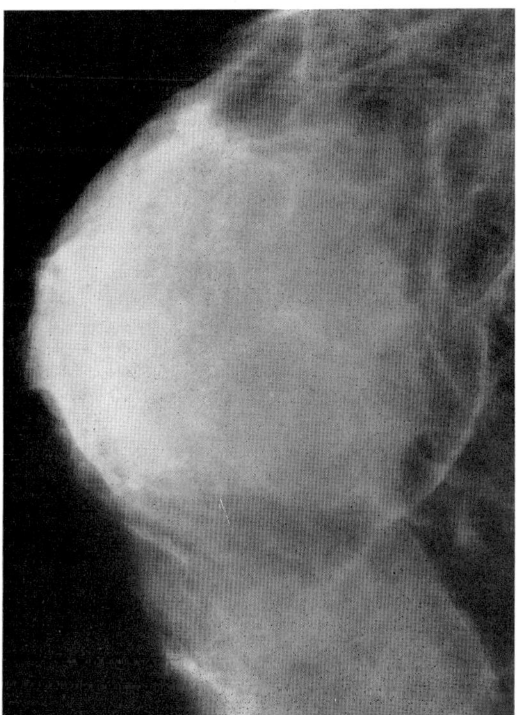

Fig. 14.4a Increased density of the subareolar parenchyma without further definitive roentgen signs. Clinically a tense fullness was palpated behind the nipple.

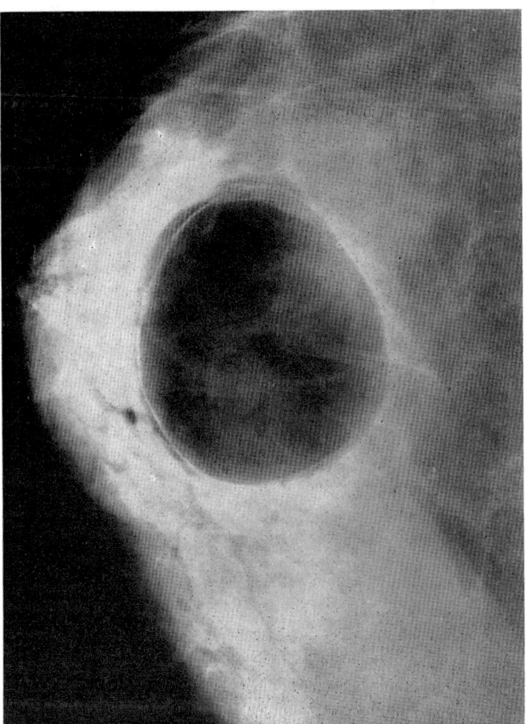

Fig. 14.4b After puncture and aspiration of 12 cc of yellow-green fluid and air instillation a cyst with smooth inner margins is demonstrated.

6a*

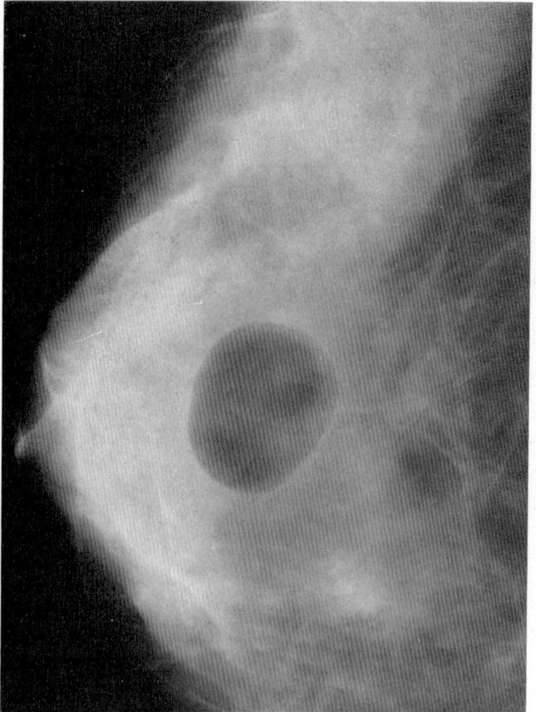

Fig. **14**.4c

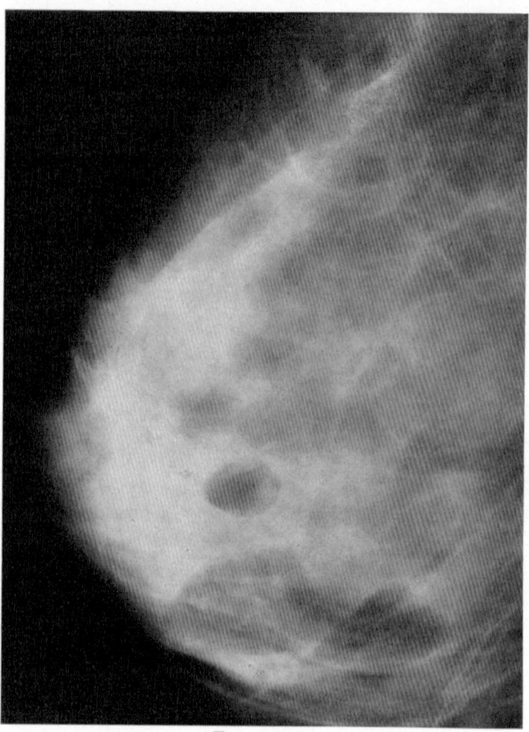

Fig. **14**.4d

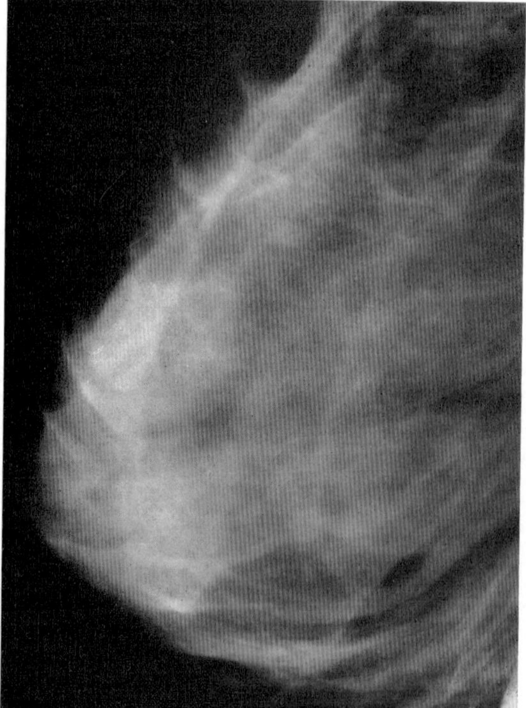

Fig. **14**.4e

Fig. **14**.4c to e Gradual decrease in size of cyst following pneumocystography during follow-up mammograms at 3-week intervals. No cytological evidence of malignancy.

performed in all diagnostically doubtful cases in order to come to some conclusion about the nature of the breast pathology when clinical, palpatory and mammographic findings are equivocal. One should avoid repeated biopsies, which are done so frequently in the dysplastic breast in order to alleviate diagnostic uncertainties. It may result in progressive scarring and deformity of the breast.

Cysts may disappear spontaneously. This, however, is uncommon (fig. **14**.8a and b). It the pneumocystogram is abnormal no time should be wasted with follow-up or control studies but immediate excisional biopsy or extirpation should be undertaken. This is particularly necessary when the wall of the cyst demonstrates nodularity either on its inner or outer borders (fig. **14**.9). At the time of the pneumocystogram the abnormal portion of the cyst wall may be punctured under x-ray control to verify whether it represents actual solid tissue or rather a small secondary, noncommunicating cyst. However, since most secondary cysts do communicate with the main cyst, such a finding of an abnormal cyst wall found on pneumocystography is strong evidence for a fibroadenoma, papilloma or carcinoma in the wall of the cyst.

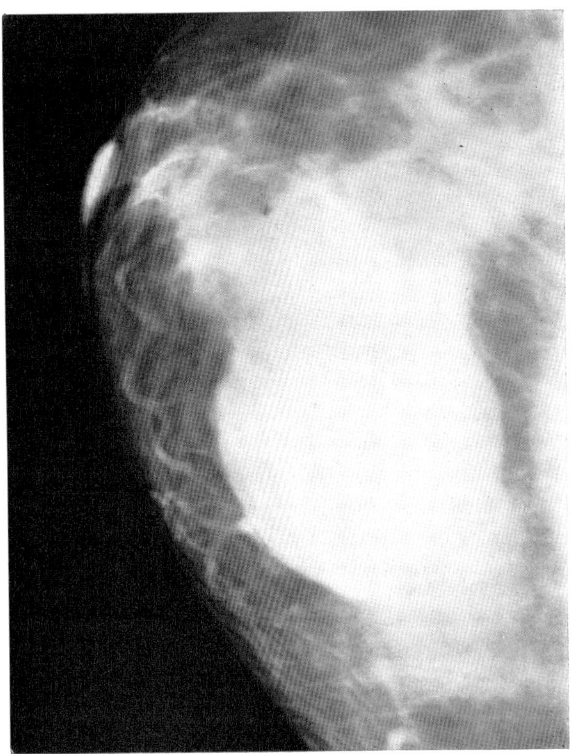

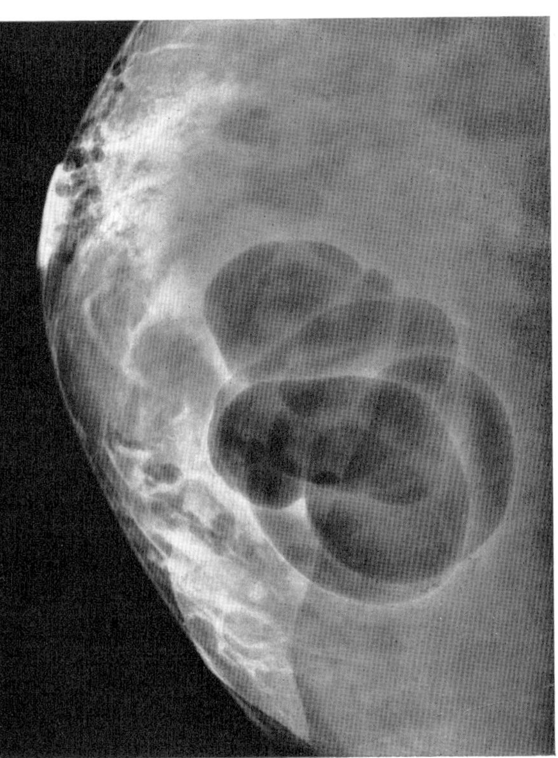

Fig. **14**.5a   Rounded, lobular mass extending into the subareolar parenchyma. No surrounding fibrosis. Serpiginous vein in the subcutaneous fatty layer (!). Clinically a tense, movable, poorly marginated mass was palpated.

Fig. **14**.5b   After puncture and aspiration of 10 cc of greenish fluid pneumocystography reveals a loculated cyst with smooth inner walls. Roentgenologically and cytologically no evidence of malignancy. Follow-up mammograms revealed complete regression.

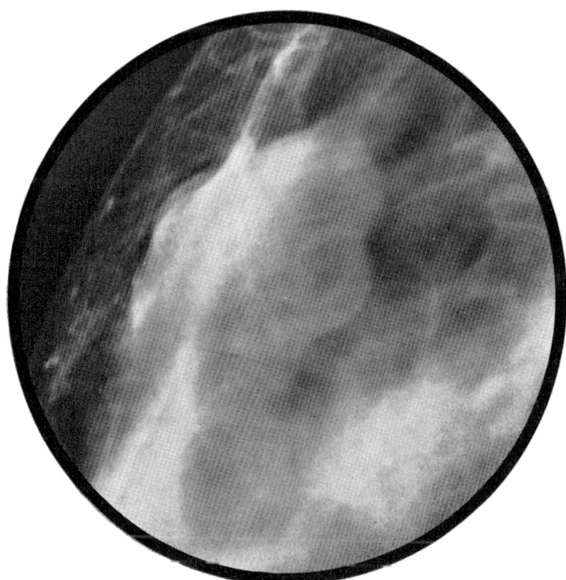

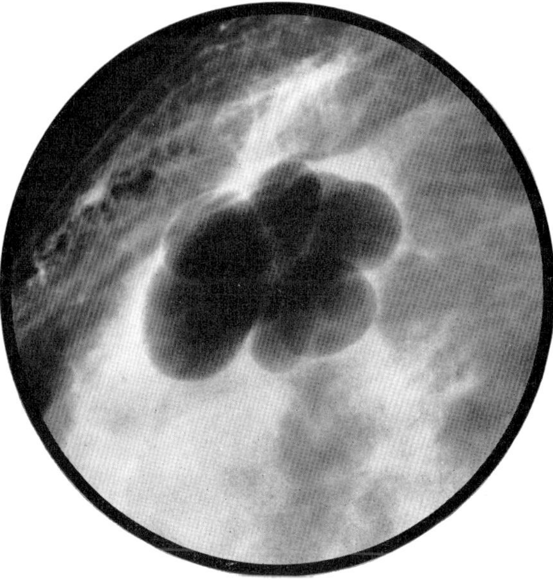

Fig. **14**.6a   Rounded, mainly smooth-contoured lobular mass 4 cm in diameter, corresponding to a hard, easily movable nodule: Fibroadenoma? Cyst?

Fig. **14**.6b   After puncture, aspiration and air instillation: Loculated cyst with smooth inner margins. Cytology: Negative. Complete regression after 3 months.

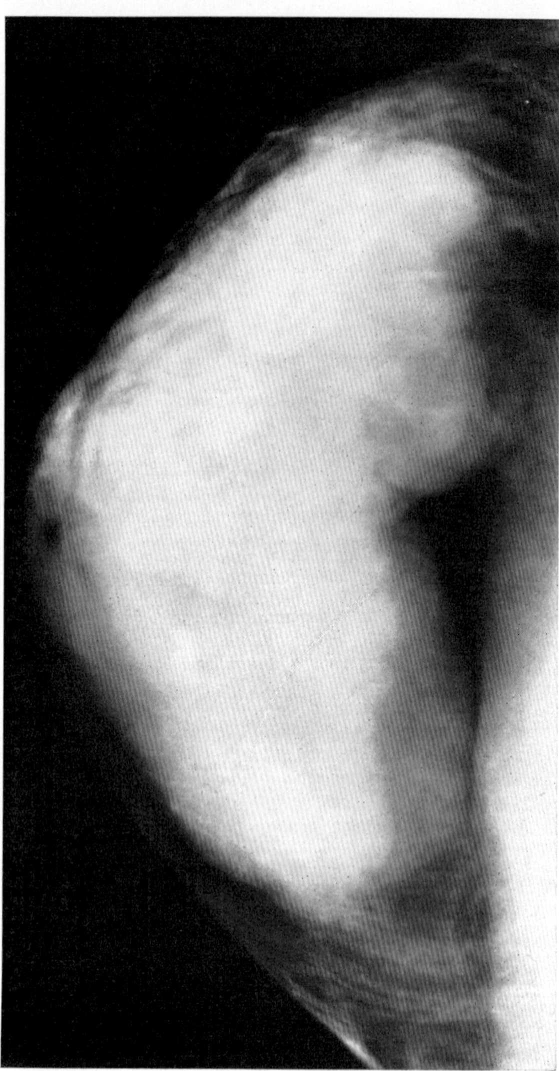

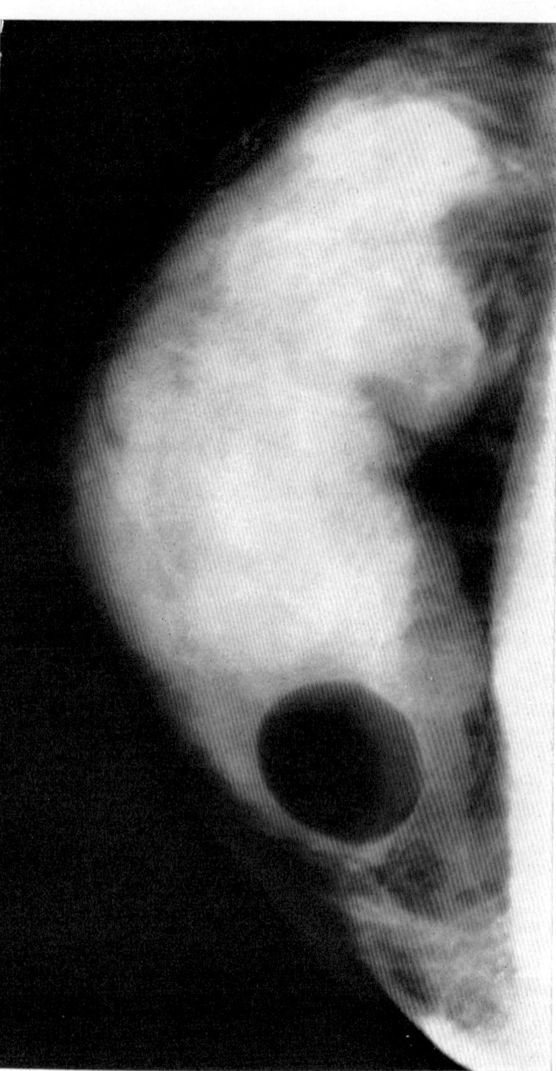

Fig. **14**.7a   Very dense nodular parenchyma. Specific masses or other lesions cannot be differentiated. Clinically a tense solitary mass was palpated in the lateral aspect.

Fig. **14**.7b   Puncture of the palpable mass revealed 3 cc of fluid. Pneumocystography reveals smooth inner walls. No evidence of malignancy at cytology. Complete regression at follow-up examination.

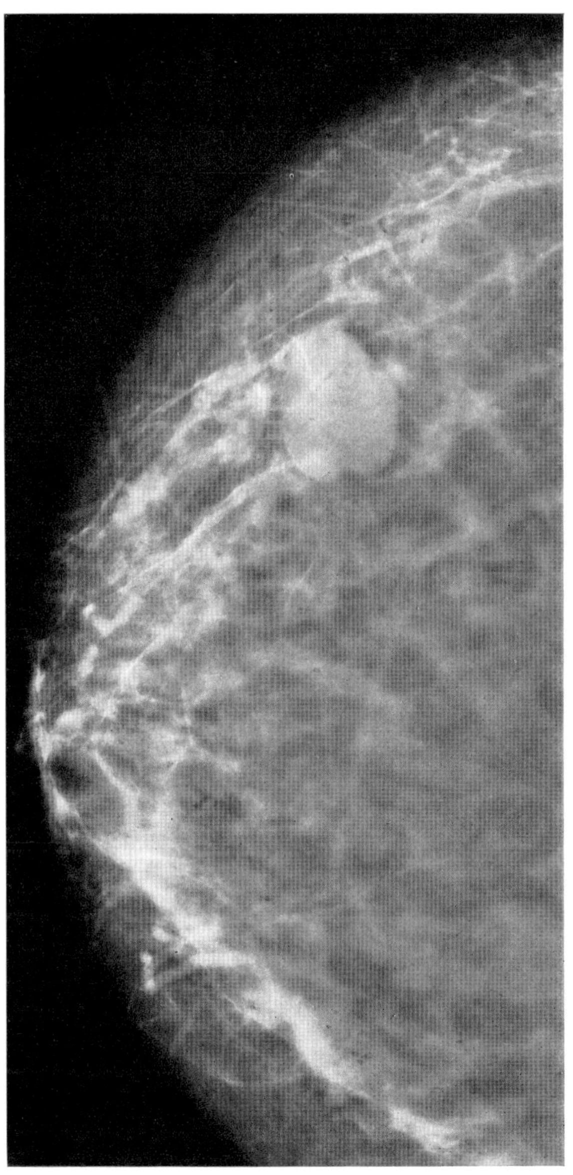

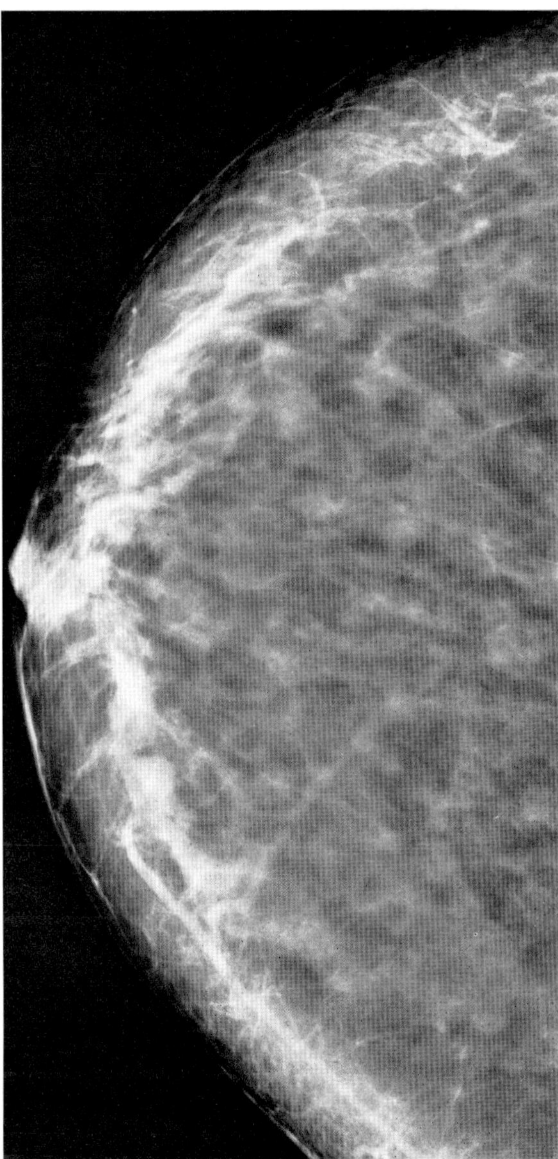

Fig. **14**.8a   Round lobular mass 2 cm in diameter with smooth borders. No palpatory findings. Presumptive diagnosis: Cyst or fibroadenoma. Follow-up examination in 3 months was advised.

Fig. **14**.8b   Follow-up examination was done after 2 years. The rounded mass is no longer visible. No surgery in the interim! Diagnosis: Cyst with spontaneous regression.

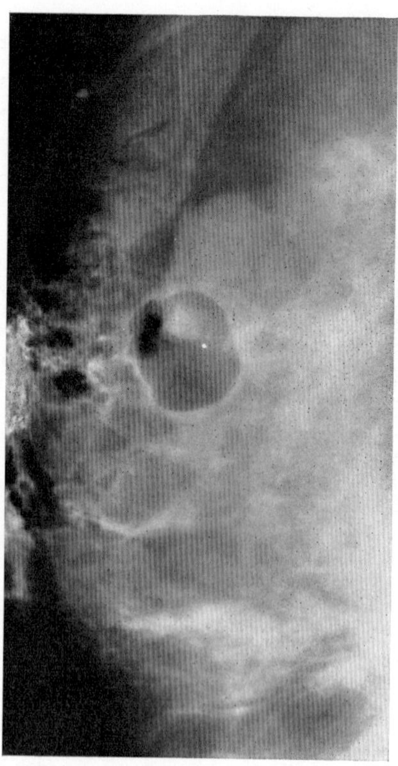

Fig. **14**.9

Fig. **14**.9 Pneumocystography after puncture of a cyst, 1.5 cm in diameter. A pea-sized soft tissue density extends into the cyst interior along its superior aspect. In spite of negative cytology excisional biopsy in such cases is indicated. Histology: Intracystic papilloma.

Fig. **14**.10a 13-year-old girl: painful paraareolar lump for 3 days with cloudy discharge from an opening in the areola. Following puncture and aspiration the cavity was filled with Conray-80. A cyst as well as delicate communicating milk ducts are demonstrated.

Fig. **14**.10b Following aspiration of the contrast material air was instilled: Loculated cyst. Diagnosis: Cystic dilatation of an accessory milk duct.

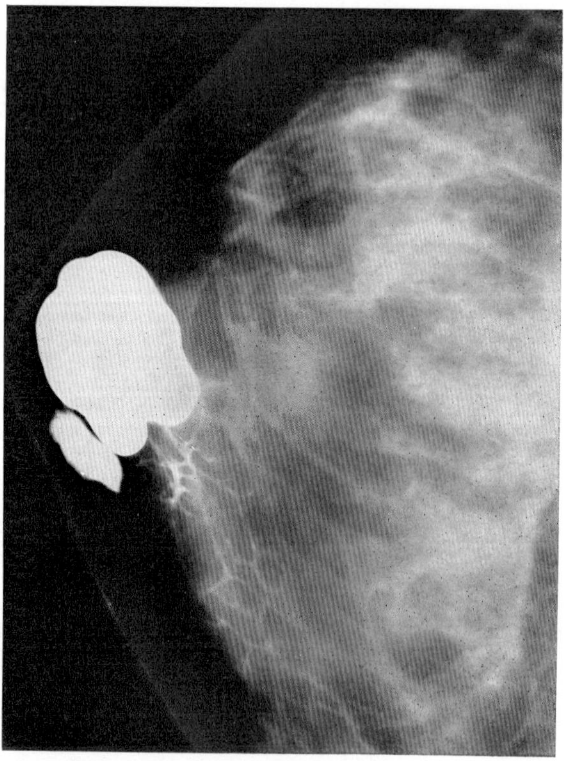

Fig. **14**.10a

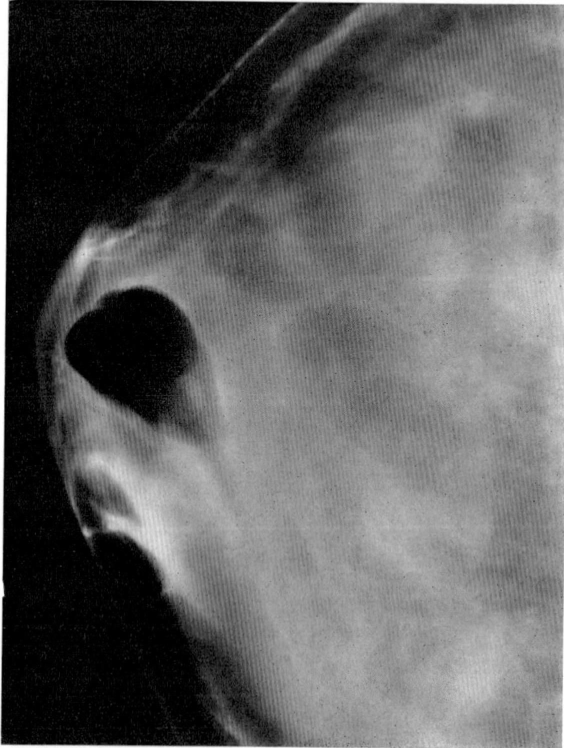

Fig. **14**.10b

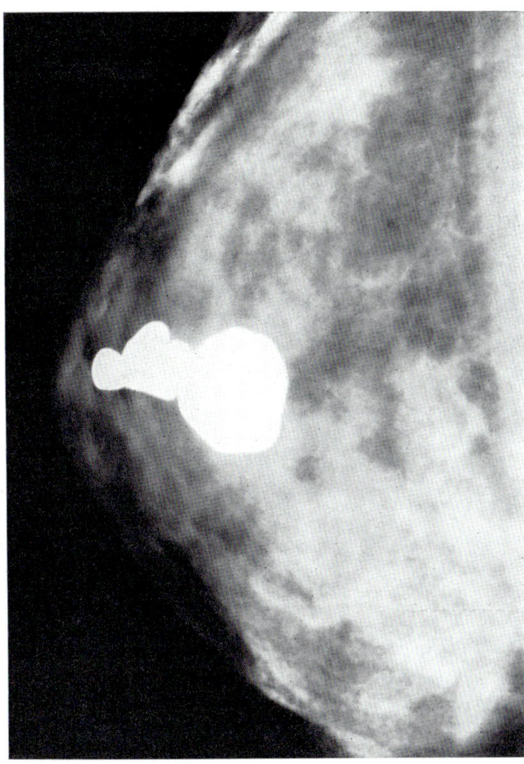

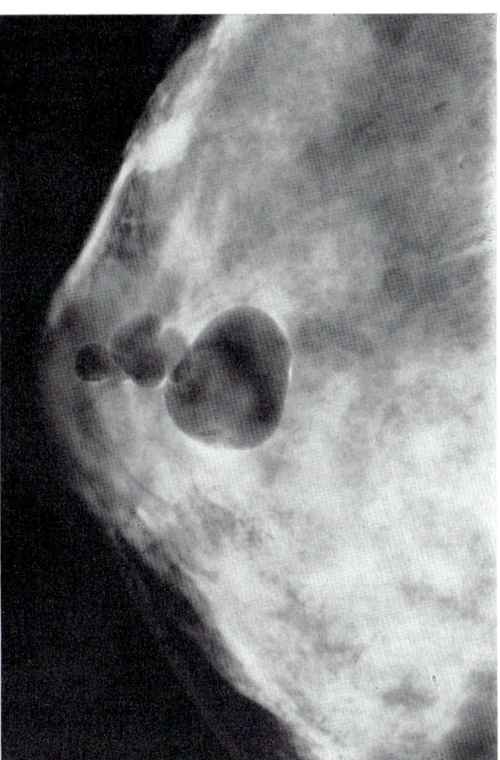

Fig. **14**.11a 15-year-old girl, painful subareolar lump for one week. Brown discolored secretion from an opening beside the nipple. Contrast instillation into this opening reveals a system of communicating cysts.

Fig. **14**.11b Following aspiration of the contrast material and secretion air is instilled (double contrast technique). Cystic dilatation of an accessory lactiferous duct.

Attention must be directed to the special case of retromammary cysts, found in young girls, which are not related to mammary dysplasia, but instead represent a developmental anomaly of accessory breast tissue. The lactiferous ducts of such accessory breast tissue empty into the areola rather than into the nipple. The openings of the accessory ducts are recognized as small secreting "fistulas" in the areola. These cysts are palpable as retromammary masses. If one punctures such a cyst, aspirates the content (fig. **14**.10), and then instills air or contrast material, one may observe the flow of the contrast from the accessory duct opening in the areola. Retrograde study using ductography with cannulation of the accessory duct, may make possible the demonstration of the retromammary cyst (fig. **14**.11). The walls of these cysts occasionally calcify in a circular, semicircular or punctate fashion (see page 258 and page 266).

Galactoceles should also be mentioned. These are cysts filled with milk that appear during or immediately after lactation (HAAGENSEN 1971;

WITTEN 1969). The contents may be semisolid due to saponification and the formation of soapy or cheesy cysts. These lesions have a radiolucent appearance in the mammogram because of their lipoid content and are therefore differentiated from the denser, water-containing cysts of the breast.

Signs of Malignancy

It has been the general expirience that large solitary cysts of the breast have no malignant potential. BLOODGOOD as far back as 1929, observed that patients who had been operated upon for "blue-dome" cysts and followed for a period over 30 years, had a lower incidence of carcinoma than an equal number of patients operated upon and followed for a similar period of time for other benign breast diseases. GESCHICKTER (1945) in a prospective study of 378 cases found only two resultant carcinomas. LEWISON and LYONS (1935), over a period of ten years, noted a 2.6% incidence of carcinoma in

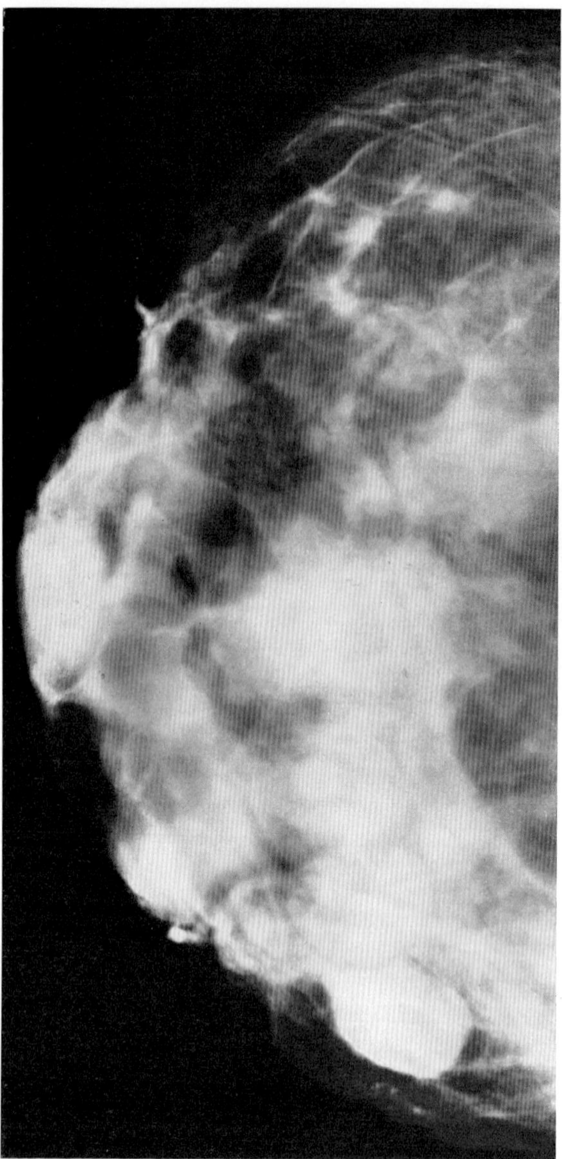

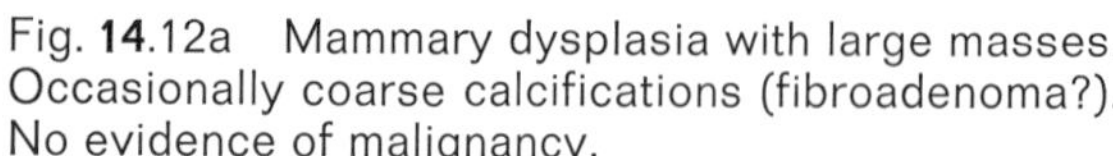

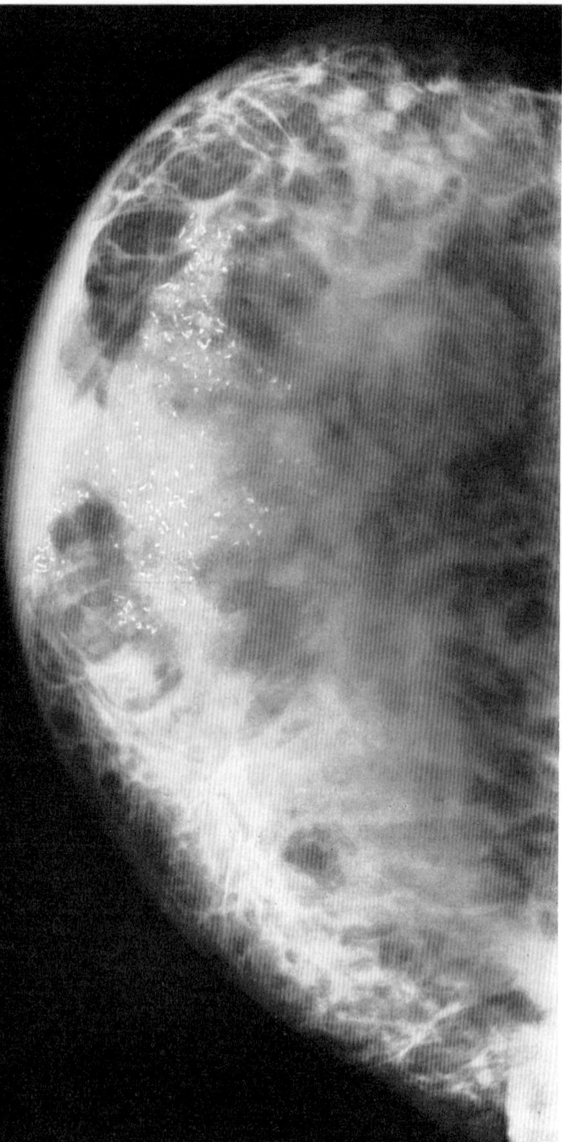

Fig. **14**.12a   Mammary dysplasia with large masses. Occasionally coarse calcifications (fibroadenoma?). No evidence of malignancy.

Fig. **14**.12b   Same case 3 years later: uncountable fragmented microcalcifications in the subareolar region. The skin of the areola and the surrounding skin are thickened, with thickening of connective tissue trabeculae. Margins are ill-defined. The sharply bordered, round masses in the earlier roentgenogram appear confluent. Mammographic diagnosis: Invasive intraductal carcinoma with lymphatic obstruction. Histologically verified.

large solitary cysts. Other prospective studies, reporting large numbers of cases, have recorded similar findings indicating the malignancy rate in women with large solitary cysts from 3.3% (CLAGETT et al 1944) to 6.5% (KIAER 1954). The difference here reflects the patient selection as well as the difference in patient categorization found among the authors (BERNDT and MARWITZ 1968; AUFDERMAUER 1969; FISCHERMANN et al 1969).

Malignant change in the inner wall of a cyst is a rarity. In the patient with solitary or multiple cysts, who has breast carcinoma, it is much more common to find that the carcinoma has arisen in a site removed from the cyst. Reports about the appearance of carcinoma following several months after excisional biopsy of a cyst are questionable and suggest that the carcinoma was missed at the operation and a nearby cyst was biopsied and removed instead, thus leading to the eventual diagnosis of fibrocystic disease.

Therefore, the risk of carcinoma in the patient with large cyst mammary dysplasia is rather small. This does not, however, mean that yearly follow-up examinations are not indicated in such patients. Such follow-up examinations, however, whether by palpation or mammography, are difficult because in the vast majority of cases the breast changes secondary to carcinoma are invariably obscured by the extensive findings of mammary dysplasia. Changes in the formerly sharp smooth borders of a documented cyst as well as the development of desmoplastic changes are more significant signs of neoplasm. The appearance, of course, of newly developed microcalcifications, many in number and collected in groups, is an easily detectable sign of malignant change (fig. **14**.12a and b).

Chapter 15

Adenosis and Sclerosing Adenosis

Adenosis

Hyperplasia of lobules and small lactiferous ducts is part of the general picture of fibrocystic disease. If adenosis is the predominating histolog-

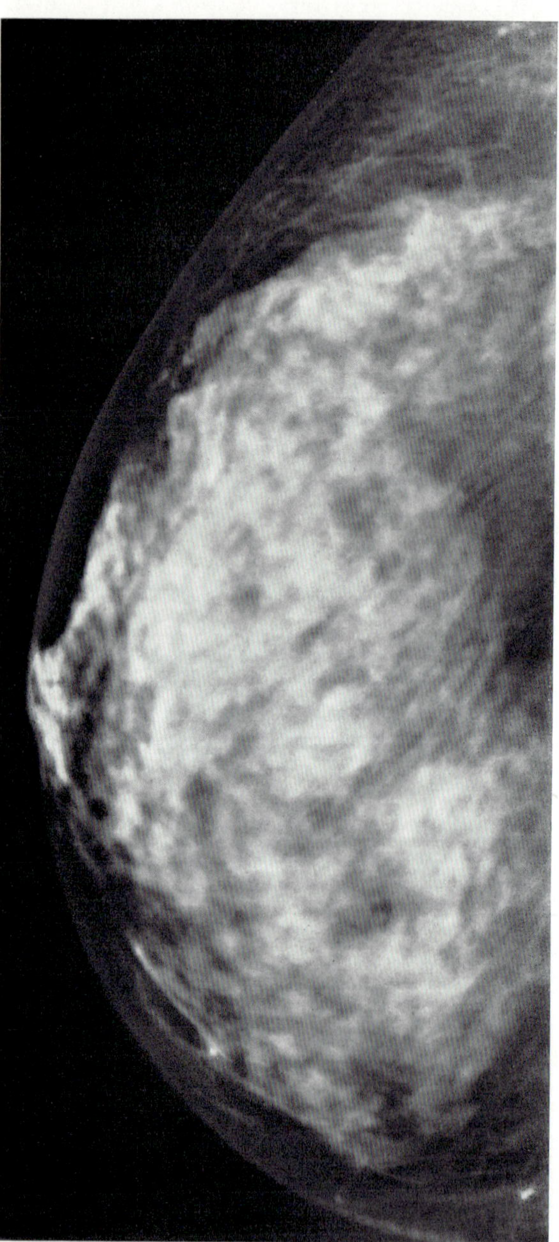

ical appearance, however, then this type of mammary dysplasia is called adenosis. In this condition the great majority of the breast parenchyma is characterized by the presence of small adenomatous nodules. Clinically this is recognized at palpation by a diffuse fine nodularity often desingated as a "shotty" breast. This is particularly easily palpated in the involuted, predominantly fatty breast. Adenosis is most frequent in middle-aged females in the premenopausal stage.

Roentgenology

In the mammogram adenosis is recognized as finely nodular (2 to 4 mm in diameter) dense shadows, fairly sharply circumscribed, separated by fatty tissue and dispersed generally throughout the breast in greater or lesser degree (fig. **15.1**). There is thickening of stromal fibers which approach a diameter of 2 to 3 mm. There may also be ectasia of milk ducts which are seen as broad radiating densities in the subareolar region.

Sclerosing Adenosis

A special form of adenosis is so-called sclerosing adenosis (HAMPERL 1939; FOOTE and STEWART 1945; URBAN and ADAIR 1949). This condition is difficult to differentiate from carcinoma histologically, particularly in frozen sections. Sclerosing adenosis consists of a special sort of myoepithelial proliferation distributed in a nodular or lobular type fashion. Solid cords of cells or nodular collections resembling parenchyma spread throughout the normal breast substance (fig. **15.2**). In some cases the epithelial proliferation

Fig. **15.1** Mammary dysplasia with numerous small nodules. It is impossible to differentiate this from numerous small cysts or adenosis (or a mixed form of mammary dysplasia). The entire breast is evenly permeated by small, slightly irregular ill-defined densities. Only interspersed fatty tissue allows definition of individual small nodules.

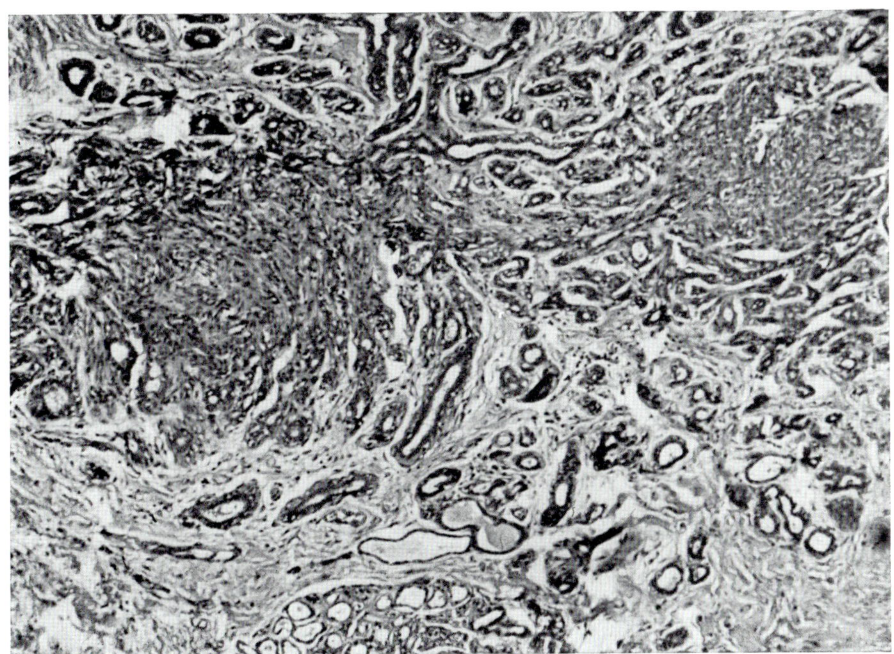

Fig. **15**.2   Adenomatous proliferation of terminal ductules associated with myoepithelial proliferation, fibrosis and hyalinization. Sclerosing adenosis.

resembles parenchyma and in others the proliferation is primarily that of an increase in connective tissue and subsequent sclerosis. Numerous small deposits of calcium are seen within the altered tissue.

The absence of mitotic figures and of bizarre-appearing cells allows differentiation from carcinoma.

Roentgenology

About half of the cases of sclerosing adenosis are detectable on mammography by recognition of calcium deposits in the area of adenomatous abnormality. These calcifications are characteristic and can be differentiated from the microcalcifications found in carcinomas. In sclerosing adenosis the calcifications are discrete but are widely distributed through the breast (occasionally bilaterally) (fig. **15**.3 a and b). They are coarse and rounded in shape, in distinction from carcinomatous calcifications which are finer, granular and somewhat more irregular. Calcifications in sclerosing adenosis are generally larger than 500 microns. These calcifications are seen within areas of connective tissue proliferation which may be diffuse or assume a very fine nodular pattern, indicating fibrosis and adenosis

(fig. **15**.4a and b). Single or multiple large cysts may be associated. Thus sclerosing adenosis may be the predominating pattern of mammary dysplasia or can be seen in conjunction with other forms of this disease. A diffuse form of sclerosing adenosis is rare. HOFMANN and BOSCHBACK (1970) indicate an incidence of 2.8% among cases of general benign disease of the breast. They reported an incidence of 4.9% in the biopsy material from patients with benign breast disease.

Sclerosing adenosis may only be recognized roentgenologically when the typical calcifications are present. This is so in about half the cases. The remaining cases cannot be differentiated in the mammogram from the predominantly fibrous type of mammary dysplasia (fig. **15**.5).

The difficulty in roentgen interpretation occurs when the calcifications of sclerosing adenosis are relatively focal within a localized region of proliferative connective tissue, especially when the latter demonstrates irregularity and indistinct margins (fig. **15**.6a and b). In such cases differentiation from carcinoma is very difficult. Biopsy is indicated to rule out malignancy. As a result, a great percentage of patients with sclerosing adenosis are subjected to biopsy because of these mammographic findings. In

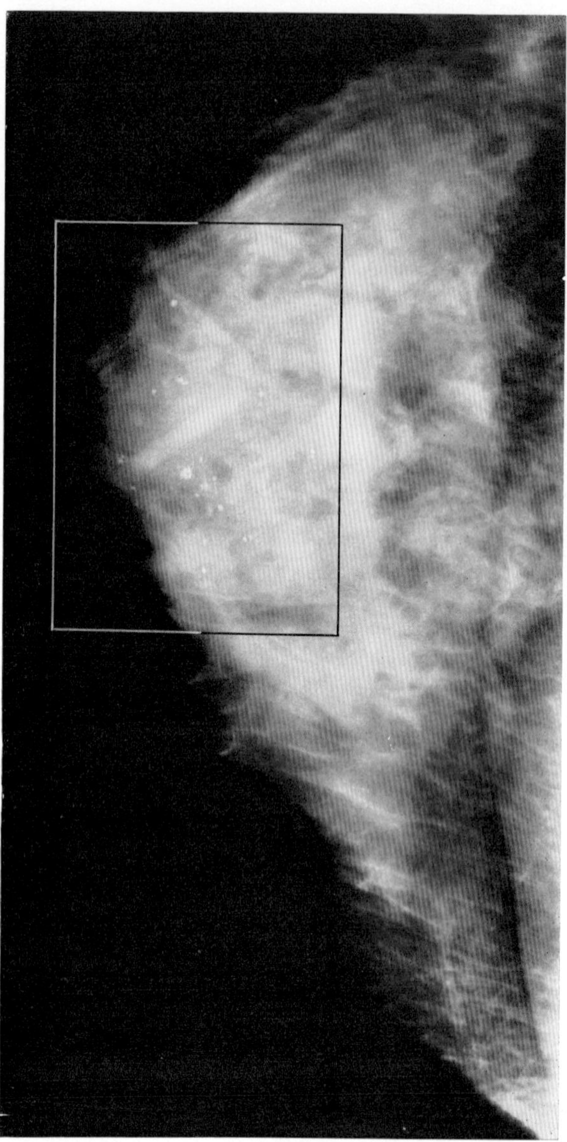

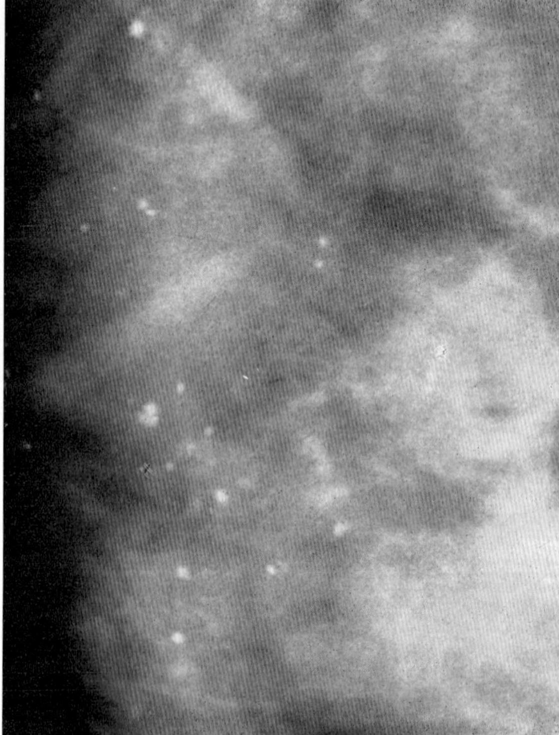

Fig. **15**.3a Sclerosing adenosis with dense sub-areolar fibrosis of the parenchyma and numerous calcifications. Similar findings in the other breast.

Fig. **15**.3b Local area magnified 2 times: coarse, rounded singular calcifications.

our patient population, however, half of such breast biopsies resulted in the diagnosis of carcinoma.

It is essentially a problem for the radiologist and pathologist. In both disciplines it is extremely difficult to differentiate certain phases of sclerosing adenosis from carcinoma. However, according to investigations by URBAN and ADAIR (1949), STEWART (1950), HAAGENSEN (1956), and CUTLER (1961) and others, as well as in our experience, there is no evidence to indicate that sclerosing adenosis predisposes to malignancy. Local excision of the abnormal tissue is sufficient. More aggressive operative procedures such as mastectomy are senseless. What is important is that if sclerosing adenosis is the suspected disease, histological examination should not be limited to frozen sections but final diagnosis should be made by routine staining and paraffin sections. Only then can one avoid what may be an unnecessary mastectomy.

Mammography is particularly important then in this condition because the differential diagnosis according to roentgenograms will be "carcinoma versus sclerosing adenosis", alerting the surgeon

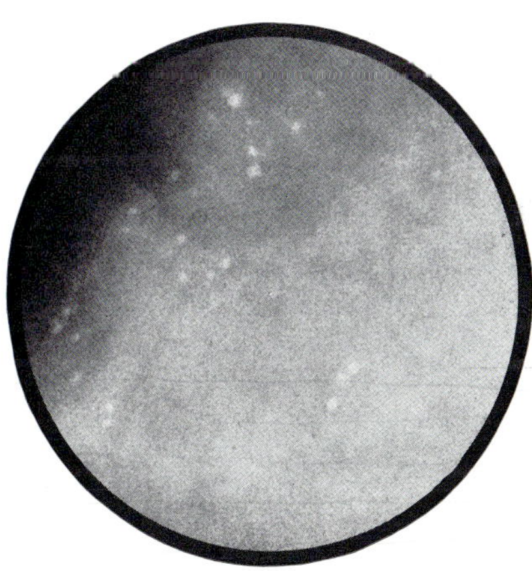

Fig. **15**.4a

Fig. **15**.4b

Fig. **15**.4a, b Local area magnified 2x in b. Sclerosing adenosis with extensive soft tissue density lateral to the areola. Numerous round but predominantly coarse calcifications both singular and in groups. Similar findings in the other breast. Excisional biopsy was performed since carcinoma could not be definitely ruled out roentgenologically. Histology: Fibrocystic disease with myoepithelial proliferation. Inspissated secretions with periductal fibrosis and siderophagic activity in lactiferous ducts.

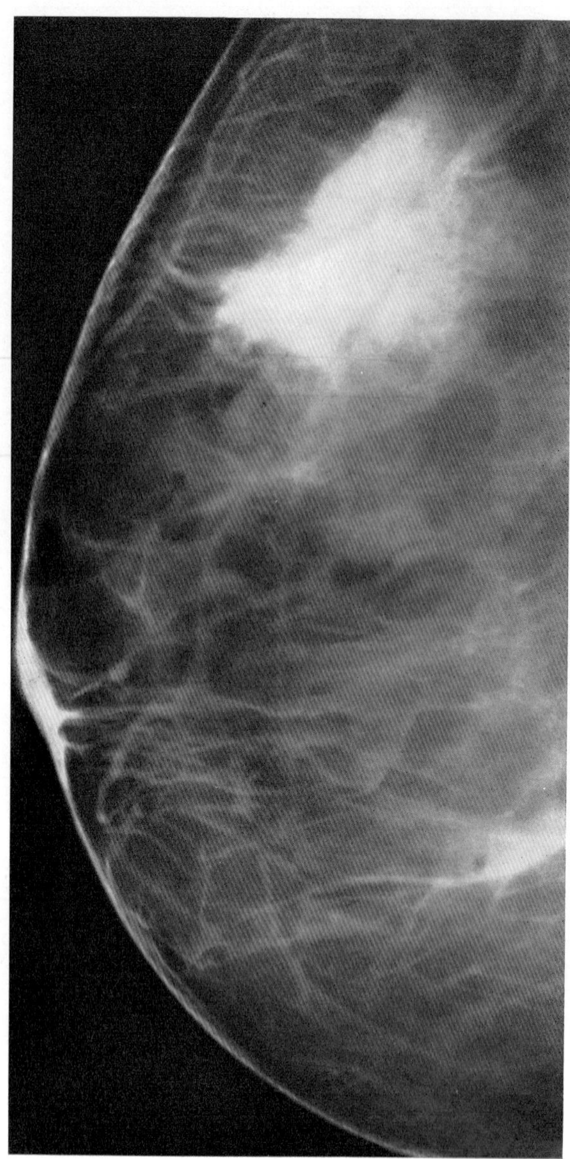

to the fact that he must allow for careful and extensive histological examination. In earlier times adenosis was a coincidental histological finding at biopsy. Currently, however, biopsy is performed specifically for this disorder, primarily because of microcalcifications noted in the mammogram. It is regrettable that the diagnosis of sclerosing adenosis made by excisional biopsy is of little significance to the patient. Nevertheless biopsy performed in this condition on the basis of mammographic findings not infrequently results in the discovery of an adjacent slow growing or early ductal carcinoma, partly of the in-situ type, especially lobular carcinoma in situ.

Clinical examination is of little help in the differential diagnosis of sclerosing adenosis from other sorts of mammary dysplasia, because the former has no specific palpatory findings.

Fig. **15**.5 The predominantly fatty breast contains a focus of residual parenchymal tissue with ill-defined contours. Clinically a mass was palpated. Mammographic diagnosis: Maderate fibrocystic disease of the residual parenchyma. No evidence of carcinoma. Histology: Sclerosing adenosis.

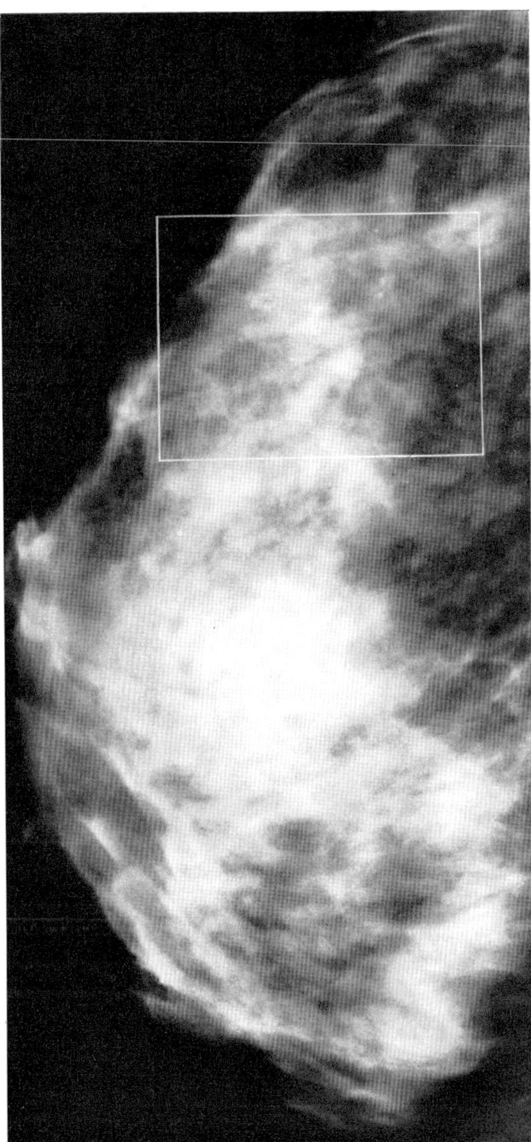

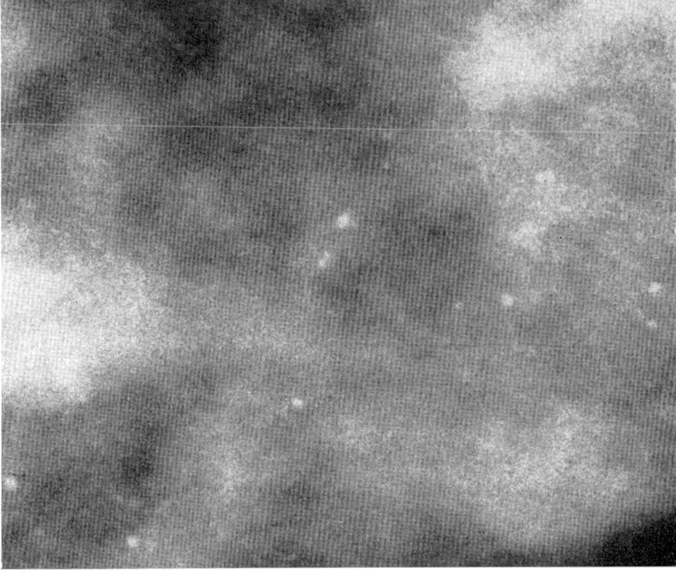

Fig. **15**.6b   Enlargement of the suspicious area 3x. There are coarse scattered calcifications.
Histology: Sclerosing adenosis.

Fig. **15**.6a   Extensive changes of fibrocystic disease with a focus of irregular structure and suggestions of stellate margins.

Chapter 16

Fibroadenoma

Definition and Pathology

Normally the hormonal influences on breast parenchyma, specifically estrogen, result in proliferation of epithelial cells in the lactiferous ducts and also in the breast stroma during the first half of the menstrual cycle. In certain disturbances of this hormonal mechanism the usual regression of such changes during the second half of the cycle do not occur. The result is the development of fibrous and epithelial nodules which become fibromas, fibroadenomas or adenomas depending on which cell type predominates (fig. 16.1a and b). Based on their histological structure fibroadenomas may be divided into intracanalicular and pericanalicular types. In the intracanalicular type there is proliferation of connective tissue into the lumen of the duct whereas in the pericanalicular type this proliferation is in the outer margin of the duct. Clinically there is no difference between the two types and in fact most fibroadenomas are of the mixed kind. It is characteristic, however, that fibroadenomas are definitely related to the menstrual cycle, pregnancy and lactation. Fibroadenoma is recognized as a breast mass most frequently seen between puberty and age 30. The lesions regress with the onset of menopause. A mucoid degeneration with hyalinization, involution of epithelial components and susequent calcification (approximately 3% calcify according to WITTEN 1969) tends to occur.

Fibroadenomas may be solitary or multiple and are frequently associated with other benign breast diseases. Therefore, small or large cysts are commonly found in the breast containing a fibroadenoma.

Malignant transformation of the solitary fibroadenoma is extremely rare. Rarely the epithelial or stromal components may degenerate into carcinomatous or sarcomatous tissue, respectively.

Clinical Findings

At palpation a fibroadenoma presents as a smooth, firm movable mass which is round, oval and occasionally lobulated. There is no skin fixation. These masses are generally first detected by the patient herself. Fibroadenomas

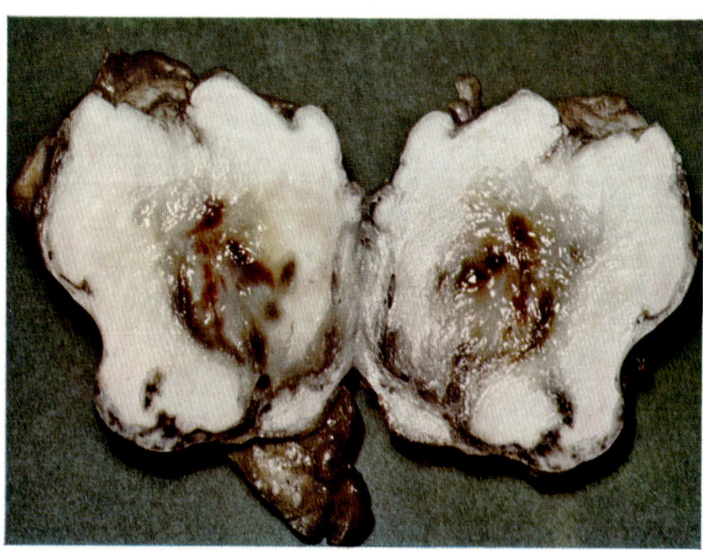

Fig. **16**.1a   Photograph of excised fibroadenoma showing regressive changes in its center.

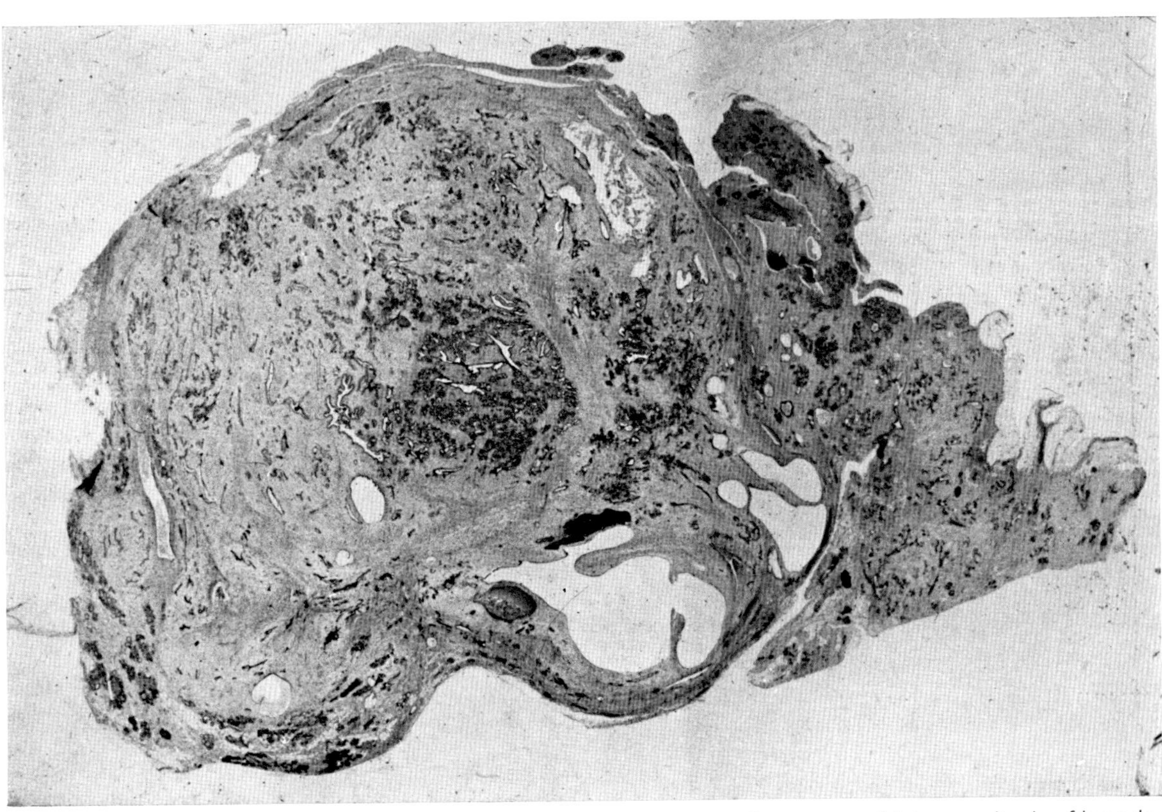

Fig. **16**.1b   Same case as fig. 16.1a. Histologically this consists of a peri- and intracanalicular fibroadenoma with microcystic changes.

grow slowly and are always influenced by hormonal changes during the menstrual cycle represented chiefly by premenstrual pain in the mass. The pain disappears with the onset of menses and begins shortly thereafter as the next cycle is begun. The size of the palpable lesion varies from 1 to 5 cm in diameter. It is typical that the size determined by palpation correlates closely with that found in the mammogram. If the palpatory size significantly exceeds that measured in the roentgenogram, carcinoma should be suspected.

Roentgenology

A fibroadenoma is round with smooth contours (fig. **16**.2). As the tumor expands in size and displaces surrounding fatty tissue it frequently assumes a radiolucent fatty border in the mammogram. This border need not be continuous and is interrupted by adjacent parenchyma or foci of mammary dysplasia. Occasionally fibrous connections to adjacent stroma may interrupt the smooth border of the fibroadenoma. Some fibroadenomas may be more angular than round.

It is impossible in the mammogram to differentiate a simple round fibroadenoma from a cyst. This can only be done by puncture and aspiration. The fact that fibroadenomas occur more frequently than solitary cysts in younger women is helpful in the differential diagnosis but is not totally reliable.

The size of fibroadenomas varies and is not correlated to the patient's age. Older women may have fibroadenomas that are as small as 1 to 2 cm in diameter some of which are in a retromammary location (fig. **16**.3); likewise, large fibroadenomas measuring 5 to 6 cm in diameter may be seen in young women (fig. **16**.4).

Fibroadenomas may have a lobular configuration (fig. **16**.5) but various and multiple shapes and sizes of this tumor may appear in one breast, as well as bilaterally (fig. 16.6a and b).

Roentgen differentiation between cyst and fibroadenoma is only possible when the latter is calcified as a result of degenerative changes. Such calcifications begin as small, irregular and bizarre-appearing deposits of calcium which are always seen within the confines of the tumor

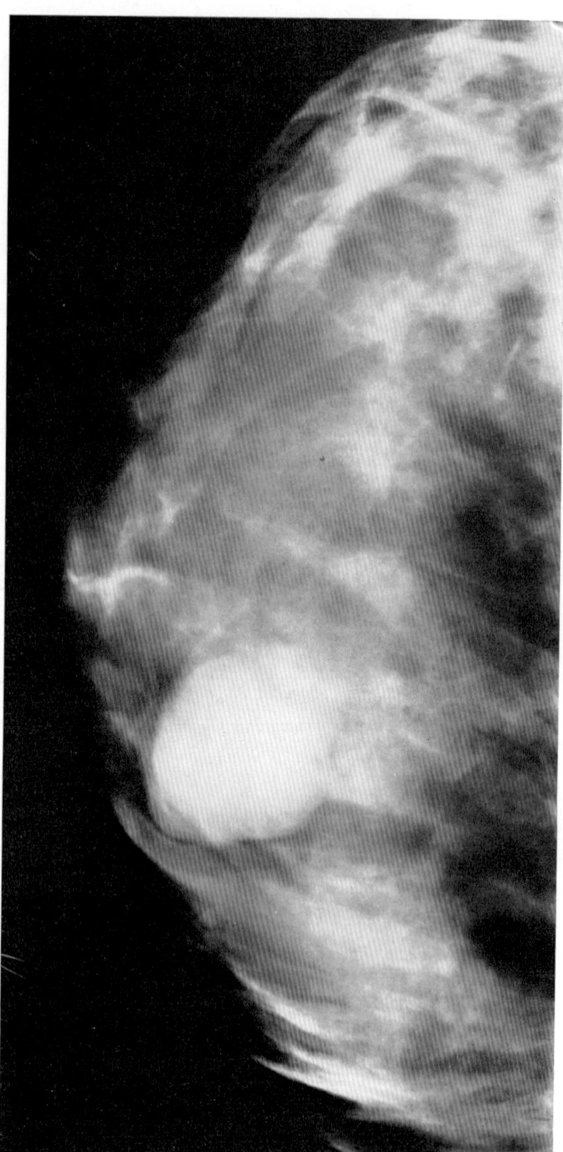

Fig. **16**.2 Clinically: Freely movable, hard mass with smooth surfaces. Mammography: Homogeneous, sharply marginated dominant mass surrounded by a radiolucent zone. Puncture revealed solid lesion. Fibroadenoma. Cytology: No evidence of malignancy.

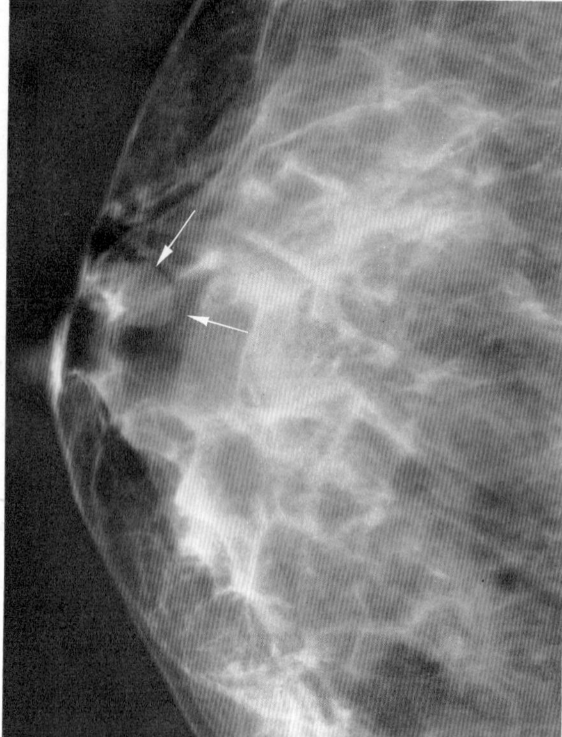

Fig. **16**.3 Subareolar fibroadenoma, 1 cm in diameter in a 50-year-old woman. Histologically verified.

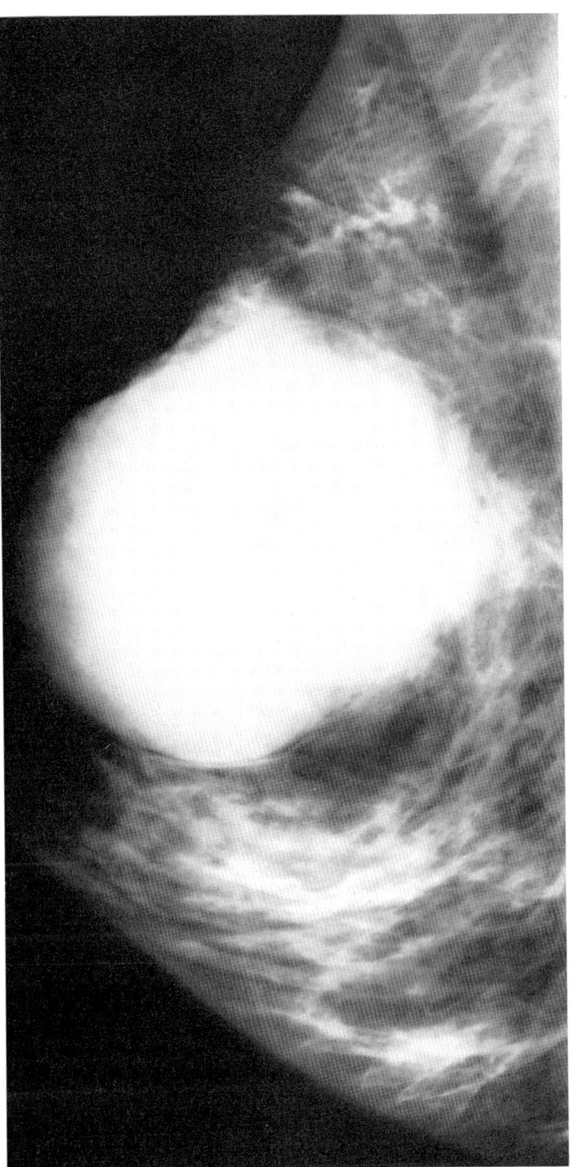

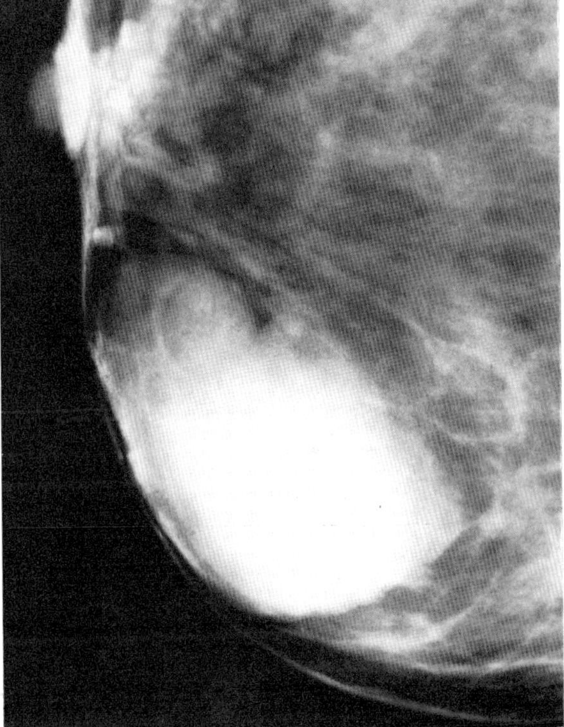

Fig. **16**.4   Unusually large fibroadenoma in a 36-year-old woman (the same case as fig. 16.1a, b). The mass is lobular but the borders are smooth and there is a radiolucent zone surrounding it. Puncture revealed a solid lesion.
Histology: No evidence of malignancy.

Fig. **16**.5   Inferior to the nipple there is a 3.5 by 5.5 cm homogeneous soft tissue density with umbilicated but otherwise sharp margins. There is a peripheral zone of radiolucency. Clinically: Freely movable smooth hard mass. Puncture: Solid. Lobular fibroadenoma verified by histology.

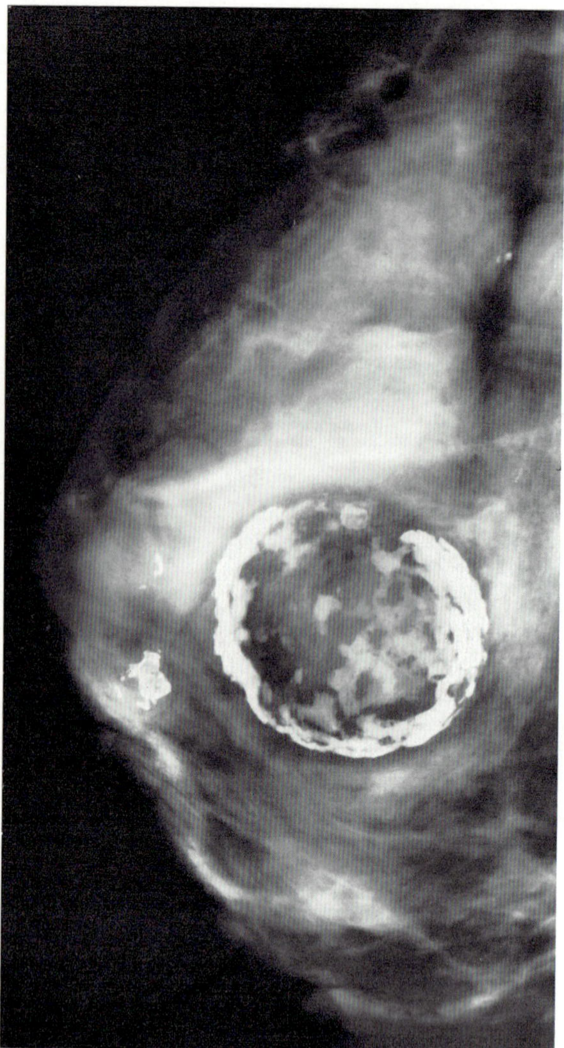

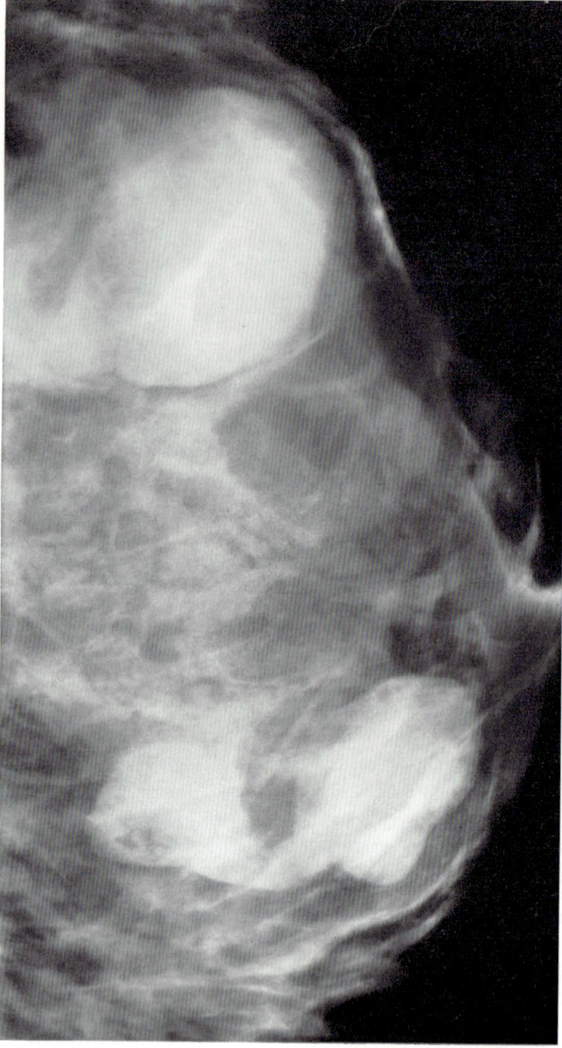

Fig. **16**.6a   Right breast of a 33-year-old woman. Large partially calcified fibroadenoma. Other fibro-adenomas in various stages of calcifications are distributed laterally and in the subareolar region.

Fig. **16**.6b   Left breast of the same patient: Three separate large lobular fibroadenomas.

(fig. **16**.7a and b). The much more extensive and coarser calcifications of a fibroadenoma allow definite differentiation from those seen in sclero-sing adenosis and particularly from the micro-calcifications of breast carcinoma. Occasionally fibroadenomas may demonstrate curvilinear calcifications as they are deposited within layers of the tumor (fig. **16**.8).

As degeneration of the tumor progresses the size and number of calcific deposits increases (fig. **16**.9 and **16**.10). Such deposits may take on a branching form and develop into large conglo-merate calcifications at many sites. The size of the fibroadenoma and the extent of degenerative calcification do not necessarily correlate. Very large fibroadenomas may occasionally contain only sparse calcifications which are not always within the center of the tumor but may be more peripheral (fig. **16**.11). Extensive and nearly total calcification of these tumors is most frequently found in the premenopausal patient (fig. **16**.12), however, occasionally a similar appearance may be seen in the mammogram of a younger patient. The appearance of extensive calcifications in a fibroadenoma has been likened to the topography seen on the surface of the moon (fig. **16**.6a).

The diagnosis of fibroadenomas is frequently obvious; however, when making this diagnosis

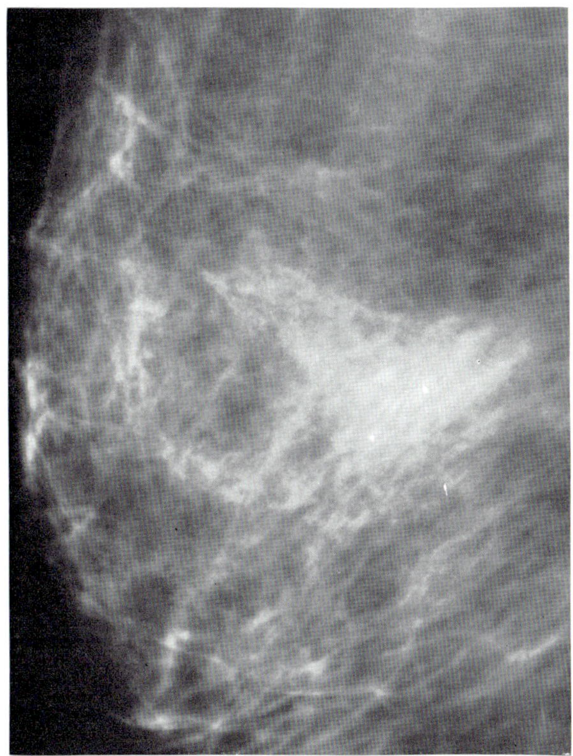 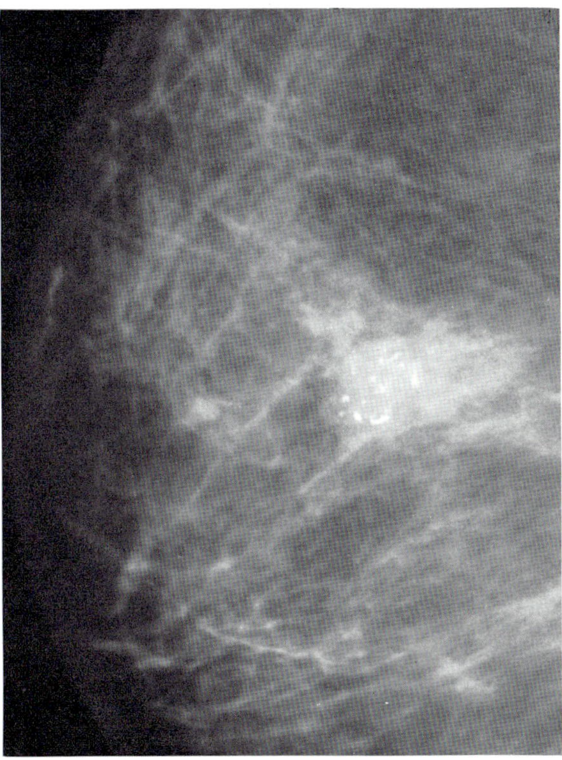

Fig. **16**.7a, b   Serial examination of a calcifying fibroadenoma. Progressive coarse calcification over a space of 2 years (localized areas).

from a mammogram one must be cautious not to overlook other diseases of the breast.

Basically fibroadenoma is a localized benign breast tumor caused by hormonal imbalance. The frequency of malignant degeneration or other complications may make excision unnecessary providing there is absolute clinical and mammographic diagnostic certainty. However, such certainty is generally only arrived at with solitary heavily calcified fibroadenomas. As a precaution therefore it is recommended that local excision be performed in most cases. This is recommended in solid nodules even after needle aspiration shows benign disease. Malignant changes, when they occur, are more common in the periphery and outside the confines of a fibroadenoma rather than in the center of the tumor. Thus mammographic evaluation should emphasize the examination of the margins of the mass, searching for microcalcification, radiating structures and desmoplastic changes.

The hyalinized fibroadenoma which is accompanied by fibrotic changes in surrounding breast tissue may cause difficulty in the differential diagnosis from scirrhus carcinoma (see page 295).

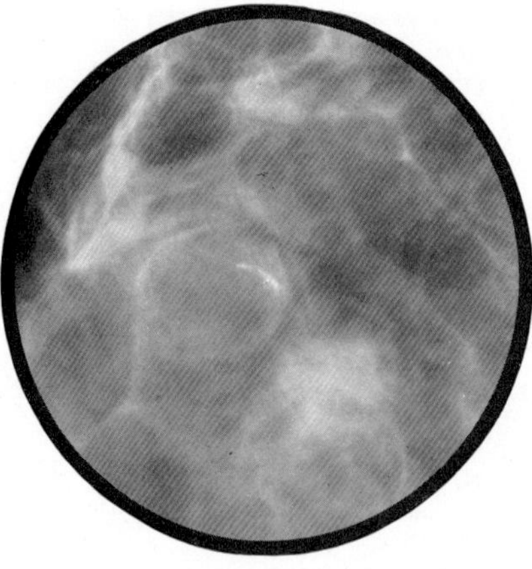

Fig. **16**.8

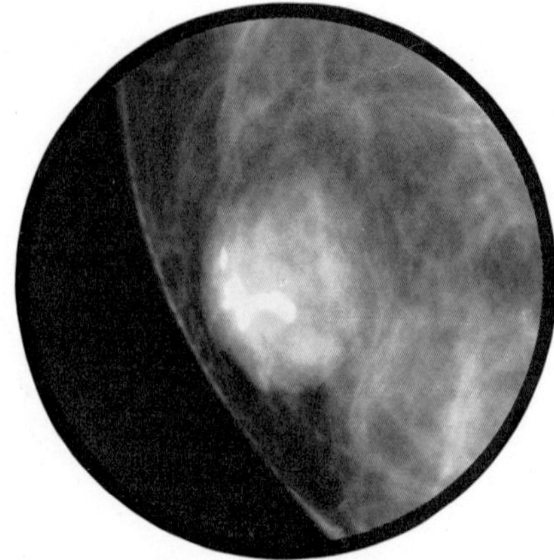

Fig **16**.9

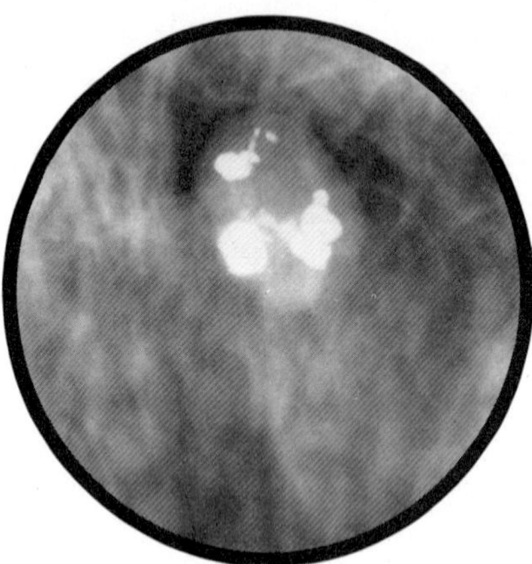

Fig. **16**.10

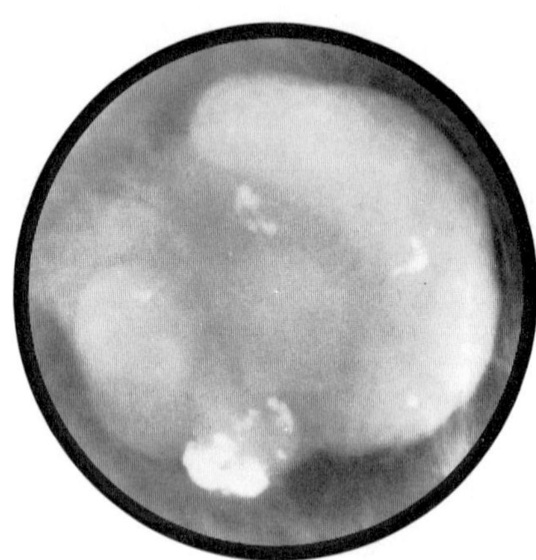

Fig. **16**.11

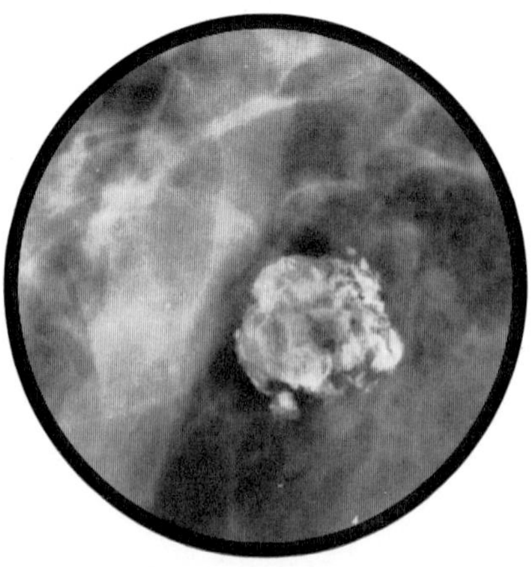

Fig. **16**.12

Fig. **16**.8—**16**.12 Mammograms (local areas) of various stages of calcification and forms of fibroadenomas (original size).

Giant Fibroadenoma or Cystosarcoma Phylloides

This tumor is in essence a very large form of fibroadenoma, but is especially designated because of its clinical findings. Giant fibroadenomas occur most commonly in middle-aged women. They are infrequent in patients following the menopause and are very rare in young women (SIMPSON et al 1969; AMERSON 1970).

Clinical Findings and Pathology

The clinical findings are often grossly obvious, with a large portion of the entire breast occupied by a large, coarse, firm mass covered by a stretched and often very tense skin. With closer examination one is suprised to note that the skin is freely movable over the entire surface of the tumor, if there has been no previous inflammation. At certain places there may be such stretching of

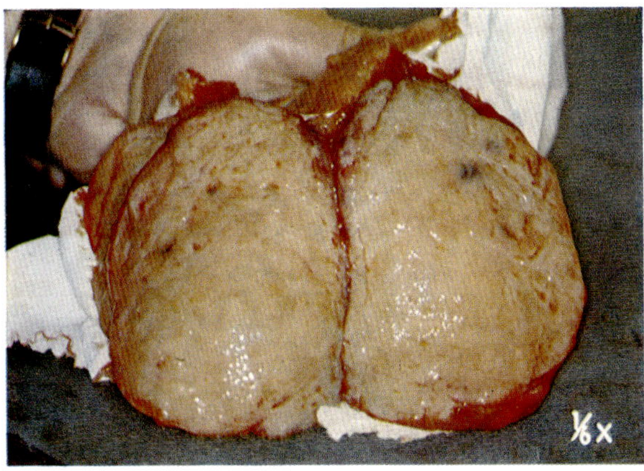

Fig. **17**.1b Surgical specimen. (From Buckmann/ Hagen and Sievert/Lethmathe).

the skin over the tumor that atrophy results and decubital ulcers may appear. However, the classical "orange peel" skin changes of breast carcinoma are not seen.

On the basis of these clinical findings the tumor was described as cystosarcoma phylloides by MÜLLER (1838). He was preceded by CHELIUS who used the term "hydatid cyst". This tumor is not related to sarcoma and this outmoded term should not be used.

The histological appearance of giant fibroadenoma is characterized by a laminar structure and cystic degeneration (fig. 17.1a). These histological characteristics have resulted in a subclassification even though overall it simply represents varying expressions of a basic fibroadenoma. Histologically, the dominant tissue may be connective or epithelial, associated with degenerative processes, resulting in cavernous structures containing mucous. Giant fibroadenomas are relatively rare and the number of published cases is not great. This is in part because the clinical and roentgen diagnosis is based primarily on the size of the tumor rather than on microscopic diagnosis. Furthermore, the typical laminar structure associated with giant fibroadenoma in the histological section, is found only in

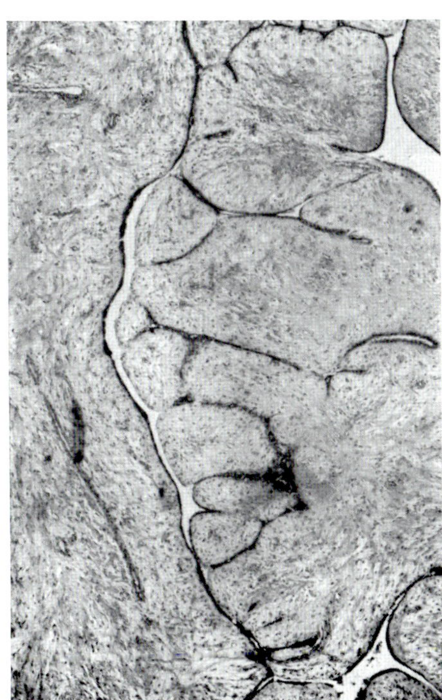

Fig. 1/.1a Histological appearance of giant fibroadenoma

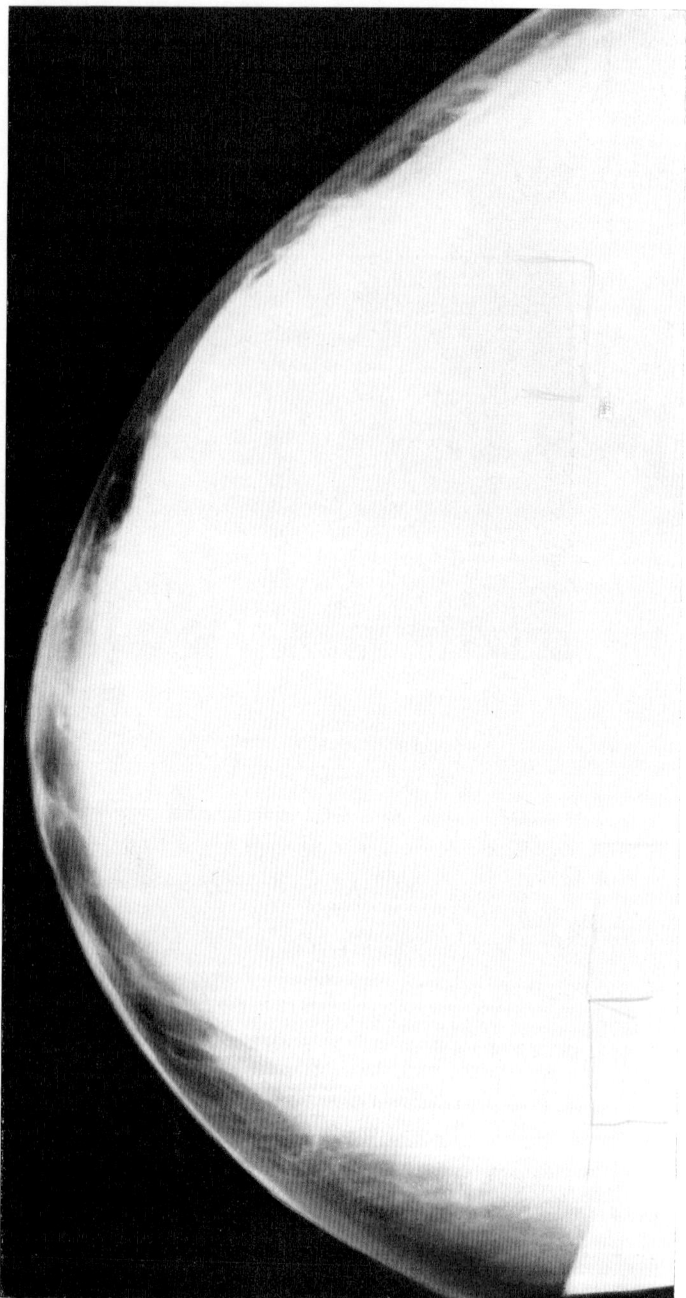

Fig. **17.1**c

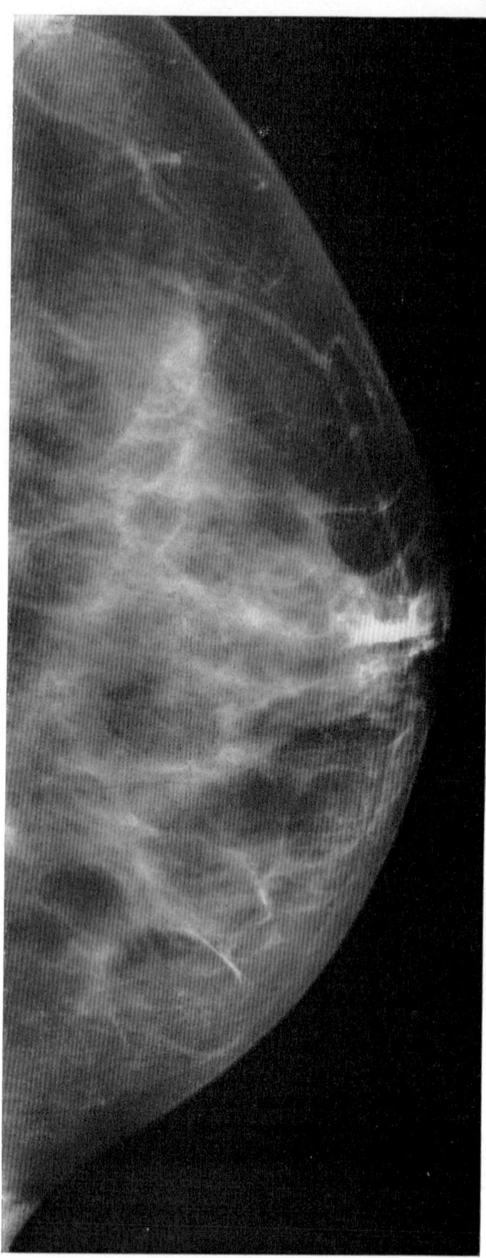

Fig. **17.**d

Fig. **17.**1c, d   Mammogram of a 33-year-old woman. Excisional biopsy (see Fig. 17.1a) 1 year before of a palpable mass. Was diagnosed cystosarcoma phylloides. The mass in the same breast grew rapidly for the last 2 months. There was an obvious difference in size between the right breast (Fig. 17.1c) and the normal left breast (Fig. 17.1d). The extremely dense homogeneous tumor mass is sharply marginated against the subcutaneous fatty layer.

certain portions of the tumor and may in fact occasionally be seen in small fibroadenomas. Thus the diagnosis of giant fibroadenoma is based on the clinical picture of a large hard tumor occupying a great portion of the breast, covered by thin stretched skin, which on histological section may reveal a basic laminar structure and multiple mucoid cyst formations. Sarcomatous degeneration of giant fibroadenomas does occur (MAIER et al 1968; ZOLTOWSKA

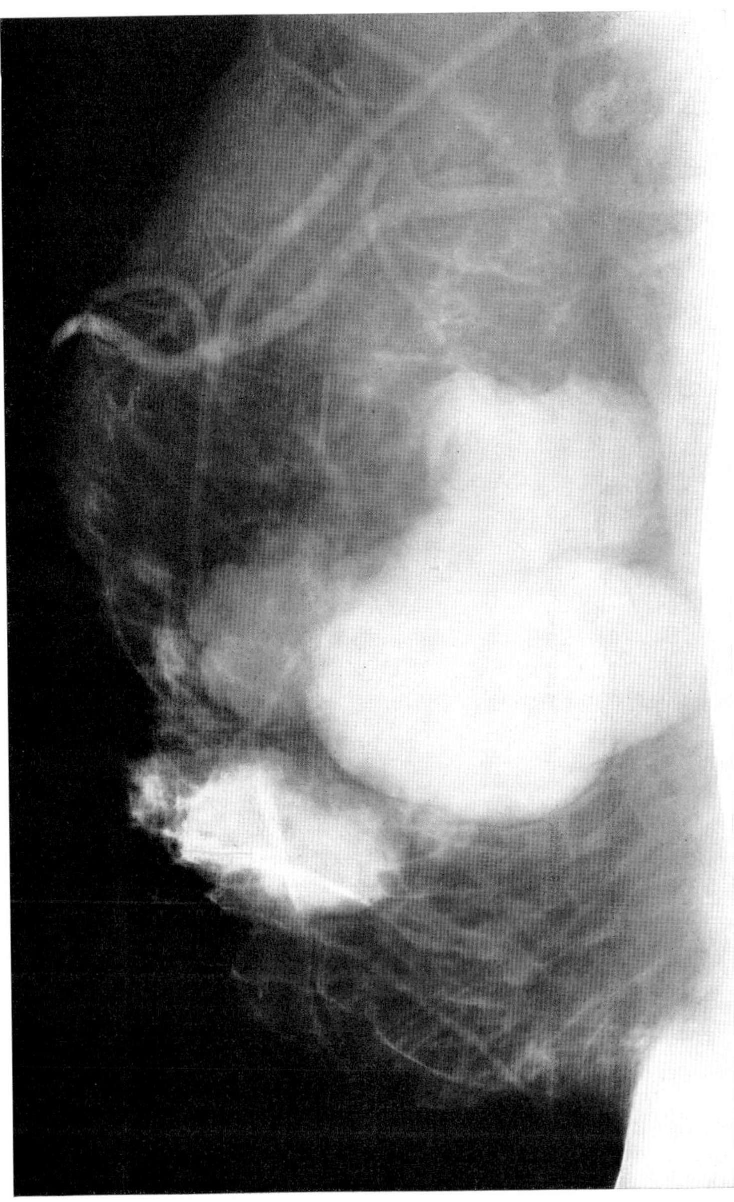

Fig. **17**.2   Giant fibroadenoma or cystosarcoma phylloides consisting of large tumor masses. A solitary fibroadenoma was removed 6 months before. Following this there was rapid growth of tumor and a mass the size of a cyst resulted. Because of clinical suspicion of sarcoma the mass was completely removed. Histology: Benign cystosarcoma phylloides.

and KOZLOWSKI 1969). We have observed several cases in which there was an apparent primary sarcomatous degeneration. Such sarcomas appear to arise from mesenchymal outgrowth of myo-epithelium. There have also been reports of carcinoma arising from giant fibroadenomas (ADAM and BARTEL 1969).

Giant fibroadenomas may grow very slowly over periods of several years or they may enlarge very rapidly over several months in which case the suspicion of sarcomatous degeneration and the designation of cysto*sarcoma* is understandable.

Giant fibroadenomas may be locally excised in order to preserve the breast; however, when the overlying skin is atrophic because of the great size of the tumor and particularly if there is ulceration of the overlying skin secondary to atrophy, mastectomy is required.

If local excision is incomplete, giant fibroadenoma will show a particular tendency to recurrence. It is therefore necessary to have complete mammographic data on the size, number and location of adjacent masses and also to perform a postsurgical mammogram for comparison. Only complete resection of the entire process guarantees against recurrence.

Roentgenology

Giant fibroadenoma consists of a solitary, extremely large, rounded mass (fig. 17.1a, b, c and d), or one may encounter a conglomerate of several individual masses (fig. 17.2). The margins of the tumor are smooth and sharp without desmoplastic changes in the adjacent parenchyma or microcalcifications. The characteristic calcifications of smaller fibroadenomas are not seen in giant fibroadenomas (GERSHON-COHEN and MOORE 1960). The skin overlying a giant fibro-

adenoma is thick and stretched; however, there may be focal areas of skin thickening as a result of inflammatory changes. To differentiate carcinomatous from postinflammatory skin thickening, however, it is important to examine the posterior border which, in the case of inflammatory skin thickening will be smooth and have a sharp margin separating it from subcutaneous fat. Dilated veins indicate increased blood flow.

Giant fibroadenoma are sharply bordered by fat and therefore easily recognized in the atrophic breast. This is not the case in the young patient, in whom the giant fibroadenoma is surrounded by dense breast parenchyma. In such cases, particularly when the tumor occupies the majority of the breast, differential diagnosis between this benign disorder and carcinoma of the breast is often impossible.

Chapter 18

Fibro-Adeno-Lipoma

Definition and Pathology

This tumor results from nodular fibrous and adenomatous proliferation within a lipoma. The entire tumor is surrounded by a connective tissue capsule. Fibroadenolipoma of the breast is rare (CUTLER 1961). PUENTE DUANY (1951 to 1961) reported three cases. Adenolipoma was described by SPALDING (1945) and HAAGENSEN (1971) who also consider these lipomatous tumors of the breast on the whole rare. The tumors described by PUENTE DUANY consisted essentially of fatty tissue into which fibrous and glandular elements were interspersed, definitely separating this lesion from a pure lipoma and adenolipoma. On histological section one or the other of these tissue components will pre-

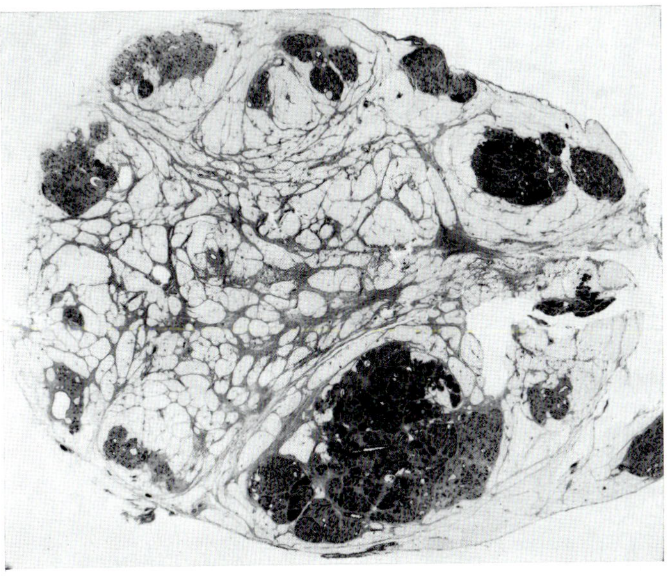

Fig. **18.**1a Extensive fatty tissue as well as nodular fibroadenomatous proliferation within a fibroadenolipoma. (Baldus, Womens' Clinic, University of Cologne).

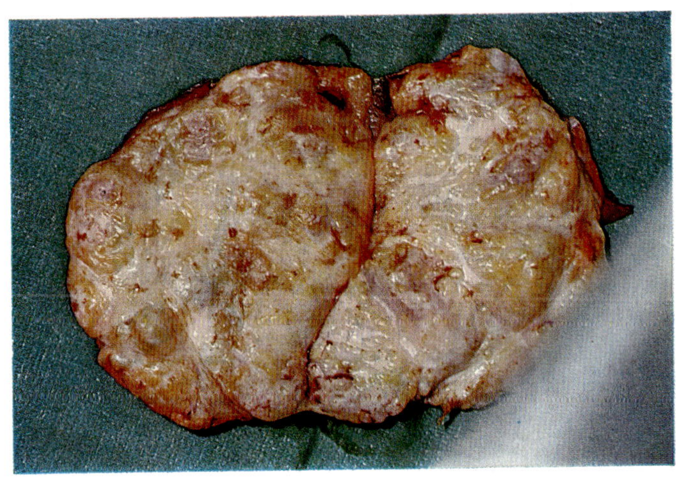

Fig. **18.**1b Surgical section of a fibroadenolipoma.

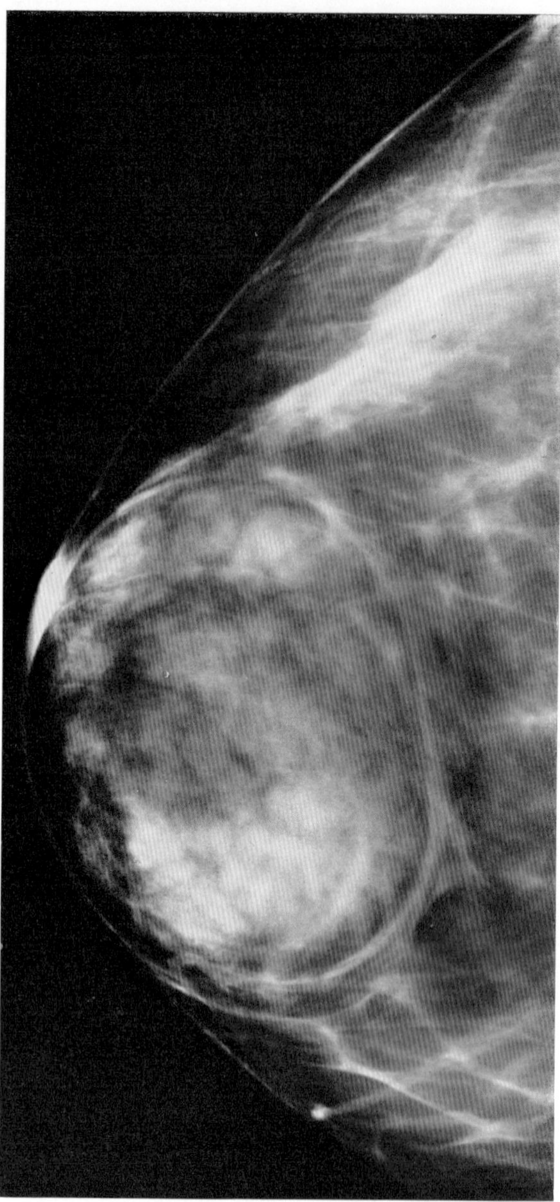

Fig. **18**.1c Characteristic mammographic appearance of a subareolar fibroadenolipoma surrounded by a fibrous capsule and containing numerous dense nodules as well as fatty tissue.

dominate (fig. **18.**1a). Most fibroadenolipomas are the size of an egg (fig. **18.**1b) but some may be larger. When they are observed it is frequently in a middle-aged or menopausal patient. It is curious that smaller fibroadenolipomas have so far not been observed.

Clinical Findings

On palpation, the findings consists of a large, soft, poorly demarcated mass, mostly in a retromammary location. Occasionally palpation will reveal a spongy mass which cannot be clearly separated from surrounding parenchyma. There is no thinning or fixation of the overlying skin. Nipple deformity or retraction has not been observed.

Roentgenology

Fibroadenolipomas possess a sharply defined, occasionally multilayered, connective tissue capsule which is easily defined in the mammogram (fig. **18.**1c). The contents of this encapsulated mass consists of fatty tissue intermixed with adenomatous masses of varying size and number. Calcification does not occur. The contents of the mass appear benign and homogeneous and the surrounding capsule is sharply demarcated along its inner as well as outer borders. There is displacement of the normal breast parenchyma by such a fibroadenolipoma. With increasing size the mass may extend to the undersurface of the skin and displace the subcutaneous fat (fig. **18.**2).

The roentgen appearance resembles a slice of sausage and the roentgen findings are so characteristic that they permit a definite diagnosis.

The treatment consists of excision of the encapsulated mass. Incomplete excision generally does not result in recurrence. There has been no report of malignant degeneration.

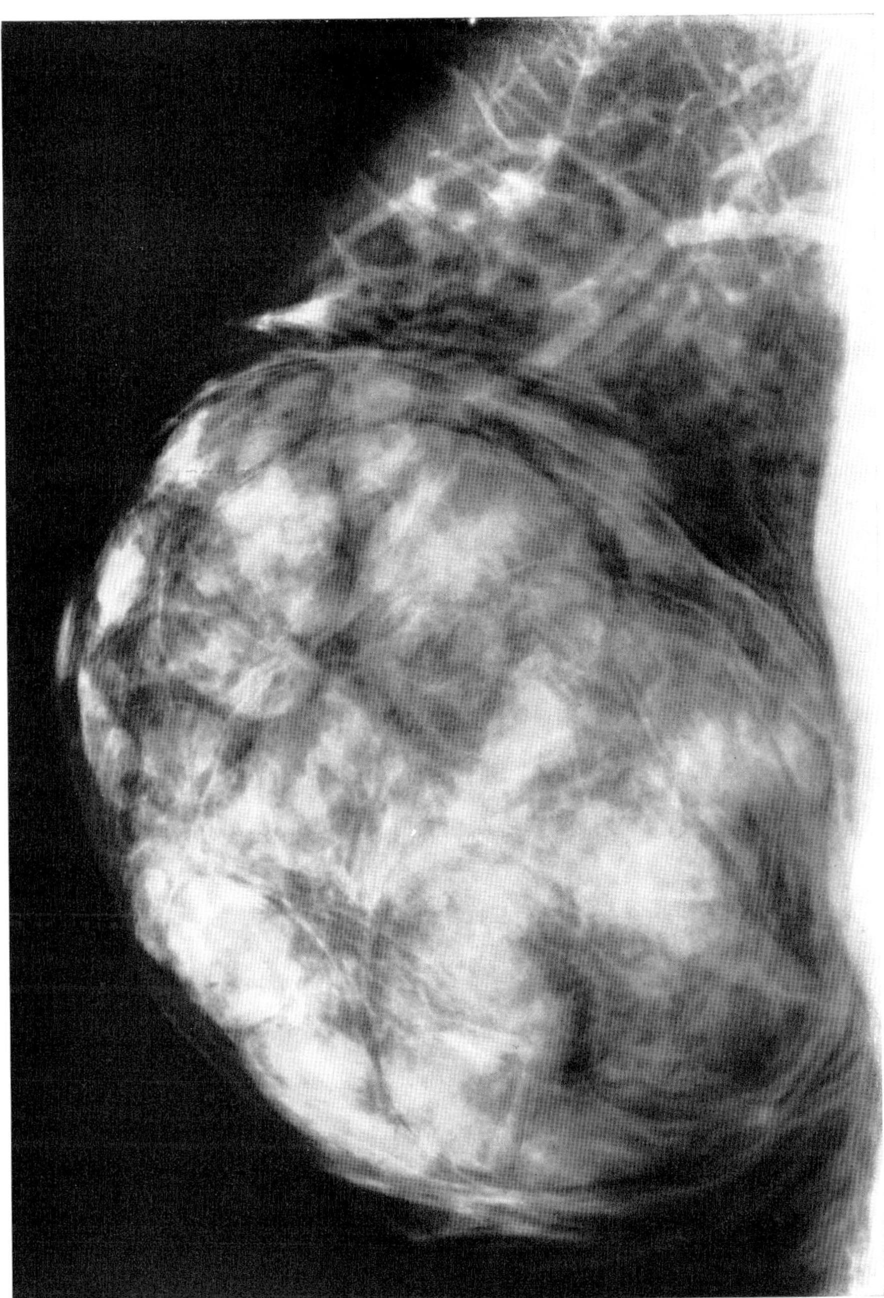

Fig. **18**.2 Large fibroadenoma surrounded by a fibrous capsule. Within are large adenomatous masses surrounded by fatty tissue and connective tissue septa. The mass occupies a large portion of the breast. Clinically: A dominant mass was barely palpable, which is in marked contrast to the obvious mammographic findings.

Chapter 19

Intraductal Papilloma
Intracystic Papilloma
Papillomatosis

Pathology

One type of proliferative mammary dysplasia consists of epithelial proliferation in the large and small lactiferous ducts. If these intraductal proliferative changes reach a large papillary form, recognizable macroscopically, the condition is termed an intraductal papilloma (fig. **19**.1).

Such papillomas are round or lobular, their surface may be flat or bordered with fine papillary fronds, and they may be large enough to fill the lumen of the milk ducts or expand the ducts as they increase in size. They may be broad-based or pedunculated to the wall of the duct and as they proliferate along the lumen may present as branched papillomatous tissues several centimeters in length. A papilloma occurring in the vicinity of the nipple may prolapse from the nipple spontaneously, or from pressure, or during the course of ductography. They are frequently the cause of sanguineous or serous nipple discharge. Papillomas may be single or multiple; the latter is called papillomatosis. HAAGENSEN (1956) is of the opinion that solitary and multiple papillomas are separate diseases. He believes that solitary papillomas are frequent and have no malignant potential, whereas multiple papillomas are less frequent and appear to represent a premalignant stage. This opinion, based on clinical and pathological evidence may be subject to revision in view of more recent experience with ductography. Galactography in patients with serous or sanguineous nipple discharge frequently demonstrates multiple but histologically benign papillomas. This discrepancy with the above stated pathological opinion

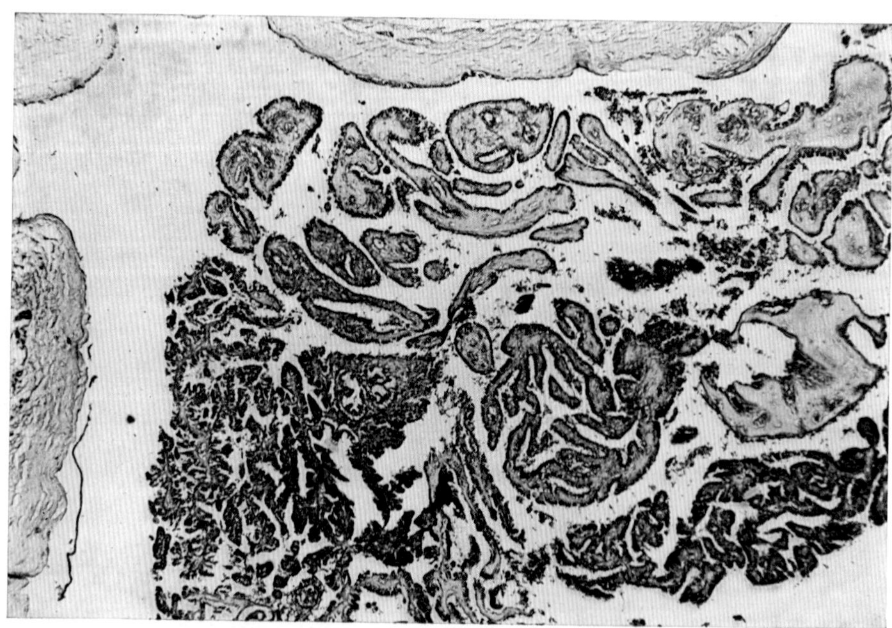

Fig. **19**.1   Histological section of a benign intraductal papilloma.

probably results from the fact that the pathologist found only the larger papillomas in the biopsy specimen, since only dilated ducts were opened on examination. Lactiferous ducts of normal size in the specimen are difficult to open with surgical scissors and therefore the small papillomas within these ducts that can be seen by galactography were overlooked by the pathologist. Furthermore, these small intraductal papillomas no doubt contracted following formalin fixation of the specimen. Therefore the more modern opinion is that papillomatosis of lactiferous ducts is frequent, that some of the papillomas may become large and others remain small, and that there is no clinical difference between solitary and multiple papillomas.

Papillomas are the most frequent cause of sanguineous and serous nipple discharge. Sixty percent of cases (in other reports over 80%) with sanguineous discharge result from one or more ductal papillomas. In spite of this, however, the clinical symptom of sanguineous discharge from the nipple should still arouse the suspicion of malignant breast disease.

The frequency of malignant degeneration of an intraductal papilloma is difficult to arrive at statistically. It is felt, however, that only a very small number of ductal papillomas undergo malignant degeneration. Papillomatosis as well as the concomitant occurrence of ductal ectasis is primarily a disease of the older patient following menopause and this is also the age of the most frequent occurrence of breast carcinoma making it difficult to exactly define whether there is or is not a relationship between such benign and malignant conditions.

A special form of intraductal papilloma is the *nipple papilloma*. In this case the papilloma develops immediately beneath the nipple, expanding the subareolar milk ducts. The tumor may prolapse from the nipple. *Intracystic papilloma* is also a special subclassification. The cyst in this case is simply an extremely dilated lactiferous duct. Pathologically there is no difference between this papilloma and other types.

Clinical Findings

Clinically *ductal papilloma* is recognized by the serous or sanguineous secretion that it produces. Serous discharge, however, may also be seen in simple ductal ectasia.

In solitary or multiple intraductal papillomatosis one is rarely able to palpate a mass. Occasionally a wormlike mass may be palpated in the region just behind the areola. This represents simultaneously occurring inflammatory changes in the duct secondary to stasis of secretions, blocked by the papilloma (the so-called "varicocele tumor" according to BLOODGOOD 1923), or it may indicate malignancy, particularly if this is the only palpatory finding in an otherwise soft breast without any relationship to the ductal papilloma.

The clinical findings of an *intracystic papilloma* are essentially the same as those of an ordinary cyst of the breast. Sanguineous nipple discharge occurs only when this cyst is in free communication with a lactiferous duct. Puncture of such a cyst will result in sanguineous aspirate and the differential diagnosis in such a case rests between an intracystic papilloma and an intracystic papillary carcinoma. Cytological examination of the aspirate is particularly difficult in our experience and often does not allow definite differentiation because involutional changes within a benign intracystic papilloma may resemble the changes found in carcinoma. Consequently resection and further histological examination are indicated.

Roentgenology

In the mammogram a ductal papilloma is only recognizable when it reaches the size of 1 to 2 cm or more, is located just behind or near the areola in a predominantely fatty breast (fig. 19.2a and b; fig. 19.3). The papilloma is then seen as a cirbumscribed, oval, beaded or spindle-shaped density radiating from the immediate areolar region (STRAX and POMERANZ 1964). Such roentgen findings in conjunction with a clinical history of sanguineous nipple discharge only permit the suspicion of the diagnosis. In the mammogram one is unable to differentiate ductal papilloma from intraductal carcinoma.

With unilateral or bilateral prolonged serous or sanguineous discharge, ductography is indicated. Only with ductography is it possible to reach a reasonably correct diagnostic opinion and simultaneously to localize the lesion in order to allow accurate surgical excision of the diseased parenchymal segment and associated ducts. Radiologist and surgeon must work closely together in this endeavor. We have frequently

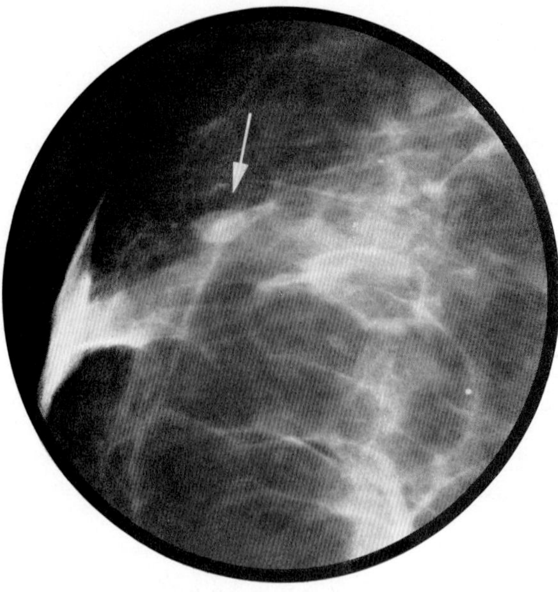

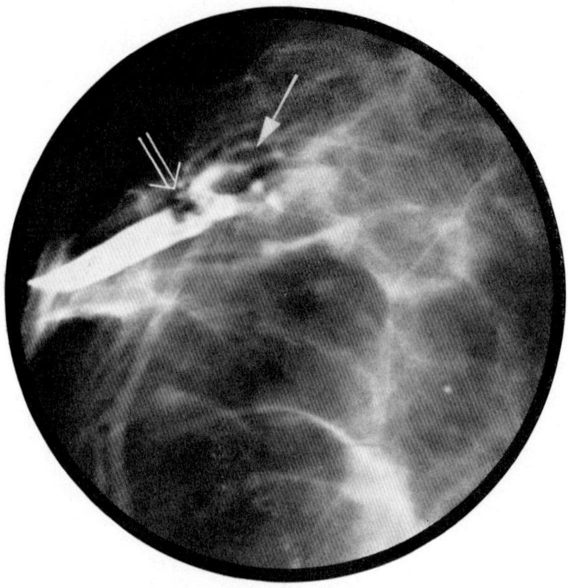

Fig. **19**.2a   Mammogram: Local area magnified 1.5x. Oval, smooth density with pediclelike extension (arrow).

Fig. **19**.2b   Ductography: The density appears as a smooth, wormlike intraductal filling defect: Intraductal papilloma. Another intraductal papilloma (double arrow), which was not visible on the plain film, is defined.

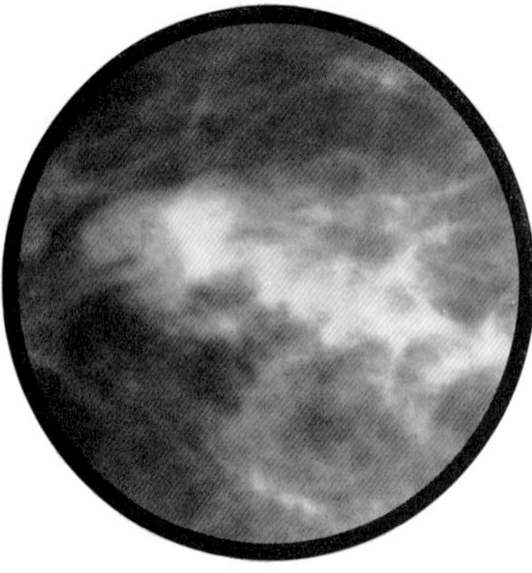

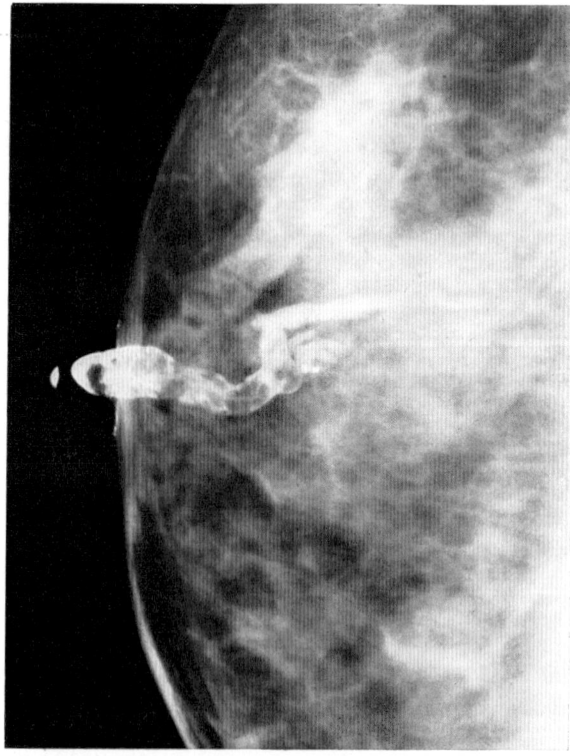

Fig. **19**.3   Coned-down view. Subareolar lobular rounded density about 8 mm in diameter. Pedicle-like extension of this tissue toward the nipple, suggesting the course of a lactiferous duct. No sign of malignancy. Clinically: Sanguineous discharge from the nipple. Cytology: Negative. Histology: Benign intraductal papilloma.

Fig. **19**.4   Ductography because of watery nipple secretion. No palpable findings. Wormy filling defect in an ectatic lactiferous duct: Lobular carcinoma extending to the nipple.

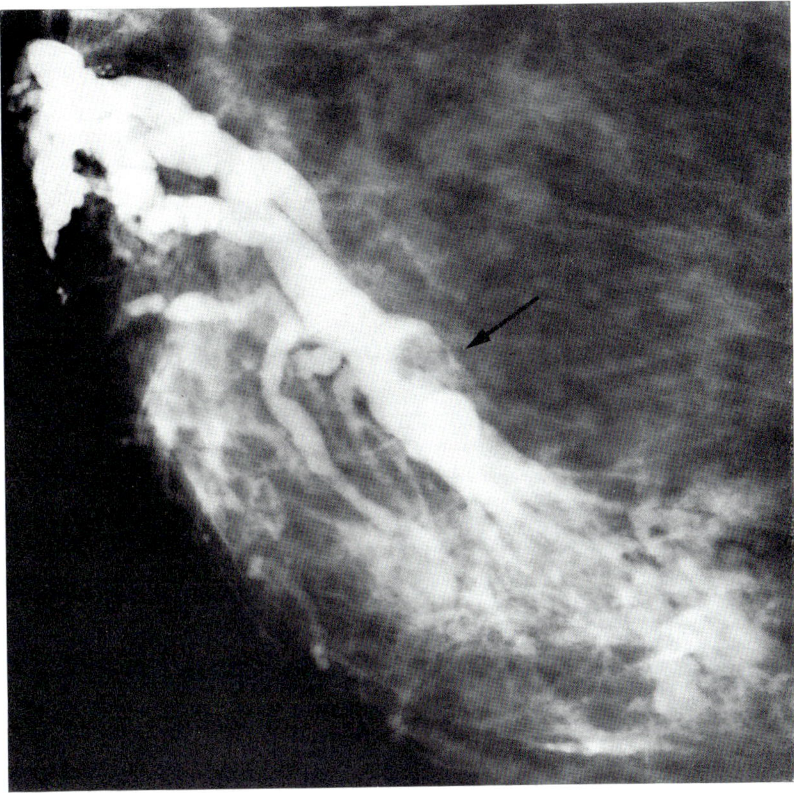

Fig. **19**.5   Large papilloma with marked ectasia of lactiferous duct.

seen the unfortunate occurrence of biopsy or excision of the wrong diseased duct in a patient complaining of sanguineous discharge. Accurate excision and biopsy is facilitated only by the use of preoperative galactography.

Surgery is made easier if the diseased ductal region can be demarcated. This can be done by injecting methylene blue into the secreting lactiferous ducts immediately prior to surgery in order to assure that the dye remains distributed either intra or periductally within the region in question and is not distributed in lymphatics over large areas of the breast.

At ductography the papilloma will present as a filling defect within a dilated lactiferous duct (fig. 19.4, 19.5 and 19.6). Occasionally the entire duct may be obstructed by the papilloma. If one is successful in injecting contrast material

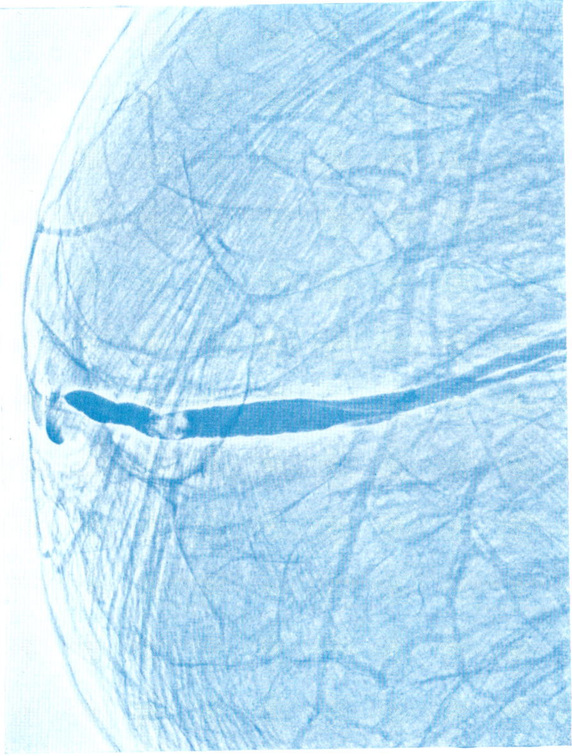

Fig. **19**.6 Galactography using the xeromammogram. Papilloma within an ectatic lactiferous duct. The halo effect obliterates perception of structures surrounding the contrast filled lactiferous duct because the concentration of contrast material was too great.

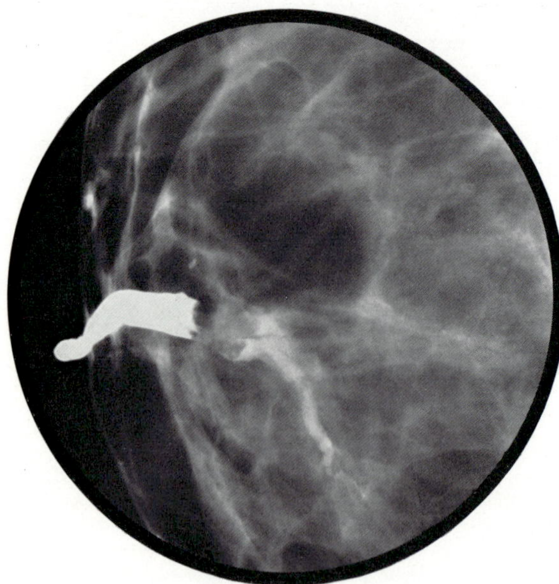

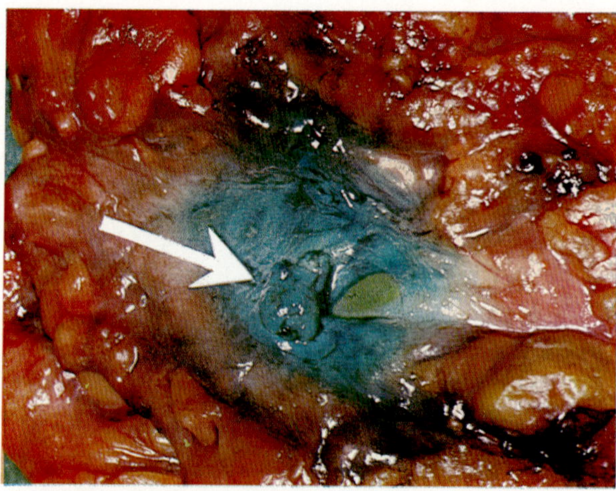

Fig. **19**.7a Moderately severe dilated lactiferous duct with oval, lobular filling defect. Proximal peripheral ducts are only faintly opacified because of contrast dilution by blocked secretions.

Fig. **19**.7b Surgical specimen stained by intraductal methylene-blue injection. The arrow indicates the papilloma.

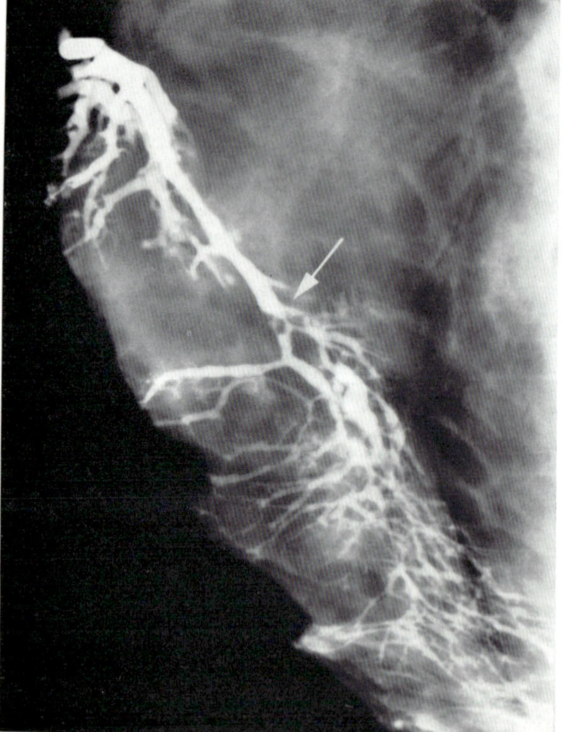

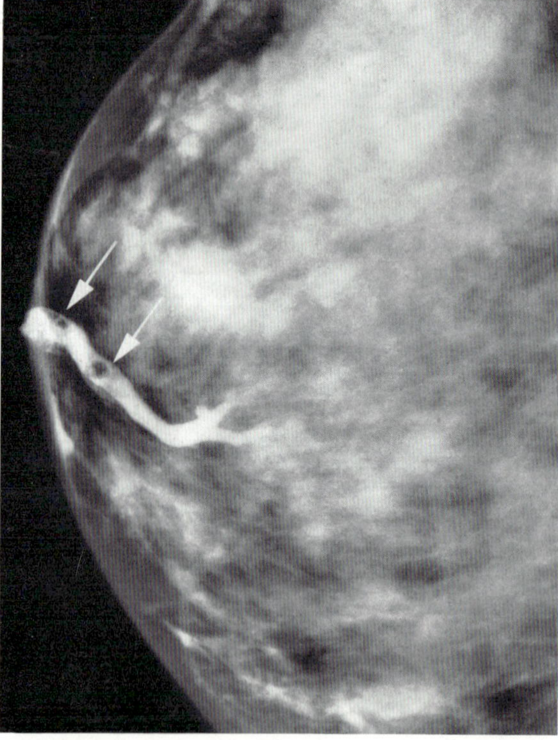

Fig. **19**.8 Filling defect caused by papilloma at bifurcation of the lactiferous duct (arrow). Contrast material goes past the papilloma.

Fig. **19**.9 Ductography because of sanguineous discharge from the right nipple. Ductal ectasia and two rounded, smoothly contoured filling defects (arrows). Mammary dysplasia of the surrounding breast tissue. Papillomatosis verified histologically.

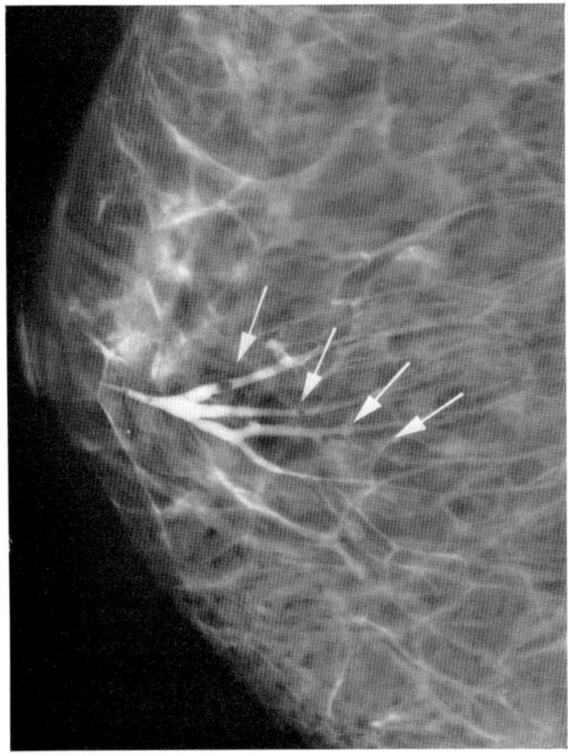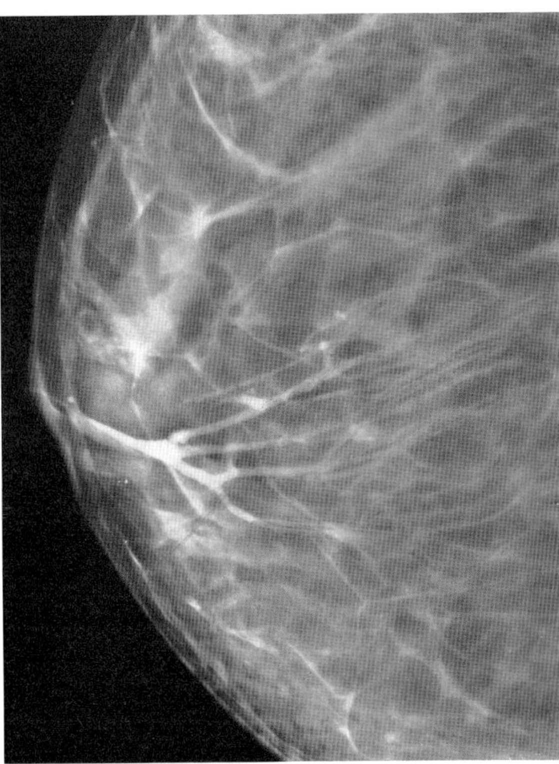

Fig. **19**.10a, b   Ductography reveals minimally dilated lactiferous ducts. Numerous filling defects (a) represent air bubbles as verified in a repeat examination (b).

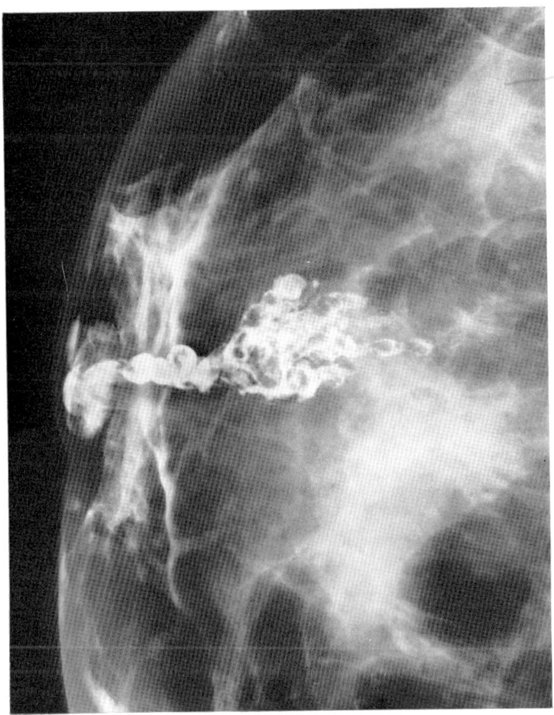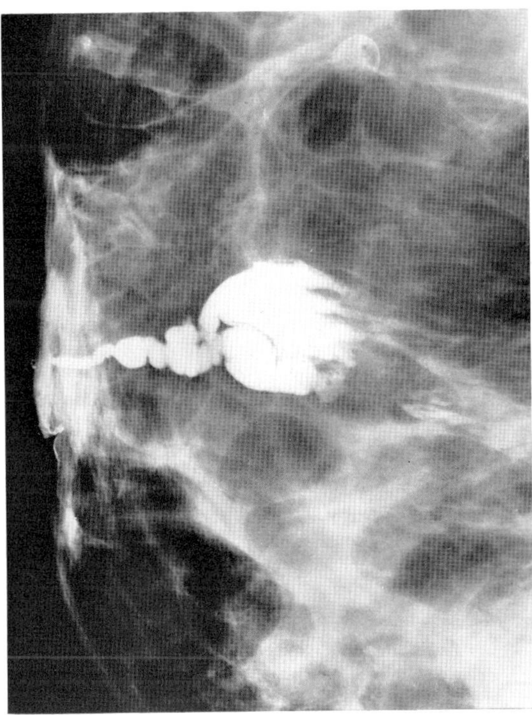

Fig. **19**.11a   Galactogram with incomplete filling of the ducts by contrast material. Residual debris is identified within the duct system.

Fig. **19**.11b   Following expression of the ductal contents complete filling with contrast and demonstration of the ductal system is possible (University Women's Clinic, Cologne).

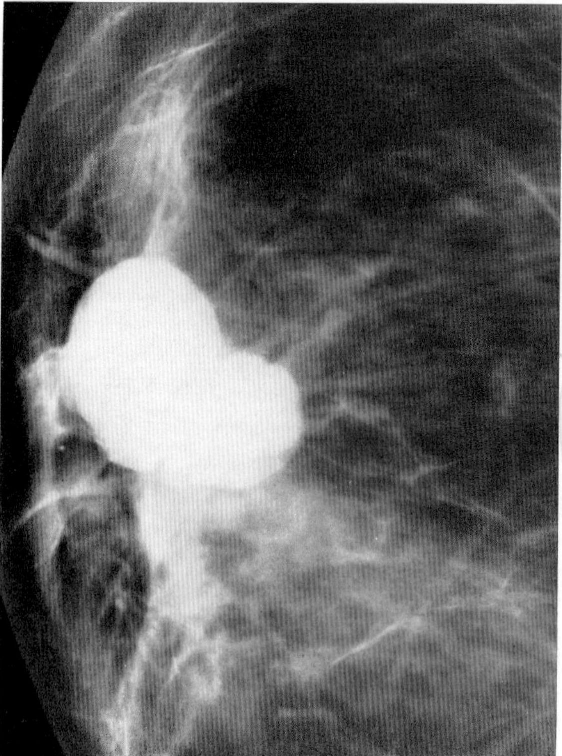

Fig. **19**.12a   Mammogram of a 60-year-old woman. Smoothly contoured oval density with umbilicated margins corresponding to clinical findings.

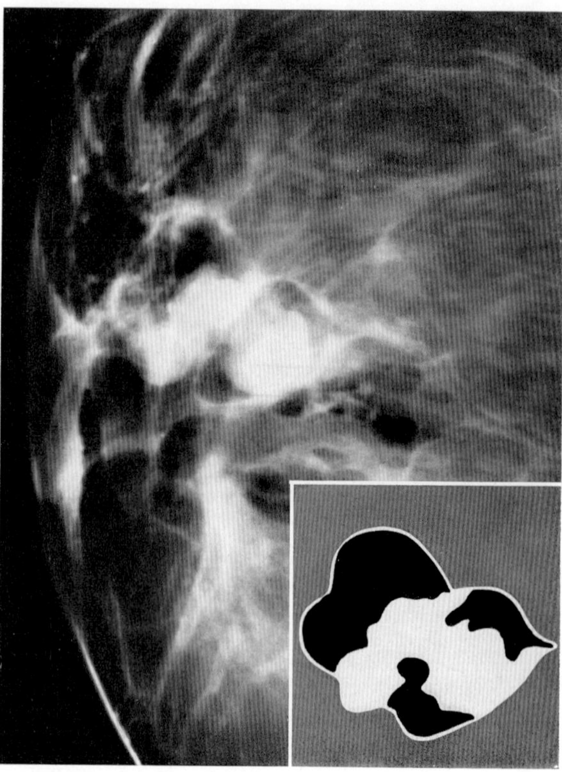

Fig. **19**.12b   Pneumocystogram revealed an irregular soft tissue density within the cyst partly free within the lumen and partly connected to the inner wall.
Cytology of the sanguineous aspirate: Suspicion of malignancy.

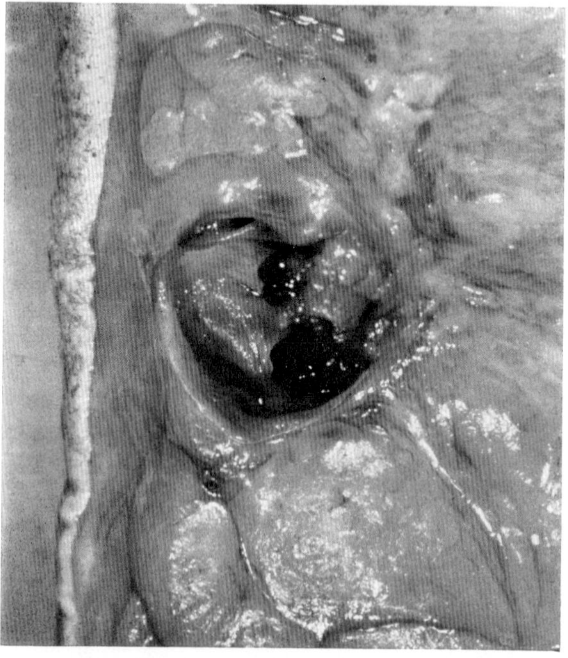

Fig. **19**.12c Surgical specimen of the intracystic papilloma with blood clots.
Histology: Benign papilloma.

beyond the papilloma into the periphery it will be possible to define the entire extent of the tumor in the mammogram. There may be dilution of the contrast material behind the papilloma by stored and blocked milk duct secretions (fig. 19.7a and b). Secondary inflammatory changes resulting from secretory stasis may be recognized at ductography. Not all papillomas are obstructive and frequently injection of contrast material allows full and complete demonstration of the parenchymal lobe served by the injected duct (fig. 19.8). Distal to the papilloma one may see marked and diffuse ductal ectasia similar to the bronchial ectasia seen distal to an intrinsic bronchial tumor. Occasionally ductal changes will include intermittent dilatation and stenosis and other alterations of caliber which raise the suspicion of multiple, pinhead-sized papillomas (fig. 19.9).

One should be wary of misinterpretation of filling defects caused by foamy contrast or by air bubbles in the contrast material. These produce

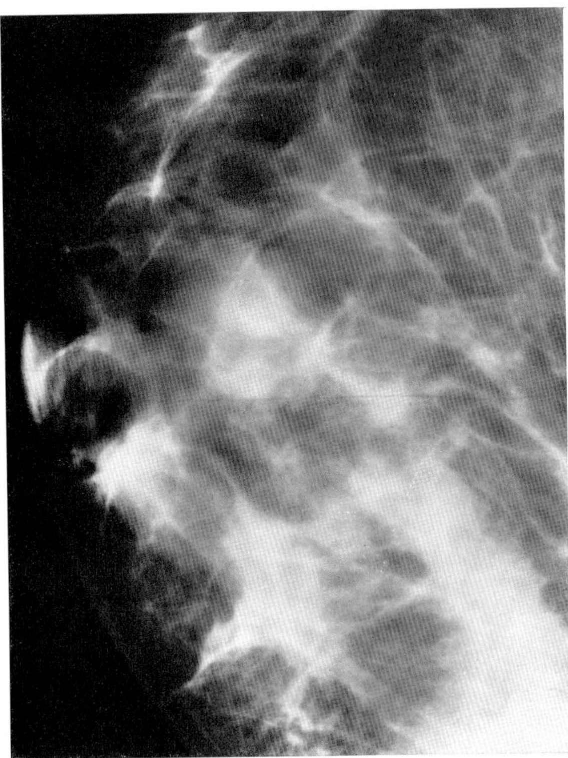

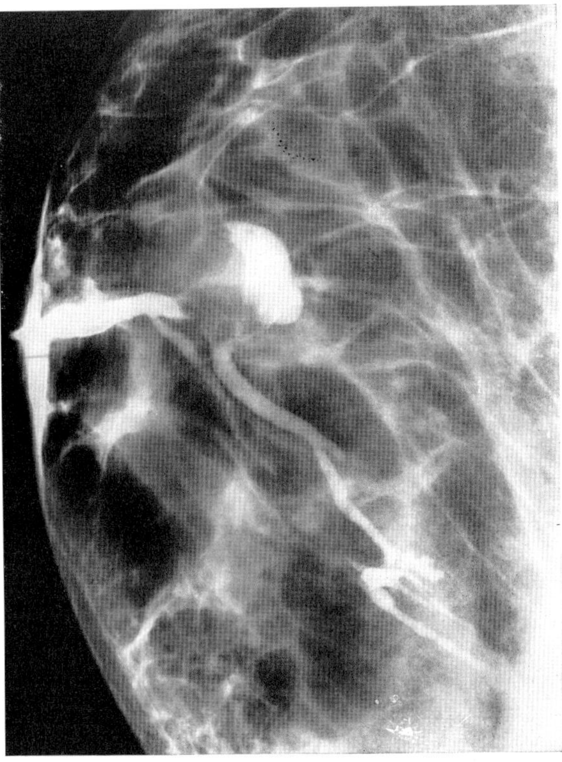

Fig. **19**.13a   Mammogram reveals a rounded sub-areolar density.

Fig. **19**.13b   Ductography reveals a dilated milk duct connecting with a cyst. A papilloma of approximately 1 cm in diameter is seen as a filling defect within the cyst.

small rounded filling defects and are very difficult to differentiate from small papillomas (fig. **19**.10a and b). Inspissated secretion within a lactiferous duct may appear as a filling defect within the contrast column during ductography and thus have the same appearance as papillomatosis (fig. **19**.11a and b). Occasionally papillomas calcify (see page 263 and page 275).
Intracystic papillomas are generally only accidentally delineated at pneumocystography. The roentgen appearance is that of a lobular soft tissue density extending into the lumen of the cyst from the inner wall (fig. **19**.12a—c).
Occasionally intracystic papillomas may be demonstrated by ductography if there is communication of the cystic dilated duct with the injected lactiferous duct system (fig. **19**.13a and b). An organized hematoma may also result in a mass density in the pneumocystogram (fig. **19**.14). Any intracystic process and any thickening of the inner wall of a cyst excludes the diagnosis of simple cyst and is an indication for complete cyst removal.

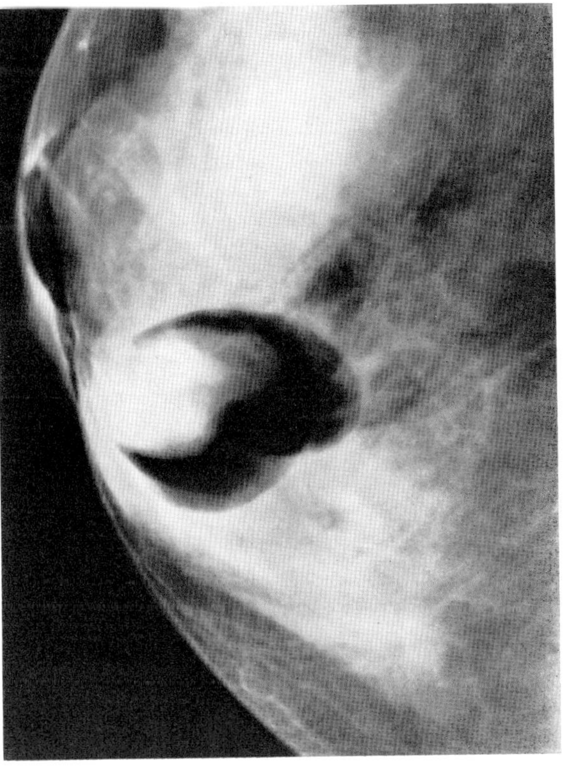

Fig. **19**.14   Intracystic organized hematoma (Dr. Seidel, Johanneskrankenhaus, Bielefeld).

Chapter 20

Lipoma

Pathology and Clinical Findings

Lipomas occur in the breast as well as in other parts of the body. The diagnosis of lipoma of the breast, an organ which contains a considerable amount of fatty tissue, can only be made by demonstration of a connective tissue capsule

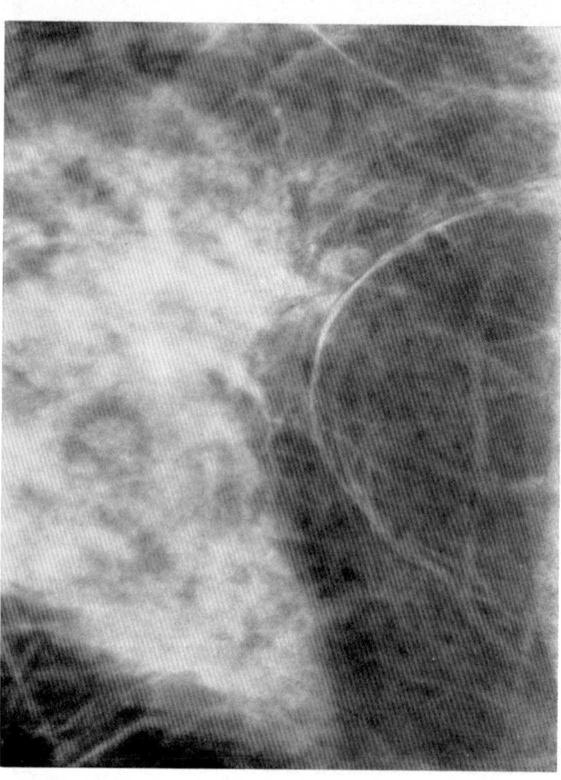

Fig. **20**.1   Clinically: Smooth hard mass the size of an orange palpated beneath the areola near the thoracic wall.
Mammography: Local area fatty tissue surrounded by a bulging connective tissue capsule: Encapsulated lipoma, verified histologically.

around a localized collection of fatty tissue. An additional requirement for the diagnosis is that the lesion is palpable. Lipomas are most common in postmenopausal and elderly women. The history will indicate that the lump has been present for a long time and has not changed. Generally a lipoma is clinically insignificant. The only importance of this tumor is that it may mimic carcinoma, sarcoma or fibrocystic disease during palpation. Surgical removal is generally not indicated.

Roentgenology

The fatty tissue of a lipoma has the same radiolucency in the mammogram as the surrounding fatty tissue. Only the identification of a surrounding connective tissue capsule allows the diagnosis of a lipoma (fig. 20.1). Most commonly a lipoma has a round or oval shape but occasionally the surface may be slightly irregular or lobular. The lipoma may contain connective tissue septa.

These roentgen findings when correlated with appropriate palpatory findings that include a soft or occasionally firm, freely movable, discrete breast mass allow a definite diagnosis of lipoma. In the absence of corresponding palpable findings one should consider that the capsule seen in the roentgenogram may in fact simply represent normal lipomatous tissue of the breast partially surrounded or septated by COOPER's ligaments. The radiologist should also convince himself that the palpable mass is present in several projections and particularly that it is not the result of displaced fat of the breast as a result of compression from the cone, before indicating that the palpatory findings represent a lipoma. Several incorrect diagnoses have occurred because of this error.

Chapter 21

Hemangioma
Lymphangioma
Subcutaneous Neurofibroma

Pathology and Clinical Findings

Hemangiomas and lymphangiomas are rare in the breast. These tumors have been reported by MENVILLE and BLOODGOOD (1933), DECHOLNOKY (1939), DAHL and IVERSON (1933), as well as MADDING and HERSHBERGER (1949). Pathologically and histologically the appearance of hemangiomas of the breast is identical to those in other parts of the body (fig. 21.1a).

Hemangiomas of the breast consist of rounded masses which can be detected as red or blue lesions through the skin (fig. 21.2a). There may be fixation of the overlying skin. Frequently the mass is somewhat soft and fluctuant. Benign hemangiomas are slow-growing and are frequently not detected by the patient until a particular size is reached; the mass .is then discovered and reported as having "suddenly appeared". Occasionally pain is reported in the mass but at least one of our patients complained of pain throughout the entire breast.

Hemangioma is a benign tumor whereas heman-

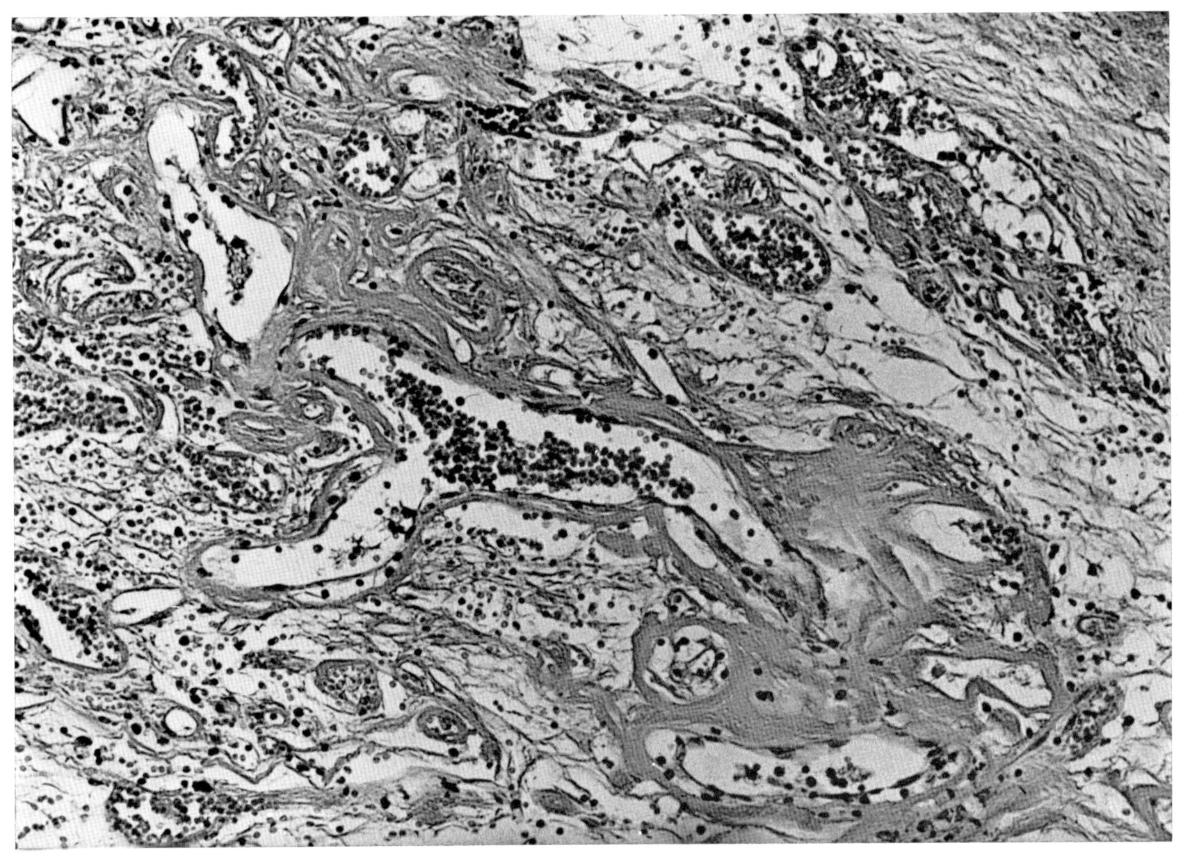

Fig. **21.**1a   Histology: Edematous, partly degenerated hemangioma of the breast.

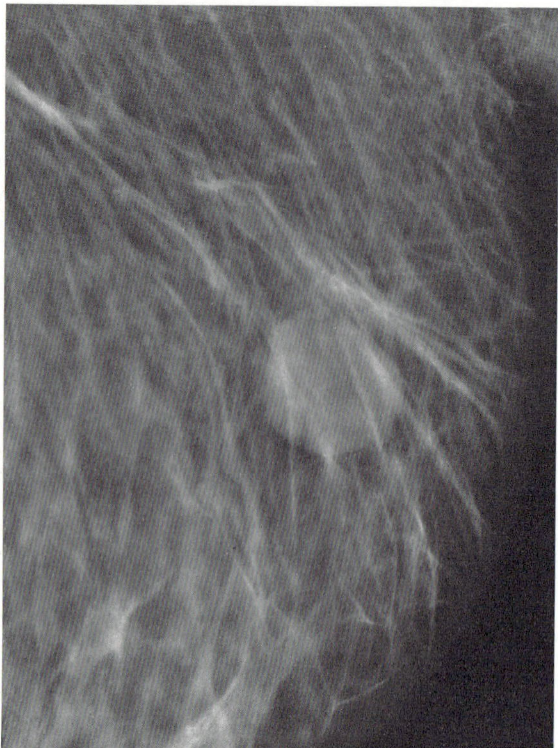

Fig. **21**.1b   Mammogram: Round mass corresponding to a palpable smooth breast lump.

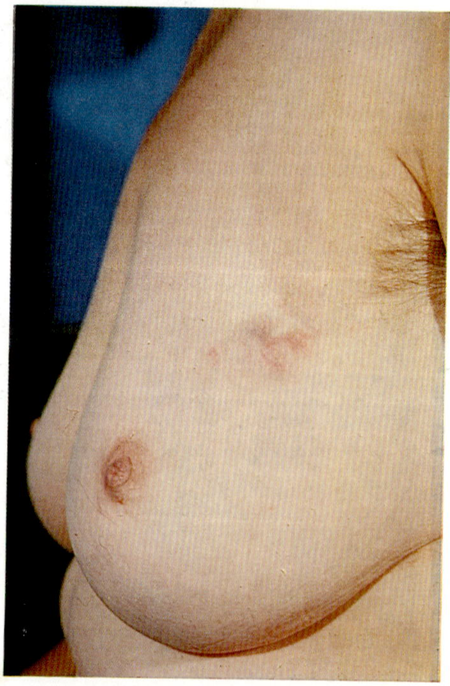

Fig. **21**.2a   Blue-tinged breast lump present since childhood and associated with skin retraction and local telangiectases.

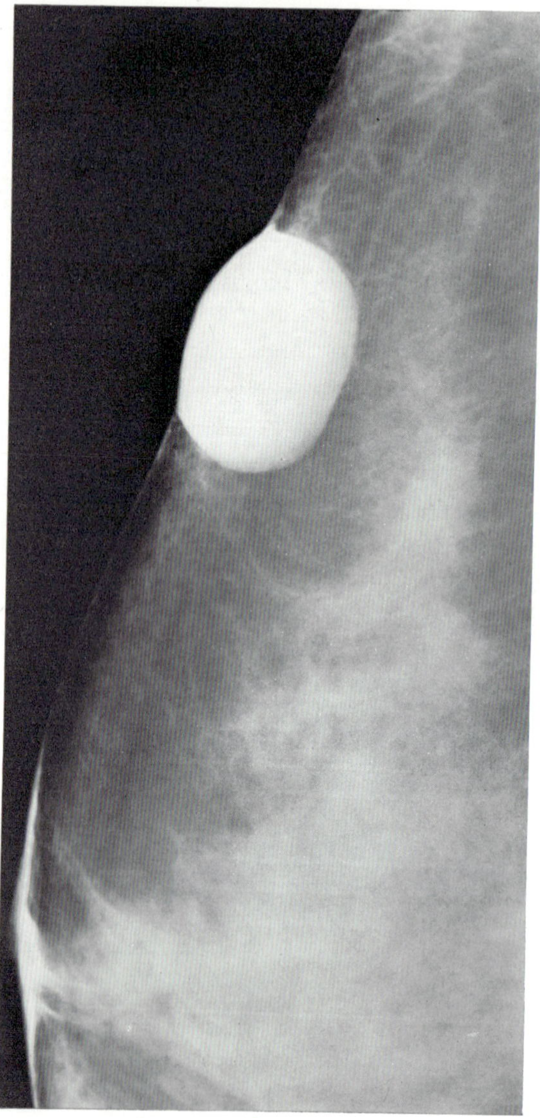

Fig. **21**.2b   Lateral mammogram: Smooth dense mass attached to the overlying skin. On the basis of the history and clinical findings it was felt that this lesion represents a hemangioma. Histological verification could not be obtained in this case.

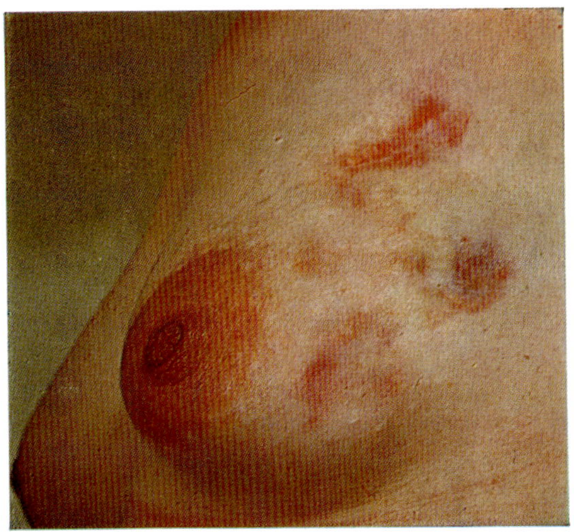

Fig. **21**.3a　Right breast following excisional biopsy. In the region of the surgical scar there is a hard bluish discolored mass 2 to 3 cm in diameter.

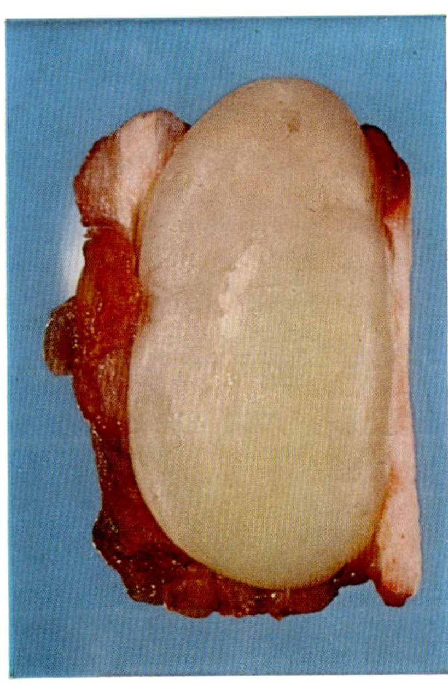

Fig. **21**.3c　Photograph of the surgical specimen. Macroscopically and histologically: Subcutaneous neurofibroma.

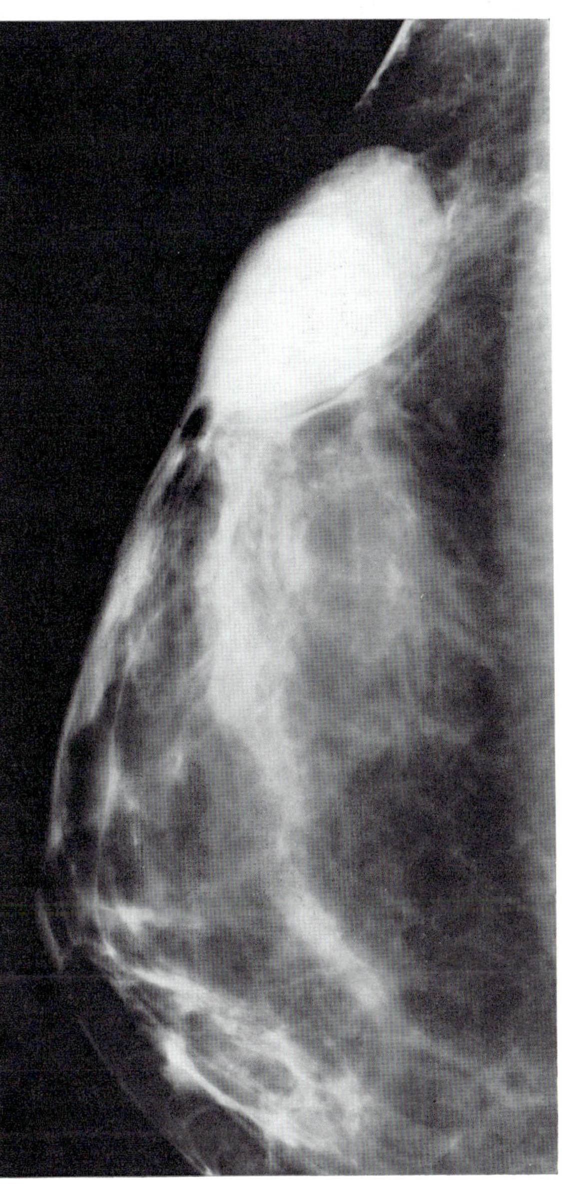

Fig. **21**.3b　Mammogram: Oval smoothly marginated directly subcutaneous mass, corresponding to palpatory findings. Puncture: Blood. Diagnosis: Hemangioma.

gioendothelioma whether benign or malignant is characterized by very rapid growth.

Under some circumstances a hypervascular and partially involuted subcutaneous neurofibroma may mimic very closely, both clinically and microscopically, a hemangioma. As a rule, however, the pathological diagnosis of subcutaneous neurofibroma is not difficult (fig. **21**.3c).

Lymphangiomas have a tendency to present more as diffuse rather than discrete dominant masses.

Roentgenology

The appearance in the mammogram is that of a smooth, sharply contoured sometimes lobular mass (fig. **21**.1b). Calcification is uncommon.

9*

Desmoplastic response in the periphery of the mass as a rule does not occur. However, there may be a connection of the hemangioma to the skin if the lesion is in an immediate sub-cutaneous location (fig. 21.2b). In such a case the appearance mimics very closely that of a subcutaneous neurofibroma (fig. 21.3a—c). Here the differential diagnosis, either clinically or roentgenologically, between hemangioma and neurofibroma is not possible. Size, shape and structure of these masses cannot be differentiated from fibroadenomas or cysts. Furthermore there is no reliable mammographic differentiation from other benign diseases of the breast.

The diagnostic puncture and aspiration reveals blood but this is not necessarily proof of hemangioma. A similar aspirate may be obtained from a cyst filled with blood, a medullary carcinoma with central necrosis or a solid carcinoma. The mass must be surgically removed and complete histological examination performed for final diagnosis.

Chapter 22

Acute Mastitis

Pathology and Clinical Findings

Acute mastitis is an infectious disease occurring almost exclusively during lactation (puerperal mastitis) and particularly in primiparas. The infection begins in the lactiferous ducts and spreads by way of lymphatics or hematogenously. Clinical symptoms consist of swelling, pain, reddening of overlying skin, and fever. Swollen and painful axillary lymph nodes occur. Abscess formations may occur, palpable as solid masses, sometimes fluctuant. If the infection is superficial the overlying skin will be inflamed and fixed. Localized edema may result in an "orange peel skin". Leukocytosis with shift to the left is found and the sedimentation rate is increased. Acute mastitis during nonlactating periods is very unusual and this diagnosis should be made only after carcinoma has been ruled out, particularly when it occurs in a woman of the carcinoma age group. The differential diagnosis to be considered is inflammatory carcinoma. This differentiation is sometimes difficult. Simple acute mastitis, not occurring during lactation, results from infection of sweat or sebaceous glands. These infections are generally superficial and confined to a specific area.

Deep breast abscesses and diffuse mastitis not associated with lactation may have a hematogenous origin or result from infection in a secreting nipple.

Roentgenology

Acute mastitis appears as an increased density in the mammogram. If mastitis occurs as is usual in a young woman currently lactating, the already hypertrophied and dense breast parenchyma may make roentgen recognition of the disease very difficult. The same is true of breast abscess occurring during lactation. Such a lesion is only roentgenologically detectable when there is sufficient interspersed fatty tissue to provide differences in density, allowing recognition of the abscess.

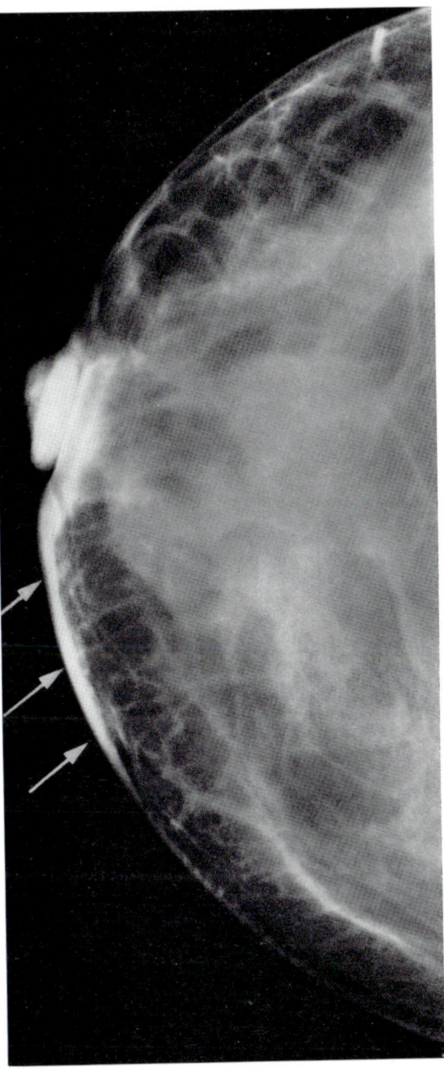

Fig. **22**.1　Skin thickening and minimal edema of the subcutaneous layer corresponding to the erythematous infiltrated skin region in a patient with acute mastitis.

Acute mastitis of lactation therefore is primarily diagnosed by clinical examination. In clinically atypical cases, however, mammography is still indicated in order to explore the possibility of underlying carcinoma. In such cases, however,

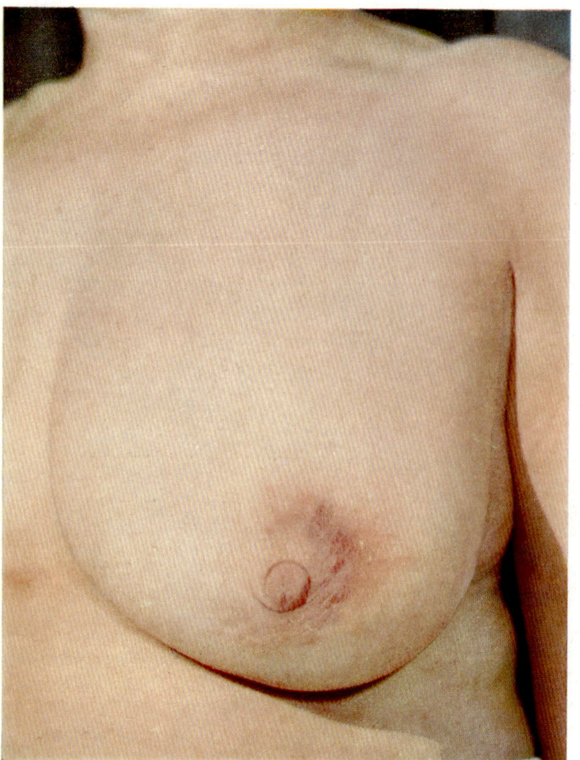

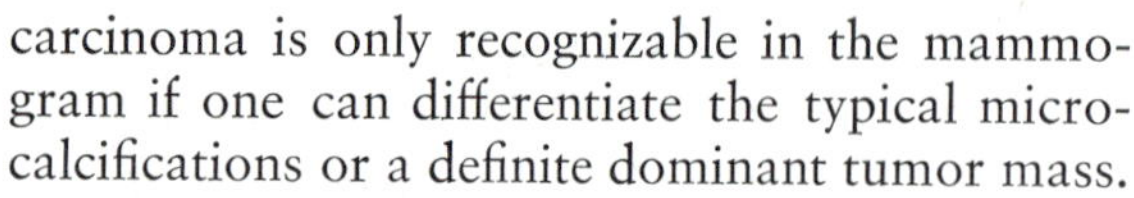

Fig. **22**.2a   59-year-old woman. Photograph of the left breast: Erythema and swelling of the skin lateral to the areola.

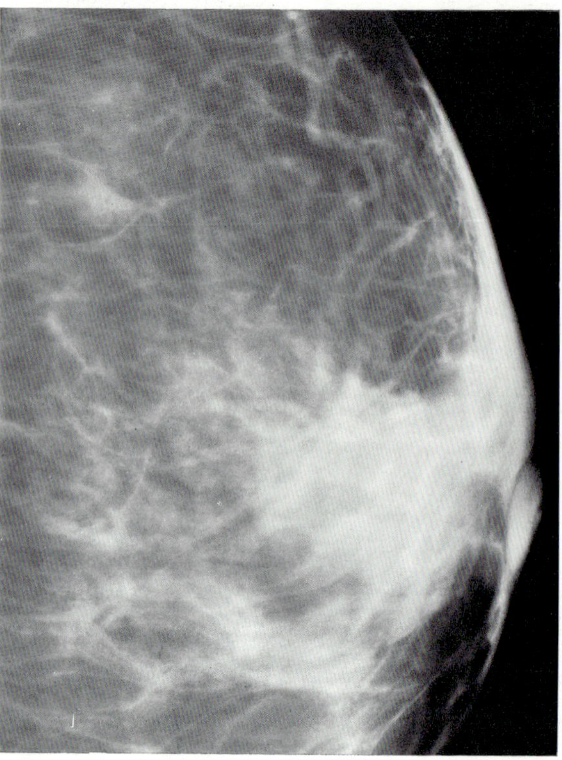

Fig. **22**.2b   Mammogram: Areola and periareolar skin is thickened; further laterally the skin thickness diminishes. Subareolar edematous changes. Normal connective tissue trabeculation, no secondary signs of malignancy.

carcinoma is only recognizable in the mammogram if one can differentiate the typical microcalcifications or a definite dominant tumor mass.

Superficial mastitis may be recognized by edema of the skin and infiltration of the subcutaneous fatty tissue (fig. 22.1). The normally radiolucent subcutaneous tissue becomes cloudy and the usual trabecular markings of connective tissue are ill-defined.

Skin thickening may be seen with acute mastitis secondary to edema but also from inflammatory carcinoma secondary to carcinomatous infiltration and/or edema of the skin. The roentgen differentiation between infiltrating carcinoma or skin edema from other causes is not completely reliable. Clinical observations, follow-up studies and therapeutic results decide the ultimate diagnosis.

Retromammary mastitis as seen in older women produces a diffuse, poorly marginated area of increased density easily localized within the predominantly fatty breast. There is edematous thickening of the overlying skin which gradually tapers to the normal skin thickness beyond the periphery of the infectious process (fig. 22.2a and b). A prominant venous pattern may be associated.

Retromammary mastitis has a tendency to spread locally in a stellate fashion ending in spiked borders or blending imperceptibly into normal breast tissue (fig. 22.3a). This differentiates the inflammatory process from carcinoma. However, the diagnosis needs to be supported by clinical findings, and response to antibiotic treatment (fig. 22.3b and c).

Abscesses may be single or multiple. In the mammogram acute abscesses will have poorly defined borders surrounding a central homogeneous density whereas mature, encapsulated abscesses are characterized by sharp borders (fig. 22.4a and b). A definite diagnosis of abscess cannot be made on the roentgenogram alone. Aspiration of pus with bacterial cultures are required for final diagnosis. Following aspiration an abscess

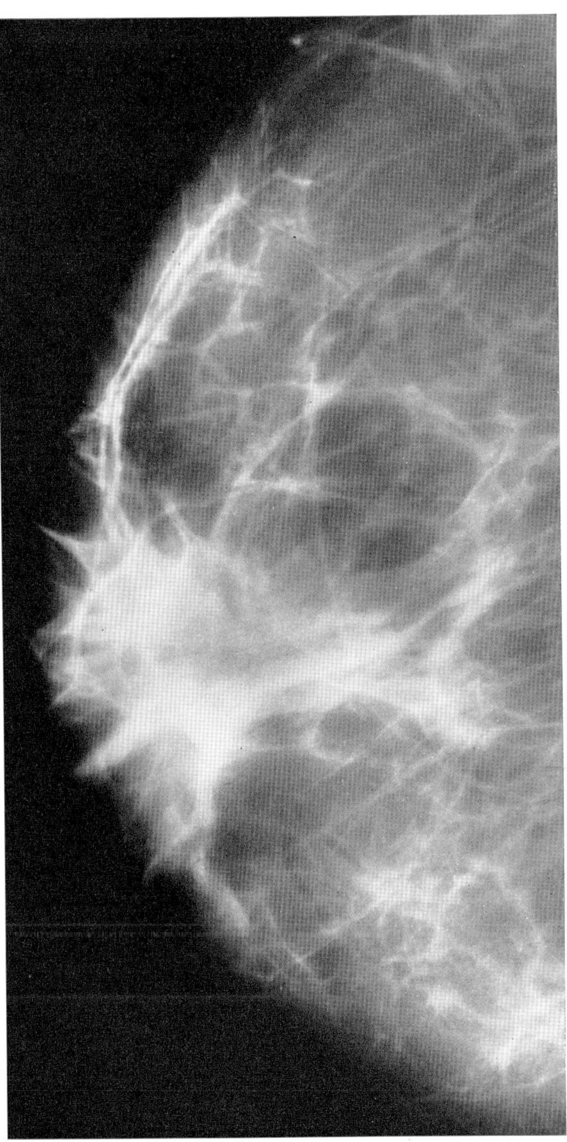

Fig. **22**.3a

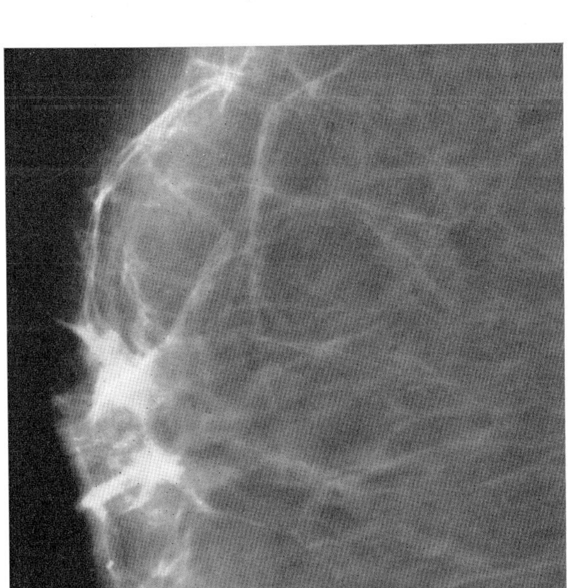

Fig. **22**.3b

Fig. **22**.3 Serial examination of subareolar mastitis.

a) Large bizarre subareolar density with radiating extensions and no definite borders. No secondary signs of malignancy. Clinically: Inflammatory process.

b) Serial examination after 1 week of antibiotic therapy: Significant decrease in size of the process.

c) Follow-up examination 1 month later: Further regression of the process with minimal residual subareolar fibrosis.

Fig. **22**.3c

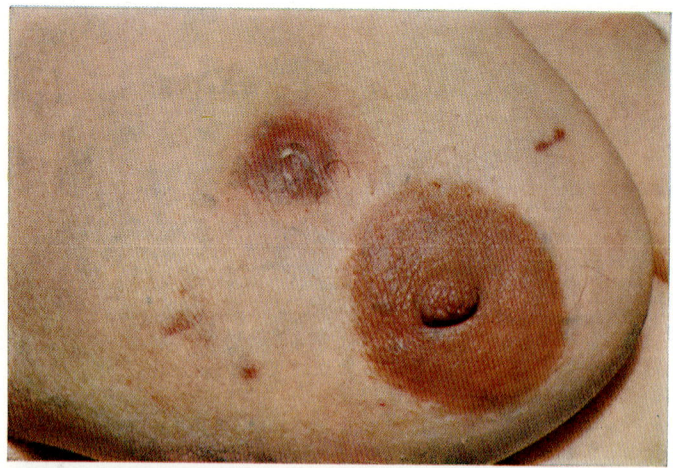

Fig. **22**.4a   Mastitis with abscess. There is blue-red discoloration of the skin at the point of perforation.

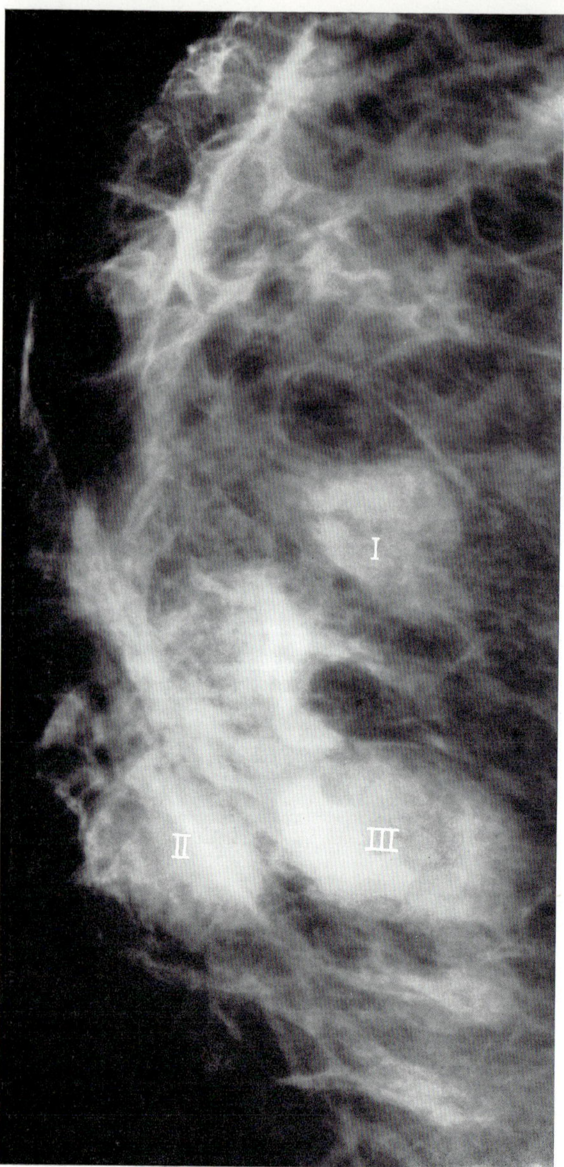

Fig. **22**.4b   Multiple abscesses in mastitis. Several rounded masses with partly smooth and partly ill-defined borders.

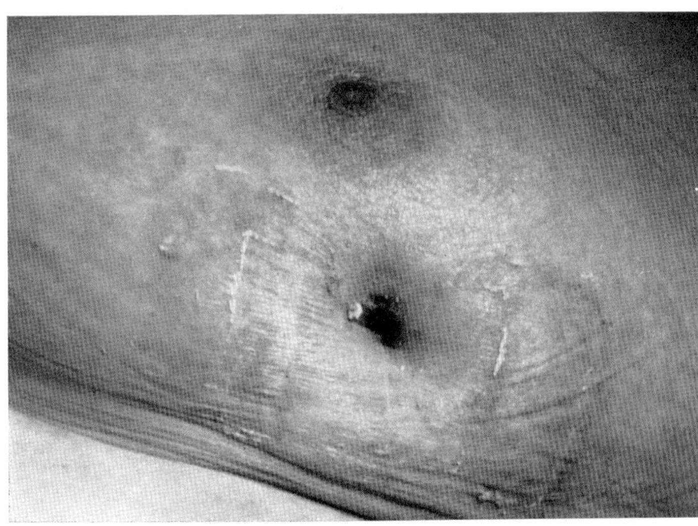

Fig. **22**.5a   Fistula inferior to the nipple recurrent over several years.

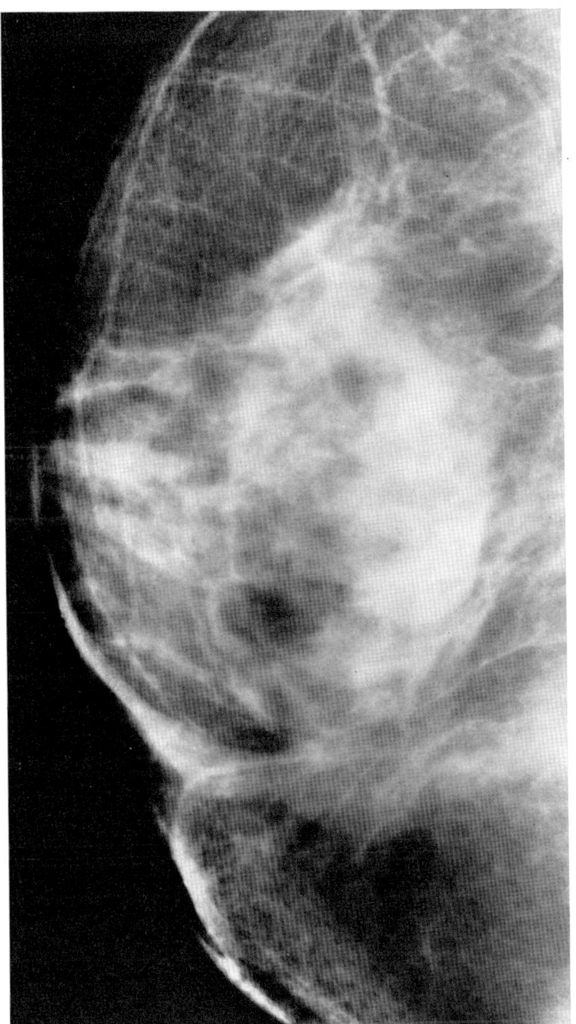

Fig. **22**.5b   Mammogram of the same case. Retraction and thickening of the skin at the site of the fistulous opening. Retractile connective tissue strands extend from the fistula towards the wall of the thorax. This indicates reactive fibrosis.

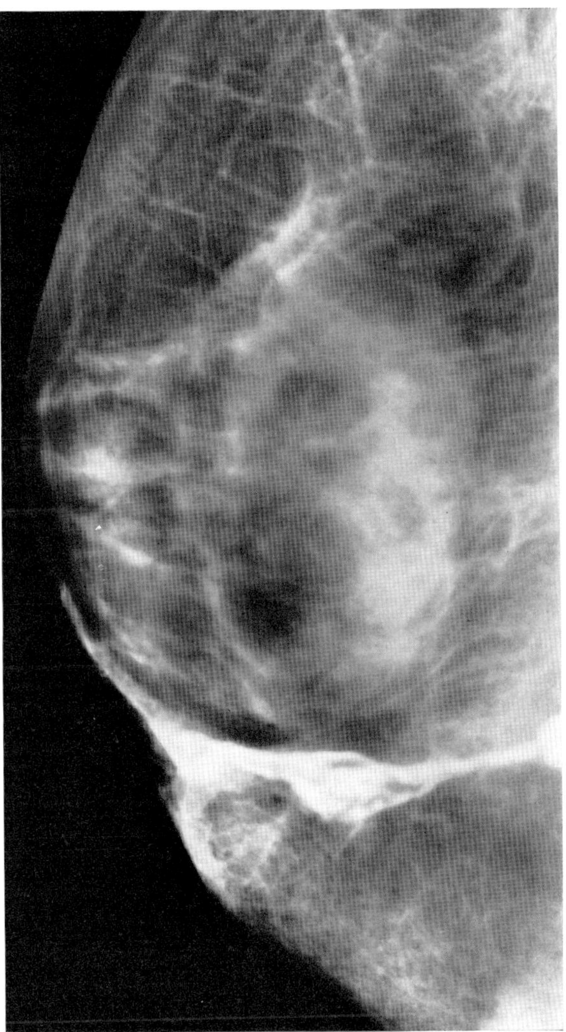

Fig. **22**.5c   Sinugram. Several irregular fistulous tracts with a "cystic" dilatation near the thoracic wall.

cavity should under no circumstances be injected with air. After aspiration the abscesses will regress if antibiotic therapy is instituted. In other cases incision and drainage is necessary.

Fistula formation in the breast appears to be rare (ATKINS 1955; INGLEBY and GERSHON-COHEN 1957, 1960).

Among other causes of mastitis one should mention chronic recurrent abscesses such as tuberculosis and chronic aseptic, so-called chemical inflammations such as plasma cell mastitis.

If a patient presents with a fistula of the breast one should determine the course and extent of the fistula by injection of contrast material (fig. 22.5 a, b and c). Fistulas opening into the areola most commonly represent secondarily infected lactiferous ducts draining acessory breast parenchyma. It is to be remembered, however, that fistulas of the breast may have their origin in an osteomyelitis or tuberculosis of the anterior ribs or in an empyema. Therefore, diagnostic examination in such cases should include roentgenograms of the ribs, sternum and chest.

Chronic Mastitis — Plasma Cell Mastitis

Pathology and Clinical Findings

Chronic mastitis is an aseptic inflammation of the breast found in elderly women. There is ductal ectasia containing calcified inspissated secretions. Connective tissue thickening in the walls of the milk ducts results in concentric or eccentric narrowing on the lumina. Histologically, numerous plasma cells and eosinophils are found (fig. 23.1). Because of this finding the term plasma cell mastitis evolved. The presumptive cause is a "chemical mastitis" which follows extravasation of intraductal secretions into the periductal connective tissue. Therefore plasma cell mastitis is a complication of so-called "secretory diasease" of the breast (GERSHON-COHEN and INGLEBY 1952). Calcific deposits which may be intraductal, within the wall, or periductal are the result of hyaline degeneration. In this disorder there are no clinical signs of inflammation. The history generally indicates serous or milky discharge from the nipple. Frequently there is retraction of the nipple. Invariably the patient will state that these changes began years ago and have progressed very slowly. On palpation one can feel subareolar thickening but a dominant mass is generally not palpated. It is important to examine the areola and adjacent breast for "orange peel skin" alterations as well as fixation of the skin, best seen when the patient flexes the spine and the breasts become pendulous, in order to assess for malignant disease. Such changes are not seen in plasma cell mastitis.

Roentgenology

In the mammogram, plasma cell mastitis demonstrates typical radiating coarse linear, round or oval calcifications (GERSHON-COHEN et al 1956). The concomitant increased tissue density is

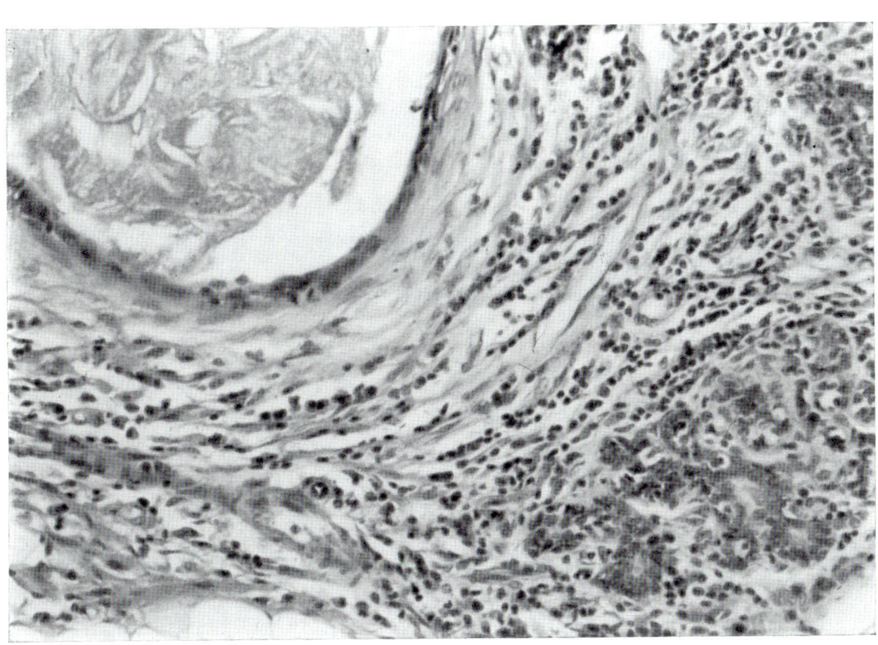

Fig. 23.1   Plasma cell mastitis, dense infiltration with lymphocytes and plasma cells in the vicinity of a dilated lactiferous duct filled with inspissated secretion.

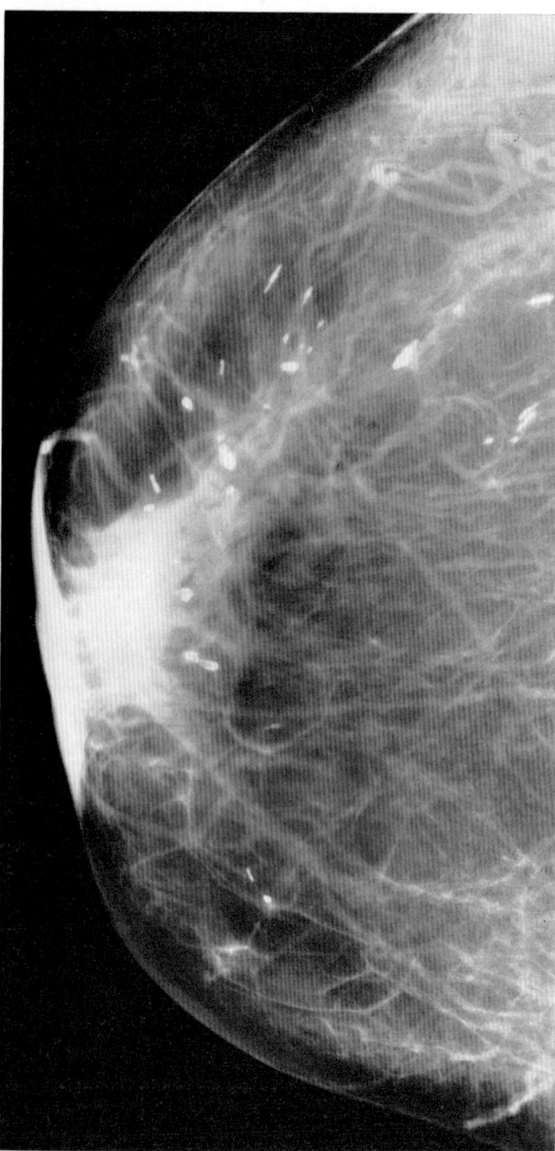

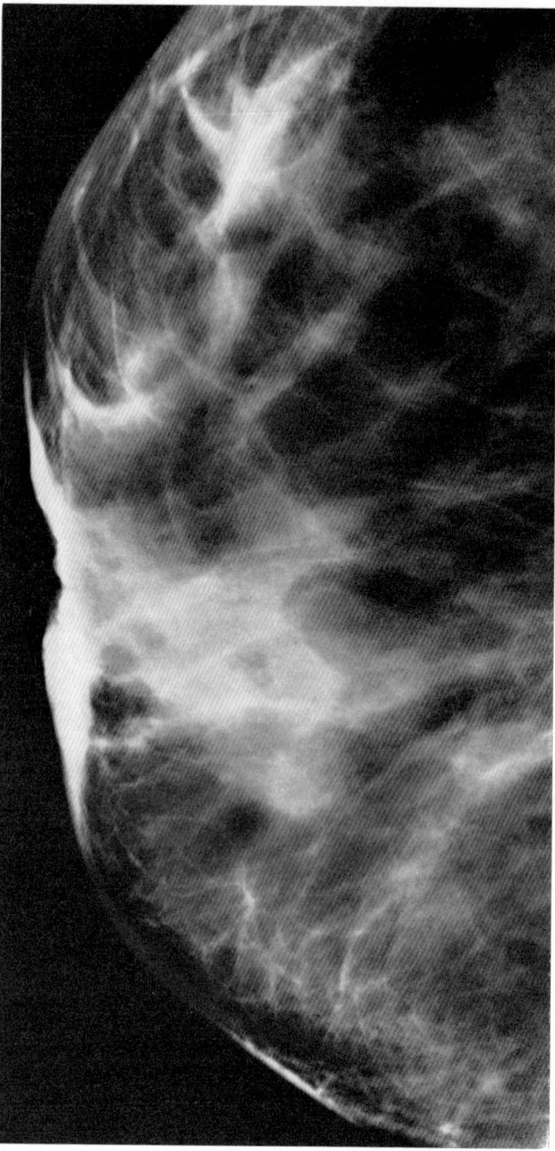

Fig. **23**.2 Plasma cell mastitis in a 62-year-old patient. Oval and linear calcifications oriented towards the areola. Triangular subareolar fibrosis. Thickening of areola and nipple. Typical plasma cell mastitis.

Fig. **23**.3 Recurrent inflammatory process in the paramamillary region for 18 months, treated multiple incisions and drainage. Gradually retracting nipple.
In the mammogram there is a triangular subareolar fibrosis without calcifications typical for mastitis. No secondary signs of carcinoma.
Roentgen diagnosis: Plasma cell mastitis? Tuberculosis? Excisional biopsy is indicated!
Histology: Plasma cell mastitis.

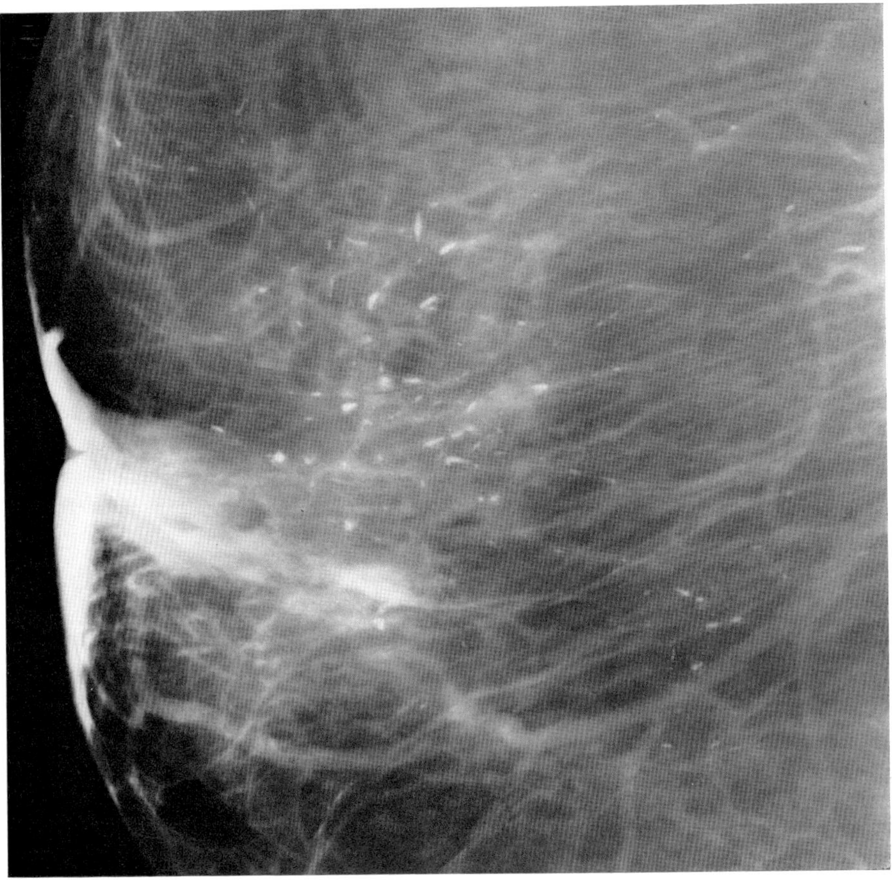

Fig. **23**.4   Typical calcifications of plasma cell mastitis. Retracted nipple secondary to subareolar fibrosis.

always subareolar in location, frequently triangular in shape with the apex of the triangle immediately beneath the nipple. There may be thickening of the areola (fig. 23.2).

Without the distinct calcifications, one cannot make the diagnosis of plasma cell mastitis in the mammogram. However, if the classical appearance is seen in one breast the diagnosis may be supposed in the other breast even in the absence of these calcifications. A subareolar triangle-shaped density even without the typical calcifications, however, should at least cause consideration of the diagnosis of plasma cell mastitis, particularly if historical data indicates gradual nipple retraction and recurrent inflammation (fig. 23.3).

In the event of advanced fibrosis and chronic inflammatory changes, retraction of the thickened areola is observed (fig. 23.4). If one recognizes the linear or rounded calcifications in the vicinity,

the diagnosis of plasma cell mastitis may be made (fig. 23.5).

Fine microcalcifications located in groups are not seen in plasma cell mastitis but instead raise suspicion of an intraductal malignancy (see differential diagnosis of microcalcification, page 261). The characteristic calcifications of plasma cell mastitis need not always be subareolar but may extend over greater portions of the breast; additional thickening or retraction of the areola and nipple are not always seen (fig. 23.6a).

The classical calcifications are seen to even better advantage in the roentgenograms of the biopsy specimen (fig. 23.6b). One can discern the spherical, periductal, ductal, as well as linear intraductal calcifications, the latter deposited within the duct secretions. The spherical calcifications probably represent areas of calcified fat necrosis (liponecrosis calcificata cystica, LE-BORGNE). The diagnostis ic more difficult if the

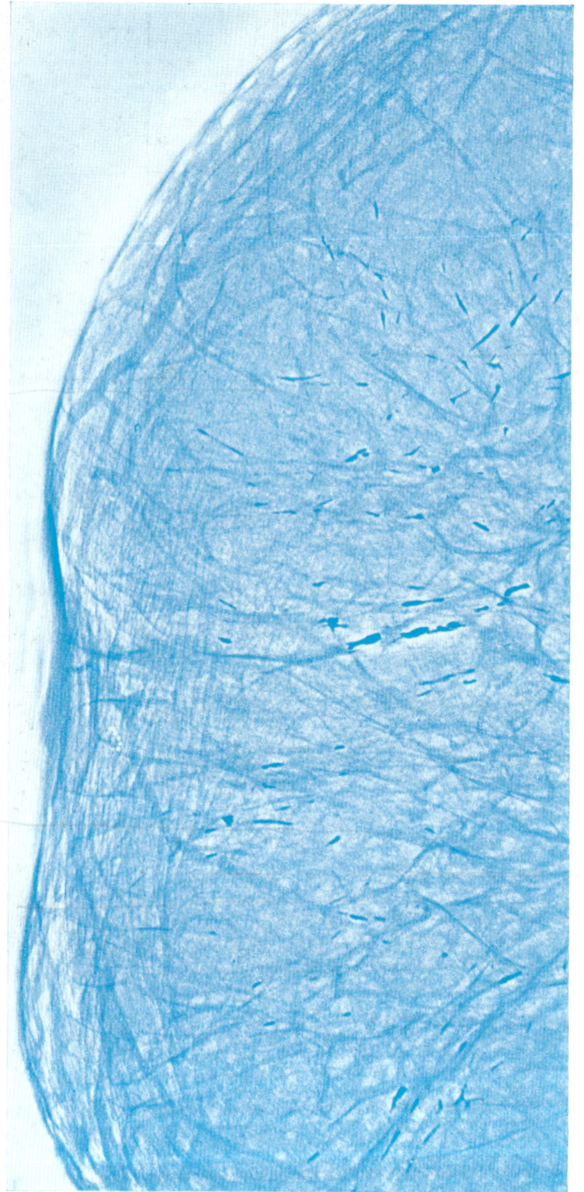

Fig. **23**.5

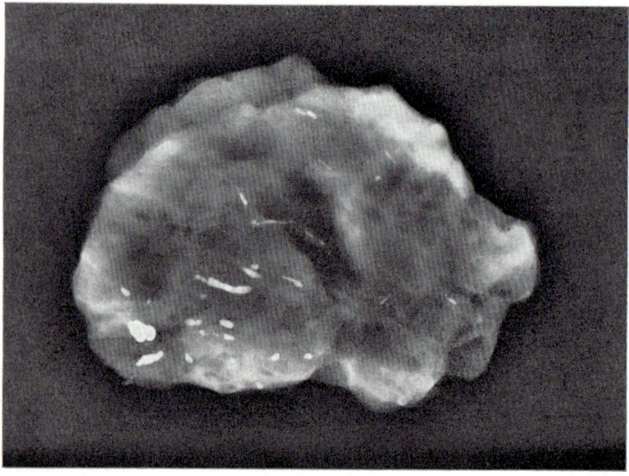

Fig. **23**.6a

Fig. **23**.6b

Fig. **23**.5   Plasma cell mastitis in a section of a xeromammogram.

Fig. **23**.6a   Plasma cell mastitis in a 65-year-old patient. Round and linear calcifications oriented towards the nipple.

Fig. **23**.6b   Roentgenogram of biopsy specimen. The typical calcifications are seen to better advantage.

disease is confined to a small section of the breast and has an atypical appearance. In this case one must carefully differentiate this condition from microcalcification of an intraductal malignancy. Invariably, however, microscopic examination allows differentiation. Vascular calcifications are not a part of the spectrum of plasma cell mastitis but instead are generally seen because most patients with this disorder are elderly women in whom such calcifications are common (fig. 23.7). Prominent veins are not associated with plasma cell mastitis and when present should alert the examiner's suspicion.

Plasma cell mastitis and carcinoma may occur together. The first report of that association and a description of the typical appearance of plasma cell mastitis was published by FINSTERBUSCH and GROSS (1934).

Plasma cell mastitis may be uni- or bilateral. The condition is not precancerous and surgical treatment is indicated only in cases of diagnostic uncertainty, to alleviate nipple retraction or to remove a cause of chronic nipple secretion. Repeat mammography after two or three months and a yearly examination thereafter are generally sufficient in following a patient with this disorder.

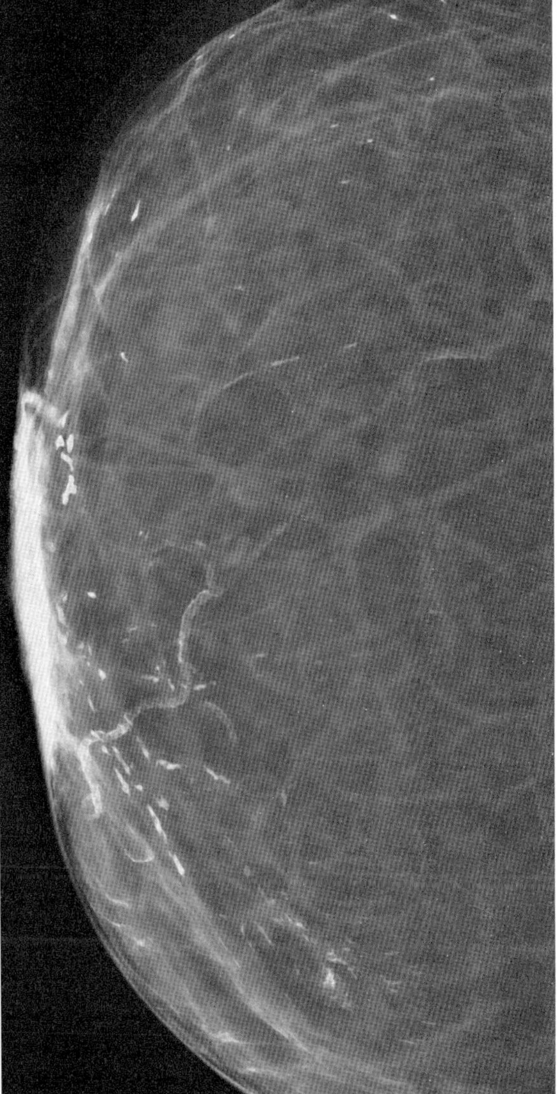

Fig. **23.**7   Plasma cell mastitis with the typical calcifications oriented towards the nipple. Subareolar arterial calcifications are also present.

Chapter 24

Mondor Syndrome

Pathology and Clinical Findings

This condition consists of a superficial thoracic venous thromophlebitis and was first described by HENRI MONDOR in 1939 and was named for him. His report was preceded by descriptions of the same condition in 1922 by FIESSINGER and MATHIEU, WILLIAMS (1931) and DANIELS (1932). Subsequent reports were made by HUGHES (1952), BRAUN-FALCO (1953), LUNN and POTTER (1954), FELDMANN et al (1954), KAPLAN and TRAPHAGEN (1957), MUSGROVE (1961), HONIG and RADO (1961), JOHNSON et al (1962), OLDFIELD (1962), and GROW and LEWISON (1963).

The Mondor syndrome may occur in young women and men as well. The thrombophlebitis or phlebothrombosis develops along the lateral thoracic wall and frequently along the lateral aspect of the breast (fig. 24.1). Occasionally several adjacent superficial veins are involved resulting in painful thrombosed cords that can be palpated immediately beneath the skin. If the skin is stretched the cords are visible (fig. 24.2 and 24.3). Occasionally the thrombophlebitis may extend along the abdominal wall all the way to the inguinal region.

Roentgenology

The inflamed veins are subcutaneous in location. They are difficult to detect in the mammogram because, unlike the thick cords palpated at

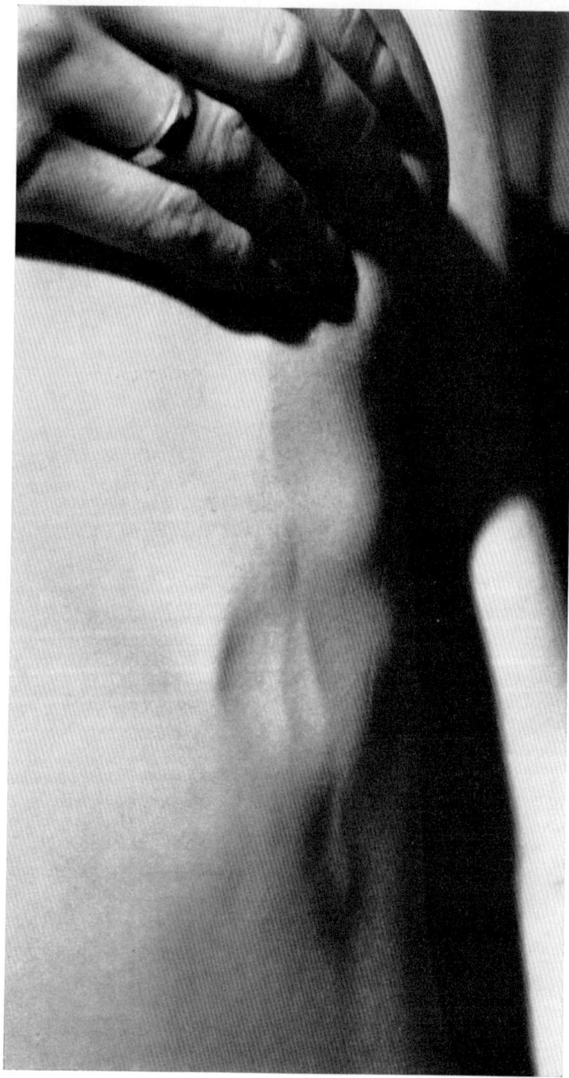

Fig. **24**.2 Mondor syndrome. Stretching the skin reveals the branching form of the thrombophlebitic cord.

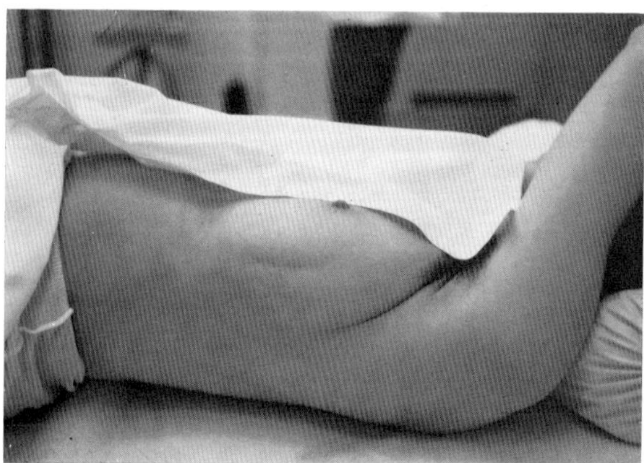

Fig. **24**.1 Mondor syndrome. Typical linear skin retraction associated with a palpable subcutaneous cord which is quite painful during the first few weeks of the disorder.

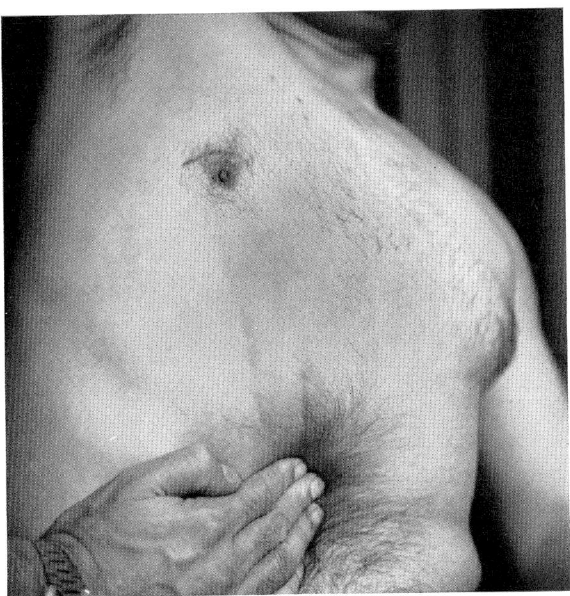

Fig. **24**.3   Typical Mondor syndrome in a male with two linear, parallel areas of skin retraction on the thoracic wall. Painful venous cords are palpable.

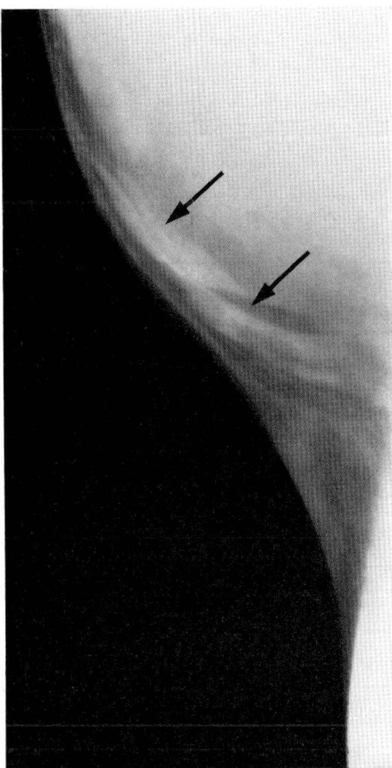

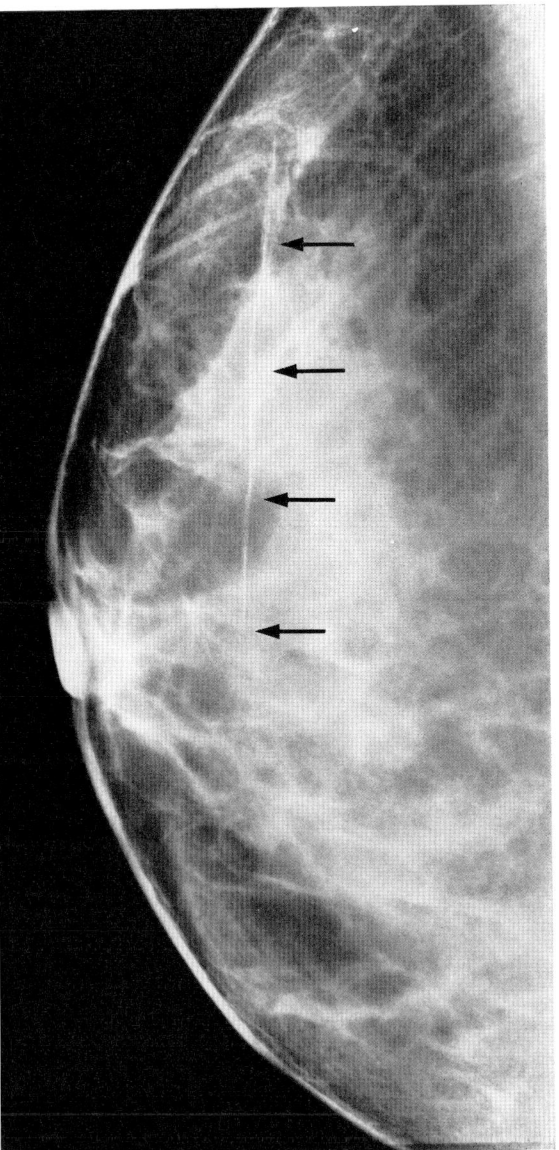

Fig. **24**.4   Mammography in a male shows a slightly thickened, branching venous cord in the subcutaneous fatty layer extending towards the anterior thoracic wall.

Fig. **24**.5   Mammogram in female shows fine, linear, elongated densities which represent the thrombosed vein (arrows).

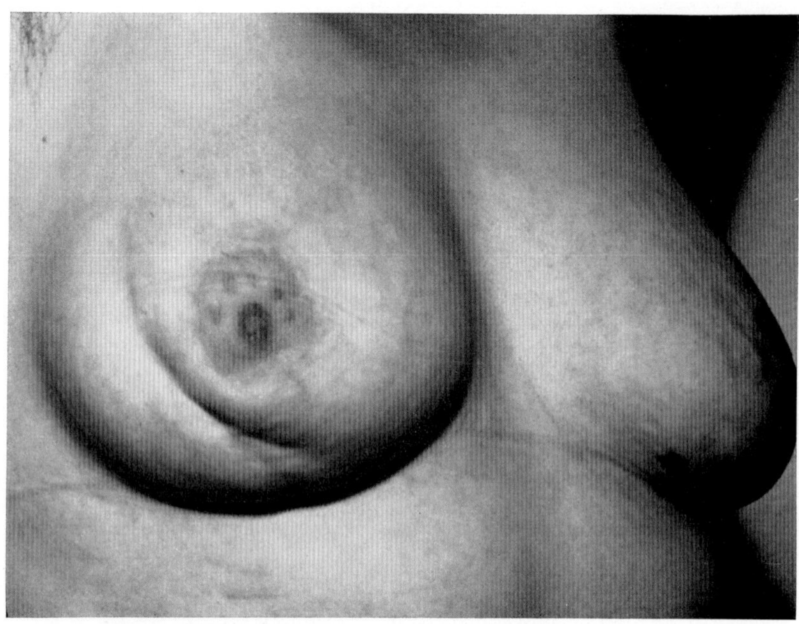

Fig. **24**.6a Unusually deep curvilinear skin retraction on the lateral aspect of the breast in Mondor syndrome. Complete disappearance after 2 weeks.

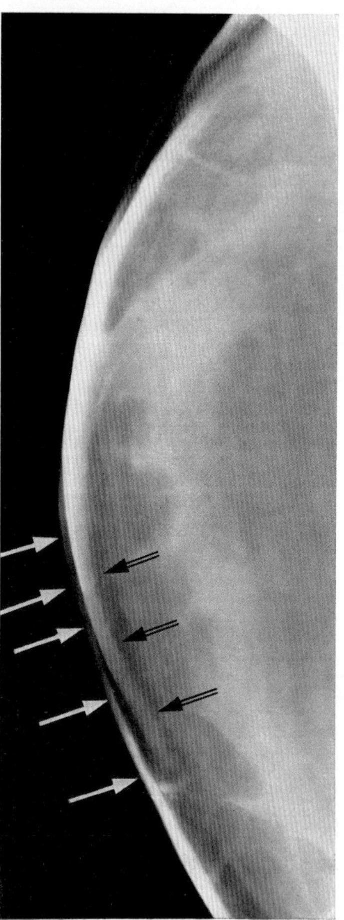

Fig. **24**.6b Mondor syndrome with retraction and thickening of the skin in the mammogram.

physical examination in the roentgenogram, they are represented as fine delicate venous stripes. Routine examination in at least two projections allows demonstration of these thin venous cords (fig. **24**.5). The exact location of the venous cords in the subcutaneous fatty layer is possible with a tangential roentgenogram using appropriate film technique (*Bipac films*) (fig. **24**.4).

Rarely there is extensive curvilinear retraction of the skin in this condition which in the roentgenogram mimics a duplication of the skin line and allows definite recognition of skin thickening (fig. **24**.6a and b). Mondor's syndrome may occur in the male; however, mammographic demonstration is not generally possible.

Chapter 25

Tuberculosis

Pathology and Clinical Findings

Tuberculosis of the breast was not an uncommon disease in previous decades. Today it is rare; 1.6% of patients with tuberculosis will have breast involvement (MESTWERDT 1969).

The source is most commonly pulmonary tuberculosis which has penetrated into the intercostal space. Involvement of the breast may occur by spread from tuberculous infraclavicular or axillary nodes. In rare cases the source is hematogenous. The clinical picture of breast tuberculosis consists of an abscess or multiple caseating nodules; the lesion is palpated as a firm, painless mass in the breast. Fluctuance of a mass generally indicates an abscess that is about to perforate the skin. There may be red or blue discoloration of the overlying skin; however, signs of inflammation are absent ("cold abscess").

Tuberculosis is not frequently considered these days when examining the breast, but this disease may mimic the findings of carcinoma especially when skin fixation and thickening accompany the tuberculous process. The correct diagnosis is made with aspiration of the tuberculous exudate and appropriate bacteriological cultures.

If there is a know focus of tuberculosis elsewhere in the body, one is more inclined to consider tuberculosis as an etiology for disease of the breast. In tuberculosis of the breast there may be secretion of tuberculous exudate from the nipple. Cytological identification of the organism,

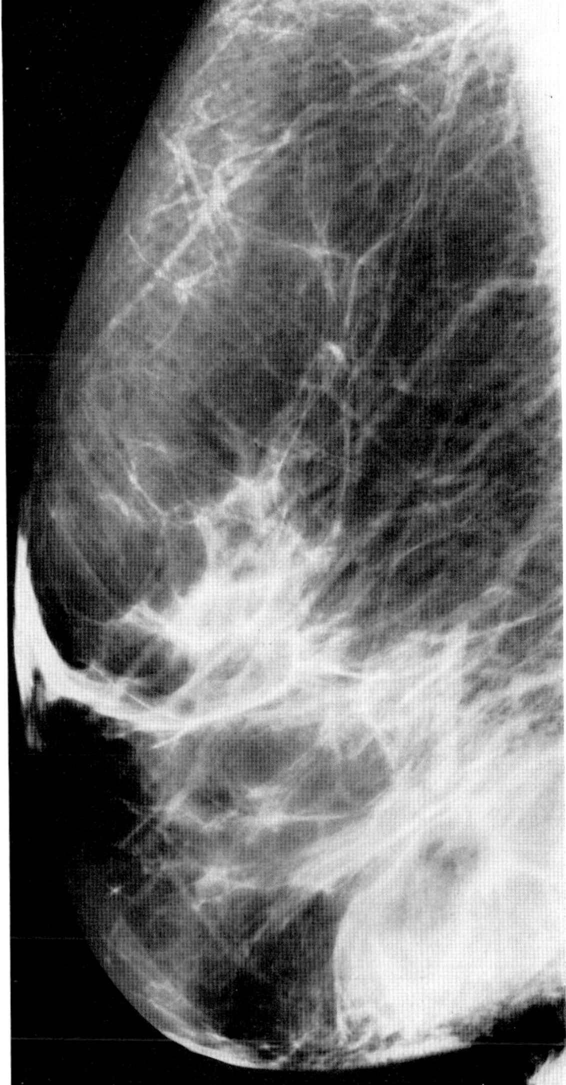

Fig. **25**.1 Clinically: Large (the size of an apple) barely movable mass close to the chest wall. Several areas of skin retraction. The impression was carcinoma.
Mammogram: A large fibrotic density corresponding to the palpated mass. There is skin thickening and the subcutaneous fatty layer is hazy. No dilated veins or microcalcifications.
Thermogram: Increased heat signal.
Radiological-thermographical diagnosis: Malignant changes.
Histology: Suspicious for tuberculosis.
Animal culture: Tuberculosis.

however, may fail if the slide preparation is not examined with a phase contrast microscope.

Roentgenology

LEBORGNE (1953) described three mammographic appearances of this disease: nodular, sclerosing and the diffuse form. Tuberculous abscesses with an ill-defined border will present as nodules. These are difficult to differentiate from routine abscesses or carcinoma.

The sclerosing form of breast tuberculosis has a stellate structure and is difficult to differentiate from scirrhous carcinoma (fig. 25.1).

The diffuse type of tuberculosis develops primarily along the base of the breast in close proximity to the thoracic wall. One may see large confluent masses. The subcutaneous fatty layer loses its sharp radiolucent appearance and there may be thickening of the overlying skin. Again it is nearly impossible to differentiate this from a diffuse infiltrating carcinoma.

Chapter 26

Actinomycosis

Actinomycosis of the breast is very rare. CUTLER (1961) reports that the disease begins as a small, very painful lump which may easily be mistaken for an ordinary abscess or a carcinoma. If the lump is incised the diagnosis is assured by observation of the typical yellow granules seen within the exudate.

No mammographic findings in this disease have been reported.

Hematoma

Fat Necrosis

Spontaneous Necrosis (Breast Infarct)

"Brassiere Syndrome"

Hematoma

Hematomas of the breast are not only the result of trauma but may also occur as a result of thrombopenia, anti-coagulant therapy, and spontaneous hemorrhage as may be seen in leukemia, or macroglobulinanemia. Spontaneous hemorrhage in the breast is occasionally the first sign of breast carcinoma. A breast hematoma without history of adequate trauma is therefore of special diagnostic significance.

Roentgen Findings

The roentgen signs of breast hematoma are: skin thickening, associate with ground-glass appearance and increase in the reticular structure of the subcutaneous fatty tissue. Another sign is diffuse increased density of the entire breast. Follow-up examination shows regression of these changes over a fairly short period of time. If the alterations persist one is dealing with a diseased breast. Circumscribed hematomas may organize and not be reabsorbed. In its earliest stages such a hematoma will have the appearance of a poorly marginated mass but later on the margins become more sharply defined and the lesion may have the appearance of a cyst.

Fat Necrosis

The breast is easily subject to injury. It is felt that fat necrosis is caused by traumatic events. In favor of this belief is the observation of *oil* cysts (see page 244) or liponecrosis with micro-cystic calcifications (see page 258) following breast surgery. Against the theory of traumatic etiology is the fact that only rarely are these lesions found after severe breast contusion.

Fat necrosis probably has several etiologies. Aside from trauma one cause could be aseptic, chemical inflammation (plasma cell mastitis) or an inflammatory process of another sort (PFEIF-FER-CHRISTIAN-WEBER syndrome). Furthermore, fat necrosis may be related to the involutional processes of the breast since it is more common in older women.

The pathological picture of fat necrosis consists of focal necrosis of fatty tissue with the development of a connective tissue capsule (oil cyst) or healing with extensive calcification.

Clinically this disorder presents as a spherical nodule which is generally superficially palpable under a layer of calcified fat necrosis. Oil cysts are identified as small nodules within the confines of a surgical scar.

A deep lying focus of fat necrosis may cause skin retraction and thus mimic carcinoma.

Deep small calcific foci of fat necrosis are asymptomatic and are not palpable.

Roentgenology

In the roentgenogram the fat necrosis appears as an area of nodular fibrosis (see page 296) or typical multiple cystlike calcifications (fig. 27.1a and b). These spherical calcifications have a diameter of 2 to 3 mm. The cystlike or ringlike calcifications occasionally contain further punctate calcifications. Such calcific foci of fat necrosis may be single, or multiple, are frequently in the superficial portion of the parenchyma, may be found within areas of fibrotic breast changes and also may appear bilaterally. LE-BORGNE (1967) termed this condition "liponecrosis microcystica calcificata".

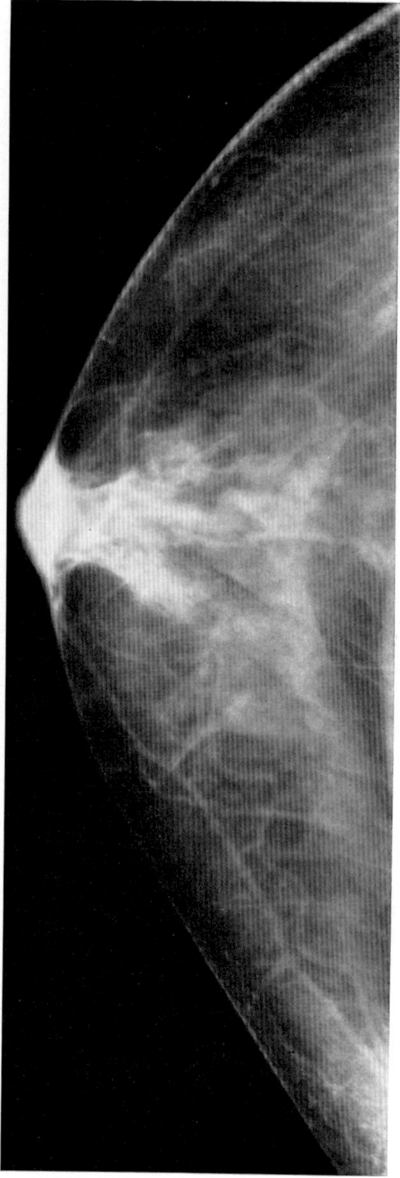

Fig. **27.**1a

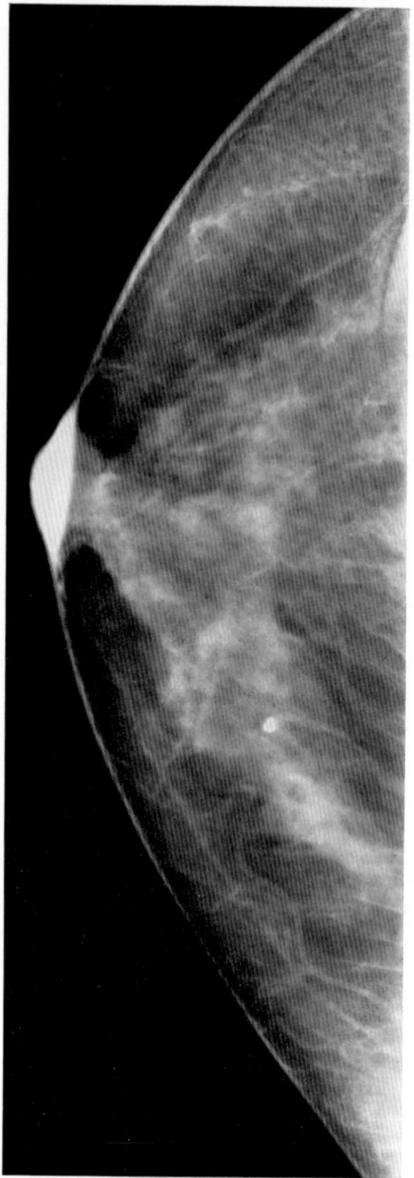

Fig. **27.**1b

Fig. **27.**1a, b   Development of liponecrosis microcystica calcificans within a space of 7 months.

In favor of a traumatic etiology in such breast calcifications is the fact that they are frequently seen after biopsies or cosmetic breast surgery (see page 242). Occasionally it may also be seen in the vicinity of a carcinoma (see fig. 32.4a).

Large cystlike calcifications which do not have the typical true spherical or ringlike shape are rarely seen. LEBORGNE has termed these variants as macrocystic calcified fat necrosis. We have seen this in calcified oil cysts (page 245).

An unusual collection of multiple small and larger calcified areas of fat necrosis was reported in both breasts of a 40-year-old woman (fig. 27.2) by ALBRING (1970). Numerous cystlike, complete or incomplete calcific rings with smooth borders sometimes of a granular consistency, most of them round, some oval, were distributed primarily in the subcutaneous fat layer and in the superficial parenchymal tissue. The history in this patient was non-contributory. There was no evidence of nipple secretion. A satisfactory explanation for the appearance of these numerous foci of fat necrosis in both breasts was not determined in this case. One can presume that it might represent the PFEIFFER-CHRISTIAN-WEBER syndrome. This disease consists of a nonsuppurative, painful, nodular panniculitis, associated with recurrent fever and distributed primarily in the subcutaneous tissues of the trunk and extremities but also in the breast (LEONHARDT 1968).

LEBORGNE (1967) has described a similar case; however, there was no histological confirmation.

Spontaneous Necrosis (Breast Infarct)

Infarction which may involve part of the breast, predominantly the lower hemisphere, or the entire breast is the result of thrombotic disease. Infarcts of this sort have included necrosis of the connective tissue and overlying skin (VERHAGEN 1954). There appears to be some connection with dicumarol therapy. CONSIGLIO et al (1967) assume that the cause of breast infarcts is based on an arteritis with subsequent thrombosis. HAAGENSEN (1971) cites a case originally reported by SUSTERSIC (1962), which occurred in a heart patient who had been taking sulfonamides and penicillin; however, the exact etiology was not determined. HAAGENSEN has not observed a case of spontaneous breast necrosis in his clinic. We have also not observed this lesion.

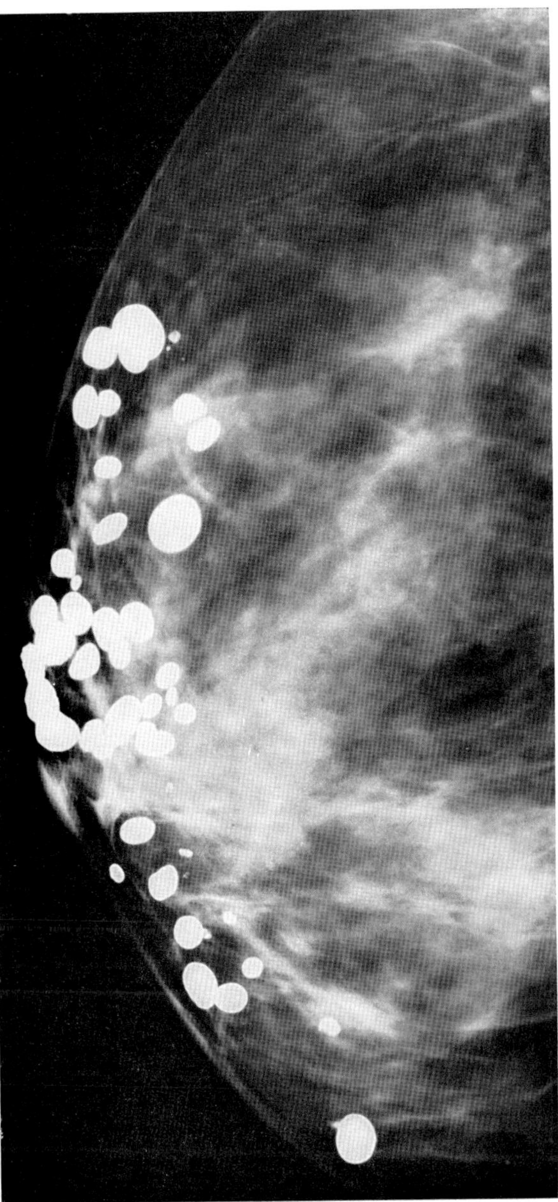

Fig. **27**.2 Numerous spherical calcifications within the subcutaneous fatty tissue: Multiple calcified foci of fat necrosis. Similar findings were present in the other breast. Nonsuppurative nodular febrile panniculitis.

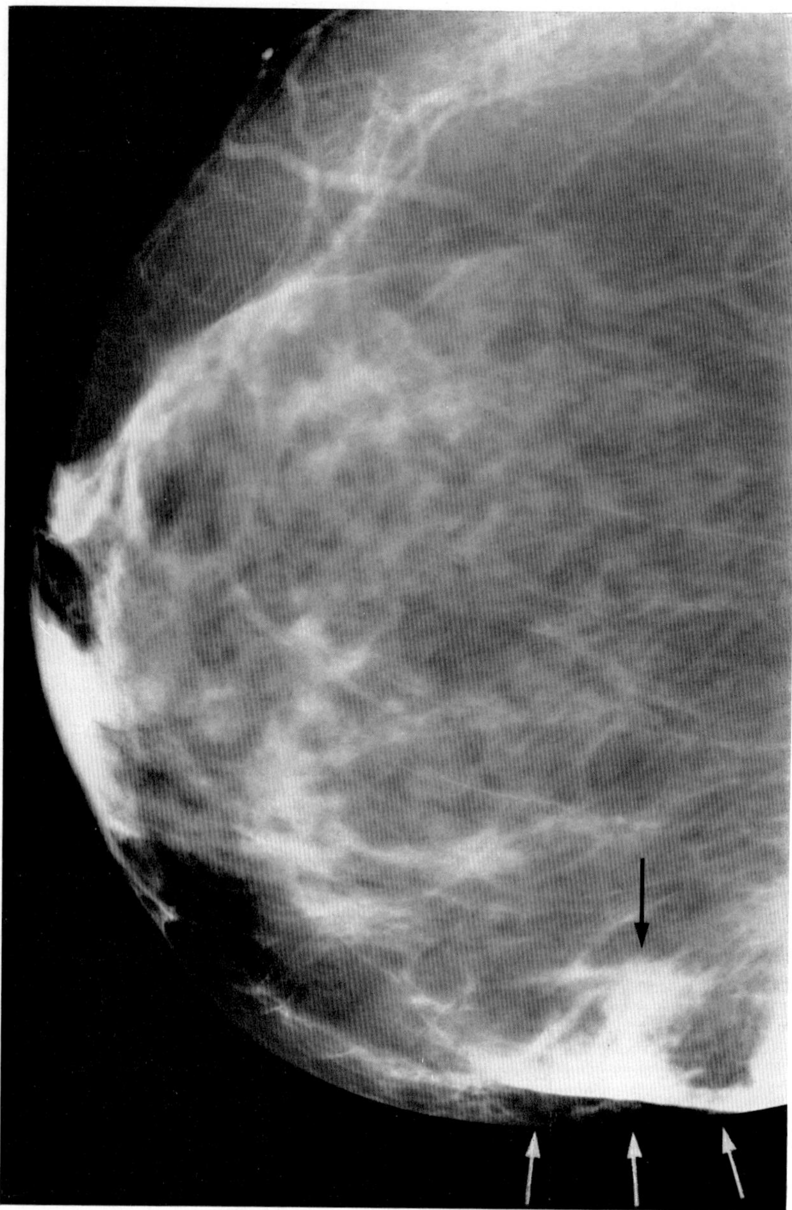

Fig. **27**.3 Round soft tissue density (arrow) with overlying skin thickening (arrows) immediately in front of the inframammary fold. No microcalcifications or increased vascularity. Serial follow up examinations showed no change. "Brassiere breast".

Brassiere Syndrome

As a result of a chronic poorly-fitting, pressure-exerting brassiere there may be thickening of the skin and subcutaneous fibrotic reaction of the breast particularly in the inferior portion. This is particularly the case in large fatty breasts. Clinically one cannot differentiate this lesion from a small carcinoma or inflammatory process with overlying skin fixation and thickening. GERSHON-COHEN (1970) called these changes "brassiere breasts".

Roentgenology

In the mammogram one notes thickening of the skin and subcutaneous connective tissue proliferation without evidence of a carcinomatous mass or microcalcifications (fig. 27.3).

This diagnosis should be verified by a follow-up examination in a relatively short period of time. If there is any question about the diagnosis a biopsy is recommended.

Chapter 28

Abnormalities of the Skin

Nevi and Fibromas of the Skin

Pigmented or nonpigmented nevi as well as fibromas of the skin of the breast when observed tangentially in the mammogram appear as sharply circumscribed skin thickening.

In the orthograde projection these lesions are seen as round or lobular densities with very sharply defined margins (fig. 28.1a and b). There may be a radiolucent halo around the lesion if it is pushed into the surrounding skin as may occur for example in a compression mammogram. These lesions may cause the misdiagnosis of intramammary cyst, fibroadenoma or even carcinoma. Clinical examination, however, allows a correct diagnosis.

The same remarks apply to neurofibromatosis (fig. 28.2a and b).

Sebaceous Cyst

Small sebaceous cysts are not uncommon in the skin. Occasionally they may be as small as 2 to 3 mm in diameter and still will be palpable. If the cyst reaches a diameter of 1 to 2 cm it can present a problem in the differential diagnosis of carcinoma. This is particularly the case since such sebaceous cysts frequently are accompanied by inflammatory complications and thus may mimic inflammatory carcinoma on clinical breast examination. Inflamed sebaceous cysts which cause fixation of the overlying skin, are seen as reddish or blueish tinged masses and may demonstrate central ulceration. Excision is the appropriate

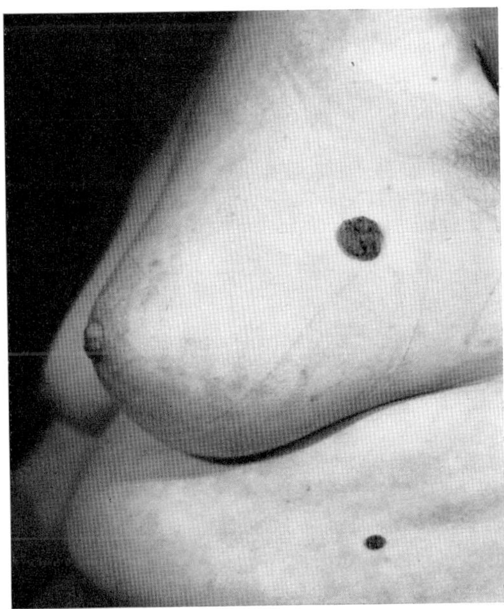

Fig. **28.**1a   Pigmented nevus of the skin.

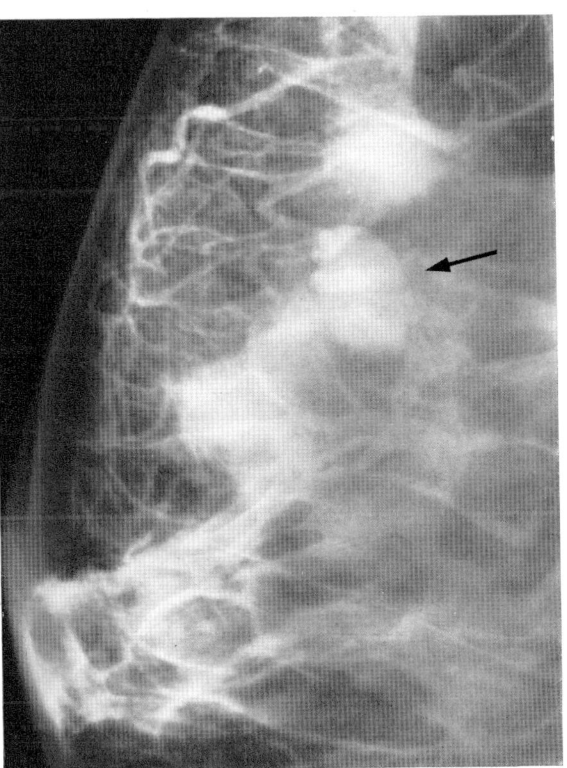

Fig. **28.**1b   Mammogram showing projection of the nevus over the breast parenchyma. This may simulate an intramammary mass.

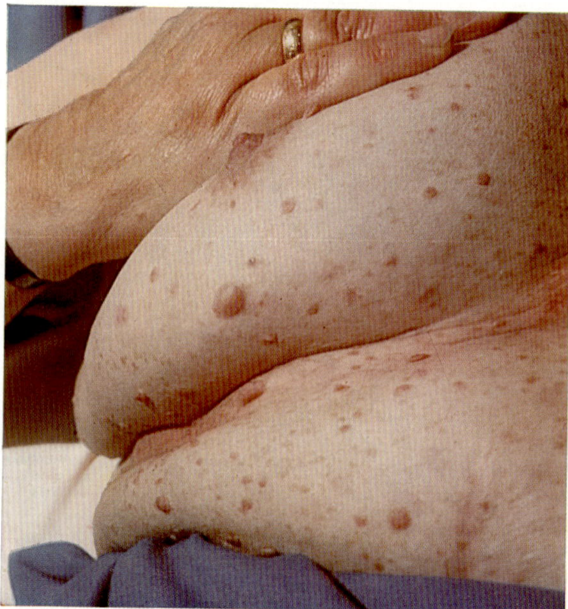

Fig. **28**.2a   Neurofibromatosis of the skin of the breast.

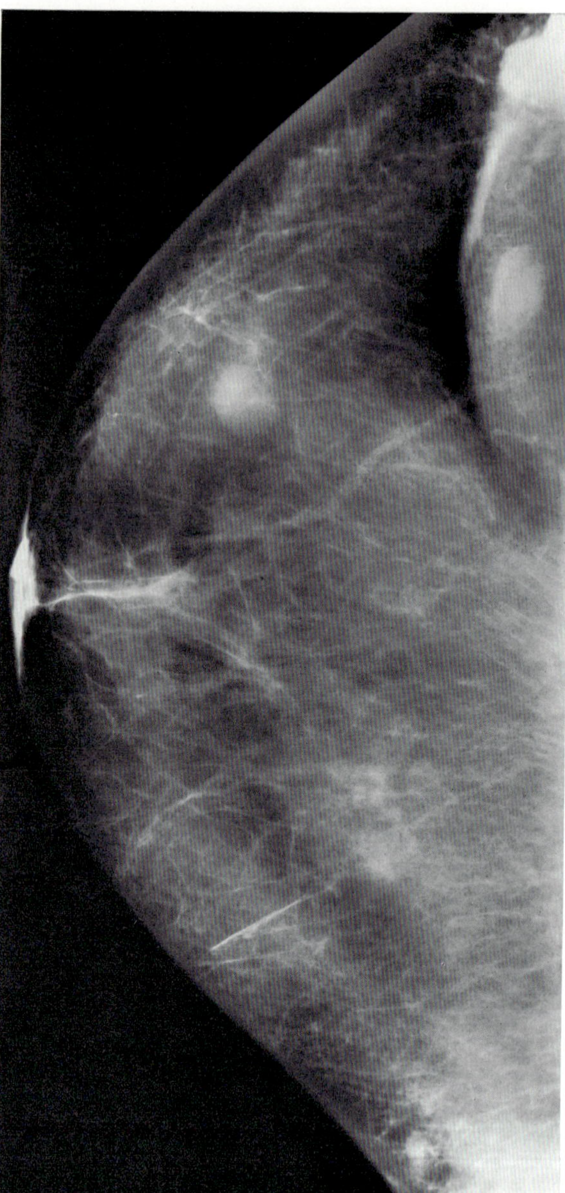

Fig. **28**.2b   The skin neurofibromas project over the mammogram simulating breast masses.

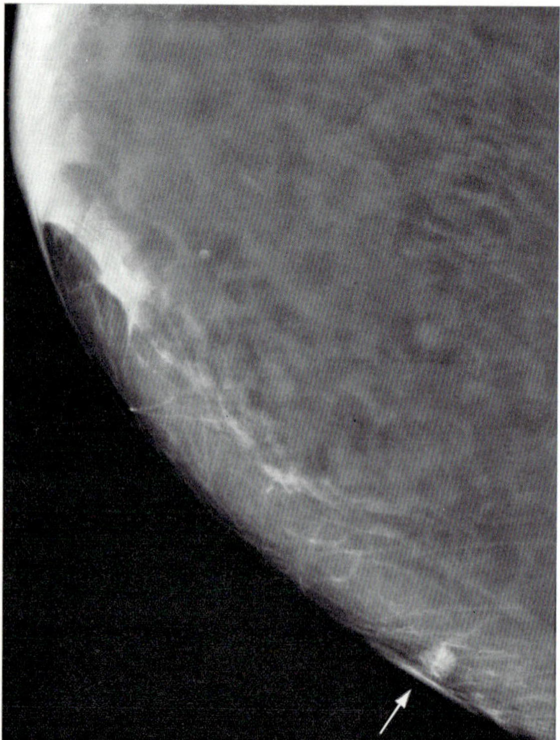

Fig. **28**.3   Inflamed skin gland. Round shadow, 4 mm in diameter, demonstrable on only one mammographic projection. There is slight thickening of the overlying skin.

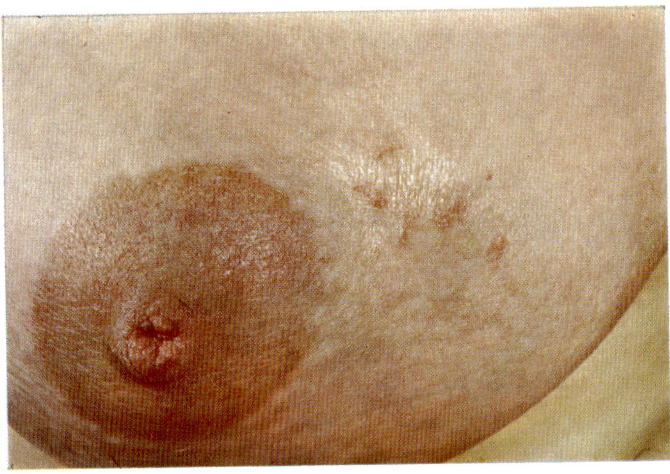

Fig. **28**.4a   White, glistening skin changes with circumscribed atrophic skin retraction.

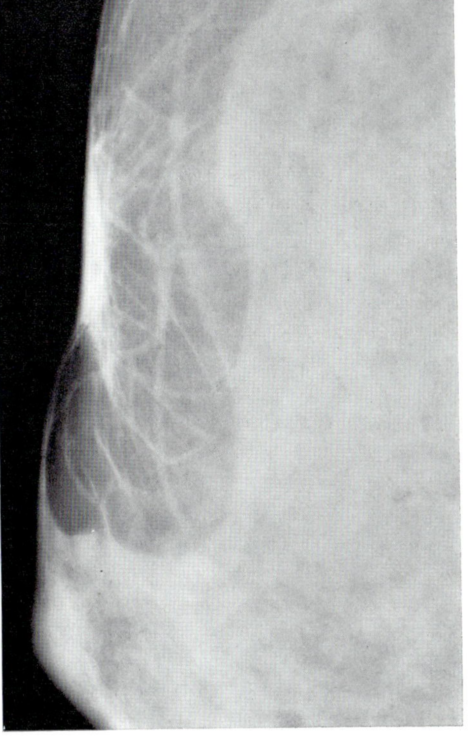

Fig. **28**.4b   Mammogram: Circumscribed form of scleroderma with localized thickening of the skin. Beneath the skin lesion there are small connective tissue strands extending through the fatty layer. No tumor mass demonstrable.

therapy. This, however, should always be accompanied by histological examination in order to avoid any chance of error.

In the mammogram, small sebaceous cysts are recognized as round or lobular masses in the immediate undersurface of the skin (fig. 28.3). They may calcify (see fig. 49.7 a). Inflammatory skin changes may accompany the lesion. Larger cysts may be difficult to differentiate from a cyst of the breast; however, the sebaceous cysts are always in close apposition to the undersurface of the skin. They are always dense since there is some calcium in the contents. This differentiates such lesions from the oil cysts previously described. The sharp margin will become indistinct if there is adjacent edema secondary to the frequently associated inflammatory changes. Under such conditions the cysts are difficult to differentiate from carcinoma as well as abscess. The diagnosis of infected sebaceous cysts is supported by the observation that the process is in close communication with the undersurface of the skin and is generally confined to the subcutaneous fatty layer.

Scleroderma

Diffuse as well as circumscribed forms of scleroderma can occur in the breast.

We have observed a localized area of scleroderma immediately lateral to the areola in a 26-year-old woman (fig. 28.4a). The mammogram revealed a sharply defined and marginated thickening of the skin associated with fine connective tissue septa traversing the subcutaneous fatty layer (fig. 28.4b). The breast was otherwise normal. In the subcutaneous tissue a delicate but otherwise normalappearing vein was observed. Histological examination of the excised skin verified the clinical and roentgen diagnosis of circumscribed scleroderma.

Malignant Disease of the Breast

The majority of malignant breast tumors are of epithelial origin (carcinoma) and only rarely arise from connective tissue (sarcoma). Other malignant diseases affecting the breast are secondary to systemic neoplasms (leukemia, lymphoma).

There are numerous ways to classify malignant disease of the breast based either on clinical or pathological characteristics. Although roentgen examination of the breast is reliable as a clinical method of differentiating benign from malignant diseases there is still a need for more exact pathological classification. The roentgen characteristics of malignant breast tumors (for example, nodular, stellate dominant masses, carcinomatous microcalcification, signs of infiltration), are not sufficient to form a method of classification because the signs are not specific enough to definitely differentiate malignant from certain benign diseases. The classification of McDivitt and Stewart (1968) also includes the pathological-anatomical characteristics of breast carcinoma. The latter classification is more suitable because it includes not only the histological structure but also the manner of development of each type of tumor.

Classification of Breast Carcinoma

Breast carcinoma arises as malignant epithelium of the lactiferous ducts or of the parenchymal lobules. Histogenetically ductal carcinoma can be differentiated from lobular carcinoma. Ductal carcinoma is by far the most frequent form. Carcinoma of the lactiferous ducts does not infiltrate in its early stages but later on it is invariably infiltrating. Commonly one sees both infiltrating and noninfiltrating processes simultaneously. As long as ductal carcinoma proliferates within the confines of the duct and its branches and there is no invasion through the basal membrane (preinvasive or so-called carci-noma in situ), there is no danger of metastases. In *noninfiltrating ductal carcinoma* two different histological types are recognized. Most commonly the neoplastic cells will proliferate and spread in an intraductal fashion (solid noninfiltrating intraductal carcinoma also known as "comedocarcinoma"). A more rare type of noninfiltrating ductal carcinoma is the fine, papillary type (papillary or cribriform, noninfiltrating ductal carcinoma). Frequently there is a mixture of both types.

In later stages the intraductal carcinoma becomes an infiltrating type (infiltrating comedocarcinoma or infiltrating papillary carcinoma).

Paget's carcinoma is a ductal carcinoma which may be in the noninfiltrating or infiltrating state, but which is associated with an intra-epidermal tumor component in the region of the areola and nipple.

Infiltrative ductal carcinoma according to macroscopic and histological criteria may be subdivided as follows: In widespread or anaplastic ductal carcinoma, in accordance with the amount of connective tissue response, one differentiates *scirrhus, carcinoma solidum simplex* and *medullary carcinoma*. In the scirrhus type the stromal proliferation of productive fibrosis is most prominent, less so in carcinoma solidum simplex. In carcinoma simplex, there is also connective tissue proliferation but it may vary more or less in the central or peripheral portions. Therefore scirrhus and carcinoma solidum simplex are combined in a single group called "infiltrating ductal carcinoma with productive fibrosis" (McDivitt et al 1968). About 80% of breast carcinomas fall into this category. In anaplastic carcinoma, not infrequently, there is found a proliferation of dysplastic adenoid structures within the tumor (anaplastic adenoid carcinoma with scirrhus or partly solidus growth characteristics).

In *medullary carcinoma* the carcinomatous epithelial growth predominates and the connective tissue component is seen only as delicate septa surrounding the complexes of tumor cells. *Colloid carcinoma* is a ductal carcinoma with excessive mucous production whereby carcinomatous cells and also dysplastic adenoid cellular formations are scattered in a mucoid mass (mucoid adenocarcinoma).

The so-called *"inflammatory carcinoma"* does not comprise a characteristic histological type of breast carcinoma but rather is a condition resembling clinical mastitis. It is secondary to carcinomatous invasion of subepidermal lymphatics and blood vessels with subsequent lymphatic and venous obstruction which produces the characteristic skin changes of the tumor.

Breast tumors originating from parenchymal acinar epithelial cells are much less frequent than those arising from ductal epithelium. This lobular carcinoma is characterized histologically by neoplastic reproduction of lobular parenchymal structure.

In the latter category one also differentiates non-infiltrating lobular carcinoma in situ from infiltrating types. Infiltrating lobular carcinoma is frequently of the mixed type, containing components of ductal epithelial carcinoma. Therefore these two tumor types are not always clearly separated.

Sarcomas of the breast include differentiated types, for example fibrosarcoma, hemangiosarcoma, liposarcoma as well as reticulum cell sarcoma and lymphosarcoma; undifferentiated types such as spindle cell, round cell and polymorphous cell sarcoma have also been observed. Such tumors are rare.

Chapter 29

Intraductal Solid Carcinoma (Comedocarcinoma)

Definition and Pathology

So-called comedocarcinoma refers to a solid intraductal carcinoma. Both noninvasive forms with intact basal membrane and invasive types exist.

Macroscopically the lactiferous ducts are filled with a yellow pastelike material which at section appears similar to the small plugs (comedos) normally expressible from the skin. This is particularly evident when the carcinoma has infiltrated into the larger lactiferous ducts. Because of this phenomenon the neoplasm was named comedocarcinoma by BLOODGOOD (1934). Histologically the ducts are filled with atypical, solid plugs of epithelial tumor with a strong tendency to necrosis (fig. 29.1). Polymorphism of cells and nuclei is prevalent in distinction from papillary ductal carcinoma. The intracanalicular cellular detritus contained within carcinomatous ducts frequently may demonstrate coarse calcifications (HAMPERL 1968).

Comedocarcinoma, when it extends into the smaller branches of the lactiferous ducts may invade the appropriate parenchymal lobule (so-called secondary lobular carcinoma according to BAESSLER 1969).

The prognosis of intraductal carcinomas is better than in most other breast cancers, providing no evidence whatever of infiltration can be demonstrated either roentgenologically or histologically. According to STAPLEY et al (1955) the five-year survival of 226 cases of comedocarcinoma in the absence of lymph node metastases was 90.8%. However, in the case of demonstrable metastases this figure diminished to 36.2%.

Clinical Signs

The clinical signs of intraductal comedocarcinoma depend on the stage of the tumor. In the noninvasive form clinical and palpatory findings are generally absent. If there is nipple discharge it is more frequently withe or clear than sanguineous. (In contradistinction, the patient with papillary intraductal carcinoma will frequently seek medical help because of sanguineous discharge, an early sign of this tumor). The noninvasive comedocarcinoma is found during routine examination or because the patient complains of pain. The sensation of insects crawling on the breast may be a clinical complaint found in this tumor.

With early invasiveness of the tumor minimal thickening of breast tissue may be palpated; however the clinical findings, without roentgen

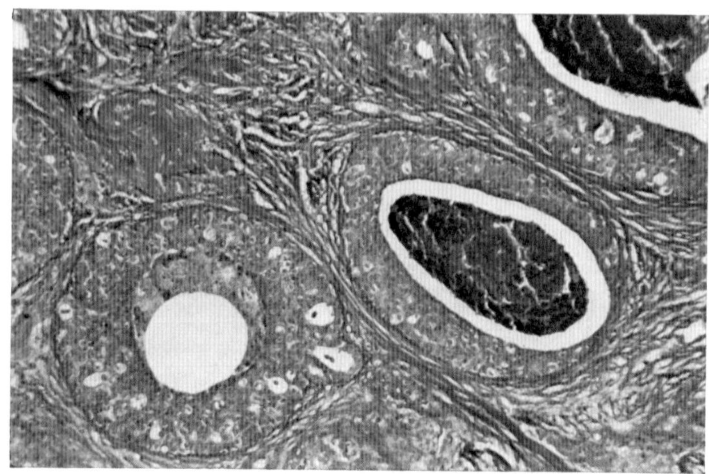

Fig. **29**.1 Comedocarcinoma: The lactiferous ducts are filled with proliferation of atypical epithelial cells surrounding a central area of necrosis.

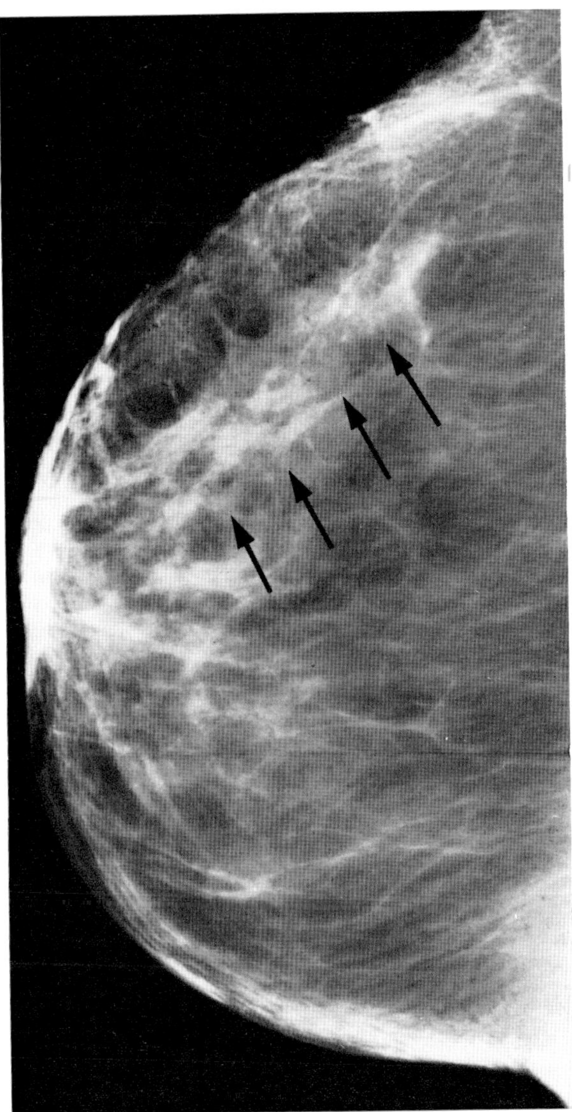

Fig. **29**.2a   Mammography of an intraductal in situ carcinoma.
Clinically: Minimal firmness palpated in the lateral aspect of the breast and observed for over $1\frac{1}{2}$ years since neither clinical nor roentgen findings were suspicious for carcinoma.

signs, usually are not impressive enough to warrant biopsy.
Only in advanced invasive stages of intraductal solid carcinoma are the usual clinical signs of breast carcinoma found (dominant masses, skin fixation, etc.).

Roentgen Findings

The most important feature of comedocarcinoma radiographically is microcalcification. Less fre-

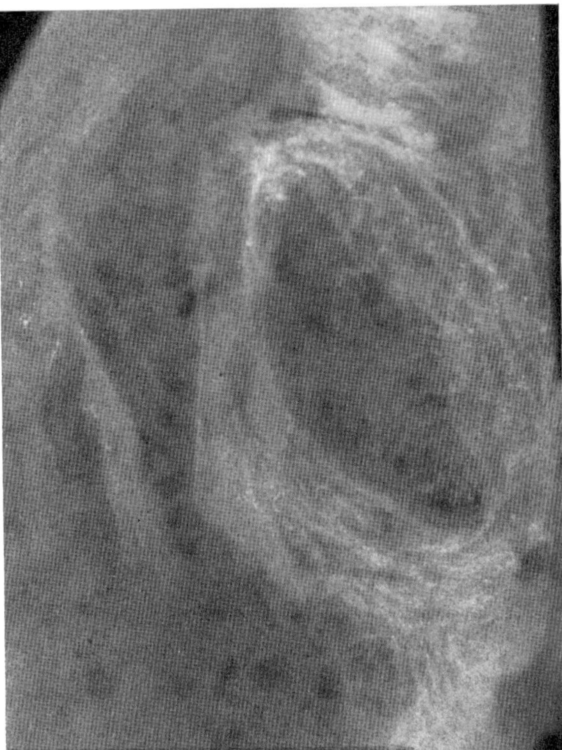

Fig. **29**.2b   Roentgenogram of specimen in paraffin block ($3\times$ magnification): Tiny microcalcifications, not visible in the original mammogram are seen.

quently cited signs are unilateral ductal ectasia or demonstration of intraductal filling defects during ductography.

Microcalcification

The first description of microcalcification in scirrhus carcinoma was written by SALOMON (1913), but the diagnostic significance of this was not recognized until 40 years later. LEBORGNE (1951) was the first to recognize microcalcification as a pathognomonic sign of carcinoma. He described the typical calcifications as "tiny, punctate or longitudinal, resembling scattered salt kernels, numerous and close together, but distributed in groups". These microcalcifications are present within or outside the tumor mass. However, they may also occur without any evidence of tumor mass at all.

According to GERSHON-COHEN et al (1962) carcinomatous microcalcifications may be distinguished from other microcalcifications because of their poorly defined borders.

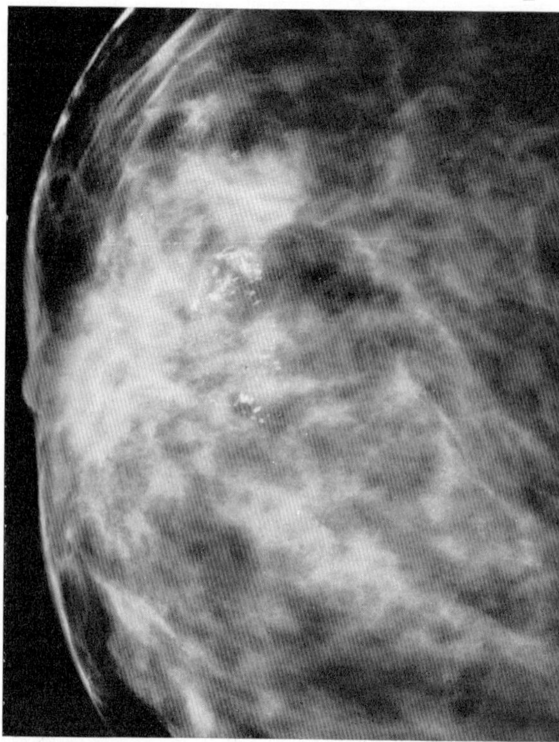

Fig. **29**.3   Subareolar tissue density with coarse and fine microcalcifications of irregular form and varying density radially distributed along the course of the lactiferous ducts. Histology: Large cell carcinoma with intra and extracanalicular invasion.

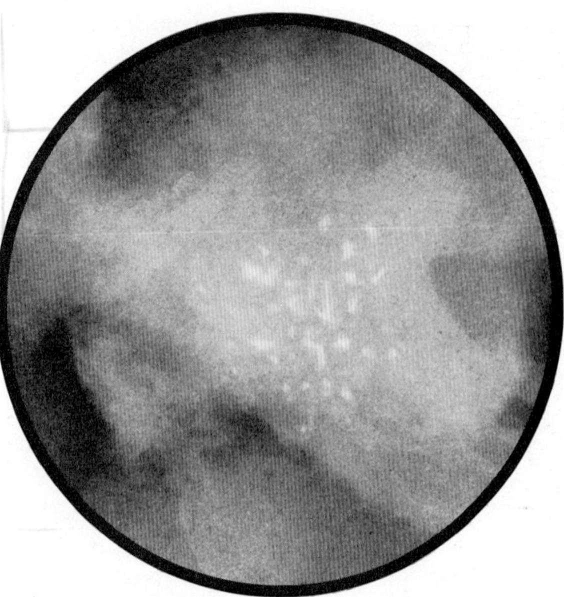

Fig. **29**.4   Roentgenogram of the biopsy specimen of an intraductal, noninvasive, clinically occult carcinoma. Magnification view reveals the typical appearance of carcinomatous microcalcifications which may be seen in noninvasive as well as invasive intraductal carcinoma.

We do not share this view of GERSHON-COHEN's and instead feel that this represents photographic unsharpness based on his experience in the premolybdenum tube era,

According to EGAN (1964) there are three requirements for the type of calcification seen with carcinomas:

1) the calcifications must be small and must not blend with one another;

2) they must be localized;

3) they must have varying density.

EGAN differentiates six types:
1) sandlike;
2) bizarre;
3) coarse and sharply bordered;
4) tear-droplike or wavy;
5) dull and round;
6) high calcific density.

BACLESSE and WILLEMIN (1967) consider microcalcifications to be typical for carcinoma when they are tiny, of varying size, round, oval or irregular, sandy or finely linear or cometlike in appearance. They may be singular or may be present by the hundreds but in general are collected in groups.

Our observations do not always agree with earlier descriptions by LEBORGNE, GERSHON-COHEN, EGAN, BACLESSE and others as regards the form, density, size, number and location of carcinomatous microcalcifications. With improvements in technique, particularly with magnification, we are presently in a better position to examine and describe these microcalcifications than was the case in earlier times. We are therefore of the opinion that only dense, crystalline, fine, sharply angulated or bizarre-appearing microcalcifications are typical of carcinoma, especially when these are located in groups, are distributed in a radiating fashion from the nipple, or are spread diffusely throughout the entire parenchyma. The typical carcinoma calcifications resemble a stone crushed by a hammer.

We have learned through our intensive studies with photographic magnification of microcalcifications that the differential diagnosis is not as simple as it seemed in earlier times. Therefore

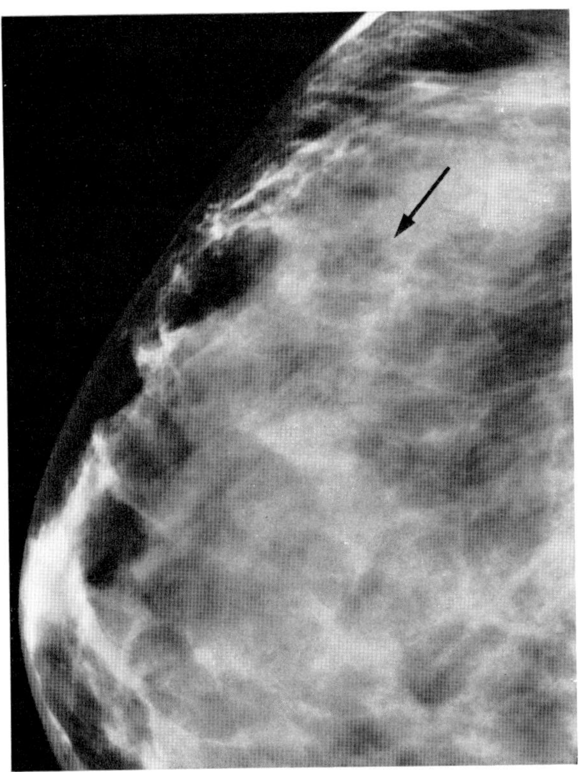

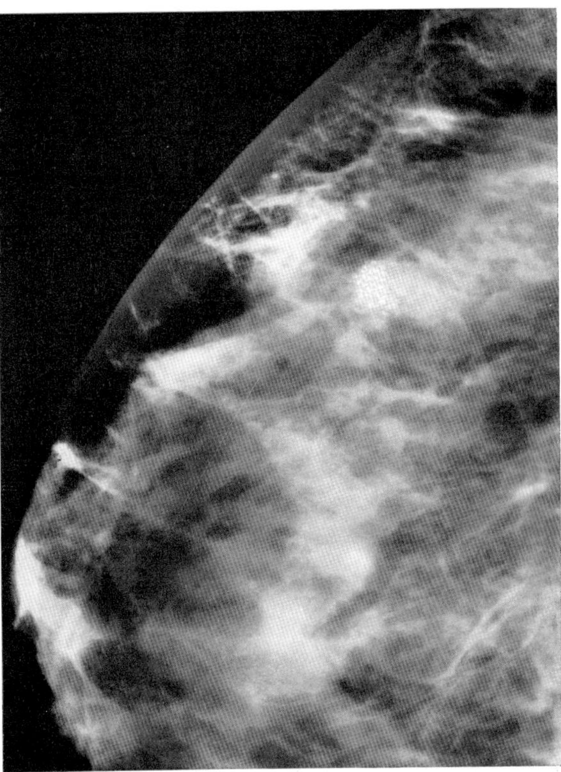

Fig. **29**.5a   Minimal increased density of a lateral portion of breast parenchyma. The arrow indicates a single calcific deposit visible with the magnifying lens. 2½ years later an intraductal comedocarcinoma was identified at this site.

Fig. **29**.5b   Microcalcifications typical for carcinoma 2½ years following the first mammographic examination. Clinically occult carcinoma.

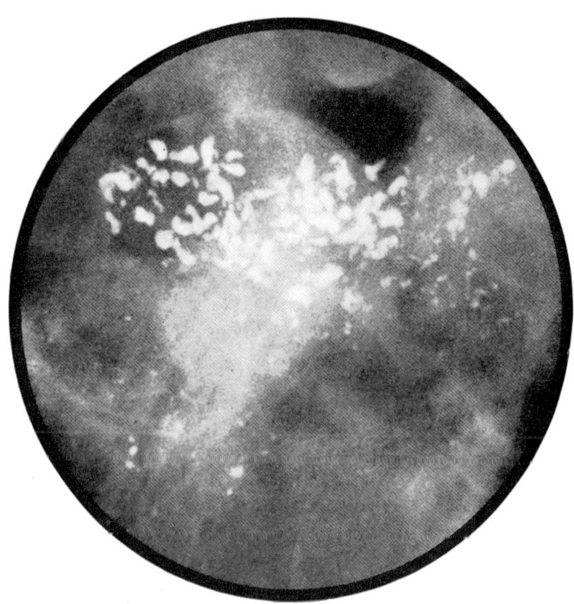

Fig. **29**.5c   Roentgenogram of the excisional biopsy specimen: Characteristic fragmented, bizarre microcalcifications within an intraductal carcinoma verified histologically.

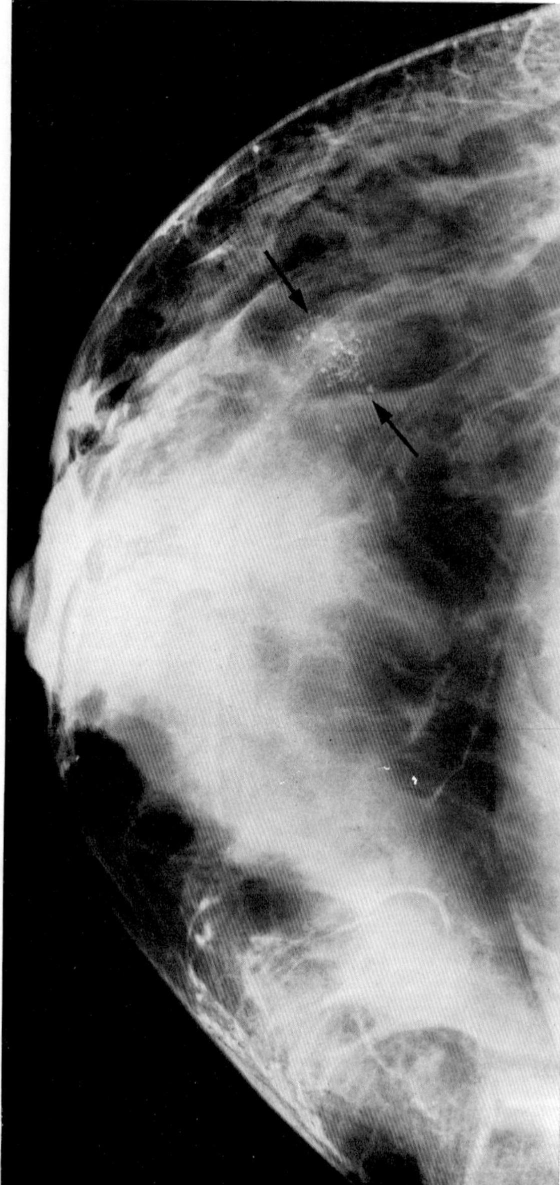

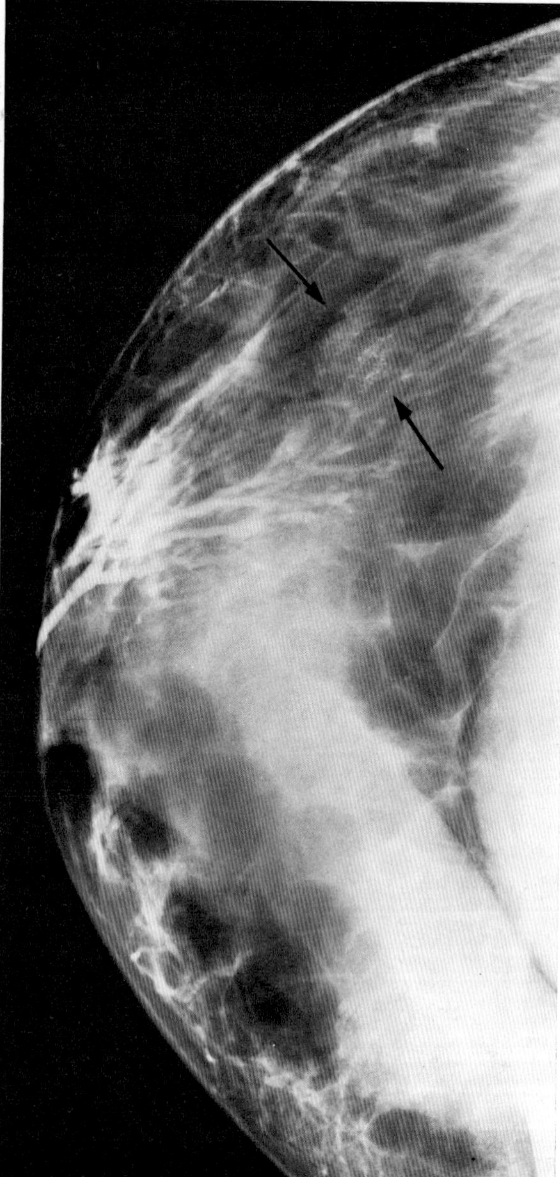

Fig. **29**.6a   Microcalcifications suspicious of carcinoma localized in a group 1 cm in diameter (arrows). Further microcalcifications are scattered throughout the parenchyma. Excisional biopsy not performed because of absent palpatory findings.

Fig. **29**.6b   Ductography: Subareolar ductal ectasia. No filling of ducts within the suspicious area (arrows).

we have included in this book a chapter on the differential diagnosis of calcification. In spite of great experience one is occasionally unable to definitely assess the importance of microcalcifications. As a rule all microcalcifications which do not give a definitely benign impression should be biopsied.

According to various authors (LEBORGNE 1953; CHAVANNE and GREGOIRE 1956; GERSHON-CO-

HEN et al 1966), about 30 to 40% of breast carcinomas have mammographically demonstrable microcalcifications. This figure increases to 44% or even 58% to 75% of the cases when paraffin block speciments of breast carcinoma are examined with mammographic technique. This difference is explainable by the difference in thickness between the breast and that of the paraffin block. According to EGAN (1963) the mammogram will also demonstrate more micro-calcifications, in the operative specimen from the breast than in the mammogram of the living patient. We found on one occasion that micro-calcification of a noninvasive comedocarcinoma could be demonstrated only in the roentgeno-gram of a paraffin block preparation of the tissue. In this case a palpable subareolar firmness and a mammographically demonstrated increase in subareolar ducts led to biopsy (fig. 29.2a and b). Such a case supports the observation frequently made that calcium deposition in a tumor occurs before infiltration by the neoplasm (GERSHON-COHEN et al 1967; STEGNER et al 1972; and others). Mammographic demonstration of micro-calcifications may be an *early sign* of breast carcinoma.

The pathogenesis of calcium deposition in the various forms of fibrocystic disease and breast carcinoma is still an enigma in spite of intensive investigations using electron microscopy, ordinary microscopy as well as chemical and radiological methods. It is certain, however, that the lactating breast has the potential of calcium secretions. Electron microscopic studies, as carried out by GERLACH and THEMANN (1965) as well as PAPE and STEGNER (1971), have shown that this metabolic activity is the result of a primary respiratory output of the mitochondria. As degenerative processes occur in the cell the intracellular calcium particles become larger by way of apposition and formation of conglo-merates and are extruded into the lumen of the lactiferous ducts or into the interstitial tissue when the cell membrane ruptures (STEGNER et al 1972). Coarse, refractive crystals can be dem-onstrated within the intraductal necrotic tumor detritus in comedocarcinoma; in scirrhus carci-noma, there are additional deposits in the fibrotic interstitium. Mammographically these calcific deposits are demonstrable when they reach a size of 0.15 mm.

Psammomatous calcifications found in various forms of fibrocystic disease are only visible microscopically. But even here it appears that these calcifications may be extruded into ductules by cells and as they aggregate, should become roentgenologically detectable. One would expect to see this particularly in blocked and inspissated secretions; however, these calcium deposits remain loose, never reaching the degree of compactness as in intraductal carcinoma, thus

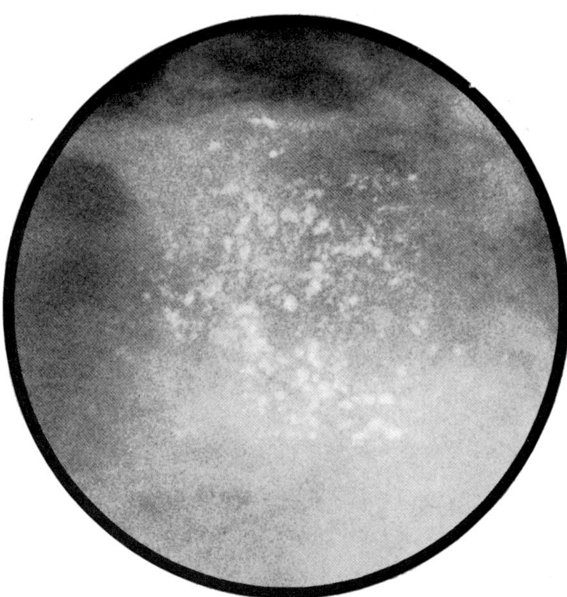

Fig. **29**.6c   2½ years later excisional biopsy per-formed on our insistence. Roentgenogram of the biopsy specimen made during surgery (magnified 5X) shows the affected area with the focus of mi-crocalcifications just as seen in the biopsy speci-men. Histology: Predominantly intraductal breast carcinoma with beginning invasion. Lobular car-cinoma in situ at several sites. Mammary dysplasia.

allowing both microscopic and mammographic differentiation between the two types of calcium deposition (STEGNER et al 1972). Why this occurs is unexplained. Different trophic influence from the proliferated connective tissue in benign mammary dysplastic states (sclerosing adenosis, diffuse interstitial fibrosis) or tumor specific factors (STEGNER et al 1972) have been discussed but these are only hypothetical concepts.
We have analyzed the chemical composition of microcalcifications from a biopsy specimen of histologically verified comedocarcinoma.
The chemical analysis of these microcalcifications was performed by Drs. L. MAROS, M. PINTER and J. MOLNAR at the Inorganic and Analytic Chemical Institute of the Eövtvös Lóránd University in Budapest. The composition of the microcalcifications was as follows: calcium, 25.4%; magnesium, 2.6%; carbonate, 5.8%; carbon, 13.8%. Spectrophotometric examination of these calcifications indicates that the calcium and magnesium ions are predominantly bound to phosphate. A quantitative determination of the phosphate content of the above preparation was not possible. Under the assumption that the cation/anion relationship to phosphate is equal

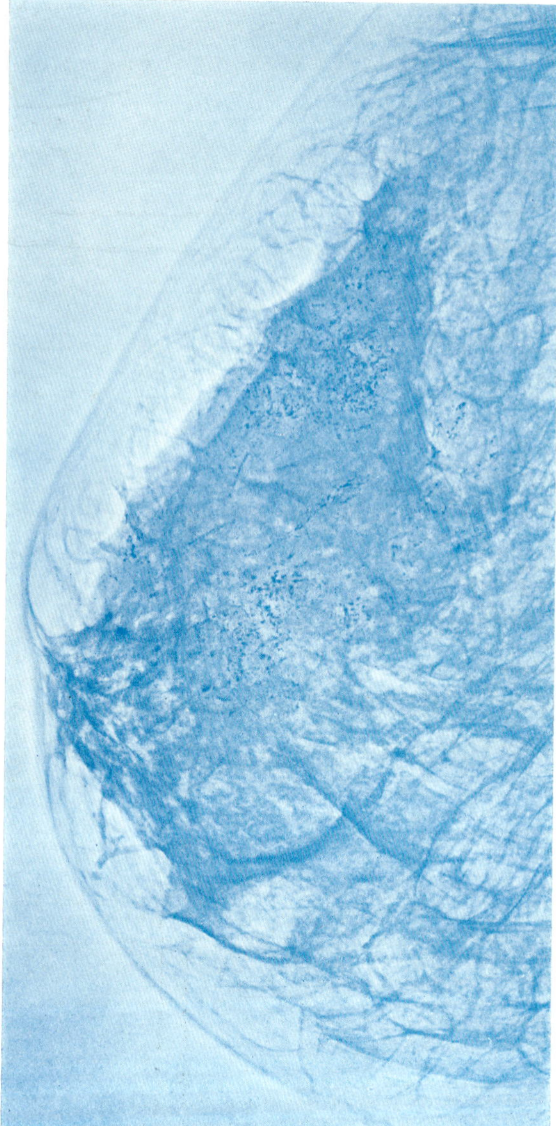

Fig. **29**.7a   Extensive comedocarcinoma shown in xeromammogram.

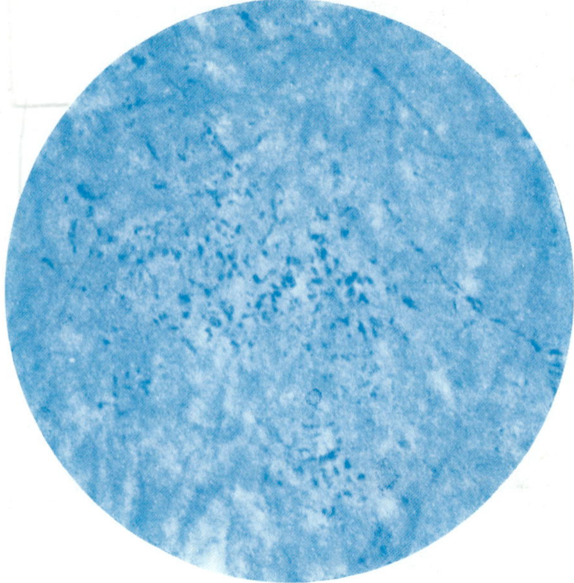

Fig. **29**.7b   Two times magnified section.

and that the carbon originates from organic bonds with amino acids of the molecular weight of 100, one may predict the following composition of the above preparation with reasonable accuracy according to this group of workers:

$$Ca_3 (PO_4)_2 \qquad 55.0\%$$
$$CaCO_3 \qquad 9.7\%$$
$$Mg_3 (PO_4)_2 . H_2O \quad 13.3\%$$
$$Albumin \qquad 22\ \%$$

In a mammogram microcalcifications are more easily detected if the film is slightly overexposed. Examination should be performed with a bright light source and magnifying glass. The demonstration of microcalcification in the mammogram does not give an indication of the degree of spread of an intraductal carcinoma since it can occur in the noninvasive stage (fig. **29**.3, **29**.4). In clinically occult intraductal breast carcinoma, microcalcification is often the most important and only roentgen sign. Experience indicates that reliable evaluation of the degree of invasiveness of a breast tumor cannot be done roentgenologically. Even in the absence of mammographic evidence of invasive changes in the vicinity of microcalcifications, evidence of invasion may be present microscopically (fig. **29**.5a, b, c). The progression of a preinvasive intraductal carcinoma to an infiltrative stage may take several years. A mammographic clue may be the observation of the appearance of a group of calcifications not observed on previous mammograms (fig. **29**.5a, b, c). Several years may elapse from the first appearance of microcalcification to the stage of widespread tumor infiltration. During this time the groups of microcalcifications may remain unchanged in form, size or distribution. Similarly there may be no palpatory findings and the real significance of these microcalcifications is dismissed. In such early cases, when biopsy is performed on the basis of the mammogram, in the absence of palpatory findings, a mammogram of the biopsied preparation during the operation is mandatory to ensure that the

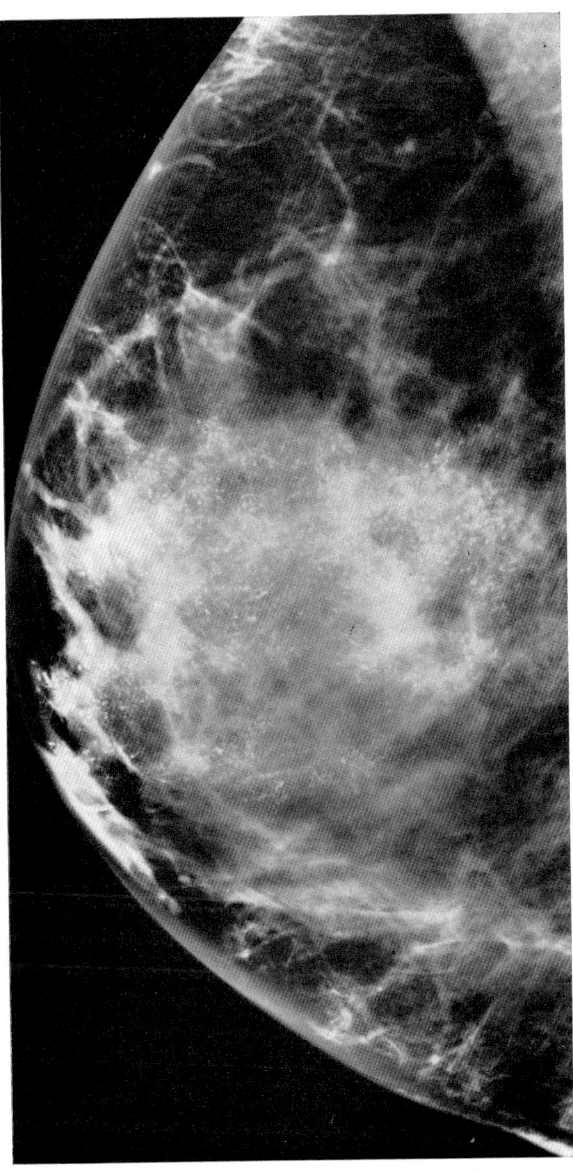

Fig. **29**.8a   Diffuse distribution of numerous irregular microcalcifications of varying size throughout the breast. Roentgen diagnosis: Intraductal carcinoma with diffuse spread through the breast.

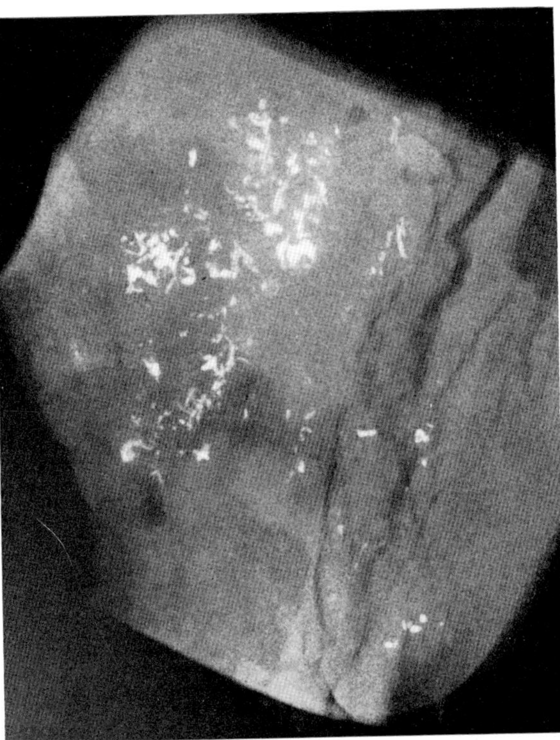

Fig. **29**.8b   Roentgenogram of the paraffin block: The irregular microcalcifications of varying size are seen to better advantage. Histology: Widespread comedocarcinoma with foci of necrosis and calcification.

removed tissue is indeed that section of the breast under suspicion (fig. 29.6a, b, c). We have not always been able to carry through such biopsies because of the absence of palpatory findings. Eventual biopsy later on invariably revealed an intraductal carcinoma. However, earlier biopsy may have allowed surgical removal prior to the tumor reaching the invasive stage. Therefore we have insisted on removal biopsy in all cases of breast calcification which do not appear to be definitely benign in the mammogram.

Our insistence on biopsy seems justified even though about 30% of such cases eventually are proved histologically to be benign breast disease (intraductal hyperplasia, intraductal papillomatosis, sclerosing adenosis, mammary fibrosis). Biopsy under these conditions has turned up lobular carcinoma in situ and noninvasive intraductal carcinoma. It is important, however, to ensure that such mammographically directed biopsies as well as the histological examination be performed exactly on that section of breast tissue which is suspect in the mammogram. If there is any doubt, one should insist that the biopsy material embedded in a paraffin block undergo x-ray examination and also that a follow-up control mammogram on the patient be performed. We will further expound on this in the chapter on occult carcinoma (see page 306).

If one sees numerous widespread branching or broken crystals of microcalcifications scattered throughout the breast parenchyma there is no doubt of the diagnosis. This is only found in comedocarcinoma (fig. 29.7a and b, 29.8a and b).

Duct Ectasia

WOLFE (1967 and 1969) was the first to call attention to the diagnostic significance of focal unilateral ductal ectasia (without ductography) in the mammogram. According to his experience the incidence of unilateral ductal ectasia is particularly great in breast carcinoma. He believes one may make the diagnosis of breast carcinoma by the observation of unilateral, circumscribed, tortuous ductal ectasia, alone. According to WOLFE these carcinomas are predominantly of the intraductal type.

We are of the opinion that ductal ectasia which appears as a subareolar density with wormy or wavy contours represents an important sign of intraductal pathology but only allows the suspicion of tumor (fig. 29.9, 29.10 and 29.11).

Not only carcinoma but also benign papilloma may produce the same mammographic appearance of ductal ectasia (see fig. 19.3).

Nipple secretion is not particularly frequent in comedocarcinoma. In the case of abnormal secretion ductography may be performed and an intraductal carcinoma can be detected even in the absence of tumor calcification.

If ductography reveals an ectatic lactiferous duct with irregular margins and intermittent complete block of its branches, then excisional biopsy is indicated.

In these cases also the differentiation of the pathological intraductal process can only be made by histological examination (fig. 29.12a and b) 29.13a, b, c; 29.14a and b). Only the presence of microcalcifications, in combination with the above findings at ductography, should arouse the firm suspicion of carcinoma as the underlying process.

The nipple secretion unquestionably must be submitted for cytological study. Exfoliative cytology is frequently positive in comedocarcinoma because the cellular elements and sometimes even pieces of tumor tissue are occasionally easily expressed from the nipple.

Infiltrating Intraductal Carcinoma

The infiltrative stage of an intraductal carcinoma may be recognized in the mammogram by the appearance of scirrhus, stellate or nodular tumor tissue next to intraductal microcalcifications (fig. 29.15 to 29.19). In such cases one may describe the roentgen findings as a ductal carcinoma with scirrhus and solid tumor infiltration or a scirrhus, solid carcinoma with intraductal invasion.

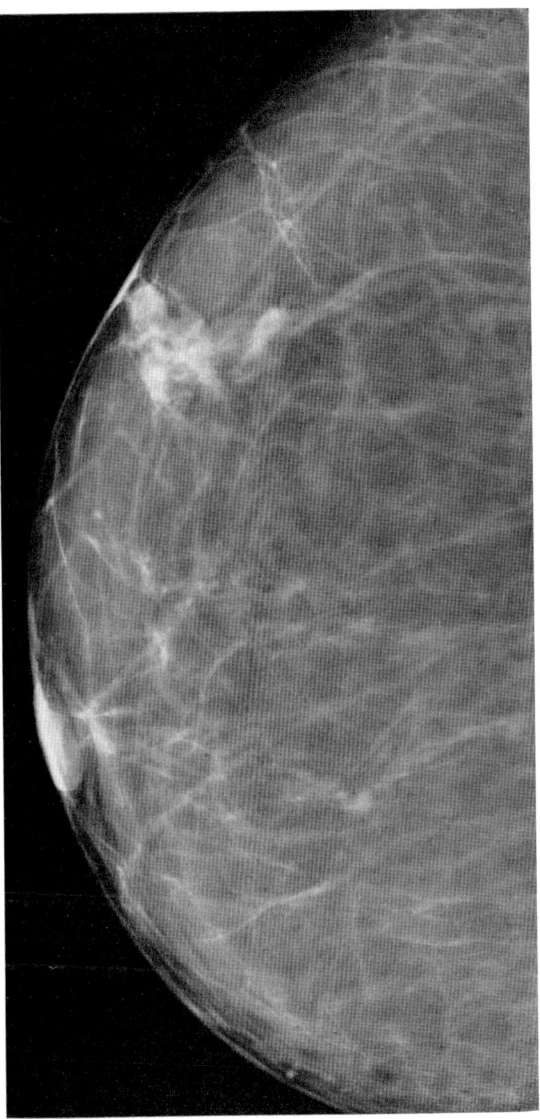

Fig. **29**.9   Irregular, lobular mass with occasional stellate extensions within the subcutaneous fatty layer. Focal skin thickening. Roentgen diagnosis: Invasive intraductal carcinoma. Histology: Invasive intraductal carcinoma with the infiltrating portion having assumed the characteristics of carcinoma simplex.

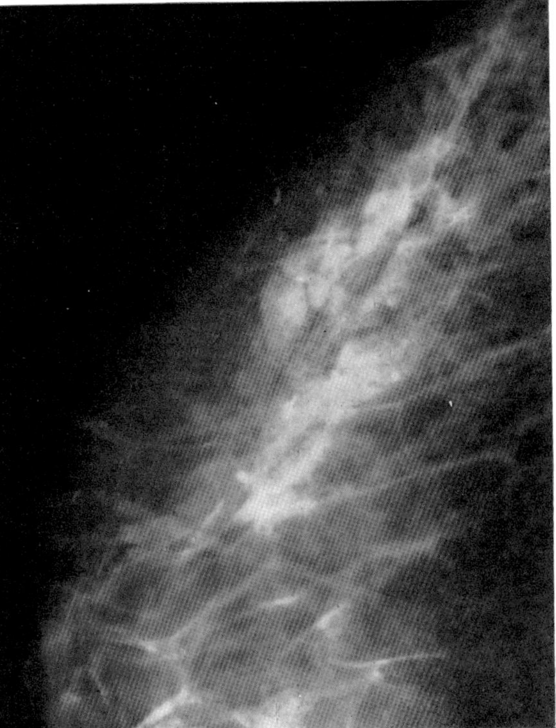

Fig. **29**.10   Dilated tortuous lactiferous ducts. No palpatory findings. Excisional biopsy was performed because of the roentgen suspicion of intraductal carcinoma. Histology: Partially solid, partially papillary intraductal carcinoma, noninvasive.

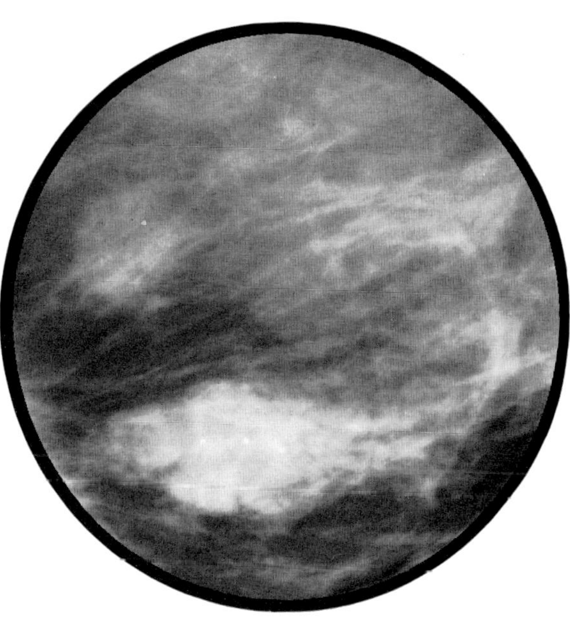

Fig. **29**.11   Soft tissue density whose margins on the whole appear smooth but there are fine umbilications along its borders. An occasional coarse calcification is seen within the lesion. The picture is similar to that in Fig. 29.10. Clinically, cordlike easily movable area of parenchymal thickening, free from the overlying skin. There was nipple secretion but cytology proved negative.
Roentgen diagnosis: Intraductal neoplasm benign or malignant. Excisional biopsy indicated.
Histology: Predominantly intraductal carcinoma.

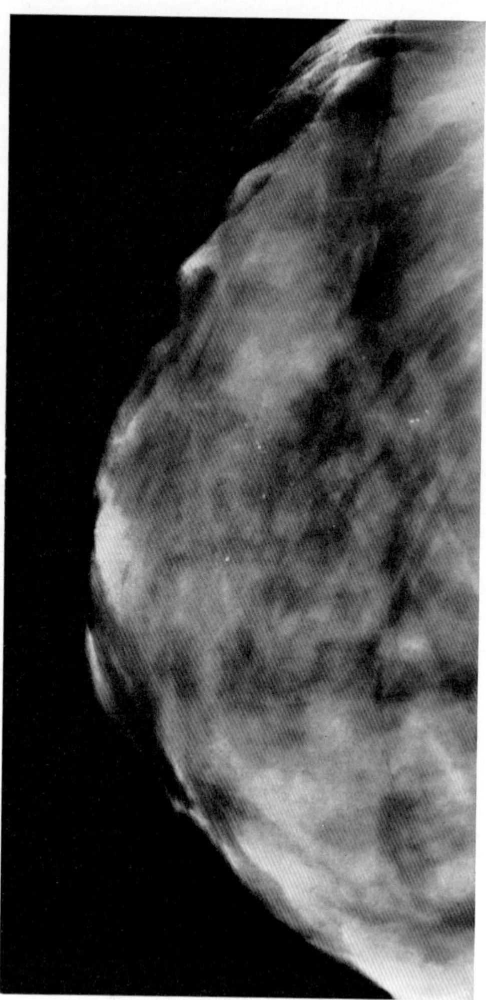

Fig. **29**.12a Several microcalcifications predominantly singular but quite dense and irregular in size and form are distributed within dense parenchyma. Mammographic diagnosis: Intraductal process: Proliferation? Papillomatosis? Carcinoma in situ or ductal carcinoma?

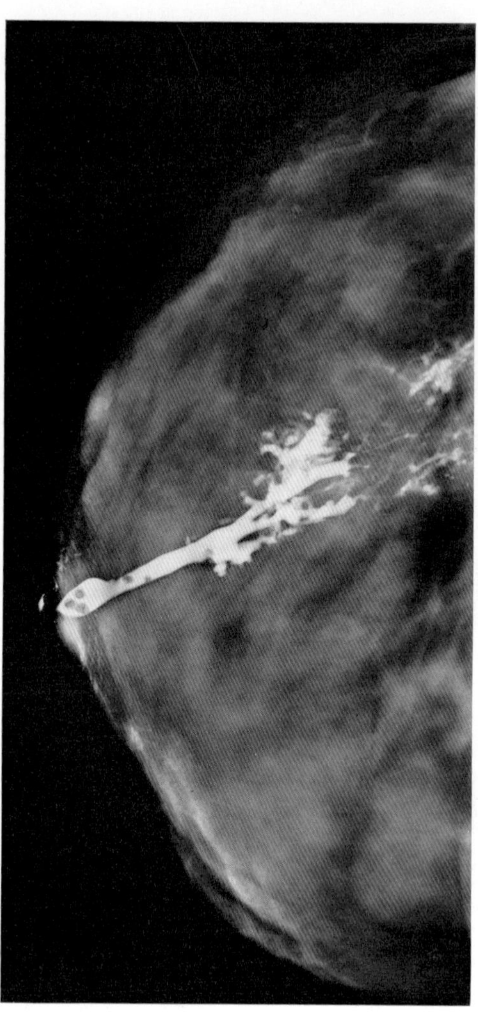

Fig. **29**.12b Ductography: Ductal ectasia with small papillomas immediately behind the nipple. Peripherally there are irregular filling defects within the milk ducts some of which have an irregular contour and reveal stenosis with mild poststenotic dilatation. Malignant degeneration of ductal papillomatosis is highly probable.
Histology: Intraductal carcinoma of the scirrhus type.

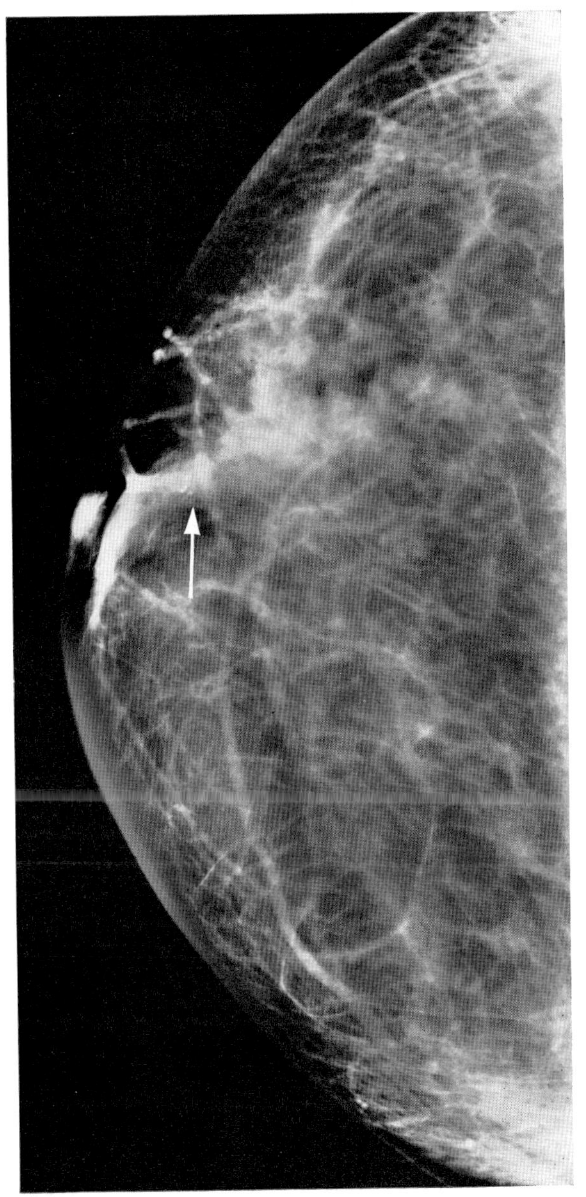

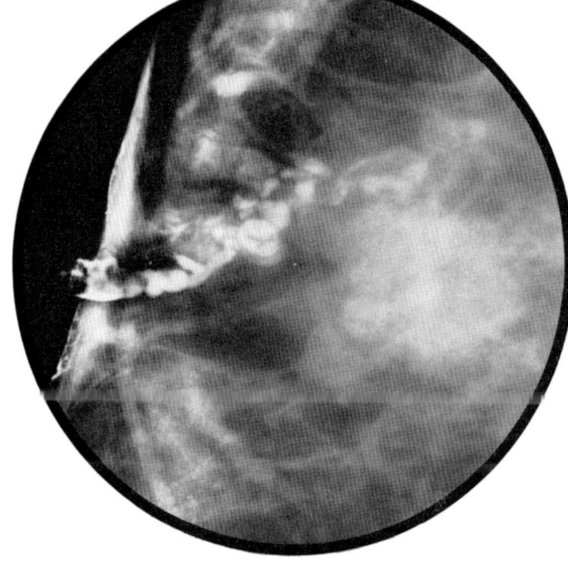

Fig. **29**.13a   Subareolar nodular tissue density with poorly defined margins and streaky extensions. Occasional coarse calcifications.

Fig. **29**.13b   Ductography: The secreting milk duct is filled by a polypoid mass indicating an intraductal process.

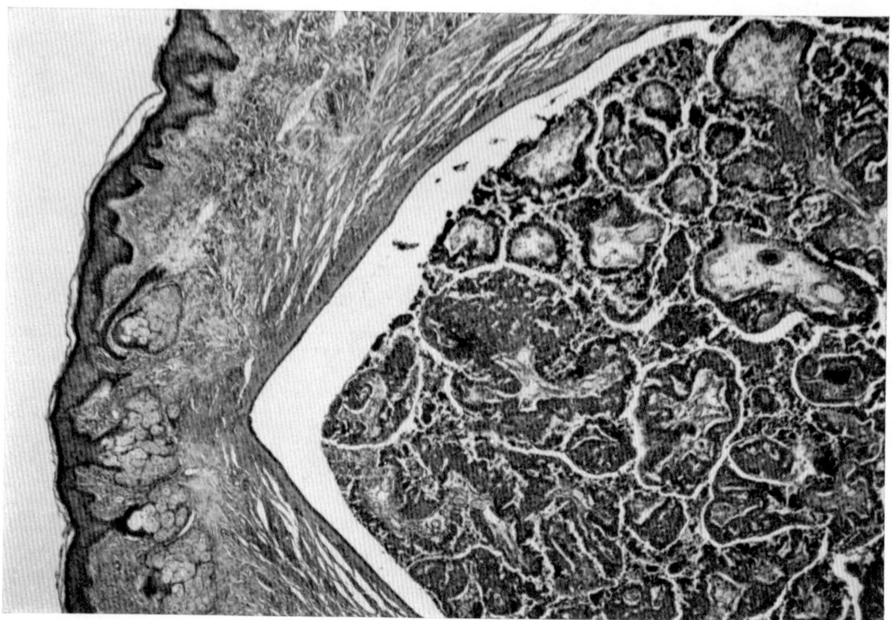

Fig. **29**.13c   Histology: Intraductal carcinoma with partly solid and partly papillary components. Papillary carcinoma identified in a dilated lactiferous duct of the nipple.

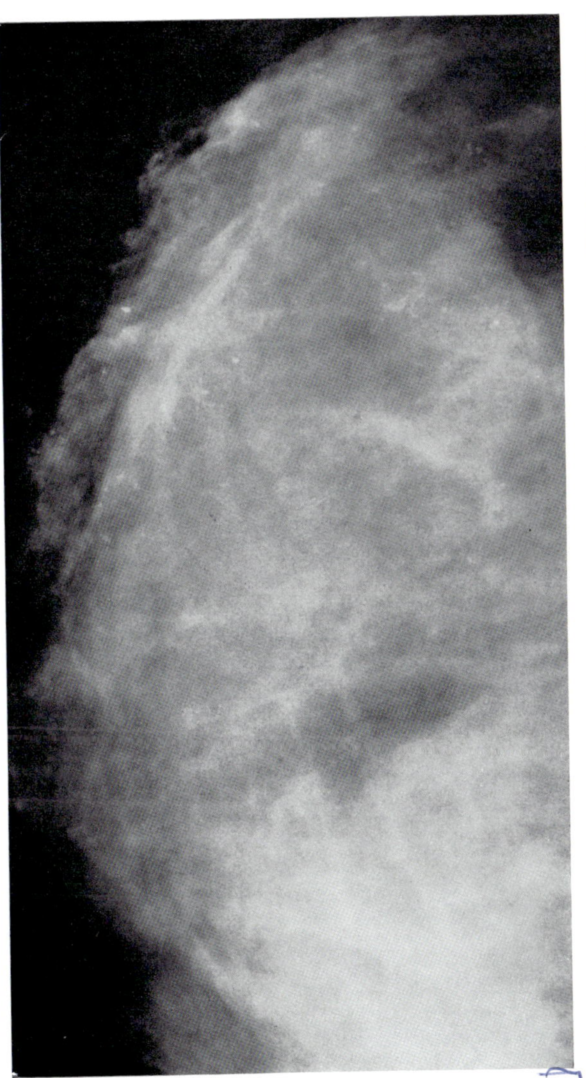

Fig. **29**.14a Numerous microcalcifications typical for carcinoma scattered throughout dense parenchyma. Dominant mass indicative of a tumor is not visible: Roentgen diagnosis: Intraductal carcinoma.

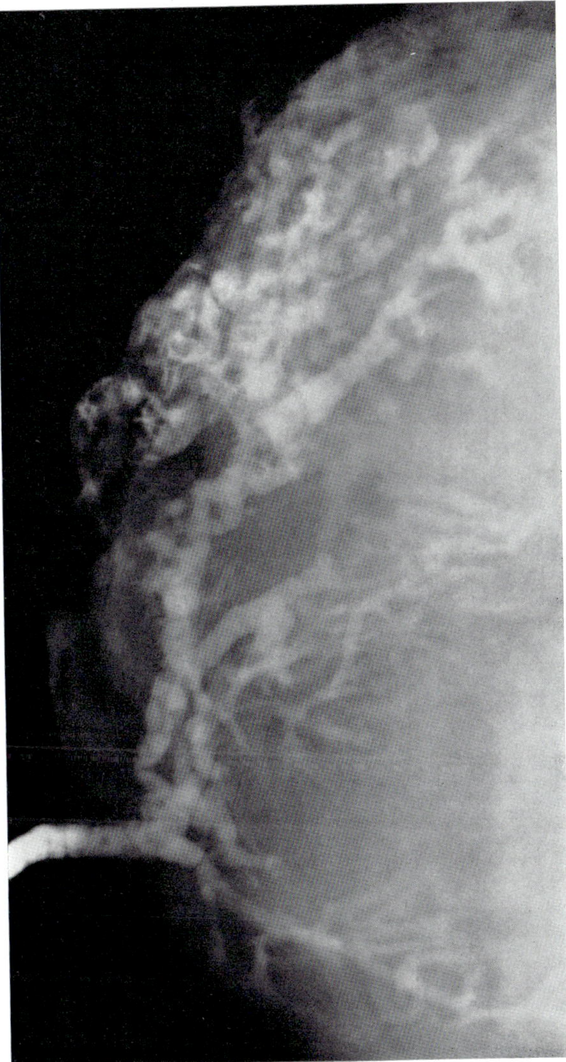

Fig. **29**.14b Ductography supports the mammographic diagnosis: several lactiferous ducts are dilated and filled with intraductal tumefactive growths. Histology: Intraductal comedocarcinoma.

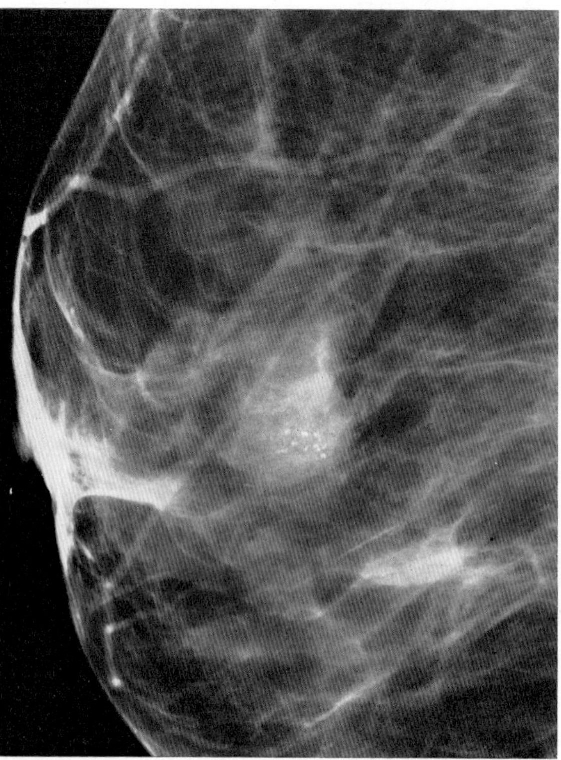
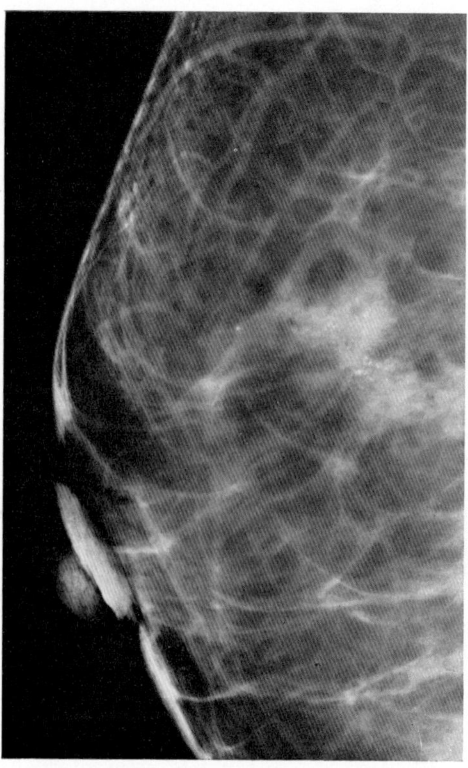

Fig. **29**.15 Irregular nodular subareolar tissue density. Focal calcifications of varying size and density within the mass. Minimal nipple retraction. Roentgen diagnosis: Invasive ductal carcinoma. Histology: Lactiferous duct carcinoma with scirrhus stromal proliferation.

Fig. **29**.16 Soft tissue nodules with stellate borders and numerous microcalcifications. Histology: Infiltrating milk duct carcinoma with adenocarcinoma and partly carcinoma simplex characteristics.

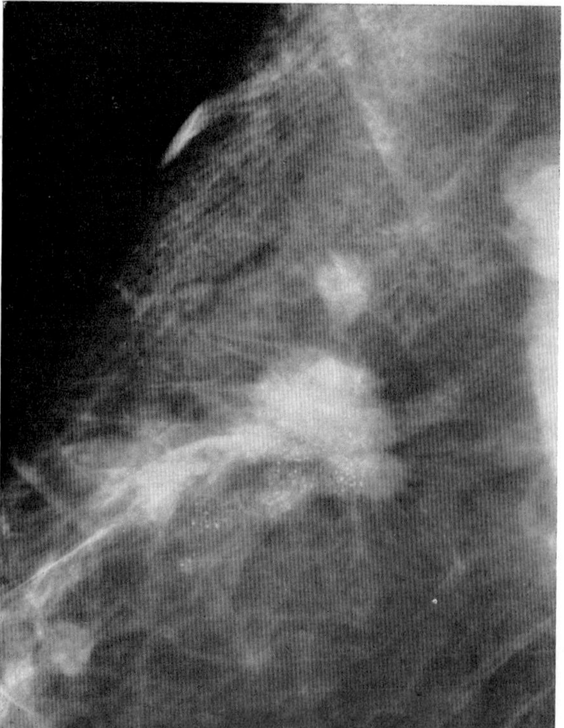

Fig. **29**.17 Irregular, lobular soft tissue mass with numerous spicules extending from its surface. Microcalcifications are seen within and outside the mass. Roentgen diagnosis: Intraductal carcinoma, scirrhus type, verified histologically.

Fig. **29**.18   Walnut-sized mass with numerous irregular microcalcifications and small spicules on its surface. The mass is much denser than the subareolar tissue. Ductography reveals only partial filling of an adjacent duct. Histology: Intracanalicular poorly differentiated adenocarcinoma with scirrhus extension.

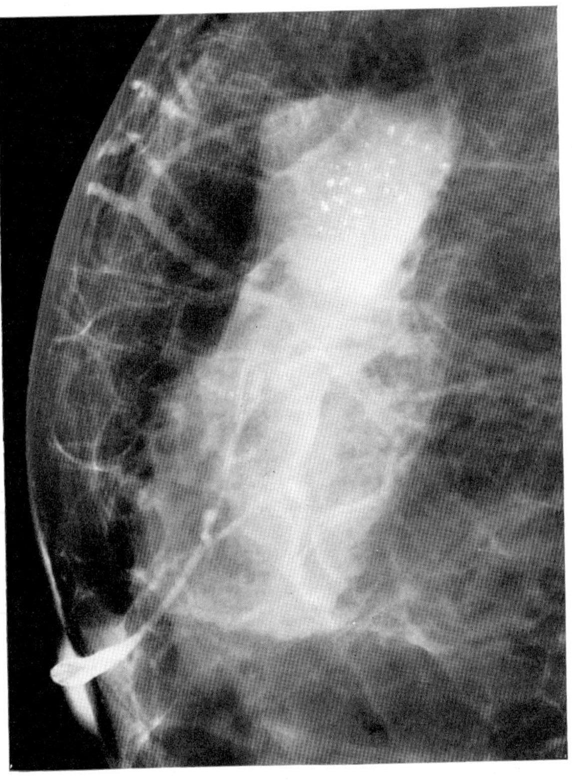

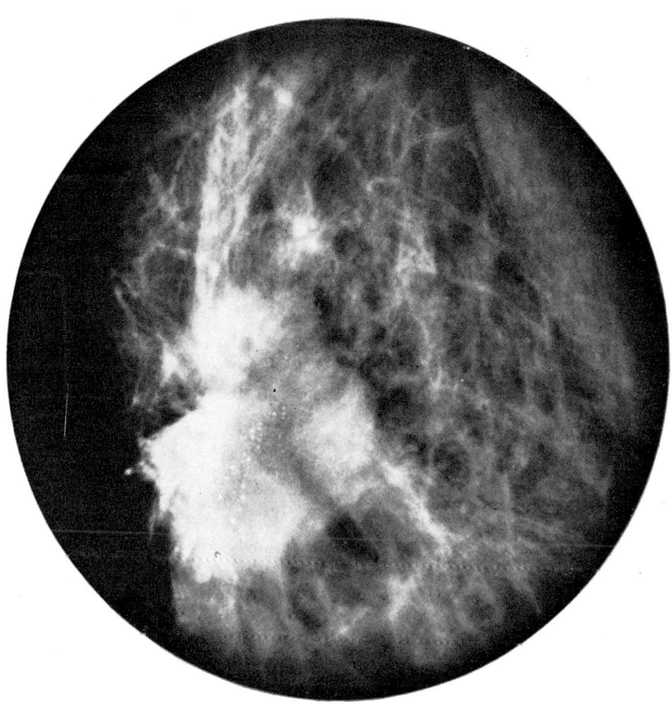

Fig. **29**.19   Local area of mammogram 2X. Numerous microcalcifications of varying size are clearly seen within the tumor mass. Histology: Intraductal carcinoma with carcinoma simplex and scirrhus extension.

Papillary (Cribriform) Breast Carcinoma

Definition and Pathology

Papillary carcinoma is recognized as exclusively or at least predominantly intraductal; more rarely it is an intracystic tumor with development of fine papillary and adenoid epithelial tissue formation.

Papillary carcinoma arises from malignant lactiferous duct epithelium. It is rare that this tumor arises from a benign ductal papilloma. However, the latter may occur in multiple intraductal papillomas (papillomatosis). According to HAAGENSEN (1971) the frequency of malignant degeneration in papillomatosis is approximately 38%. HAAGENSEN therefore considers papillomatosis as a precancerous condition. This concept has been previously discussed on page 82 and page 120.

Early papillary carcinoma is a noninfiltrating intracanalicular or intracystic tumor.

Intracystic carcinoma, however, is rare (GROS 1958; HAAGENSEN, 0.3%, 1971). Macroscopically intracystic carcinoma is characterized by a white, gray or gray to red-colored lobular and fine papillary ingrowth into the cyst. There may be intracystic hemorrhage.

Microscopically the cellular elements contain hyperchromatic nuclei with relatively little alterations of shape or size. These cells combine to form a fine papillary, occasionally adenoid, cribriform structure with almost complete absence of connective tissue (fig. 30.1). This characteristic histologic appearance persists even when the tumor becomes invasive.

The typical histological changes in infiltration, however, are not a predominant pattern in this tumor and the pathologist must rely primarily on the appearance of the stroma and the cells to determine the stage of the tumor. This can result in difficulties of differential diagnosis.

An important differential sign between noninfiltrating intraductal papillary carcinoma and

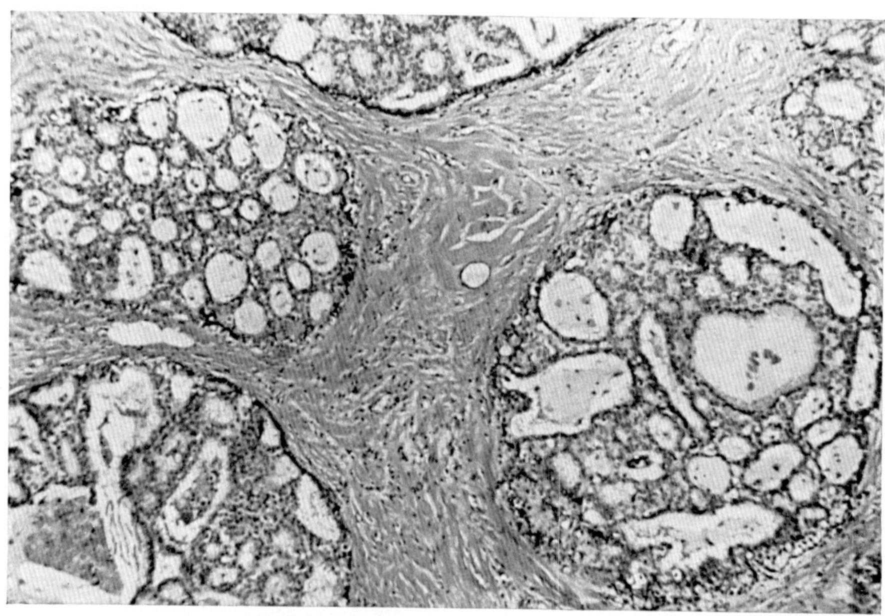

Fig. **30.1**   Cribriform intraductal carcinoma: Adenoid and papillary proliferation of a relatively atypical epithelium within a milk duct resulting in a cribriform structure.

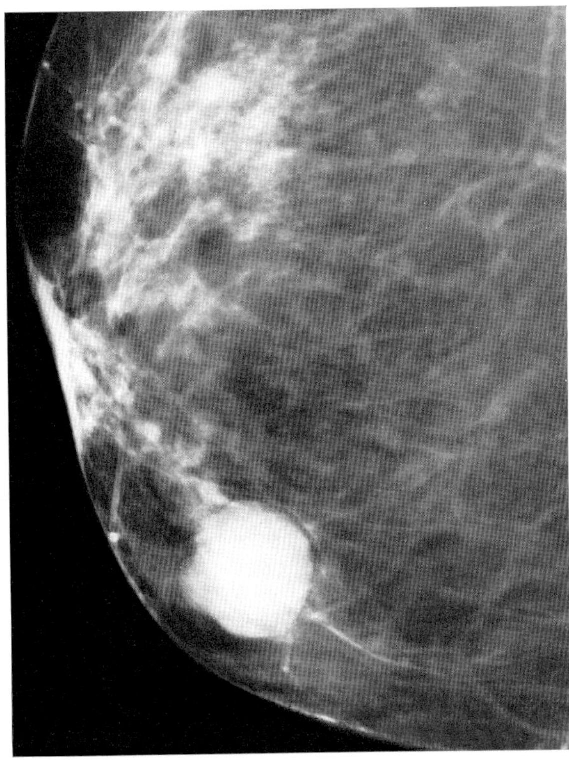

Fig. **30**.2a   Lobular but smoothly marginated mass in a 51-year-old woman, which was palpable clinically. No skin changes or surrounding fibrosis. Puncture: 4cc sanguineous material.

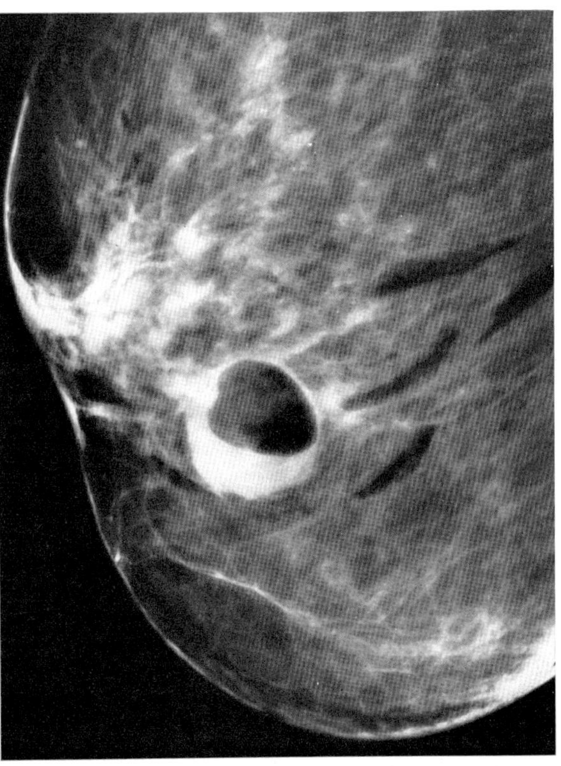

Fig. **30**.2b   Pneumocystography: Definite thickening of the inner wall of the cyst. Slight irregularity of the wall raises suspicion of intracystic papillary carcinoma.

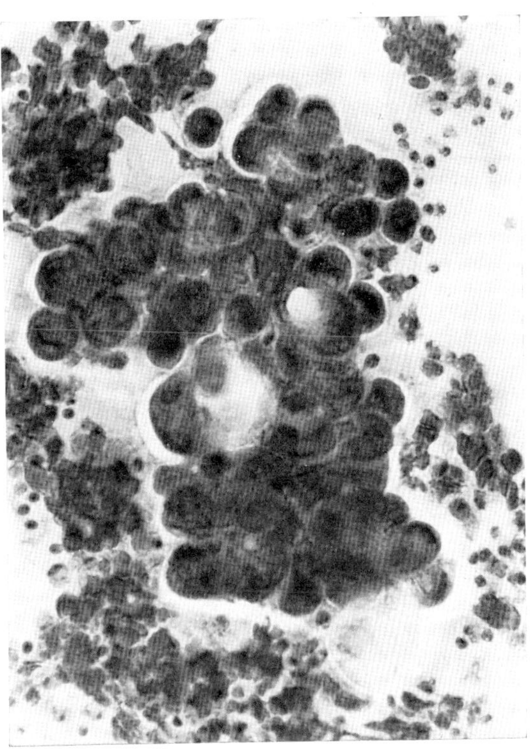

Fig. **30**.2c   Cystology: Group of atypical, malignant tumor cells. Histology: Intracystic papillary carcinoma.

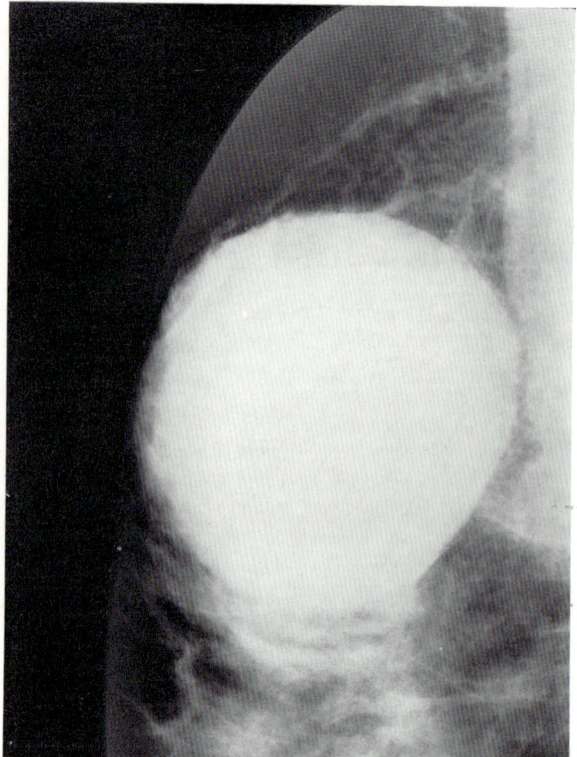

Fig. **30**.3a Solitary, round density with smooth contours, palpable as a firm, movable lump.

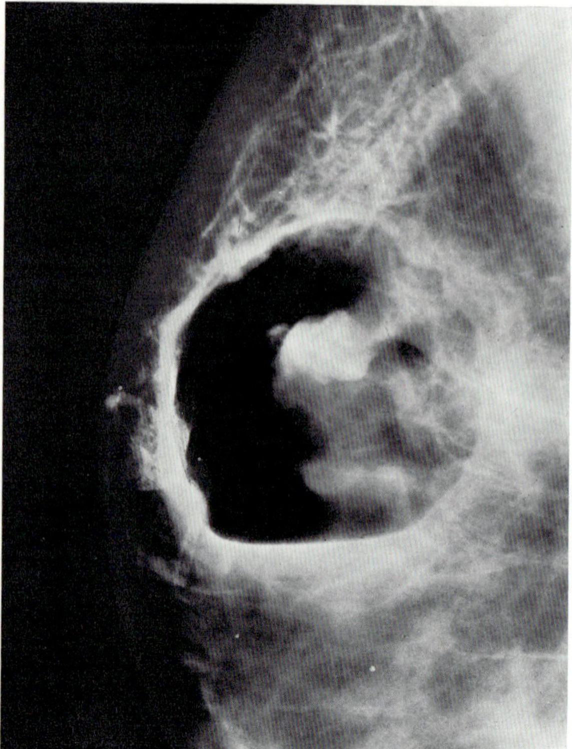

Fig. **30**.3b Pneumocystography: Endocystic tissue proliferation. The inner margin of the cyst is irregular.

benign papillomatosis of the lactiferous ducts is the frequent absence of associated stromal proliferation and the almost invariable absence of myoepithelial proliferation.

It must be remembered, however, that before the diagnosis of a noninfiltrating, intraductal, or intracystic carcinoma is made, that there is always the possibility of "microinfiltration" of the stroma which may be too subtle to be recognized on histological examination.

Because of the diminished or absent stromal proliferation papillary carcinoma demonstrates a strong tendency to necrosis; however, this is not as great as in the purely solid form of intraductal carcinoma, in other words comedocarcinoma.

Clinical Findings

Intraductal or intracystic papillary carcinoma is relatively rare (1.5 to 2% of all breast carcinomas) GATCHELL et al (1958) found 48 papillary carcinomas in 9,000 cases of breast cancer. KRAUS and NEUBECKER (1962) have reported 21 cases.

HAAGENSEN (1971) reported 130 cases from his own patient population. The description of this carcinoma rests on a few special diagnostic characteristics which indicate its significance as to prognosis.

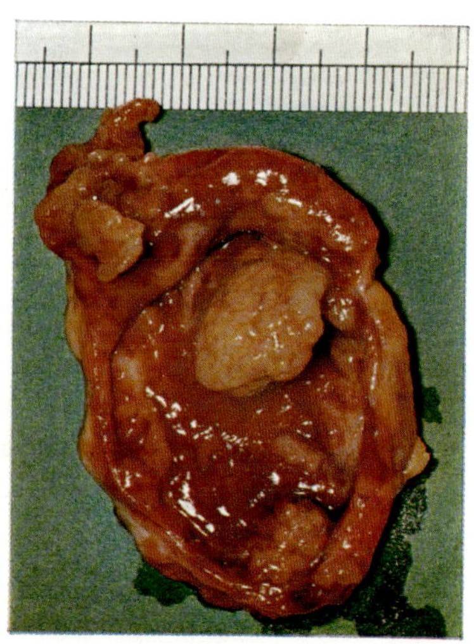

Fig. **30**.3c Tissue diagnosis: Endocystic carcinoma.

With *intraductal* papillary carcinoma sanguineous nipple discharge is the earliest clinical sign. Such a discharge, however, is not always due to a malignant papilloma but may occur with the benign form. A preoperative differential diagnosis is not always possible even on cytological examination of the secretion.

Occasionally papillary carcinoma may be palpated as a small, firm, well circumscribed mass particularly in its early intraductal stages. It can be easily mistaken for a benign fibroadenoma. Intraductal papillary carcinoma is most frequent in the subareolar region and there may be skin changes in this area as the invasive stage of the tumor is reached. There may be blue or red discolored nodules under the skin with central ulceration, frequently described by the patient as furuncles. The experienced physician, however, should have no dificulty in recognizing a carcinoma by the firm consistency, the absence of surrounding inflammatory reaction and the peculiar blue-red coloration. A special variant is multiple intraductal papillary carcinomas which may cause a difffusely nodular or "buckshot" appearance of the overlying skin.

Intracystic papillary carcinoma is clinically indistinguishable in its early stages from a cyst of mammary dysplasia or a fibroadenoma. Only after invasion through the wall of the cyst by the tumor can one recognize fixation of the mass, immobility, poorly definable borders and, in advanced cases, infiltration of the overlying skin. This process may proceed to ulceration.

The prognosis of papillary carcinoma is relatively favorable. GATCHELL et al (1958) have reported an 83.3% five-year survival.

Roentgenology

Noninvasive, purely *intraductal* papillary carcinoma cannot be diagnosed in the plain mammogram in its early stages. In the case of sanguineous or serous nipple discharge the intraductal process may be detected during ductography.

At ductography one finds ductal ectasia. In the dilated duct, single or numerous intraductal, irregular and often poorly defined filling defects are seen. One cannot, however, differentiate papillomatosis from papillary carcinoma.

As the tumor invades, however, this may be detected in the plain mammogram as ill-defined, unsharp contours of dilated milk ducts.

Intracystic papillary carcinoma is only recognizable in the mammogram when invasion beyond the wall of the cyst has occurred. Before this stage the diagnosis can only be made with cyst puncture, cytological examination of the aspirate and pneumocystography. In the pneumocystogram one may see a thickening (fig. 30.2a—c) or "papillomatous" soft tissue ingrowth into the inner portion of the cyst (fig. 30.3a to c). One cannot differentiate this from a benign papilloma. In the case of papillary carcinoma the cyst aspirate may be bloody and frequently pieces of tissue can be aspirated.

As tumor infiltration beyond the cyst wall occurs the sharp contours of the cyst are lost because of surrounding edema and infiltration. One may also see "comctlike" tumor or connective tissue extension from the cyst. If there is nearby skin thickening one has further evidence of an intracystic carcinoma.

In the differential diagnosis one must recall that a similar appearance can be seen with an infected cyst. Likewise inflammatory fibrosis in the vicinity of a simple cyst may give a similar appearance. Therefore a positive diagnosis of invasive intracystic carcinoma is not possible in the plain roentgenogram but only with pneumocystography.

Chapter 31

Paget's Carcinoma

Definition and Pathology

Paget's carcinoma is a variant of intraductal breast carcinoma. The tumor arises "in situ" either in a superficial, subareolar or in a deeper lactiferous duct and grows in the direction of the nipple, spreading into the intraepidermal region of the nipple and areola (INGLIS 1946; MUIR 1935). Paget's carcinoma therefore is not a primary tumor of the skin of the nipple and areola but a special type of ductal carcinoma. Furthermore the lymph node metastases of Paget's carcinoma are those of an intraductal tumor rather than those of a skin cancer.

On microscopic examination typical "Paget cells" are seen in the epidermis. These are relatively large cells with light-colored cytoplasm and a large round or polymorphic nucleus containing various amounts of chromatin (fig. 31.1). Occasionally Paget's cells may contain scanty amounts of melanin and may resemble melanocytes causing some difficulty in differen-

tiating this disease from *melanosis circumscripta* (DUBREUILH, McDIVITT, STEWART, BERG 1968).

One condition that resembles Paget's carcinoma very closely is Bowen's disease. This disorder includes a destruction or retraction of the nipple with concomitant weeping, crusty skin lesions which both clinically and in some cases histologically, may be difficult to differentiate from Paget's carcinoma.

Clinical Findings

Clinically this disease resembles an eczema of the nipple and areola as first described by JAMES PAGET 1874. Clinically these eczematous changes of the nipple and areola are always the first sign of this special type of ductal carcinoma. Erosive and ulcerative nipple changes predominate (fig. 31.2a, 31.4a, 31.5a). Paget's carcinoma is relatively rare (HAAGENSEN: 2.5% of all breast carcinomas).

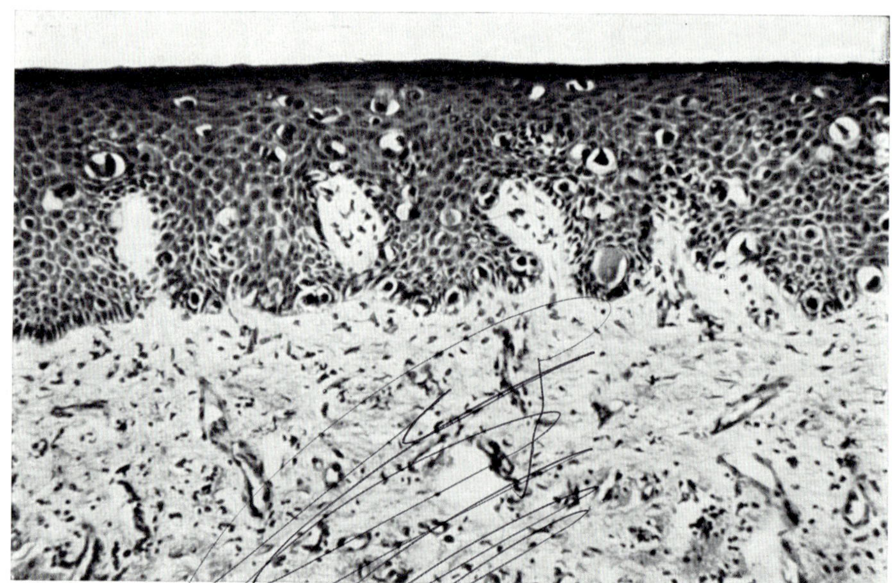

Fig. **31.**1   Paget's cells with clear cytoplasm and polymorphic nuclei within the epidermis of the areola (Paget carcinoma).

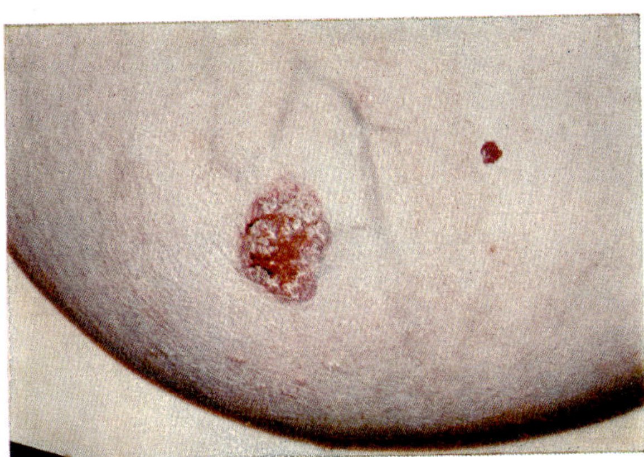

Fig. **31**.2a Nipple eczema of 1 year duration in a 50-year-old woman. The nipple is erythematous, crusty and thickened. Periodic sanguineous discharge. No palpatory findings.

Paget's carcinoma occurs in an older age group than the rest of breast cancers. Invariably the patient is beyond 50 years of age.

The differential diagnosis from a benign inflammatory eczematous condition of the nipple is often very difficult clinically because positive palpatory findings are frequently not present. The carcinomatous mass may be quite deep or embedded in a mass of benign fibrotic breast tissue and thus not palpable. The suspicion of Paget's carcinoma must be entertained if an areolar and nipple eczema fails to improve following four weeks of therapy. In such a case cytological examination of the secretion should be performed. This may not be positive for carcinoma since the primary tumor may be very deep. Likewise, if there has been prolonged treatment with tinctures and other topical medications cytology may be negative.

Mammography is definitely indicated. It will invariably detect a deep or immediately subareolar ductal carcinoma. It is therefore medical negligence to conservatively treat a nipple or areolar eczema over a period of several months without mammographic evaluation.

In the event of a negative mammogram and a therapeutically resistant eczema, histological examination is indicated.

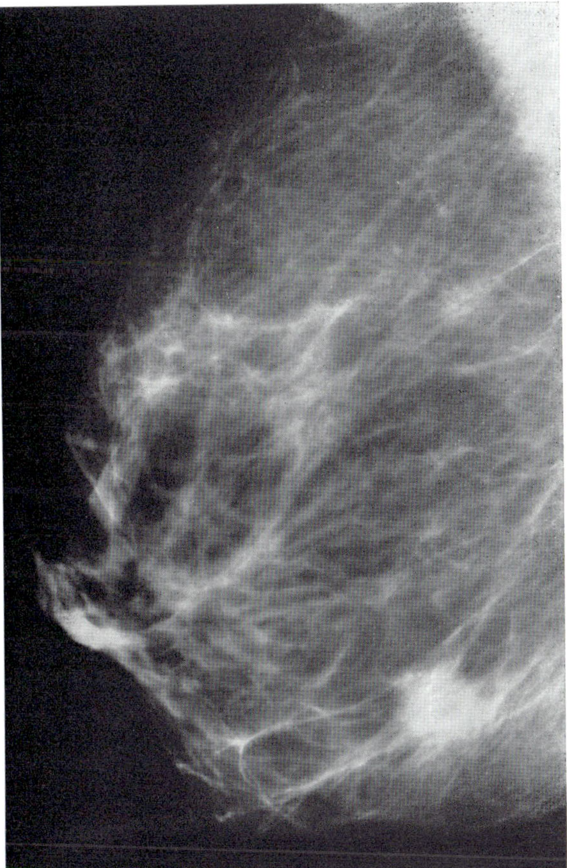

Fig. **31**.2b Roentgenogram: Subareolar milk duct thickening. Deep within the breast there is a carcinoma measuring about 1.5 cm in diameter with central microcalcifications and peripheral tumor spicules.

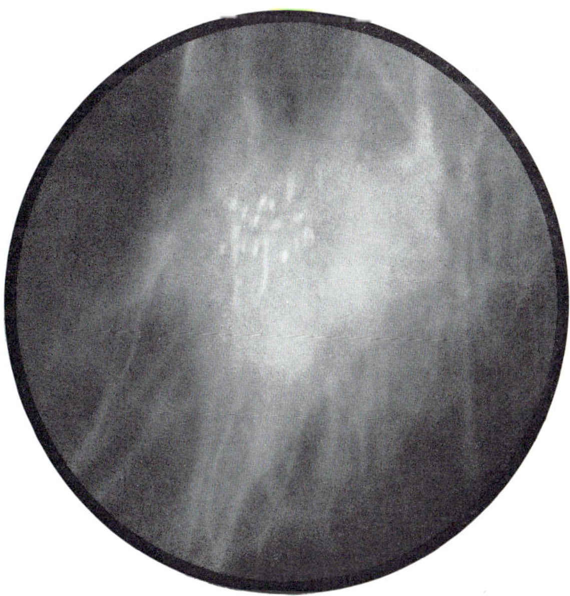

Fig. **31**.2c Section from the same case. Magnification brings the microcalcifications into better definition.

12*

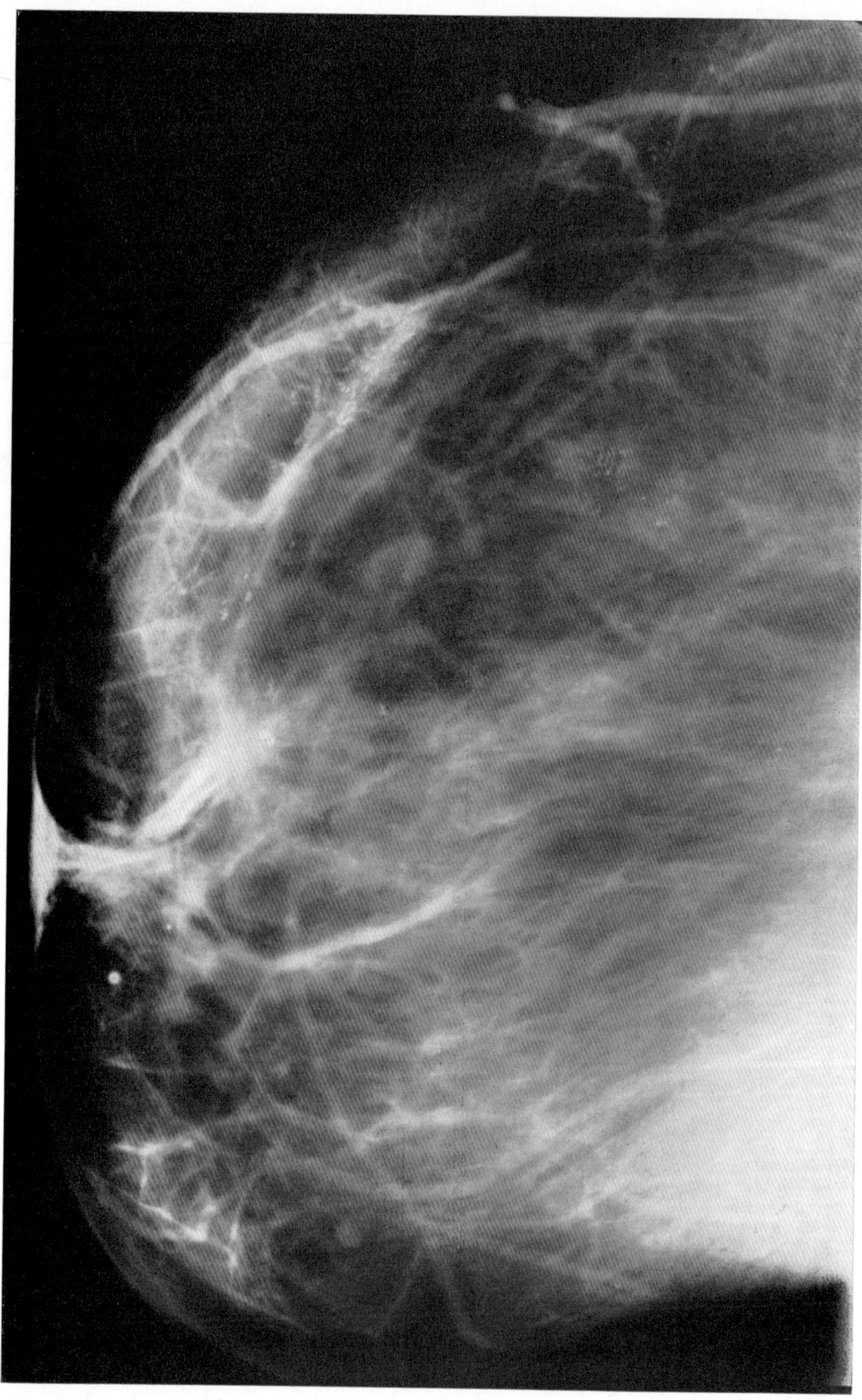

Fig. **31**.3a Clinically: Nipple eczema. Roentgenologically: Minimal skin thickening of the areola and enlargement of subareolar lactiferous ducts. Numerous microcalcifications which are particularly obvious in the magnification of a coned-down roentgenogram (Fig. 31.3b). Roentgen diagnosis: Intraductal carcinoma which in association with eczema of the nipple and areola represents Paget's carcinoma. Histologically verified.

Without doubt nipple eczema is the most important clinical sign of Paget's carcinoma; however, correlation is not total. KISTER and HAAGENSEN (1970) in evaluating 159 cases of Paget's carcinoma reported 68 cases in which the manifestation was exclusively eczema of the nipple and areola. In 49 cases there was no eczema but a dominant mass on palpation.

The survival of patients with Paget's carcinoma depends on the length of existence of the tumor, the degree of spread into the deeper portions of the breast and the presence or absence of metastases. Large series of cases are not available for analysis because the absolute number of Paget's carcinomas is relatively small. HAAGENSEN noted axillary lymph node metastases in 66% of his patients. This percentage is higher than that of breast carcinomas in general. The number of 10-year survivals among his patient population is also less than among other cases of breast carcinoma.

The prognosis of Paget's carcinoma is ultimately dependent on the presence or absence of invasiveness. The prognosis is good as long as the basal membrane of the epithelial layer of the involved duct is intact. The prognosis is poor when there has been tumor invasion beyond this membrane and/or if a dominant mass is palpable.

Roentgen Findings

The areola may be thickened as a result of the eczematous changes or of tumor infiltration. This thickening is not always very impressive. Thus one cannot conclude that areolar eczema is benign simply because the skin thickening observed in the roentgenogram is minimal.

In its classical form, the mammogram reveals in addition to the thickening of the areola, radiating densities in the subareolar region indicating thickened milk ducts. Occasionally one may identify a solid tumor mass deep in the breast far removed from the areola, and not clinically palpable (fig. 31.2a—c). If one can indentify microcalcifications either in a punctate or linear arrangement in the area of the lesion, one may make the diagnosis of ductal carcinoma with considerable certainty.

Ductal carcinoma of the comedo type may occur elsewhere in the breast and still present with Paget's disease of the nipple (fig. 31.3a and b).

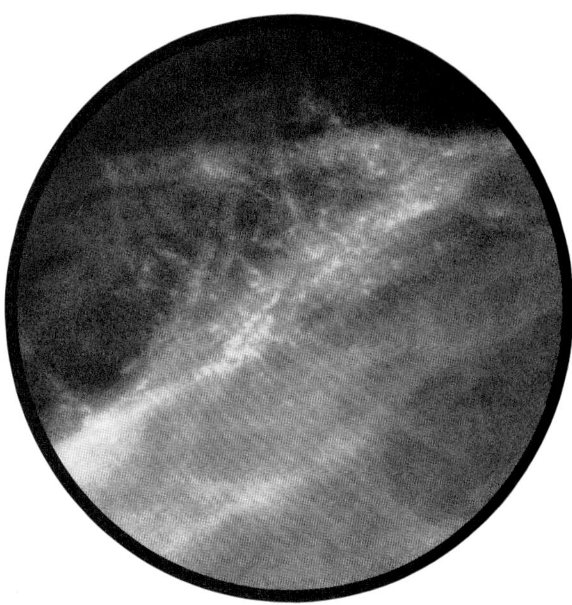

Fig. 31.3b

Essentially any form of lactiferous duct carcinoma may produce Paget's disease of the nipple through epidermal invasion by tumor. One should always be very careful to search for fine, intraductal calcifications in the immediate subareolar region. These calcium deposits may not always be of the microcalcific type such as are typical for carcinoma. Instead they may manifest themselves as linear, typically intraductal calcifications, occasionally appearing in association with more coarse benign calcifications (fig. 31.4b and c). The carcinomatous thickening of the lactiferous ducts may not be particularly marked and in some cases may be absent in the mammogram.

In any case of areolar or nipple eczema the entire breast must be carefully examined. A carcinoma may only be recognized by calcification or an increase in connective tissue proliferation within the parenchyma (fig. 31.5b and c). It is of fundamental importance that in any case of protracted areolar or nipple eczema the entire breast and retromammary tissue should be suspected of harboring a carcinoma and that the most minimal abnormality of breast tissue should be subjected to accurate excisional biopsy with intraoperative mammography of the biopsy material.

A negative mammogram in the presence of suspicious areolar or nipple changes does not rule out the diagnosis of Paget's carcinoma!

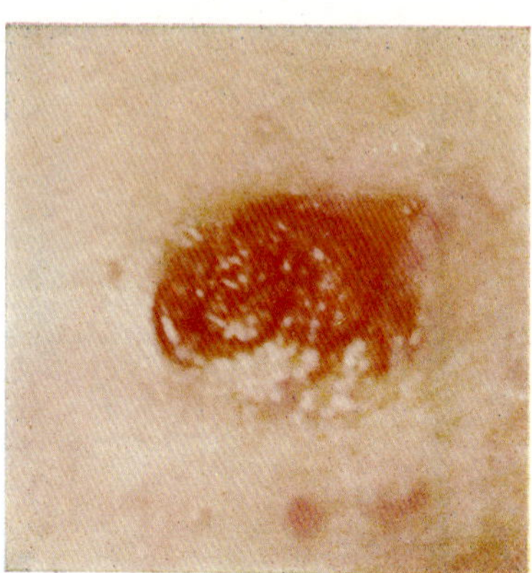

Fig. **31**.4a Gradually progressive nipple eczema over a period of several months with erythema and thickening of the areola.

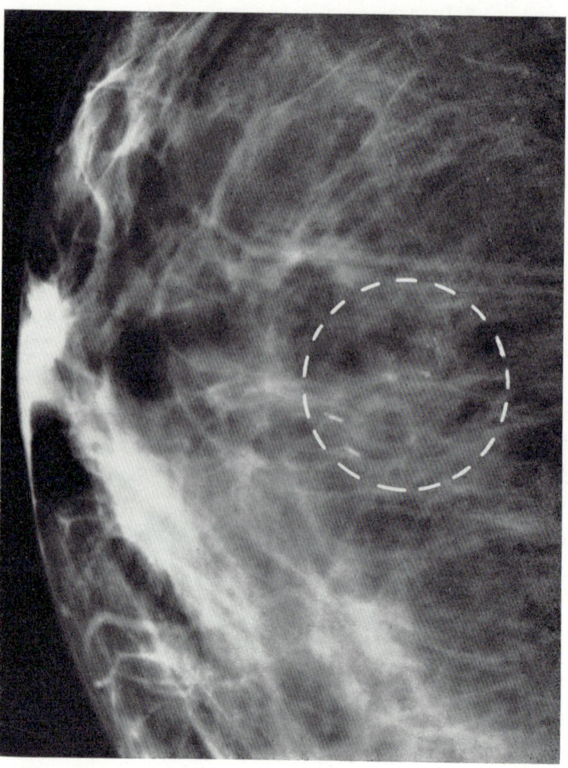

Fig. **31**.4b, c Mammography: Skin thickening of the areola is not present; however, there is enlargement of the subareolar lactiferous ducts. An occasional linear and somewhat coarse calcification is identified to better advantage in a magnification of the local area (Fig. 31.4c). This roentgen finding in correlation with the nipple changes suggests Paget carcinoma. Histologically verified.

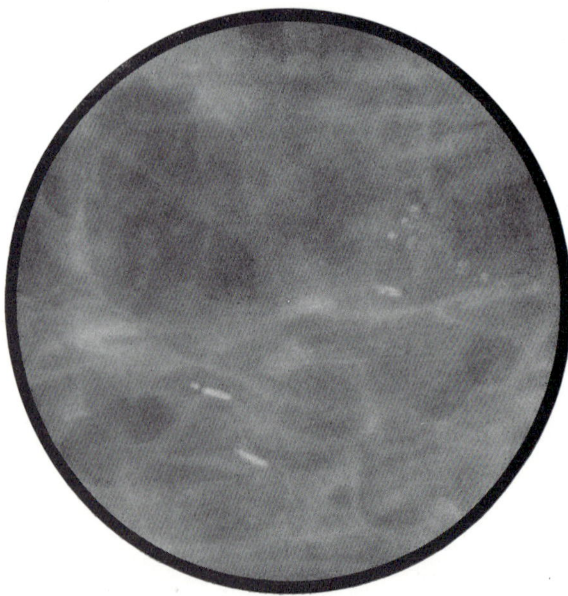

Fig. **31**.4c

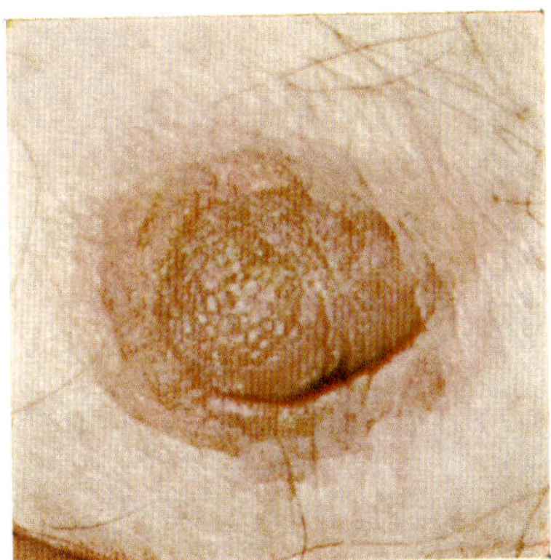

Fig. **31**.5a   Noncharacteristic nipple changes which are more suggestive of local benign inflammation. No palpatory findings.

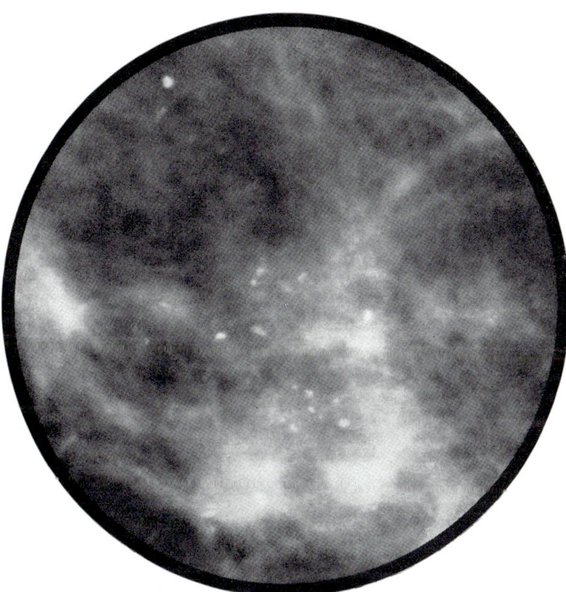

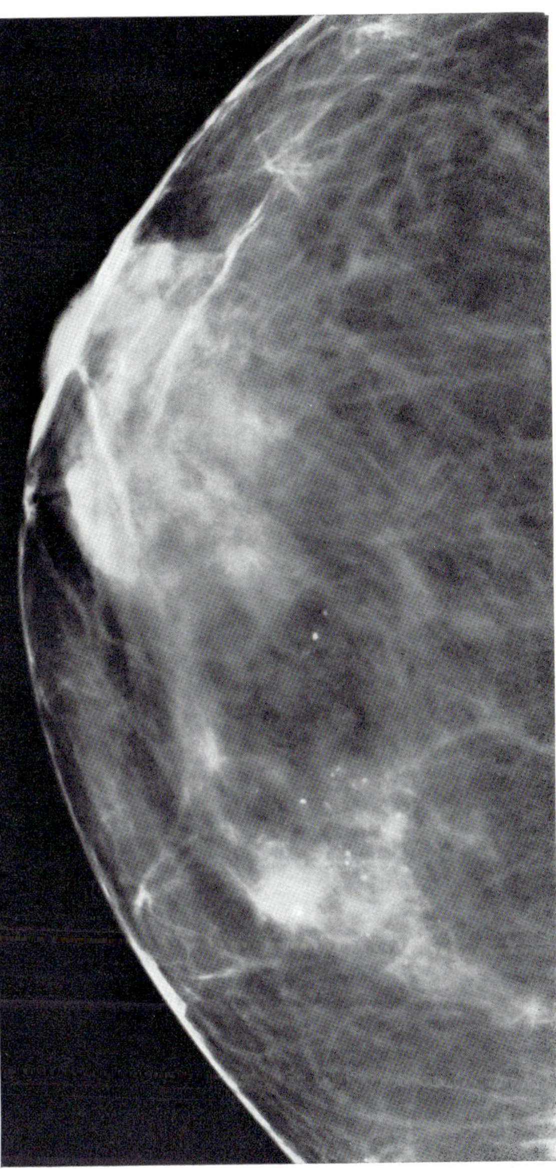

Fig. **31**.5b, c   Increased density of the subareolar tissue, microcalcifications deeper in the breast. The calcifications are very dense, vary in size and form and appear somewhat fragmented. The surrounding tissue is of increased density. Roentgen diagnosis: Infiltrating lactiferous duct carcinoma; in view of the nipple changes represents Paget's carcinoma. Histologically verified.

Chapter 32

Carcinoma Simplex

Definition and Pathology

As the name indicates carcinoma simplex consists of a regularly structured carcinomatous tissue growth associated with much stromal proliferation (fig. 32.1). At operation this whitish-gray or grayish-red, moderately firm tumor mass is relatively well circumscribed (fig. 32.2). If there is much proliferation of stromal tissue the border between tumor and surrounding breast parenchyma is less sharply defined. Carcinoma simplex not uncommonly and particularly within the central confines of the tumor mass, evokes a productive fibrosis giving the appearance of a scirrhus carcinoma on histological examination. Because the differentiation between carcinoma simplex and scirrhus carcinoma is not always clear microscopically it has been suggested that these two types of breast carcinomas be included in one group under the name "infiltrating ductal carcinoma with fibrosis" (McDivitt, Stewart, Berg 1968). About 75% of breast carcinomas fall into this category.

Clinical Findings

The clinical findings in this type of breast carcinoma are variable. In one case the productive fibrosis and in others the proliferative carcinomatous growth is the predominant finding. In the case of predominating fibrotic changes, as in those cases which are mostly scirrhus, the clinical findings are tumor fixation, nipple retraction, and skin retraction and fixation. In tumors with lesser stromal proliferation the primary palpatory findings will be an irregular, nodular, coarse dominant mass connected to or displacing the overlying skin. In advanced cases the tumor may ulcerate. Puncture and biopsy may yield positive cytological diagnosis.

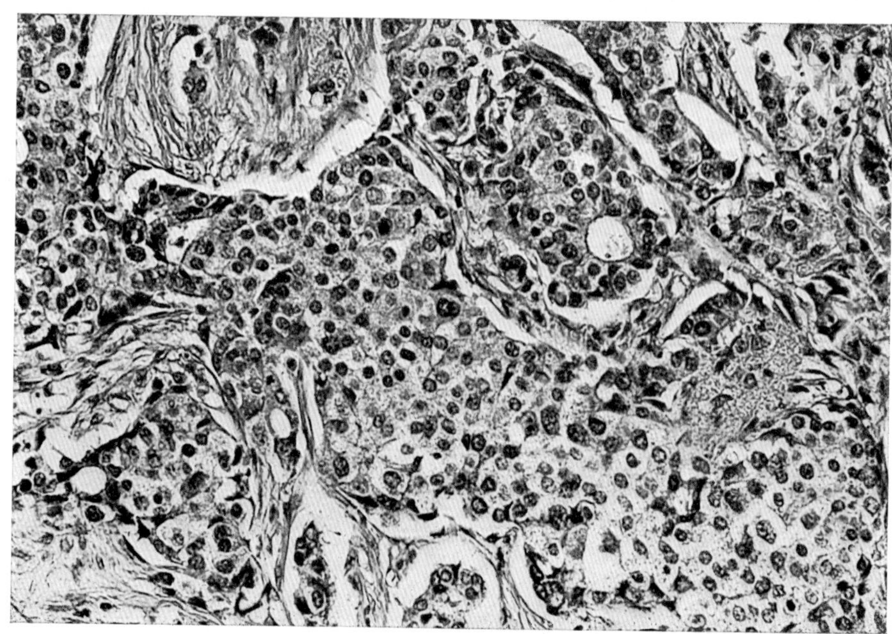

Fig. **32**.1 Carcinoma simplex: Solid strands and clumps of atypical epithelial cells with polymorphic and hyperchromatic nuclei, asscciated with stromal proliferation.

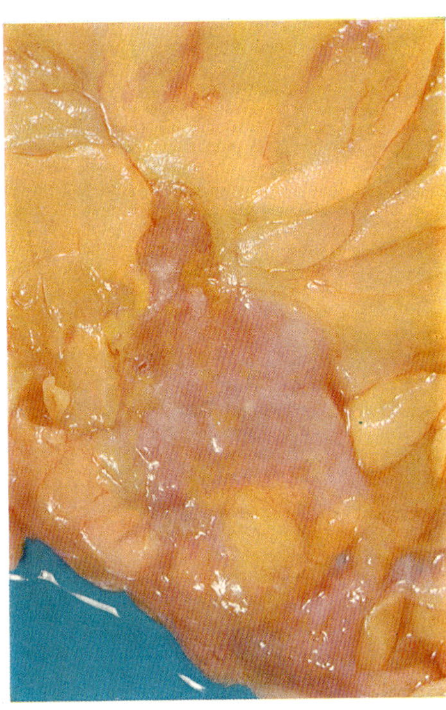

Fig 32.2   Carcinoma simplex with relatively sharp differentiation from surrounding fatty tissue.

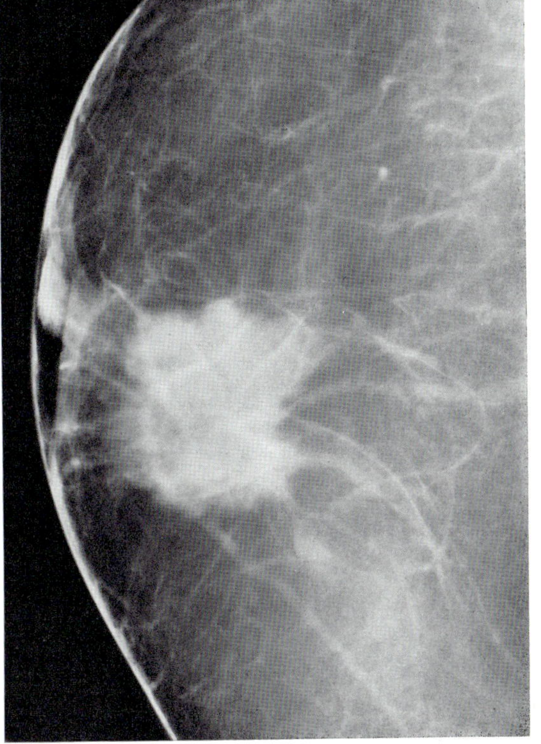

Fig. 32.3   Subareolar mass 2.5 cm in diameter. Tumor margin is nodular. Small spiculations as well as several "tail of the comet" extensions are seen. No calcifications. There is nipple retraction and thickening of the areola. Histology: Carcinoma simplex.

Roentgenology

The infiltrative ductal carcinoma of the simplex type presents as a nodular dominant mass in the mammogram. The extensive connective tissue reaction in the vicinity of the tumor, frequently seen in scirrhus carcinoma, is not present. The solid mass has a nodular poorly defined contour with occasional short, fine connective tissue extensions. More peripherally the breast tissue appears normal and without reactive changes. There may be increased vascularity with tortuous, "cork screw" dilated veins. Calcification of this tumor is less frequent than in the scirrhus or other types of ductal carcinomas. When it does occur it is more likely to exhibit coarse, irregular calcific deposits rather than the fine punctate microcalcifications typically seen in intraductal and scirrhus carcinoma. The coarser calcifications of carcinoma simplex result from tumor necrosis. These calcifications are not as dense or as bizarre as those seen in fibroadenomas, but instead are more chalky and ropelike and are distributed in the area of tumor necrosis. There is a definite difference in the calcification of carcinoma simplex, compared to that in fibroadenoma (fig. 32.5).

In the surrounding area of the tumor mass one frequently finds the ringlike calcifications indicative of liponecrosis microcystica calcificans (LEBORGNE). Infiltration in the subcutaneous fatty tissue and edematous or infiltrative skin thickening is rare in carcinoma simplex. The overlying skin may be deformed by large tumor masses when the carcinoma is in the periphery of the breast. Only in the later stages when there is direct adhesion of the skin to the carcinoma and beginning ulceration will thickening be observed.

The roentgen signs of carcinoma simplex (fig. 32.3; 32.4a and b) are as follows:

1) Irregularly contoured, nodular mass;

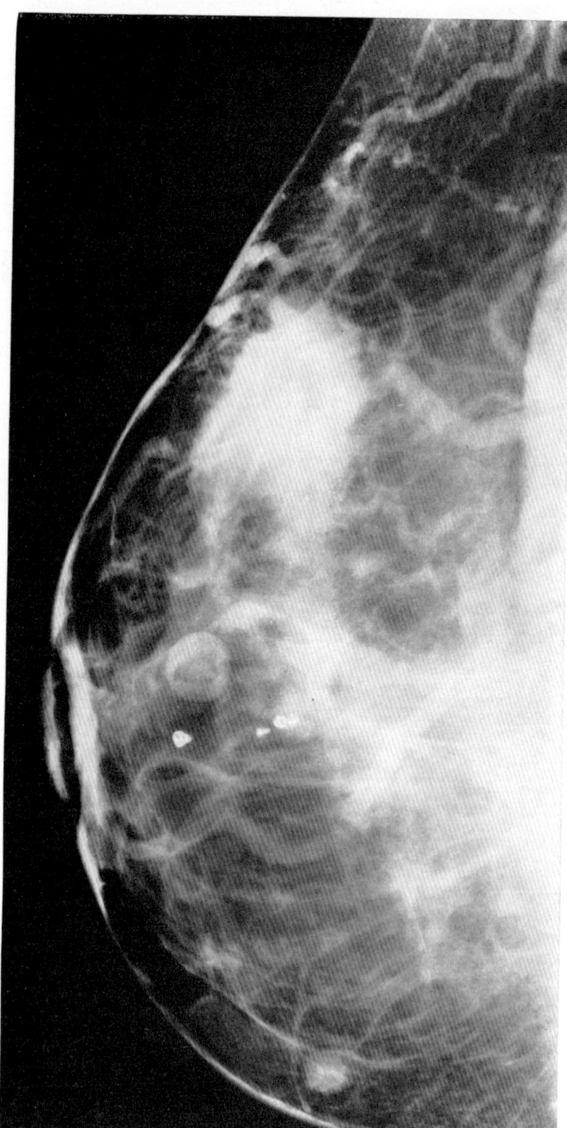

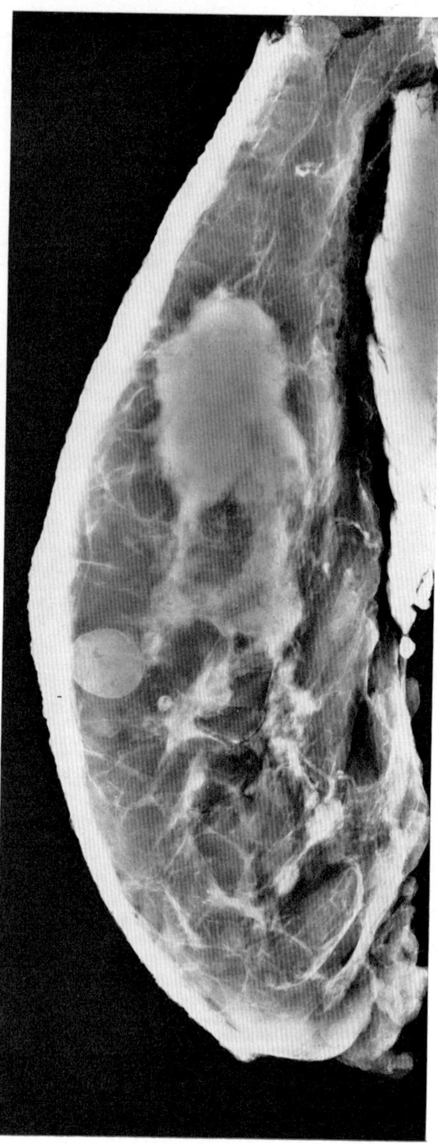

Fig. **32**.4a   Irregular mass about 1.7 × 2.5 cm in size above the nipple immediately underneath the skin. Tumor surface is ill-defined, lobular with spicules. Several tortuous, dilated veins are seen in the vicinity of the mass. There is only minimal infiltration of the subcutaneous fatty layer. No skin thickening. There is an area of linear infiltration connecting the tumor mass to the subareolar region and there is thickening of the areola. In the immediate subareolar region a cyst 5 mm in diameter and numerous cystlike calcifications are observed (fat necrosis, Leborgne).

Fig. **32**.4b   Roentgenogram of the biopsy specimen. The solid carcinomatous tumor mass is seen to better advantage with its irregular borders and tumor spicules. The cordlike carcinomatous infiltration from tumor to the areola is particularly evident. Histology: Carcinoma simplex.

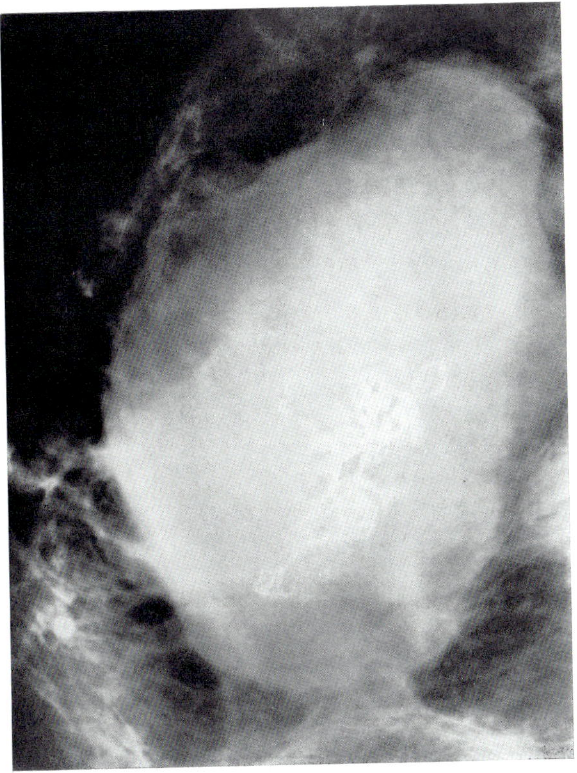

Fig. **32**.5

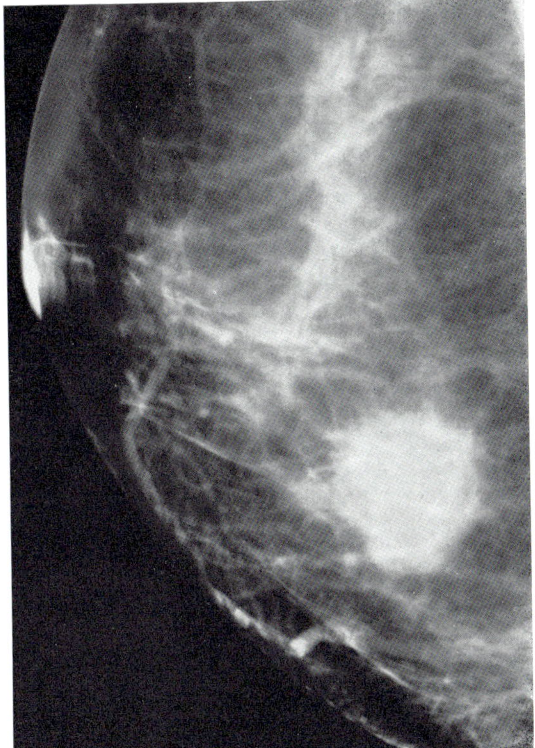

Fig. **32**.6

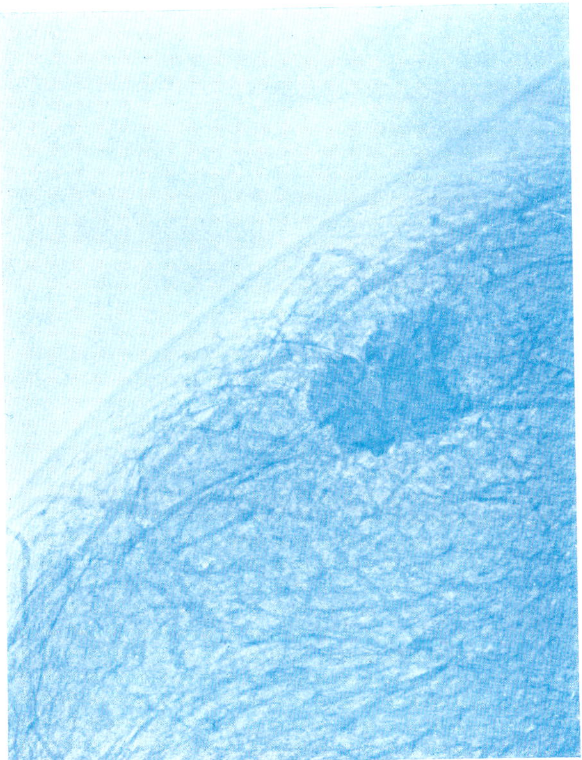

Fig. **32**.7

Fig. **32**.5 Unusually large carcinoma simplex with a diameter of 7 cm. Tumor surface is lobular with a few spiculated extensions and there are central bizarre, stringy calcifications of relatively low density. These are clearly different from the bizarre, highly dense calcifications of a fibroadenoma.

Fig. **32**.6 Tumor mass, 1.5 cm in diameter. Lateral borders appear relatively smooth. The margin of the tumor facing anteriorly is somewhat ill-defined and small spicules can be recognized with a magnifying glass. Dilated veins are present in the subcutaneous fatty tissue. Histologically verified carcinoma simplex.

Fig. **32**.7 Nodular mass with irregular margins but no spiculation. Histological diagnosis: Carcinoma solidum simplex.

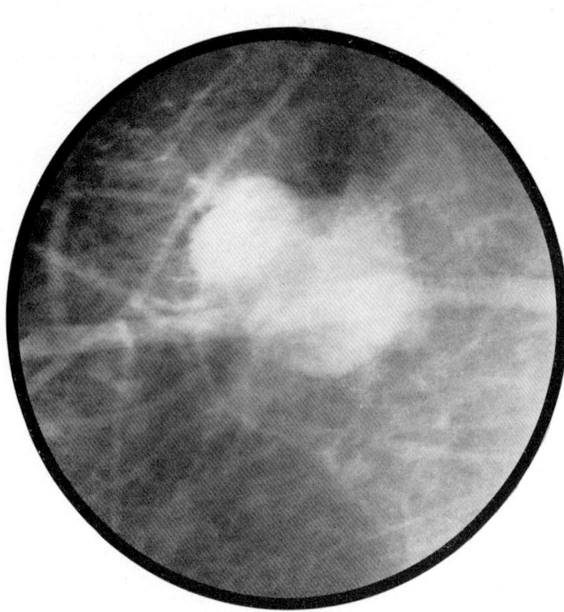

Fig. **32**.8 Smoothly marginated mass. Lobular fibroadenoma? loculated cyst? carcinoma simplex? medullary carcinoma?
The dilated vein extending across the tumor nodule is the only sign suggesting carcinoma.
Puncture: Fragmented, sanguineous tissue.
Cytology: Typical carcinoma cells. Histology: Carcinoma simplex.

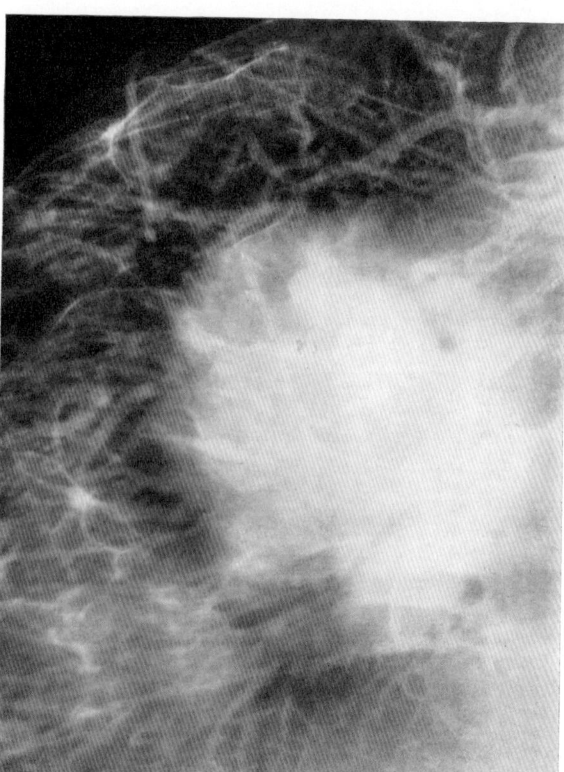

Fig. **32**.9 Tumor mass 4 × 5 cm in size. Margins of the tumor are unsharp because of numerous small spicules. Histologically verified carcinoma simplex.

2) ill-defined blurred border with fine sawtooth contour;

3) increased vascularity in the region of the tumor with dilated and corkscrew-type veins;

4) streaky connective tissue thickening between the tumor mass and subareolar region; thickening and retraction of the areola; infiltration of the subcutaneous fatty layer and skin in the immediate vicinity of the tumor mass;

5) occasionally coarse and irregular calcifications. Typical microcalcifications within the tumor mass are rare.

The greatest diagnostic difficulty ensues when the tumor mass is only minimally dense and its borders are relatively smooth and sharp (fig. 32.6, 32.7).

In such cases the tumor mass of carcinoma simplex cannot readily be differentiated from a fibroadenoma or loculated cyst (fig. 32.8). A medullary carcinoma may have a similar roentgen appearance. In the absence of other signs of carcinoma only puncture and aspiration of the tumor mass may yield further diagnostic evidence. This should be performed in all cases in order to make an accurate preoperative diagnosis. Carcinoma simplex may achieve a relatively large size but always retains its irregular borders with very fine "saw-toothing" and small connective tissue adhesions (fig. 32.9). If there is an increase in the amount of connective tissue proliferation with carcinoma simplex then there may be complete obliteration of the margin of the tumor and only large coarse septa are seen in the periphery of the mass. Such thickened strands of fibrous tissue that course directly through nearby breast parenchyma or normal fibrous stroma, particularly in a radiating fashion from the central mass, are always a sign of carcinoma (fig. 32.10).

The histological structure of carcinoma simplex is reflected in the mammogram in that, on the

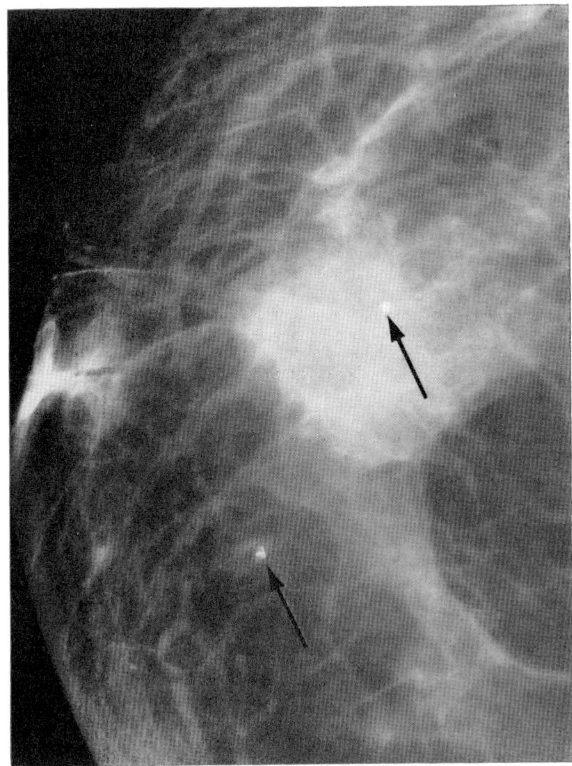

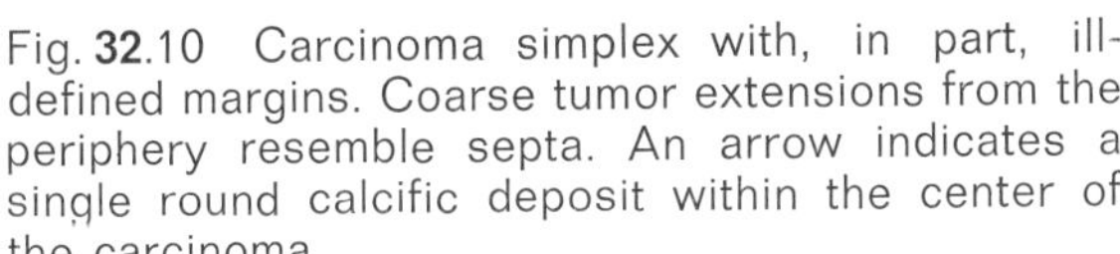

Fig. **32**.10 Carcinoma simplex with, in part, ill-defined margins. Coarse tumor extensions from the periphery resemble septa. An arrow indicates a single round calcific deposit within the center of the carcinoma.
A second calcification consists of a conglomerate of several irregularly formed calcium flecks. These are within the fatty tissue and far removed from the tumor mass and are not diagnostically significant in terms of indicating the specific type of tumor.
Of more significance roentgenologically is the septation of the tumor surface and the surrounding fatty tissue.

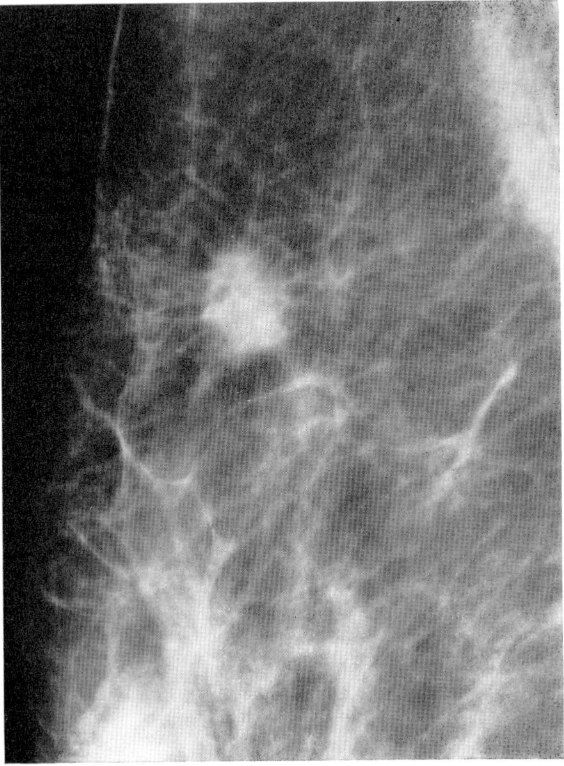

Fig. **32**.11 The tumor mass (1 × 1.5 cm in size) consists of a central nodule and numerous fine surface extensions which reach far into the surrounding fatty tissue. This characterizes the scirrhus nature of this carcinoma simplex.
Histology: Infiltrating ductal carcinoma the extension of which was characterized in part as carcinoma simplex and in part as scirrhus carcinoma.

surface of the tumor, radiating connective tissue extensions or septa are found which may reach through the subcutaneous fatty layer of the breast to the skin or to the thoracic wall (fig. 32.11).

If the tumor is subareolar, retraction of the nipple may be expected which can progress very rapidly and thus provide a clinical sign of carcinoma (fig. 32.12). If carcinoma simplex is deep within dense breast parenchyma diagnostic difficulties arise (fig. 32.13). Here one should search for a nonhomogeneous increase in tissue density noting particularly any tendency towards a nodular form with superficially distributed fine connective tissue septa. These are unequivocal roentgen signs of carcinoma.

In certain cases the histologists may have difficulty in identifying the exact type of tumor and may have to be satisfied with diagnosing a carcinoma and identifying the predominating type of tissue. There may be tumor tissue in the periphery or in other parts of the carcinoma which may not be of the same type as that of the central dominant mass. One should be cautious therefore in trying to give a histological diagnosis on the basis of roentgen morphology. Should the histological diagnosis of the type of carcinoma differ from that given by the roentgenologist one may be accused of overdiagnosis. However, it is still worthwhile to remember that, in the majority of cases, it is possible to differentiate the tumor type on the basis of roentgen morphology just as well as the pathologist is able to do this on the basis of examining the macroscopic preparation.

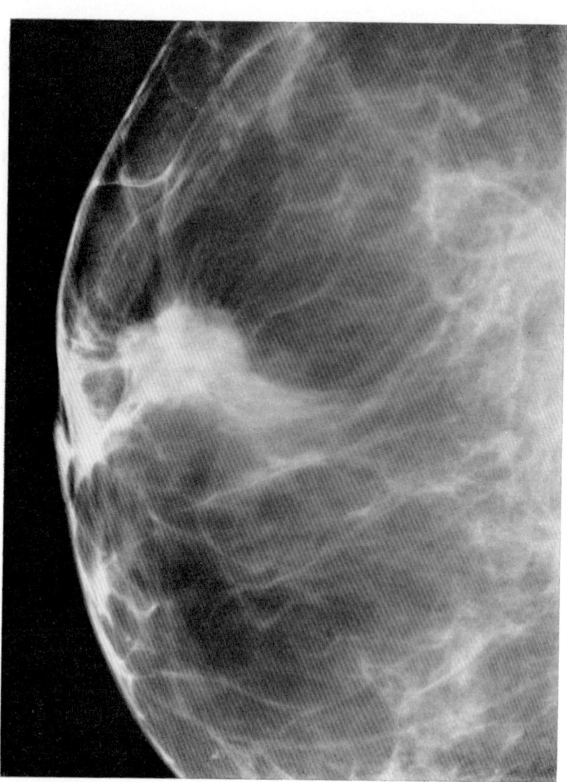

Fig. **32**.12   Tumor nodule 1.5 cm in diameter situated 1 cm above and deep to the areola. Tumor surface is nodular and numerous spiculations extend from here to the subcutaneous layer and subareolar region. Roentgenologically this picture is overwhelmingly that of a carcinoma simplex with scirrhus components. Verified histologically.

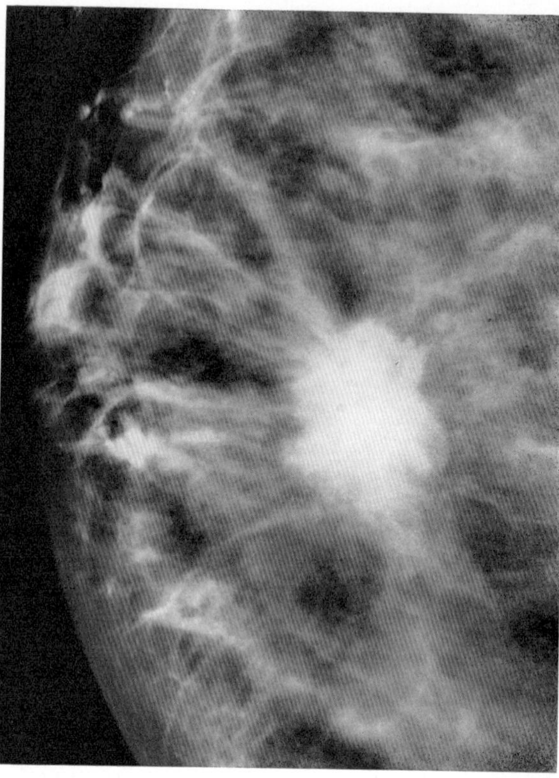

Fig. **32**.13   A masslike density of about 2 cm in diameter is identified within an area of dense breast parenchyma. Contours of the mass are ill-defined with numerous spicules extending from the tumor mass into the surrounding parenchyma.
Carcinoma simplex with scirrhus extension, verified histologically.

Chapter 33

Scirrhus Carcinoma

Definition and Pathology

Scirrhus carcinoma is a type of ductal carcinoma with particularly extensive connective tissue proliferation (productive fibrosis).

Microscopically the fibrosis is the primary presentation with extensive hyalinization of connective tissue. There may be calcification. The carcinomatous cells are found in narrow files, frequently as strands in single rows (fig. 33.1). Not uncommonly they may be dissociated within the hyalinized stroma. The carcinomatous tissue may be anaplastic or there may be a tendency towards differentiation into adenoid structures, and therefore the histological picture may be that of a partly differentiated scirrhus adeno-carcinoma. Aside from the extensive infiltrative tumor growth one may also note intraductal tumor tissue with a tendency towards necrosis and calcification.

Macroscopically scirrhus carcinoma is recognized as an irregular, white, coarse, connective tissue growth with poorly defined borders, spreading in a stellate or radiating fashion into the surrounding breast (fig. 33.2). The stellate fibrous extensions are called "cancer feet". This is not actual tumor tissue but rather a fibrotic reaction of adjoining breast tissue to the carcinoma. With extensive spread, however, even these fibrotic hyalinized bands of connective tissue may be invaded by tumor cells. So far there is no satisfactory explanation why such a desmoplastic response is elicited by scirrhus carcinoma or what may be the histochemical or immunologic cause for this response.

Clinical Findings

Scirrhus carcinoma is the most frequent form of breast cancer. The classical clinical signs of

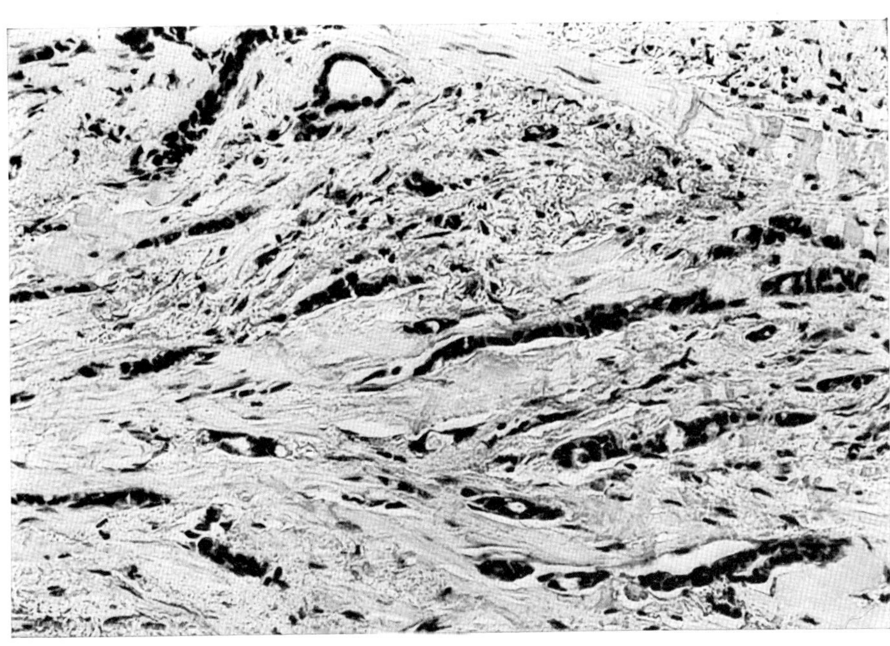

Fig. **33**.1.   Scirrhus carcinoma: Atypical epitelial cells mostly arranged in single cell rows and surrounded by extensive fibrosis with some hyaline degeneration.

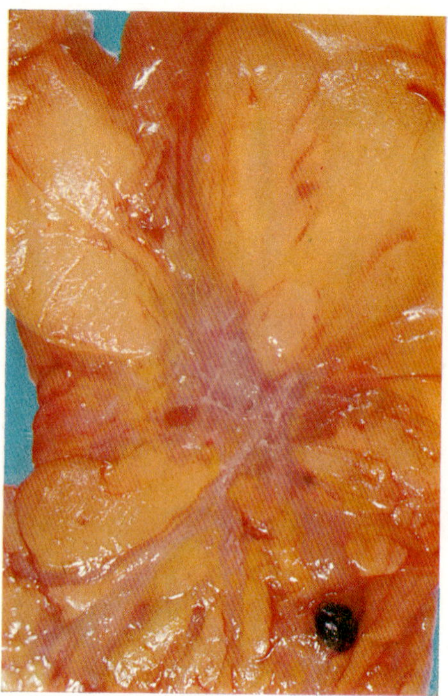

Fig. **33**.2   Scirrhus carcinoma with radiating extension into the breast tissue.

scirrhus carcinoma consist of a firm nodular, frequently nonmovable mass with fixation, as well as flattening of overlying skin and nipple retraction.

The size of a scirrhus carcinoma may vary from a few millimeters in diameter to that of a tumor involving the entire breast.

Large and deep-lying scirrhus carcinomas may grow into and be fixed to the thoracic wall.

Superficial tumors often cause extensive skin retraction; however, this same sign may be seen as a result of an infiltrative shortening of Cooper's ligament by a small and deeply placed scirrhus carcinoma. This so-called "plateau sign" however, is not pathognomonic for a fibrosing carcinoma. Similar skin fixation may be found in fat necrosis following trauma. The plateau sign can often only be elicited with the help of a special hand maneuver (fig. 2.12).

Fixation and retraction of the nipple are most frequently the consequence of a subareolar scirrhus carcinoma, but may also be caused by a benign fibrosis of the breast (although in these cases the nipple retraction takes place over a period of years).

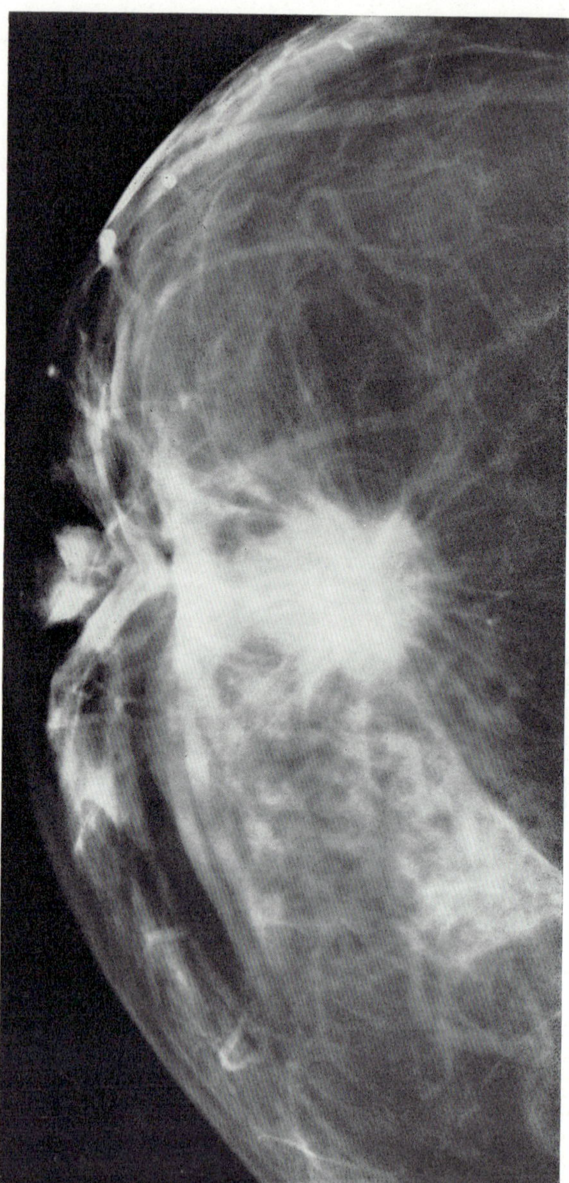

Fig. **33**.3   Scirrhus carcinoma with a central tumor mass 2.5 cm in diameter. Stellate tumor margins consisting of fine spiculated extensions surrounding the entire tumor and extending up to 3 cm into the peripheral tissues. The nipple is thickened and retracted. No microcalcifications. Clinically the tumor was felt to have a diameter of about 5 cm. The difference in size between palpatory findings and that recorded an the roentgenogram is characteristic for scirrhus carcinoma.

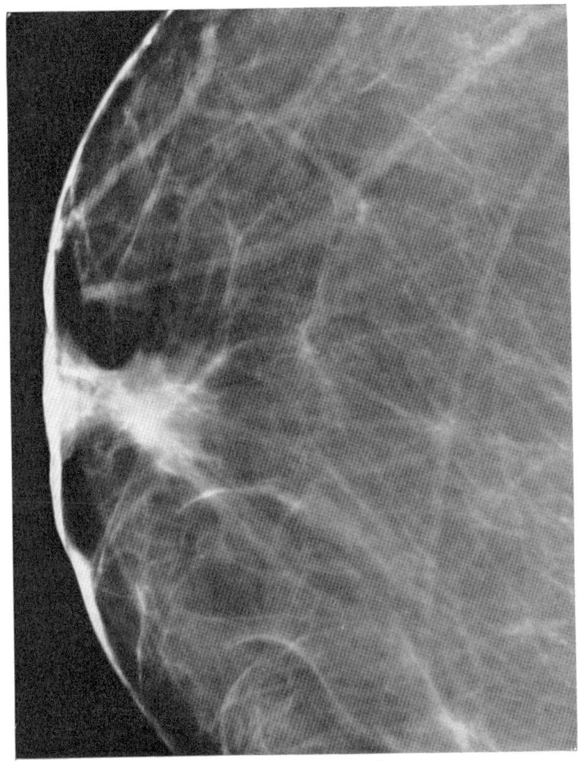

Fig. **33**.4

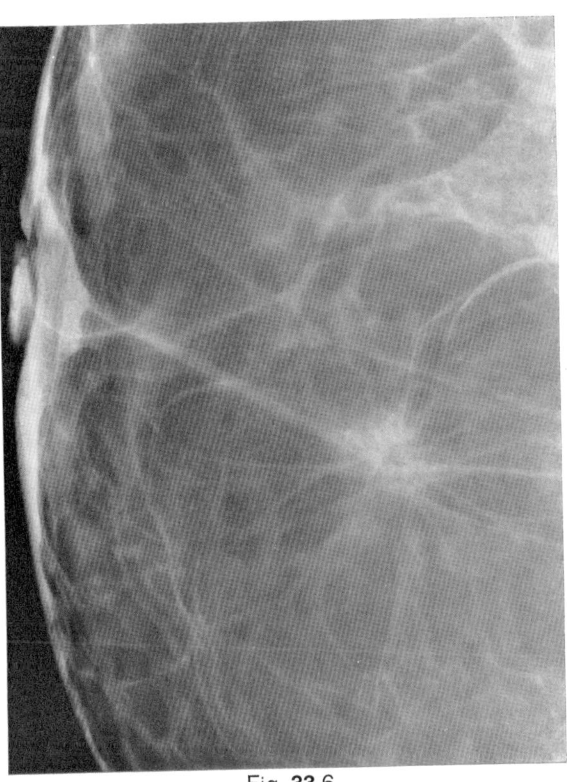

Fig. **33**.5

Fig. **33**.4   Small subareolar scirrhus carcinoma measuring 10 mm in diameter with a few coarse spicules. These radiate outward and result in minimal retraction of the nipple seen as a triangular density in the immediate subareolar area in the mammogram.

Fig. **33**.5   Thickening and flattening of the skin of the areola is observed. Careful inspection reveals a stellate structure in the immediate subareolar region with extension through the normal connective tissue. This is a small subareolar scirrhus carcinoma.

Fig. **33**.6   Deep in the breast, 5 cm behind the nipple there is a small scirrhus carcinoma with radiating spicules extending from its surface with a broader zone of fibrotic infiltration connecting the lesion to the posterior surface of the areola ("warning streaks").

Fig. **33**.6

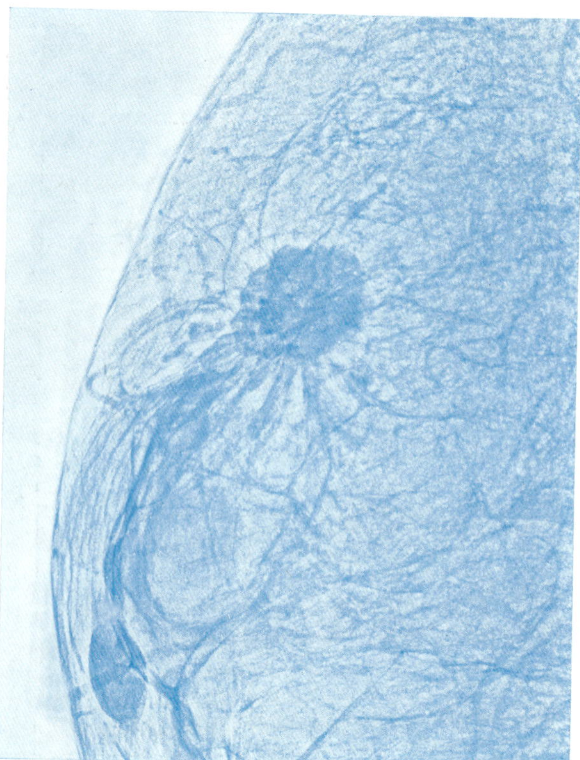

Fig. **33**.7 Scirrhus carcinoma. Nodular mass with typical spiculation. Several microcalcifications are seen within the confines of the tumor. Suspicious spicules of connective tissue extend from the tumor mass to the nipple. There was skin fixation over the mass on palpation.

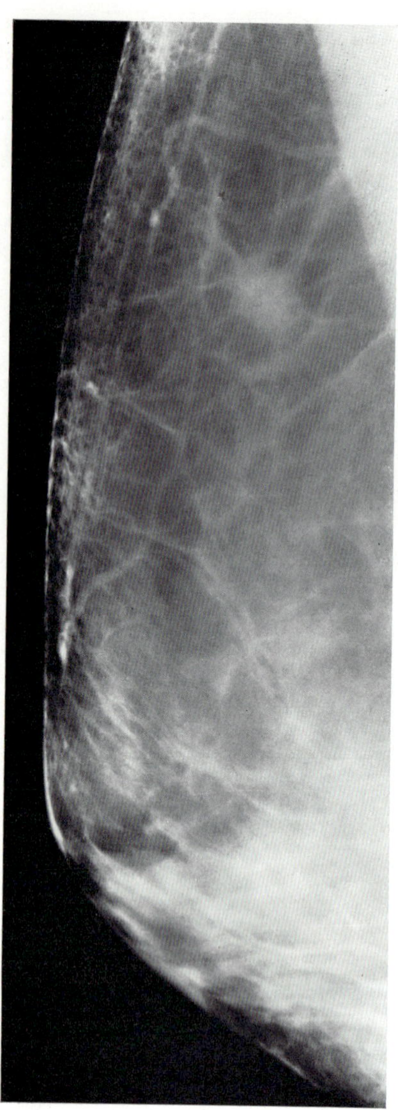

Fig. **33**.8 Small mass of low density and measuring 7 mm in diameter in the lateral aspect of the breast near the axillary fold. This distance from tumor to skin is 2 cm. It is a clinically occult scirrhus carcinoma of the left breast. A right mastectomy has been performed in the past for carcinoma. The diagnosis is verified histologically. There were no lymph node metastases in this case.

If scirrhus carcinoma is confined to the lower half of the breast then the usual curvilinear contour of the breast may become irregular.

In advanced cases scirrhus carcinoma may cause extensive shrinking or other marked deformity of the breast.

Sanguineous nipple discharge is relatively rare in this tumor.

Roentgenology

Scirrhus breast carcinoma is recognized in the roentgenogram primarily on the basis of the surrounding fibrosis.

A typical case of scirrhus carcinoma consists of a central mass with lobular and ill-defined contours from which numerous fibrous strands extend into the surrounding tissue (fig. 33.3). These fibrous extensions from the surface of the tumor are also called "cancer feet" in the mammogram.

The roentgen diagnosis of scirrhus carcinoma is relatively easy in the involutional, fatty breast. It is more difficult, even in the involutional breast, when the carcinoma is situated in a retromammary location. In older women ectatic lactiferous ducts may extend in normal fashion towards partially fibrotic residual parenchymal tissue resembling a stellate structure. Recognition that this may be a normal appearance, however, should not cause one to overlook a small carcinoma in this area. Disorganized, newly formed fibrous strands that appear to permeate all normal breast tissue whether parenchymal or connective tissue should make the radiologist suspicious (fig. 33.4).

Occasionally the diagnosis of a discrete, small retromammary scirrhus carcinoma can only be made by correlation with the clinical history, the latter indicating recent onset of nipple retraction (fig. 33.5). Careful observation of the mammogram, including the use of a magnifying glass is indicated and may reveal the fine stellate connective tissue proliferation which signifies carcinomatous changes.

In deeply located scirrhus carcinoma occasionally there are found long, linear fibrous connections with the areola and nipple (fig. 33.6), which because of their length and extent should arouse the suspicion of carcinomatous origin. GERSHON-COHEN (1970) called these fibrous connections "sentinel strands". We call them "warning strands" (fig. 33.7). Such fibrous strands are particularly suspect when they do not follow the normal subareolar radiating pattern of the lactiferous ducts.

One must also be careful to search for stellate soft tissue shadows in the periphery of the breast. Following involution of the breast parenchyma such parenchymal rests should no longer be present in the outer margins of the organ. Stellate densities such as are depicted in fig. 33.8 should immediately arouse suspicion of scirrhus carcinoma. Increased vascularity or desmoplastic response may be detected only by very careful examination. The surrounding tissue reaction may not be always as extensive as in the classical description of scirrhus carcinoma.

Occasionally slight irregularity of the tumor margin and an occasional small calcific deposit in the periphery may be the only signs which indicate the possibility of a malignant process (fig. 33.9). Scirrhus carcinoma does not always include a central tumor mass; occasionally the tumor substrate may be only a linear density, which may be connected to the subareolar region and resemble dense parenchymal tissue. If one is able to verify irregular, fine septa that course through normal connective tissue in a stellate fashion, this is a characteristic sign of scirrhus desmoplastic response (fig. 33.10, 33.11).

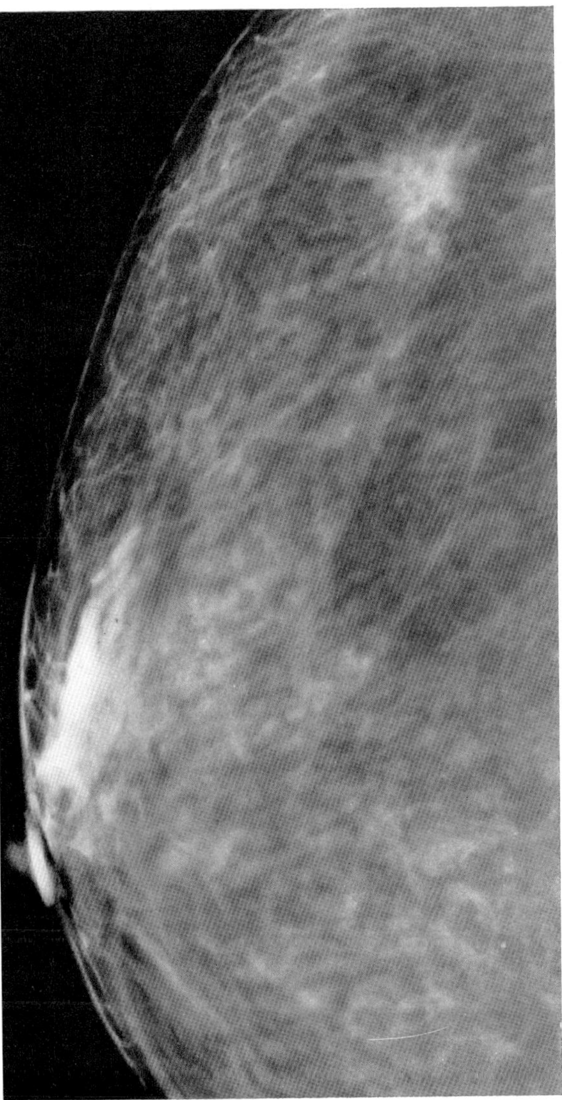

Fig. **33**.9   In the periphery of the lateral aspect of the breast parenchyma there is a tumor mass measuring 8 mm in diameter with both coarse and fine peripheral spiculations.
Histology: Ductal carcinoma predominantly of the scirrhus type. Axillary lymph node metastases were present in spite of the small size of the primary tumor.

Scirrhus changes in the vicinity of a ductal carcinoma are very difficult to recognize in the breast of a younger woman in which the normal parenchyma persists (fig. 33.12). In such a case the primary sign to look for is a proliferation of spicules of fibrous tissue permeating the subcutaneous fatty layer (fig. 33.13). Here a comparison view of the other breast becomes important. Frequently this is the only way to differentiate a

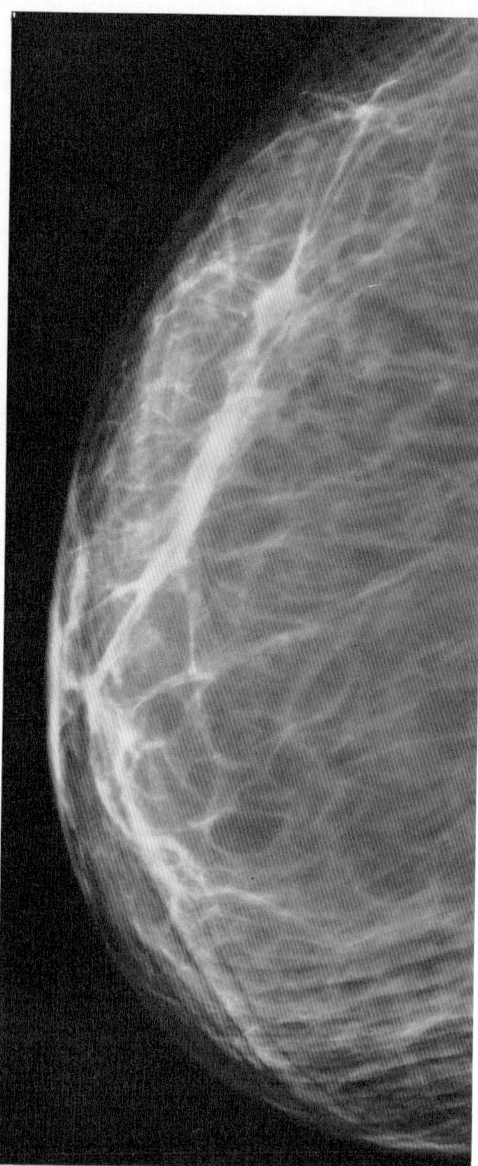

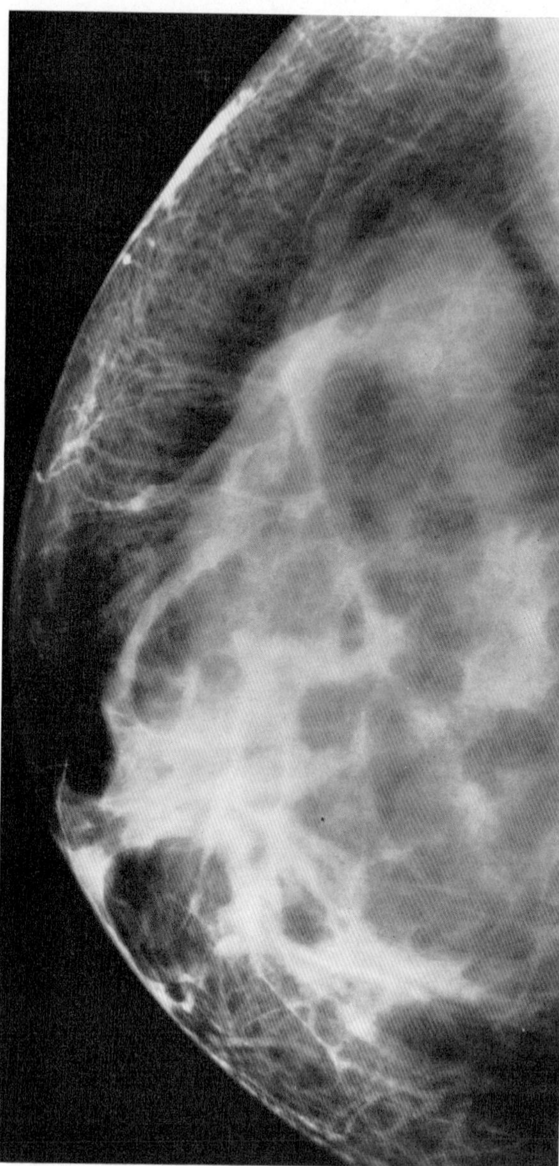

Fig. **33**.10   Involutional breast with fibrous parenchymal rests which appear to widen proximally (!)
and are associated with small fine septa extending
from the surface. These septa extend into the subcutaneous tissue and do not appear to fellow the
normal course of connective tissue septa (!).
Roentgen diagnosis: Scirrhus carcinoma, verified
histologically.

Fig. **33**.11   Scirrhus carcinoma in the upper breast
of a 71-year-old woman. Clinically: Palpable lump
with skin fixation. Mammography: The carcinoma
has infiltrated the residual parenchymal tissue in
the upper breast and has fine, scirrhus extensions
into the subcutaneous tissue. There is focal skin
thickening. Again broad linear infiltrative extensions
from the carcinoma to the subareolar region ("warning streaks") are seen.

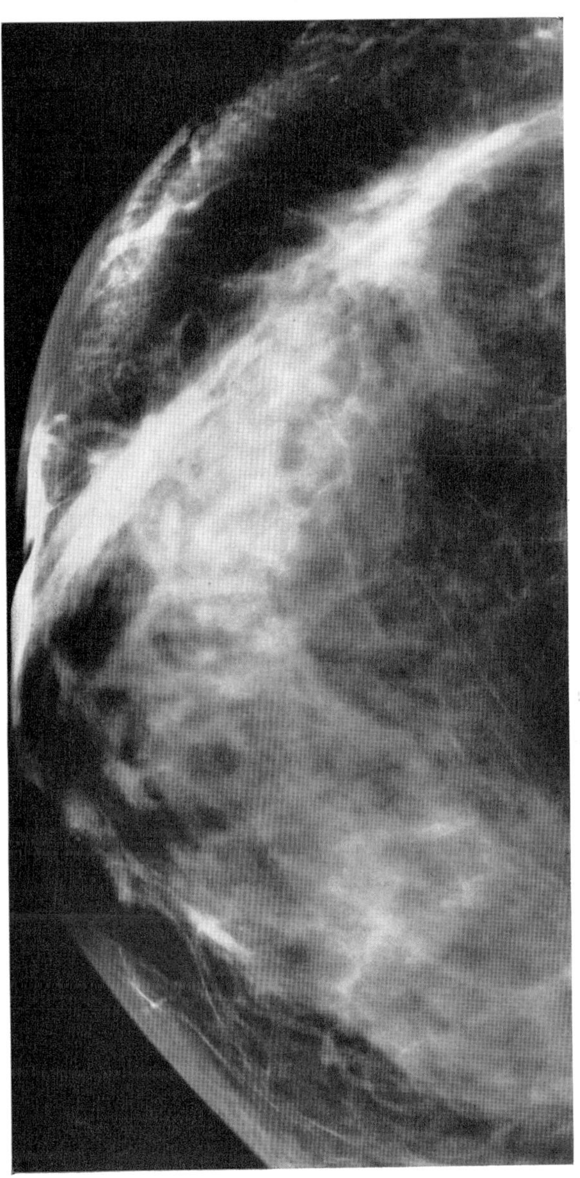

Fig. **33**.12 Scirrhus carcinoma medially. Linear infiltrative connection between carcinoma and sub-areolar region. This case clearly illustrates how infiltrated Cooper's ligaments retract the overlying skin immediately adjacent to the nipple.

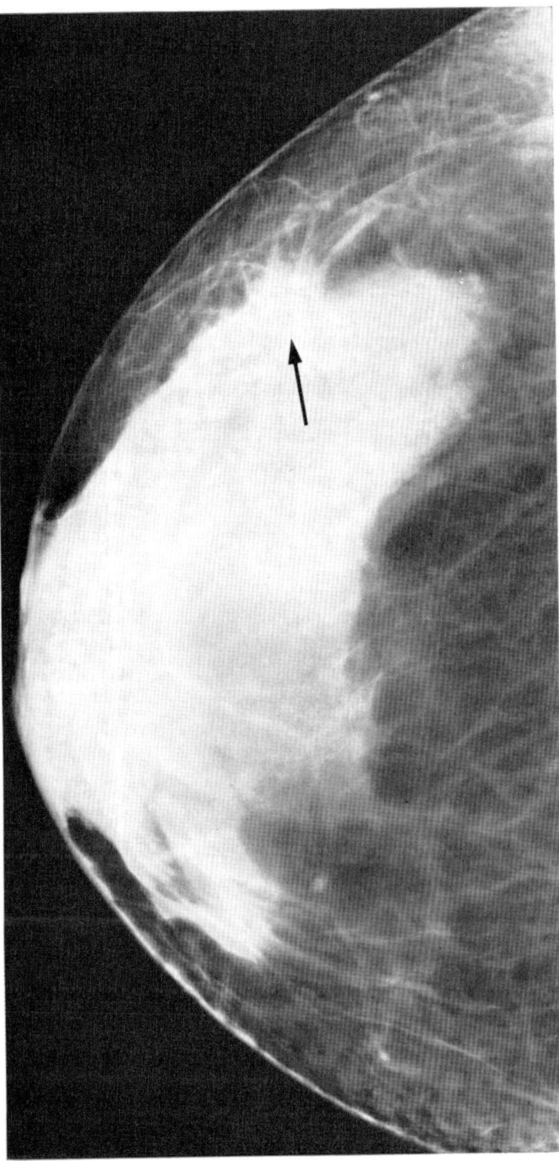

Fig. **33**.13 32-year-old woman with slightly painful firmness in the upper outer quadrant of the breast without skin abnormality. Mammography: There is considerable parenchymal residual but along the upper outer margin of the parenchyma, fine septated connective tissue extensions are seen. No skin thickening.
Roentgen diagnosis: Scirrhus carcinoma (based essentially on the changes in the contour of the parenchyma as described above). Diagnosis verified histologically.

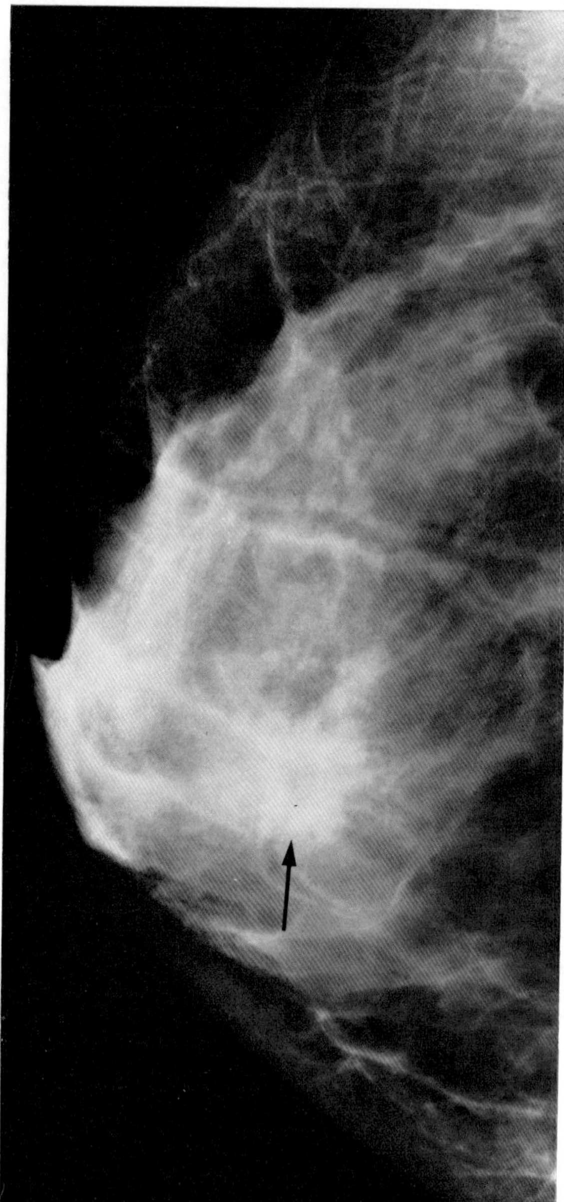

Fig. **33**.14a Irregular increased density within dense parenchyma of a 34-year-old woman (arrow).

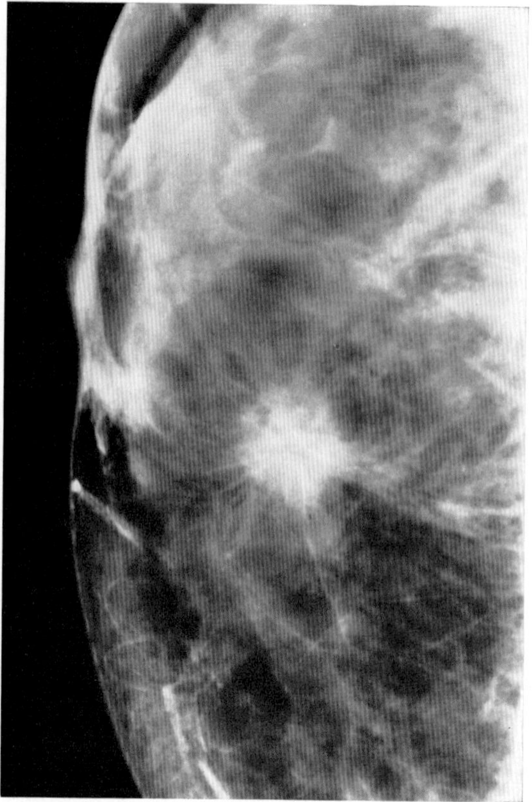

Fig. **33**.14b Coned-down compression examination of the area reveals an obvious scirrhus carcinoma. This diagnosis was verified histologically.

benign fibrotic process from the reponse to a scirrhus carcinoma.

It is important in such a case that the mammogram be heavily exposed in order to achieve as much contrast as possible between the parenchyma and sparasely interspersed fatty tissue. Even with minimal suspicion of structural changes within a dense parenchyma an additional overpenetrated mammogram using compression technique in the appropriate area should be performed (fig. 13.14a and b).

Every Stellate-Sharped Structure is a Suspect for Scirrhus Carcinoma

In the differential diagnosis between scirrhus carcinoma and mammary dysplastic fibrosis a rule of thumb is "a cancer possesses a body as well as legs, but mammary dysplasia possesses only legs". This rule, however, applies only with reservations. With some exceptions we have, in this chapter, considered the differential diagnosis of stellate-shaped breast changes. In principle all stellate breast lesions, insofar as these are not obviously the result of summation shadows of connective tissue structures, should be removed. Only in cases completely unsuspected of malignancy where there is also an absence of clinical suspicion is three months observation and repeat mammography justified.

According to GERSHON-COHEN approximately 35% of scirrhus carcinomas contain micro-

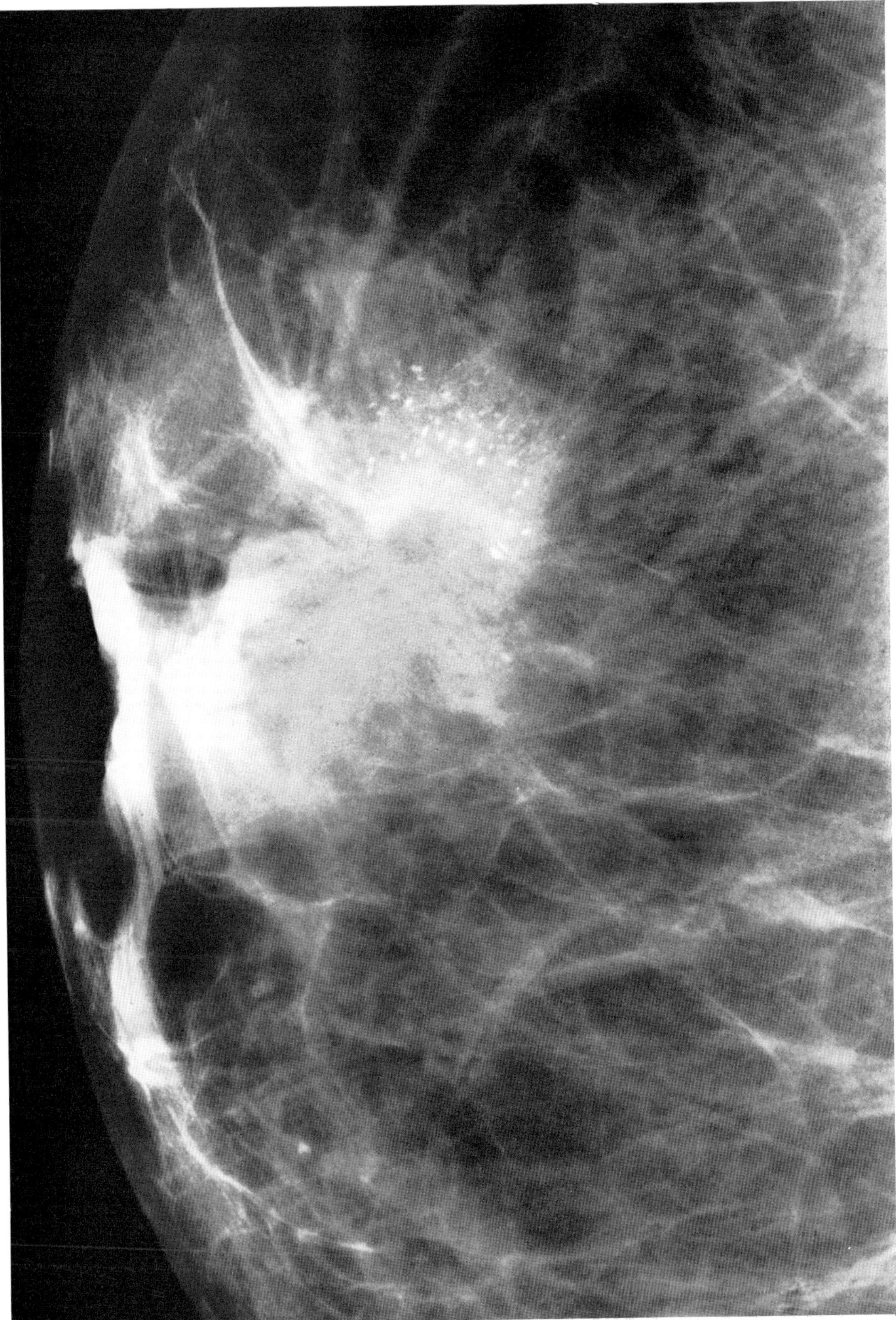

Fig. **33**.15.   Mammogram magnified 2 X. Scirrhus carcinoma with numerous typical microcalcifications. Retraction and thickening of the areola and nipple.

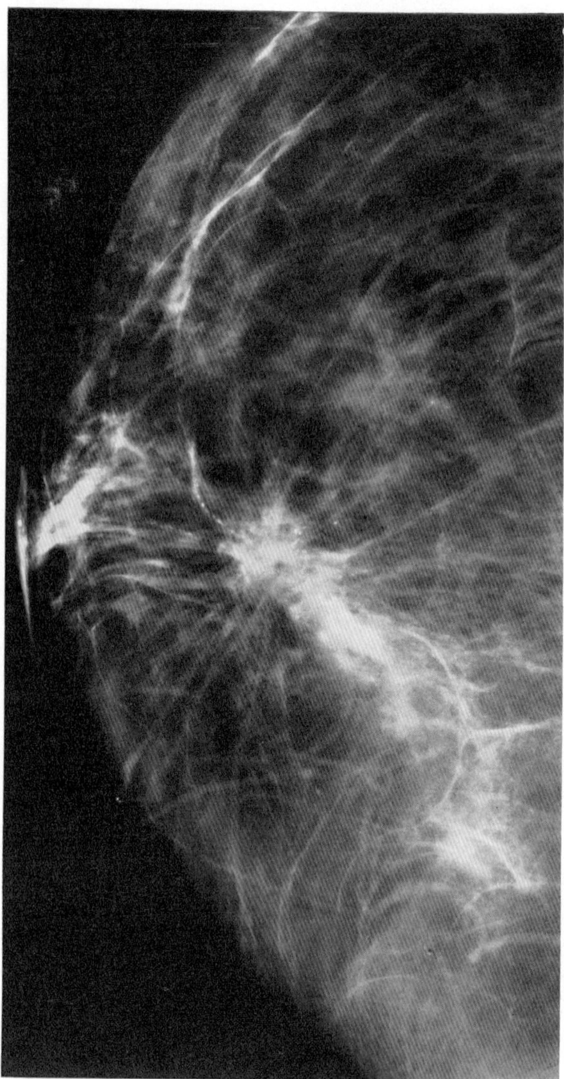

Fig. **33**.16a   Small scirrhus tumor nodule with surrounding stellate desmoplastic reaction. Microcalcifications.

calcifications. These exist within the tumor mass or in the immediate vicinity. The typical calcifications are very fine, "crystalline", extremely dense to radiation, varying in size and shape, appear "broken" (fig. 33.15, 33.16a). When extensively distributed over a large area they may resemble an "out-pouring" of the lactiferous duct (fig. 33.16b).

The veins in the vicinity of a scirrhus carcinoma are either stretched and travel through the scirrhus mass or are typically tortous, dilated and have a corkscrew appearance. Helpful again is a comparison view of the corresponding site in the other breast.

Scirrhus carcinoma by evoking a strong desmoplastic response has a tendency to involve the subcutaneous fatty tissue and result in early skin fixation (fig. 33.17a and b). The classical clinical picture results. The mammographic findings, however, precede the clinical appearance because the stellate spicules in the subcutaneous connective tissue are visible before plateau formation or retraction of the skin are clinically obvious. Similarly the skin thickening is detectable earlier in the mammogram than clinically.

It is therefore very important to evaluate the connective tissue in the subcutaneous fatty layer and also to take careful note of the skin thickness. The periphery of the breast must be carefully evaluated with a bright light source and a magnifying glass. The first sign of tumor infiltration may be a haziness of the subcutaneous fatty layer.

It is characteristic of scirrhus carcinoma that there generally exists a marked difference in tumor size as estimated by palpation and that seen in the mammogram. The mammographic tumor size is more likely to correspond to the actual diameter of the mass in the pathological specimen.

Attempting to verify the diagnosis of scirrhus carcinoma by puncture and aspiration of the tumor mass often results in negative findings. Very few cellular elements exist within the firm scirrhus tissue. Guided excisional biopsy with accurate localization of the tumor by mammography is perferable.

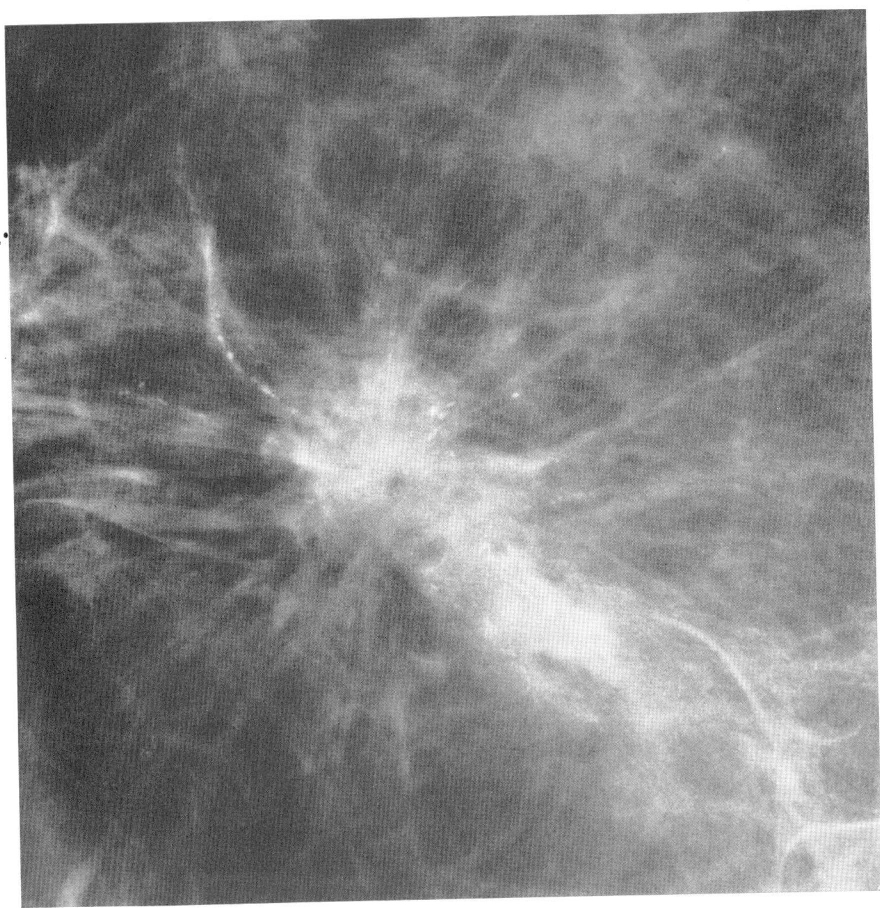

Fig. **33**.16 b.   Same case (enlarged 2 X). Adjoining the carcinomatous microcalcifications within the tumor nodules one can recognize linear intraductal calcifications.

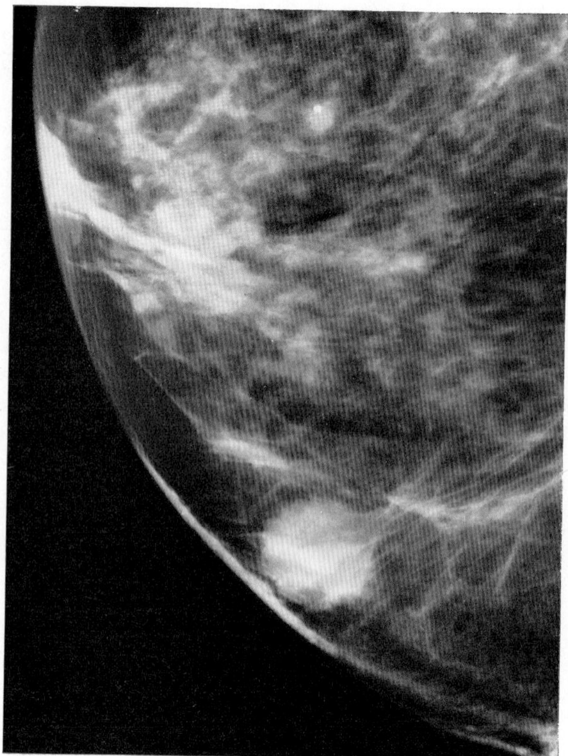

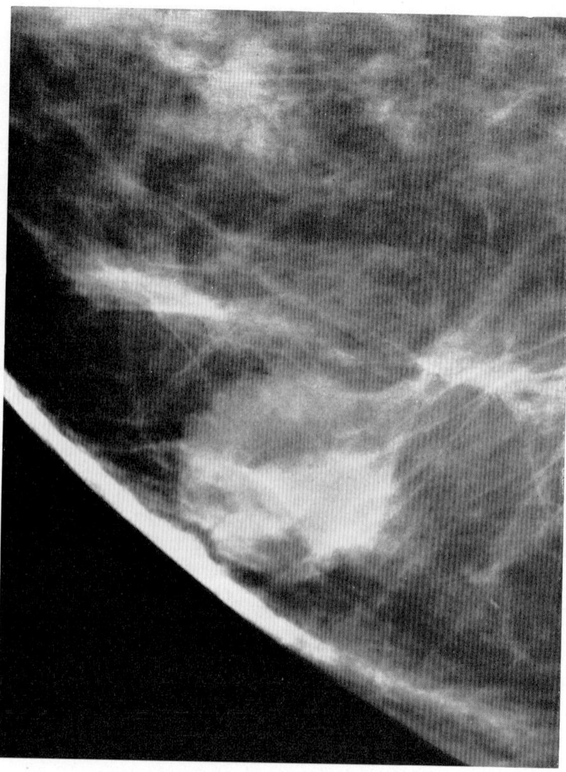

Fig. **33**.17a   Tumor mass 14 mm in diameter. Overlying skin thickening. Cometlike extension and irregular border of the mass suggests malignancy. Roentgen diagnosis: Scirrhus carcinoma or carcinoma simplex. Histology: Scirrhus carcinoma.

Fig. **33**.17b   Fig. 33.17a enlarged two times.

Chapter 34

Medullary Carcinoma

Definition and Pathology

The medullary type of ductal carcinoma is a densely cellular tumor containing large round or oval, frequently pleomorphic, tumor cells with light staining nucleii (fig. 34.1). There are numerous mitotic figures. Stromal development is sparse and more commonly there is dense lymphoid-plasma cell infiltration ("medullary carcinoma with lymphoid stroma"). Even in advanced cases the macroscopic appearance of this tumor is that of a well-contained and almost encapsulated mass. However, this "encapsulation" on microscopic examination presents as a zone of peripheral fibrosis or lymphoid-plasma-cellular infiltration. The center of a medullary carcinoma is frequently necrotic as well as hemorrhagic (fig. 34.2).

Clinical Findings

Medullary carcinoma is relatively rare. HAAGEN-SEN noted 146 cases of medullary carcinoma in 3,000 patients with breast cancers between 1915 and 1950, representing an incidence of 2.5%.

The average history of medullary carcinoma is shorter than in other breast cancers. The age of occurrence is slightly lower than the average breast cancer age.

Skin fixation over the mass is infrequent. Medullary carcinoma may occasionally reach large proportions and may have a diameter of up to 10 cm. In these large centrally necrotic masses the overlying skin is frequently red.

Bilateral occurrence of medullary carcinoma is more frequent, but axillary lymph node metastases are less frequent than in the more common types of breast carcinoma. Because of the relatively decreased incidence of axillary lymph node metastasis an improved cure rate for this tumor has been assumed. This is incorrect. HAAGENSEN reports the following 10-year survival rates: 98 cases of medullary carcinoma: 54%; 626 other types of breast carcinoma: 57%. According to

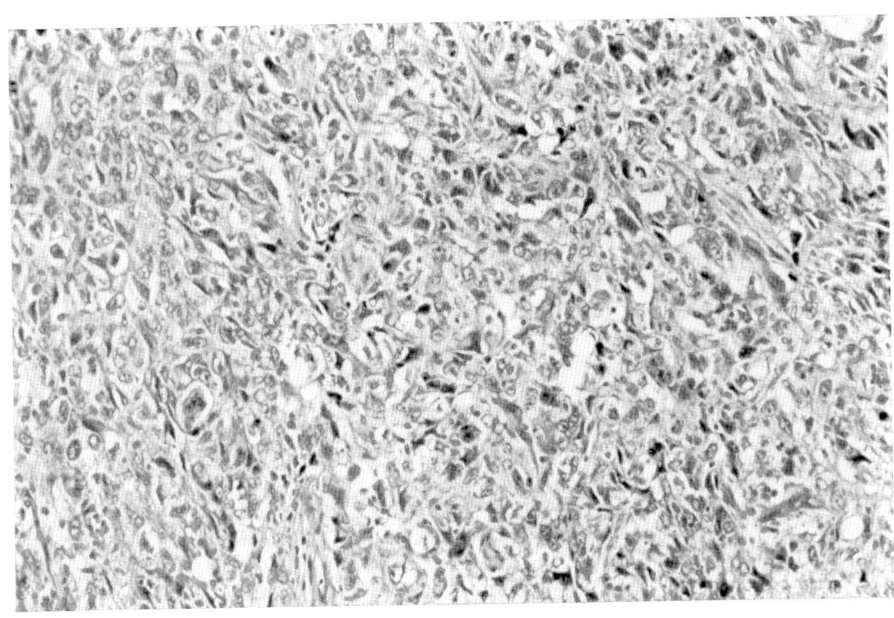

Fig. **34.**1.   Medullary carcinoma: Dense concentration of atypical epithelial cells with polymorphic nuclei; very little stroma.

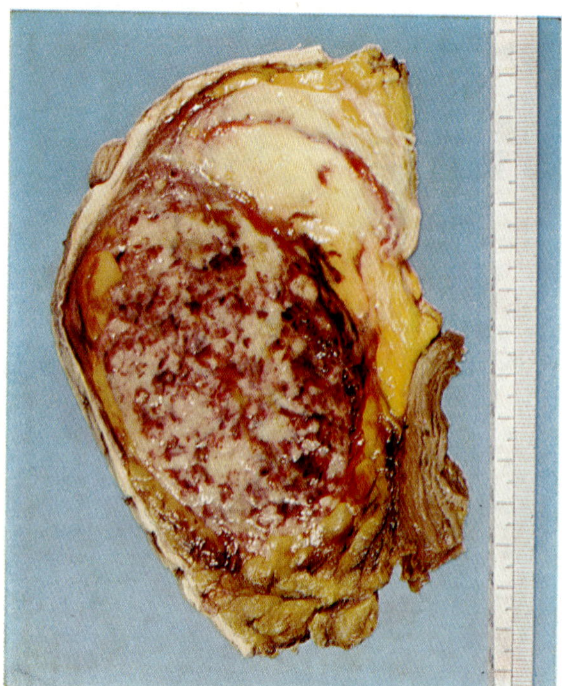

Fig. **34**.2 Unusually large medullary carcinoma with necrosis, hemorrhage and relatively sharp margins.

these figures the results following radical mastectomy for medullary carcinoma are neither better nor worse than those of other breast carcinoma.

Roentgenology

In the mammogram, medullary carcinoma presents as a rounded, oval or lobulated circumscribed mass. This reflects the macroscopic, pathological appearance.

It is easy to mistake this tumor for a benign fibroadenoma or a cyst in the mammogram (CHARDOT et al 1970). This is one of the reasons why the tumor is misdiagnosed at mammography. The margins of the tumor are occasionally very smooth and round (fig. 34.3, 34.4). Careful observation, however, invariably reveals that even this smooth contour is not completely

uniform and in various places one can detect adjacent edema. In other cases the margin of the tumor is lobulated, or scalloped (fig. 34.5). Cometlike connective tissue strands are occasionally seen in the adjacent parenchyma or in the subareolar region (fig. 34.6, 34.7). These reflect a circumscribed fibrotic reaction of adjacent tissue to the presence of the tumor.

In the periphery of a medullary carcinoma the spread of the lesion may assume a scirrhus nature. In such a case radiating connective tissue septa can be detected on the surface of that tumor (fig. 34.7).

In larger medullary carcinomas the usual secondary roentgen signs such as subcutaneous fatty tissue infiltration, skin thickening and increased vascularity are visible (fig. 34.6, 34.7, 34.8).

If the roentgen findings are equivocal, the differential diagnosis usually is not assisted by the clinical examination for on palpation the mass also may suggest a benign tumor.

If the tumor size is smaller in the mammogram than that determined by palpation (fig. 34.9), as in other carcinomas, this represents a significant sign suggesting its malignant nature.

In order to avoid costly mistakes it is wise to think of medullary carcinoma in any benign appearing breast mass when portions of the borders are ill-defined.

Clarification of each palpable and mammographically demonstrable, smooth, round breast mass must be obtained either through puncture and aspiration or excisional biopsy.

Puncture and aspiration of medullary carcinoma frequently produces a hemorrhagic material. The cytological examination invariably yields cells suspicious of malignancy and occasionally the exact diagnosis of medullary carcinoma can be made. In other cases the aspirate may be milky, mushy or contain solid bits of tissue. In these cases also cytology rarely fails to make the diagnosis.

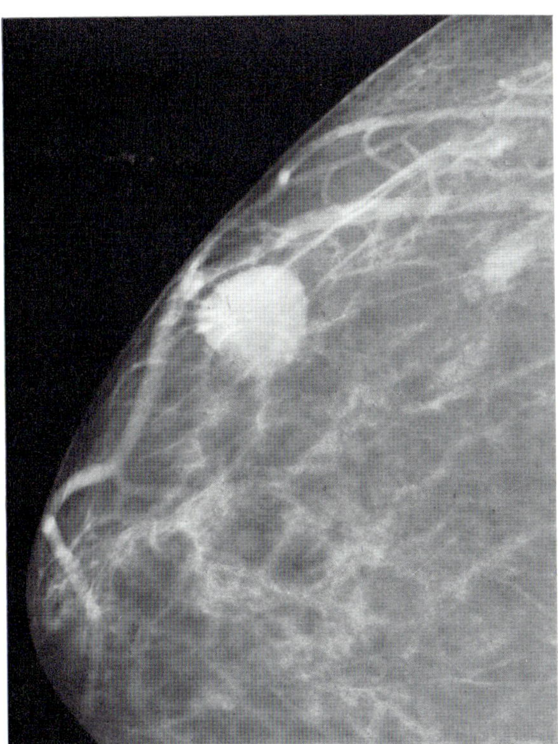

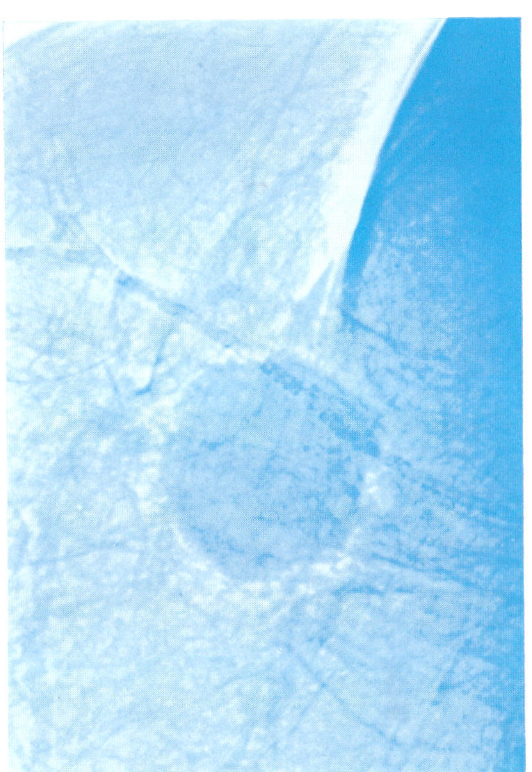

Fig. **34**.3 Rounded mass, 1.5 cm in diameter. The margin of the mass is irregular in one location. Here there are small spiculations ("warning streaks").
Palpation: Firm smoothly marginated mass corresponding in size to that seen in the roentgenogram. Puncture: Hemorrhagic tissue. Cytology: Suspicious for carcinoma. Histology: Medullary adenocarcinoma of the breast undifferentiated.

Fig. **34**.4 Xeromammogram: Round mass with relatively sharp margins and no spiculations, which is typical for medullary intraductal carcinoma.
Histological diagnosis: Medullary carcinoma. (Courtesy of John N. Wolfe, M.D., Hutzel Hospital, Detroit).

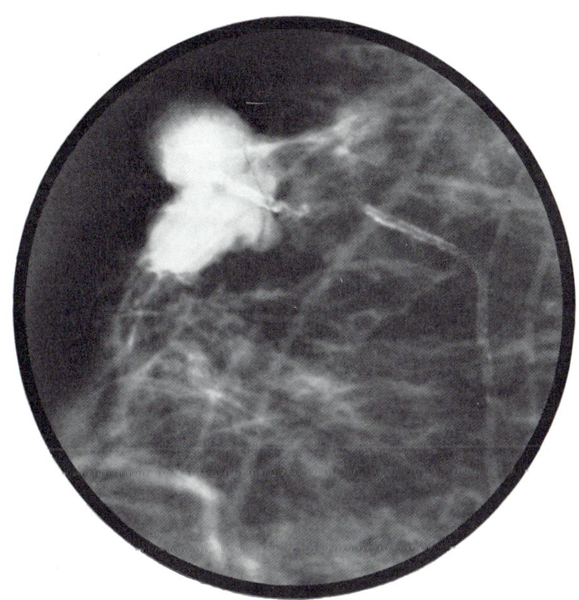

Fig. **34**.5 Lobulated mass with smooth borders measuring 1.5 × 2.0 cm. Fibroadenoma? Malignancy cannot be excluded with certainty therefore excisional biopsy is indicated. Calcified artery. Histology: Breast carcinoma, in part, of growing medullary type.

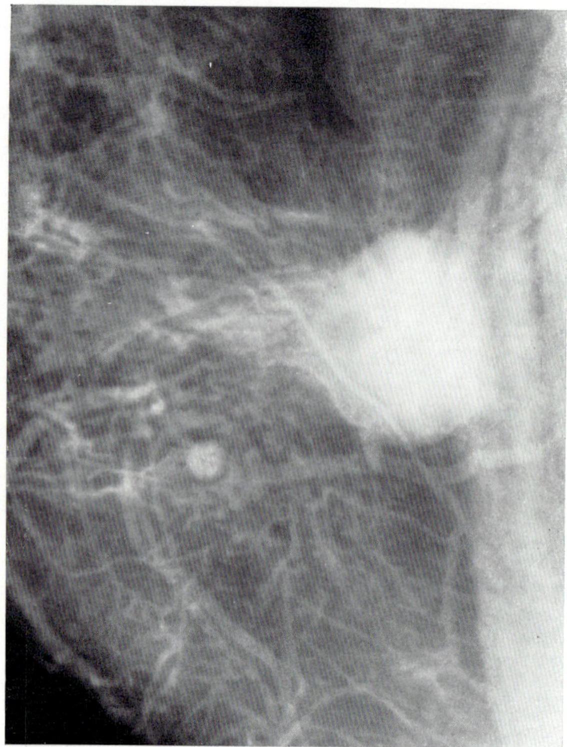

Fig. **34**.6a

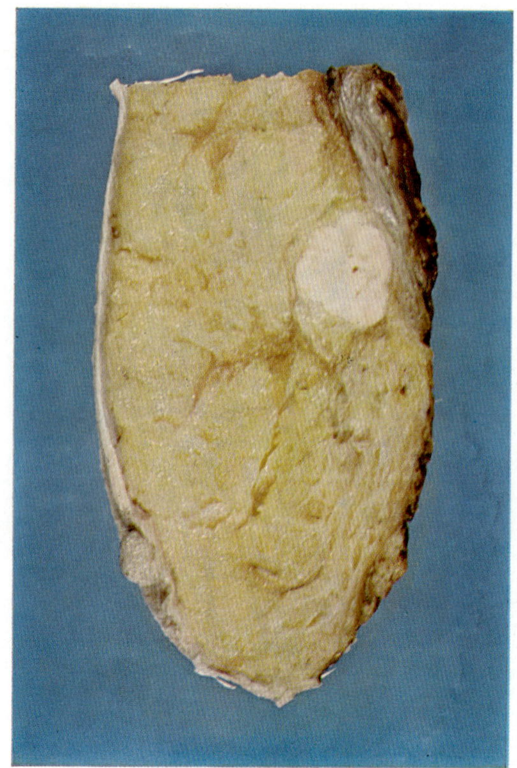

Fig. **34**.6b

Fig. **34**.6a Tumor mass 2.5 cm in diameter with mostly sharp contours. "Cometlike" tumor extension at one point. Dilated, tortuous veins. The mass was not palpable clinically. Histology: Undifferentiated, solid, growing, large cell medullary carcinoma. No lymph node metastases.

Fig. **34**.6b Surgical specimen: The almost completely marginated white tumor mass lies just in front of the pectoralis fascia.

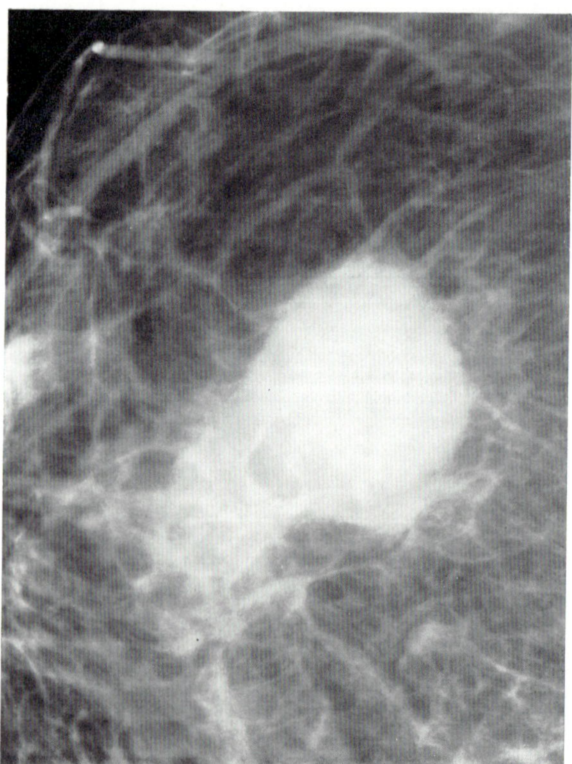

Fig. **34**.7 Rounded mass 2.5 cm in diameter with a finger-thick "cometlike" extension. Small spiculations are seen at various points. Palpation: The mass is palpated to be larger than that indicated in the roentgenogram. Puncture: Fragmented tissue. Cytology: Carcinoma. Histology: Large cell medullary carcinoma.

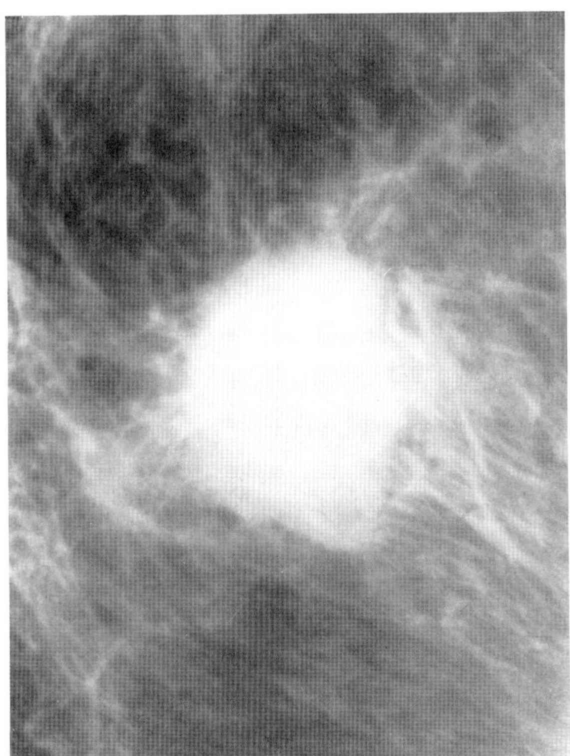

Fig. **34**.8   Rounded mass, 3 cm in diameter, with slightly lobular margins and numerous fine spiculations some of which have the "tail of the comet" appearance. Palpation: Firm freely movable mass the size of an egg. No skin involvement. Diagnosis: On the basis of the estimated size difference between palpatory findings and that on the roentgenogram as well as the unsharp contours and spiculations of the mass the roentgen diagnosis of malignant tumor is certain. Histology: Medullary carcinoma.

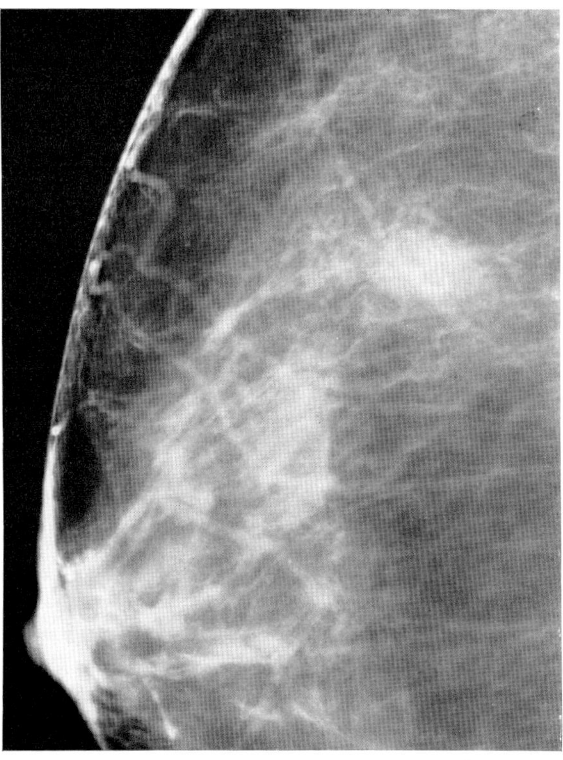

Fig. **34**.9   Small, poorly marginated nodule 0.5 to 1 cm in diameter. No increased vascularity. A significant difference between the size of the lesion at palpation and in the roentgenogram leads one to suspect carcinoma. Puncture: Relatively soft mass. Cytology: Medullary carcinoma. This was treated with radiation therapy using Cesium-137 because the patient was 82 years old and in generally poor health. Follow-up examination after 1 year: Radiation fibrosis without evidence of tumor nodule.

Chapter 35

Mucinous or Colloid Carcinoma of the Breast

Definition and Pathology

The frequency of so-called colloid carcinoma (mucinous carcinoma) among cancers of the breast is about 2—3% (McDivitt et al 1968). Colloid carcinoma on section even in the infiltrative stage appears as a circumscribed tumor with a moist, glassy surface (fig. 35.1). The tumor is of soft consistency. Macroscopically this carcinoma can resemble myxoid fibroadenoma!

In advanced stages the epithelial and partly adenoid differentiation of the tumor cells is progressively lost on microscopic examination. At this stage tumor cells are scattered or distributed in small groups within great quantities of mucin. Intracellular mucinous changes also occur resulting in signet cells. The intraductal form of the tumor leads to bare cells which produce mucinous secretions which fill the greatly dilated lactiferous ducts (fig. 35.2). The prognosis in colloid carcinoma is generally better than in other breast cancers. The greater the mucinous component of the tumor the better the prognosis. Five-year survival rates are in the range of 70—75% and approximately 60% for ten-year survival. Only about 33% of the cases demonstrate lymph node metastases at the time of surgery.

Clinical Findings

Colloid carcinoma presents as a benign, smooth, not particularly firm mass at palpation. On the

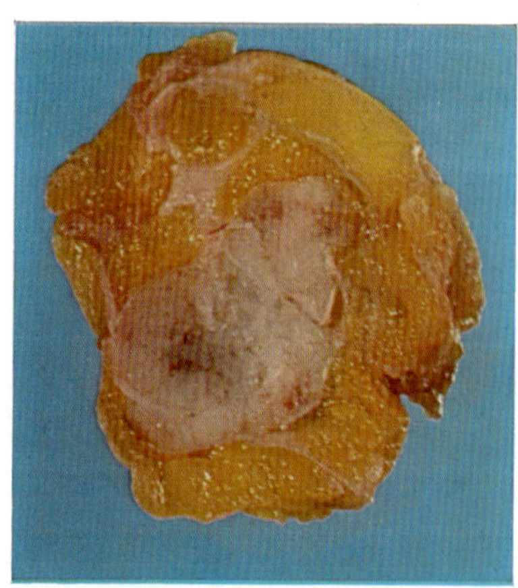

Fig. **35**.1   Specimen photograph of colloid carcinoma.

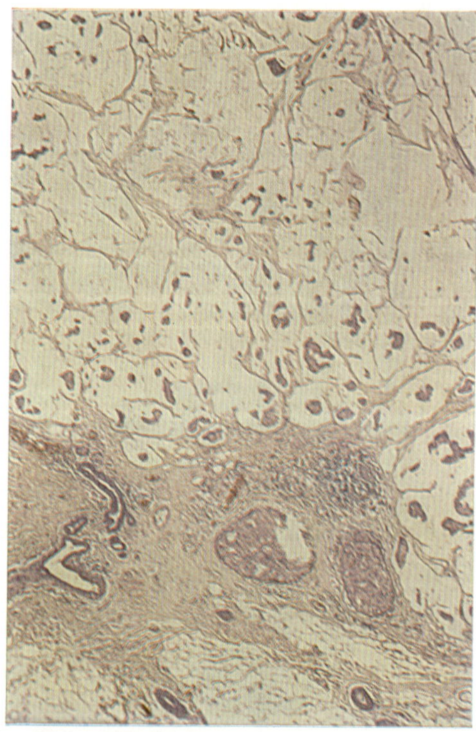

Fig. **35**.2   Histological section corresponding to Fig. 35.1.

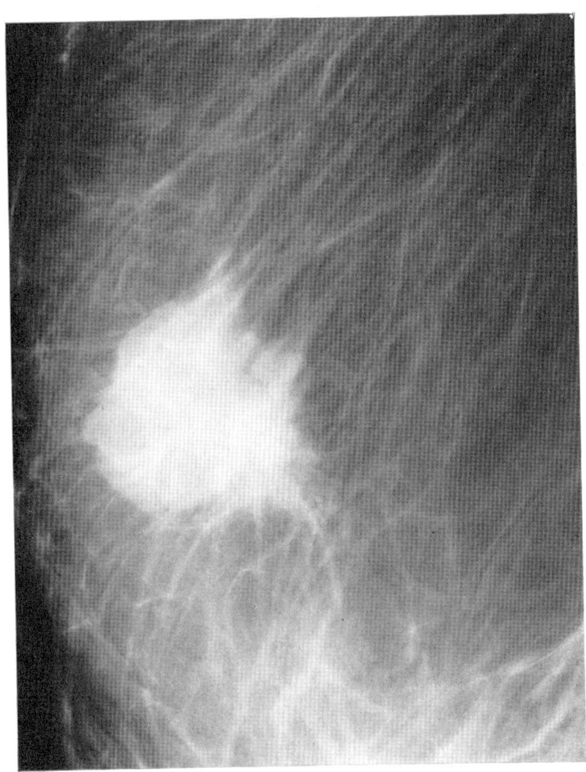

basis of the pathological characteristics of the tumor, plateauing and fixation of the skin is not to be expected.

Roentgenology

In the mammogram colloid carcinoma presents as a smoothly contoured mass, which resembles a benign tumor roentgenologically just as it does macroscopically (fig. 35.3). Calcification and signs of infiltration are not present. Puncture and aspiration is the only method of diagnosis to differentiate this tumor from a benign fibroadenoma or cyst.

Fig. **35**.3 Mammogram: Smoothly marginated lobular mass with occasional spiculated extensions. Clinically and radiologically this mass indicates signs of malignancy. Histological diagnosis: Colloid carcinoma.

Chapter 36

Diffuse Carcinoma, Inflammatory Carcinoma

Definition and Pathology

Diffuse carcinoma in histologic section presents all carcinomatous types such as scirrhus carcinoma, carcinoma simplex, medullary, intraductal, and mucinous carcinoma as well as others. It is characteristic that there is diffuse spread of the disease with capillary invasion and involvement of the lymphatics of the skin. Lymph stasis results from the extensive obstruction of lymphatics which are loaded with cancer cells. If the diffuse carcinoma involves a large portion of the thoracic wall the condition is called cancer en cuirasse. A particular from of diffuse mammary carcinoma is the so-called "inflammatory carcinoma" which is associated with red discoloration of the skin. This is not a histologically different tumor type but rather a particular clinical picture which simulates inflammatory disease of the breast. In earlier days it was called "mastitis carcinomatosa" implying that this subclass of breast carcinoma arose during pregnancy or lactation. This is incorrect. Inflammatory carcinoma is a disease of middle-age and older. Its occurrence during gestation is rather rare. The breast involved with this type of carcinoma is frequently very large.

Clinical Findings

The clinical picture of diffuse carcinoma consists of widespread skin edema ("peau d'orange"), in an enlarged, hard and heavy breast (fig. 36.1). These signs are not exclusively found in diffuse carcinoma but may also be seen in other diseases associated with diffuse breast edema such as lymphoma, leukemia, cardiac anasarca, or diffuse axillary lymphatic block. The development of inflammatory carcinoma is very rapid, the course very short.

The coloring of the skin is frequently not fully red but more or less pink and in certain cases may not be uniform but present in a geographical distribution with interspersed areas of normal colored skin. Sometimes the discoloration of the skin is not uniform but consists of small singular red blotches (fig. 36.2).

The nipple may be retracted or become very plump and firm if much edema is present.

Ignorance of this type of carcinoma not infrequently results in the assumption that these patients have mastitis and the institution of conservative therapy with antibiotics and topical methods.

It is important to note that patients with inflammatory carcinoma do not have fever or leukocytosis. This is important in the differentiation from mastitis. There may be an increase in sedimentation rate. Some patients do have pain and a feeling of tension in the breasts.

Inflammatory carcinoma has a particularly poor prognosis. It is generally felt that surgical therapy with radical mastectomy is useless. Some attempts have been made, however, to treat this carcinoma surgically but the survival rates are discouraging and the chance of survival is essen-

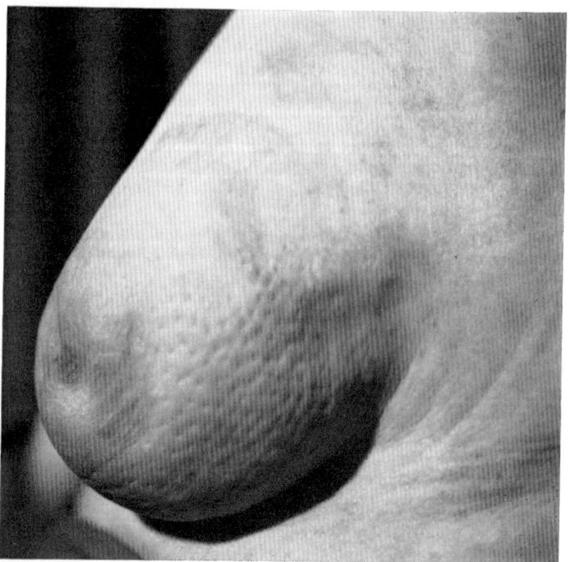

Fig. **36**.1 Extensive "peau d'orange" in diffuse carcinoma.

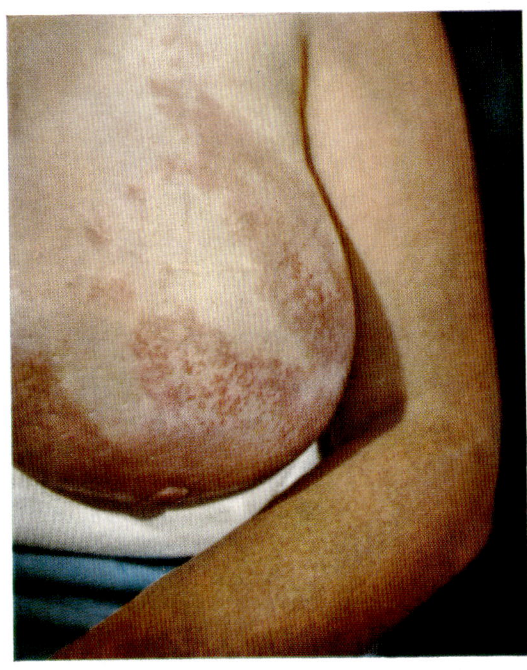

Fig. **36**.2 Topographical skin erythema with relatively sharp margins, associated with occasional smaller focus of erythema. The breast is large and edematous. No improvement with antibiotic therapy. Inflammatory carcinoma.

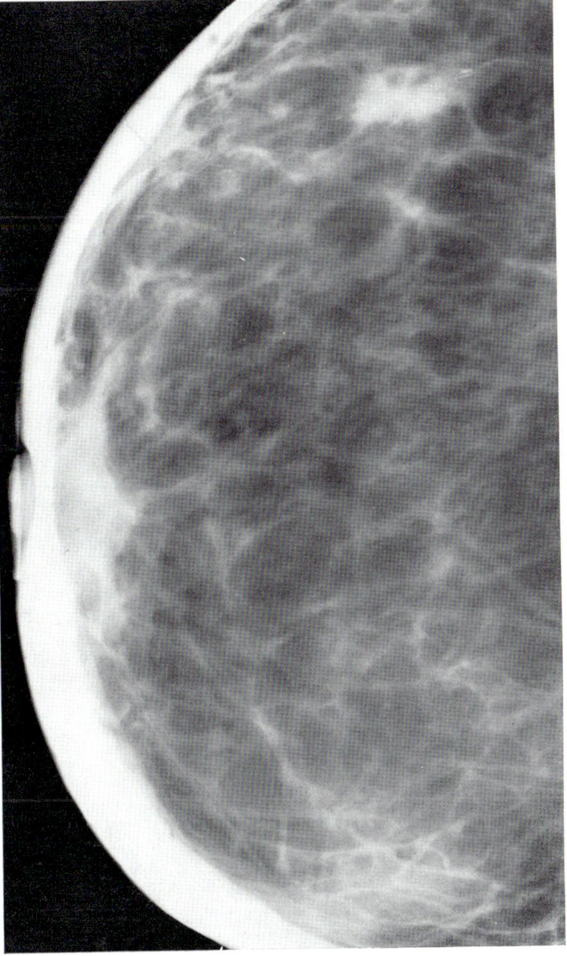

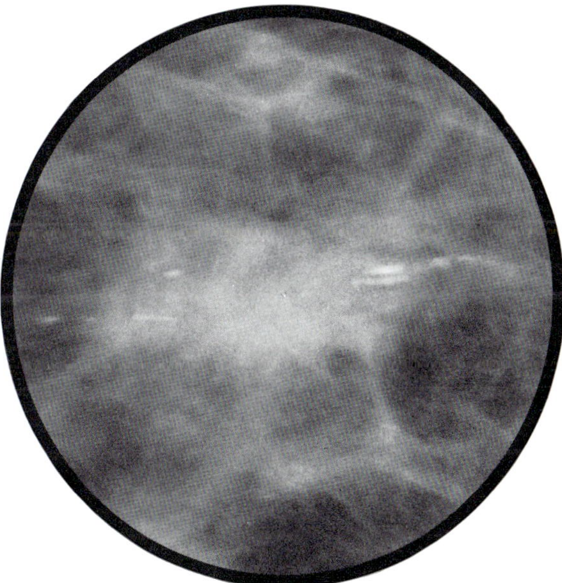

Fig. **36**.3b Local area magnified 3 ✕. Linear calcifications. Spicules are noted along the margins. Scirrhus carcinoma was verified histologically.

Fig. **36**.3a Mammogram (slightly minified): Extensive skin thickening but the posterior border of the skin is sharply defined. Reticular infiltration of the subcutaneous fatty layer is observed. The entire breast is characterized by a reticulated increase in connective tissue. Lateral mammogram reveals a 1 by 2.5 cm mass.

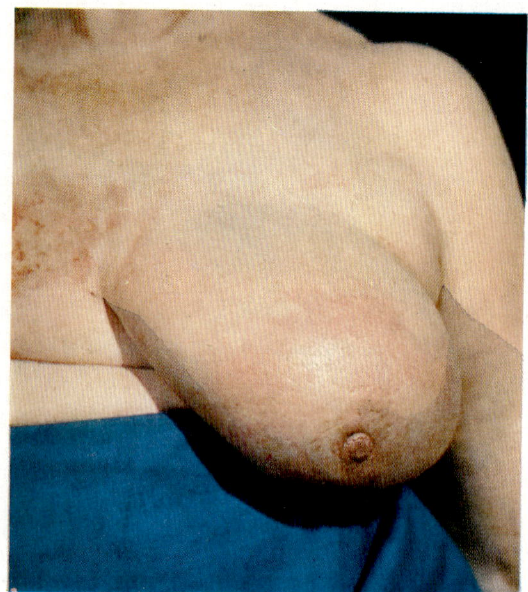

Fig. **36**.4a   Clinical findings: Diffuse erythematous changes in the center of the breast. Skin thickening is noted in the areola and that portion of the skin immediately surrounding it.

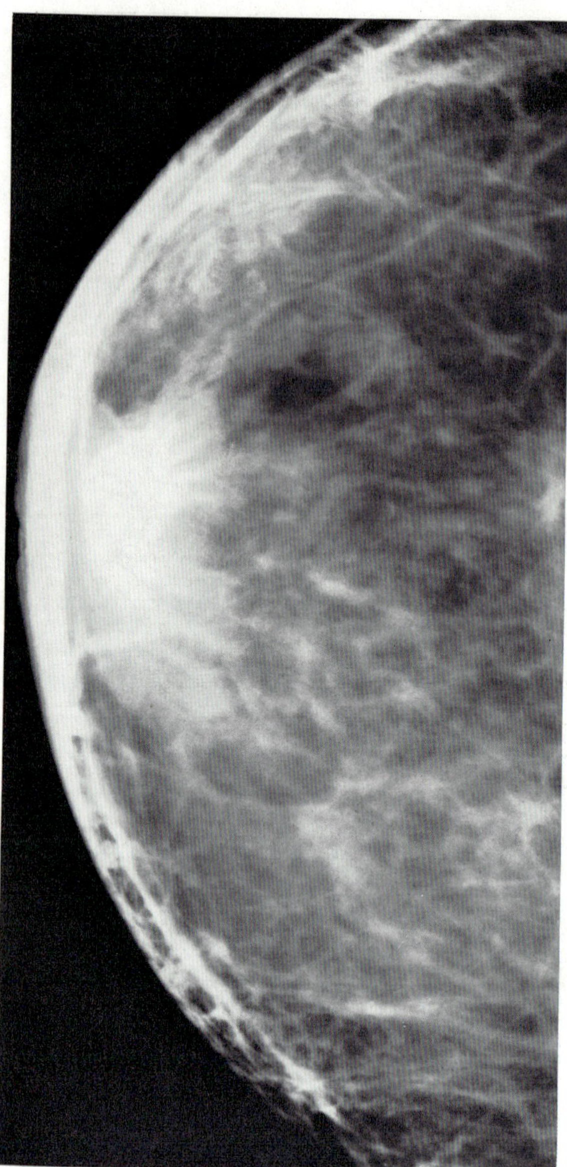

Fig. **36**.4b   Mammogram reveals not only areolar and paraareolar thickening of the skin but diffuse infiltration of the subcutaneous area in a reticular fashion.

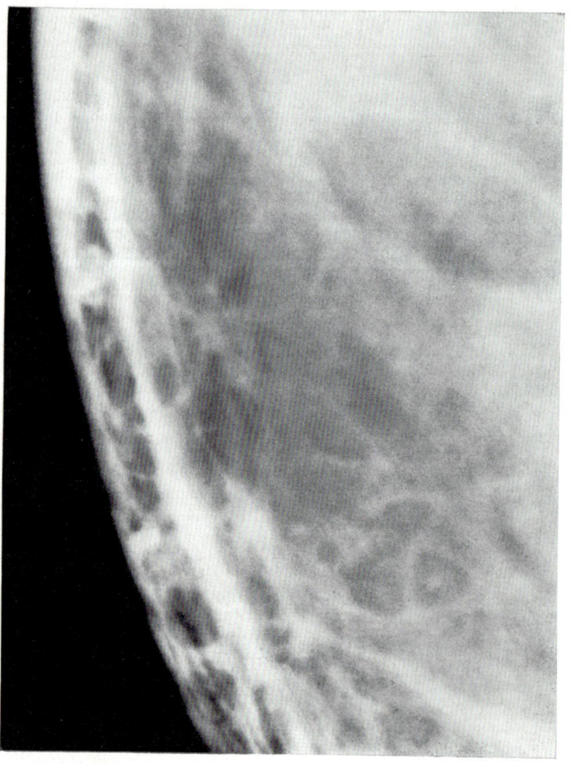

Fig. **36**.4c   This reticular infiltration of the subcutaneous tissue is seen to better advantage in this local area magnified 3 ✕.

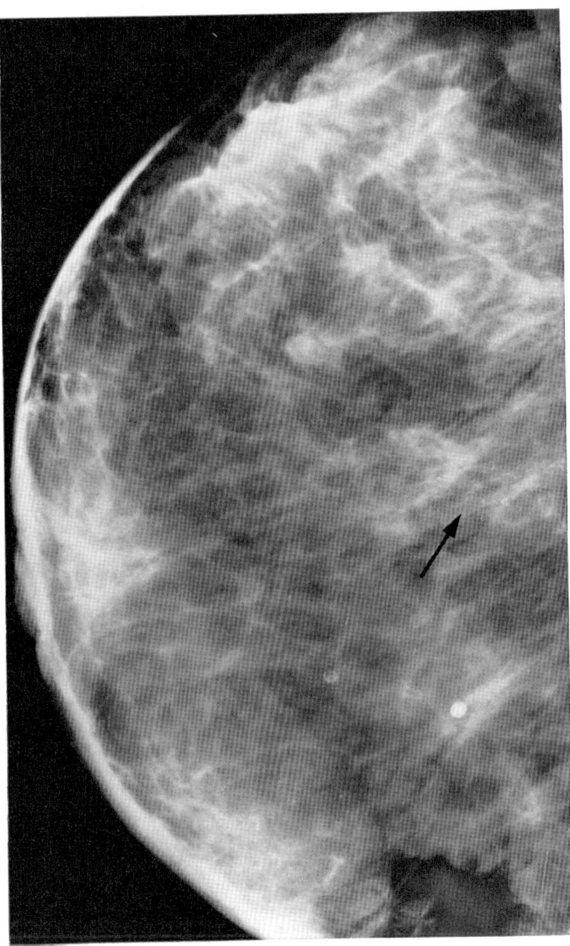

Fig. **36**.5a Extensive skin thickening in the area of the areola and medially. The posterior margin of the thickened skin is sharply defined. There is diffuse reticular infiltration of the entire breast. In the center of the breast a group of microcalcifications (Fig. 36.5b magnified 3×) is seen within an area of increased density (arrow). Two cystic calcifications are observed (liponecrosis microcystica calcificans). Histologically verified diffuse carcinoma; the primary tumor was an intraductal carcinoma.

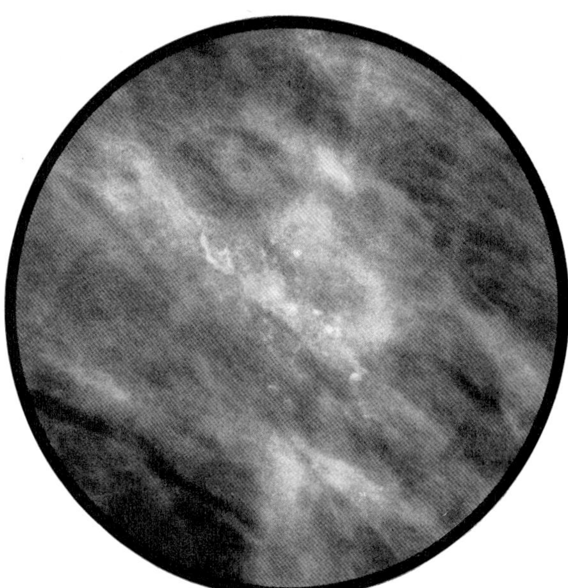

Fig. **36**.5b

tially nil. Following radical mastectomy local resurrence is inevitable and frequently this appears to lead to an almost explosive massive metastasis. Lymph node metastases are palpable or histologically demonstrable in about 90% of patients with inflammatory carcinoma, even at the first examination.

The therapy of choice today is intensive radiation combined with hormonal treatment. The treatment is only palliative; however, the remaining life span of the patient is longer and more pleasant than after attempts at radical mastectomy.

Roentgenology

Diffuse and "inflammatory" carcinoma are characterized by generalized skin thickening in the mammogram. The subcutaneous fatty layer as well as the reticular connective tissue scattered throughout is not as cloudy or ill-defined as in inflammatory mastitis; rather these structures remain fairly sharply defined (fig. 36.3a). The entire subcutaneous fatty layer and the diseased portion of the breast demonstrates a reticular proliferation of abnormal tissue of increased density (GROS and BURG 1957; BERGER 1962), as is illustrated in fig. 36.4a—c.

Occasionally one may find a dominant tumor mass from which the diffusely spreading carcinoma originates (fig. 36.3a and b). This local carcinomatous mass may be sharply circumscribed and nodular resembling carcinoma simplex or possess numerous stellate extensions as in the case of scirrhus carcinoma.

Calcifications may be present in linear or intraductal form, or appear in the five groups of microcalcifications typical of breast carcinoma (fig. 36.5a and b, 36.6).

Thus the mammographic appearance of the tumor is variable just as it is on histological examination.

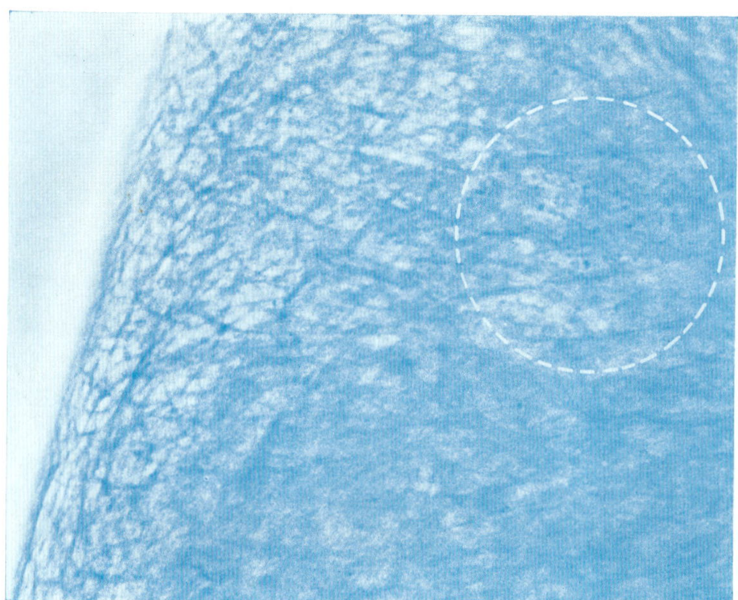

Fig. **36**.6   Clinical findings: Erythema of the skin of the breast for approximately four weeks. Peau d'orange. A discrete firm area was palpable. Does this represent mastitis or inflammatory carcinoma? Xeromammogram: Skin thickening. Increased density of breast tissue. Reticular pattern in the subcutaneous fatty layers. Microcalcifications typical for carcinoma. These microcalcifications are not visible on film mammography (Structurix D 7 / Gevaert) because they were washed out due to excessive scattered radiation.

Mammographically it may not be easy to differentiate acute mastitis from inflammatory carcinoma. The latter, however, may evoke a diffuse, reticular proliferation of connective tissue within and surrounding the diseased breast parenchyma including the extension of numerous connective tissue spicules into the stroma. These nearly always remain sharply defined within the subcutaneous fatty tissue and also produce a skin thickening, but with sharply defined subepidermal border. In contradistinction, inflammatory mastitis produces a generalized loss of sharpness of structures and a diffuse haziness of the diseased area as a result of the inflammatory edema and infiltration by inflammatory cells. These differential diagnostic signs, however, do not allow a definite differentiation between "mastitis carcinomatosa" and pure inflammatory mastitis. The roentgenogram, on the whole, permits a much more accurate determination of the extent of the tumor and of the skin infiltration and thickening than does the clinical examination.

Chapter 37

Lobular Carcinoma In Situ (Lobular Neoplasia)

Definition

FOOTE and STEWART, in 1941, were the first to describe and provide an exact definition of lobular carcinoma in situ and to differentiate this tumor from the proliferative changes of mammary dysplasia and invasive carcinoma. In accordance with the view of most American authors this disease consists of an early form of lobular carcinoma of the breast which begins in and is limited to the parenchymal lobules. The basal membrane is not invaded and there are no signs of infiltration. Secondary involvement of an adjacent terminal ductule and subsequently of a neighboring parenchymal lobule may occur. Multiple growths of lobular carcinoma in situ in various sections of the breast are not rare (CUTLER, STEWART, WARNER, FARROW, BAESSLER).

Recently KAUFMANN et al (1971) as well as HAMPERL (1971) have reported their observations on 17 cases in the German literature. We were involved in the mammographic examinations of these patients. HAMPERL and KAUFMANN are not convinced that every lobular carcinoma in situ will eventually become an infiltrating tumor.

Pathology

In the excised specimen, carcinoma in situ is neither visible nor palpable. Frozen sections are not suitable for the diagnosis of lobular carci-

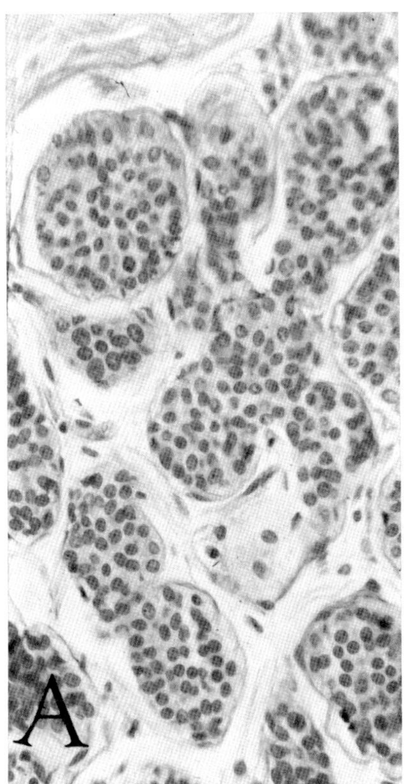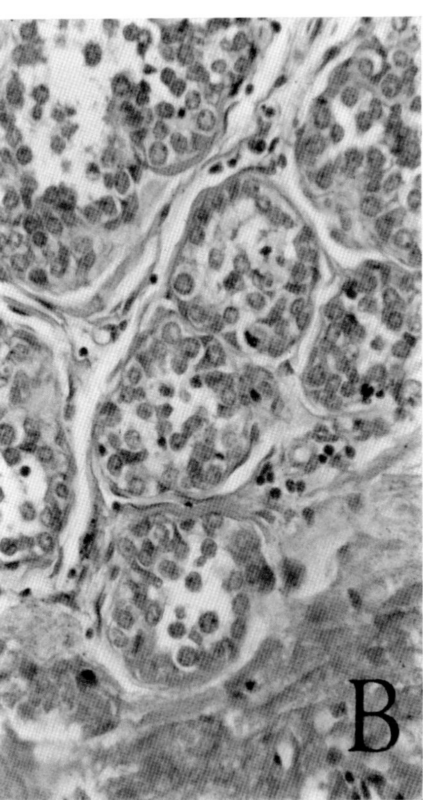

Fig. **37**.1.   Histological section of lobular carcinoma in situ type A and B, (Citoler, Women's Clinic University of Cologne).

noma in situ. Careful histological examination of the biopsy specimen should result in a detection rate of more than 90% (LAMBIRD and SHELLEY, 1969).

The pathologist's search is made easier when a preceding roentgenogram of the biopsy material has been made and the region containing suspected microcalcifications (see page 314) is demarcated.

In the histological preparation, lobular carcinoma in situ is often discovered near an area of sclerosing adenosis but also in the midst of unequivocal fibrocystic disease, as well as in regions where proliferating milk ducts are observed. Interestingly enough the tumor is also seen in the vicinity of an infiltrating carcinoma. Lobular carcinoma in situ has a diameter of several millimeters at most. There is enlargement of the lobule in which the carcinoma in situ is developing. Acini and ductules in the vicinity are filled with epithelial cells. Some of these cells have single large vacuoles in the cytoplasm. The cells are light-colored with pale nuclei and vary little one from another in size and shape. They resemble the light-colored cells of Paget's carcinoma and have therefore been called "pagetoid" basal cells, derived from the myoepithelium.

HAAGENSEN (1962, 1971) who recently has introduced the new term "lobular neoplasia" for lobular carcinoma in situ suggests a histological subdivision of these changes (fig. 37.1). His type A consists of cells with uniform round or oval nuclei. Mitotic figures are not visible. Type B consists of cells with large nuclei varying in size and shape and containing coarser chromatin deposits. Mitotic figures may be seen. Whether this subclassification produces any differences in prognosis has not yet been determined.

Localization

American authors have stated that lobular carcinoma in situ is more frequently found in the upper outer quadrant of the breast (LAMBIRD and SHELLEY). This observation may be related to the fact that the upper outer quadrant is the area in the involuted breast where residual parenchymal tissue is most likely to persist and in which, in the middle-aged or older patient, there is an increased tendency for the development of carcinoma.

In our own cases of lobular carcinoma in situ the lateral localization in the breast was the most frequent.

Bilaterality

The tendency of bilateral development of lobular carcinoma in situ poses a particular problem. This may occur simultaneously or successively. Earlier figures of a 20% rate of bilateral involvement appear a little too high today but the frequency is at least 15% (WARNER, 1969).

Because of the frequent bilaterality and the common lateral localization of this tumor, American authors have recommended that in the event of discovery of lobular carcinoma in situ in one breast, it is obligatory that a blind biopsy of the upper outer quadrant of the other breast be performed.

Frequency of Incidence

Lobular carcinoma in situ is more frequently discovered today than in preceding times. On the whole, according to WARNER (1969), at least 475 cases of lobular carcinomas have been published about half of which were noninvasive carcinoma in situ. According to the most recent literature the incidence of lobular carcinoma in situ among breast carcinomas examined per year in several pathological institutes is about 5% to 6% (NEWMAN 5% in 1,436 breast cancers, HUTTER 6%; in contrast MILLER and KAY only 1.5%, BORDEN and GERSHON-COHEN less than 1%). With increasing understanding of the histological appearance, more intensive histological workups and diligent search of biopsy material and in particular through the use of mammography, the discovery of this early form of lobular carcinoma will be more frequent.

Age and Predisposing Factors

Lobular carcinoma in situ is most commonly found in women between ages 40 and 50 (FARROW, GERSHON-COHEN, WARNER, NEWMAN, and our own observations). Affliction in younger patients including a 29-year-old woman have been reported. There are reports of occurrence at age 70 and 80. LEWISON (1965) is of the opinion that the peak of incidence of lobular carcinoma

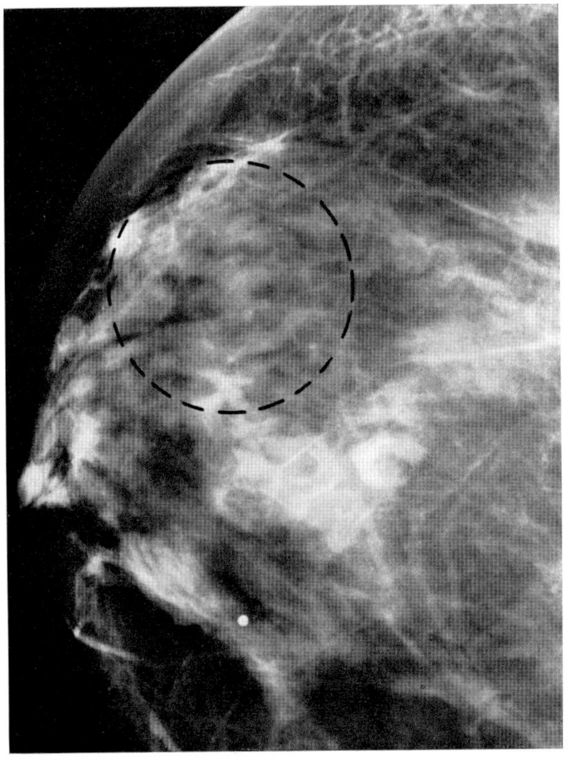

Fig. **37**.2a Mammogram of the **right** breast: Mammary dysplasia with occasional scattered calcifications.
Roentgen diagnosis: Mammary dysplasia with fibrosis.

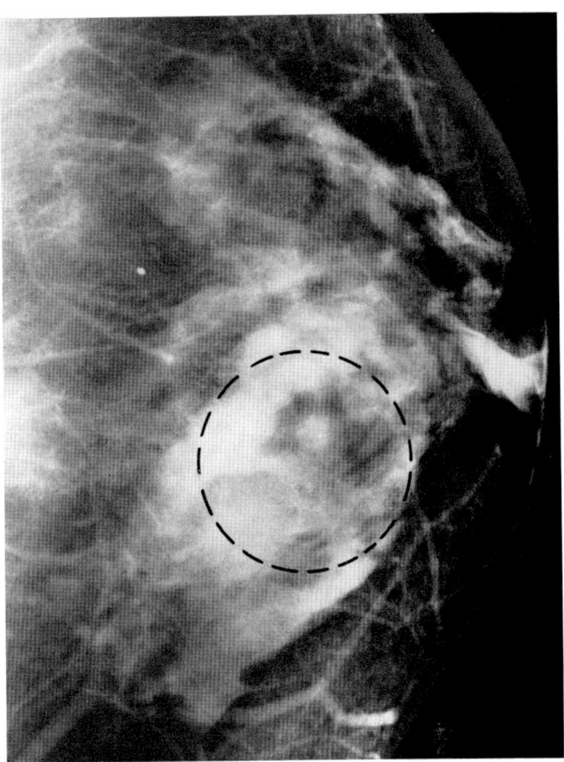

Fig. **37**.2b Mammogram of the **left** breast: Numerous, very dense microcalcifications lying in close proximity to one another.
Roentgen diagnosis: Mammary dysplasia, predominantly fibrous type, with suspicion of intraductal process.

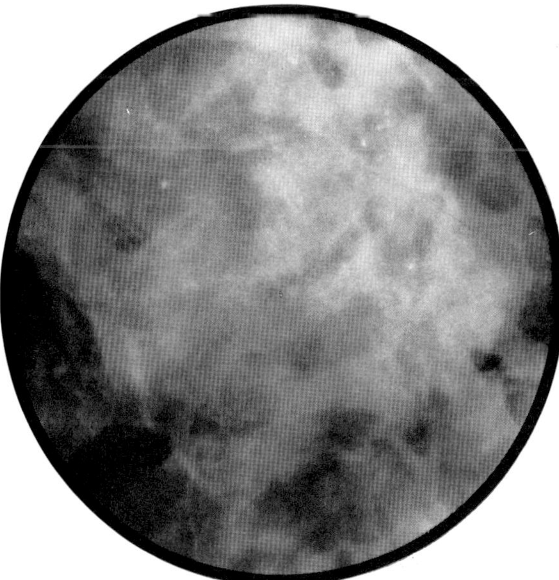

Fig. **37**.2c Roentgenogram of the surgical specimen **right side:** Within the area containing the microcalcifications more numerous microcalcifications are seen in the section, which could not be appreciated in the mammogram.
Histological diagnosis: Fibrous mastopathy.

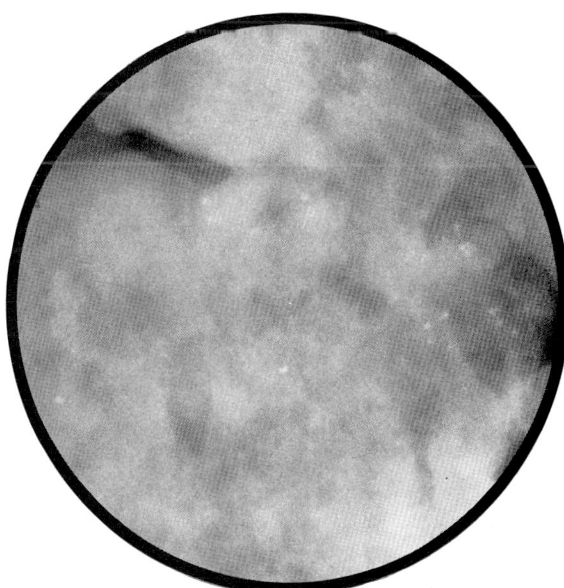

Fig. **37**.2d Roentgenogram of the surgical specimen **left side:** Numerous microcalcifications of varying size and shape, concentrated in groups.
Histological diagnosis: Fibrocystic mastopathy. Four conglomerates of lobular carcinoma in situ.

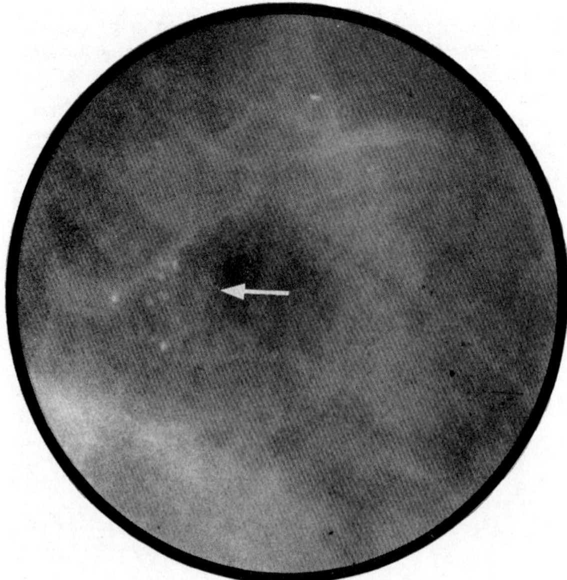

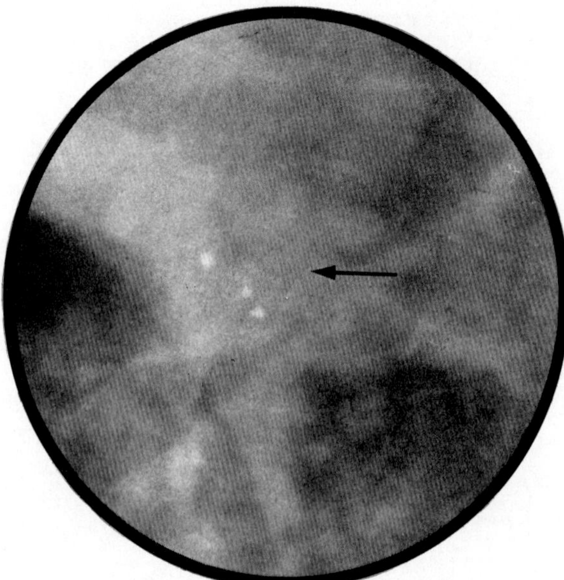

Fig. **37**.3 Mammogram of a 41-year-old woman reveals a group of microcalcifications within an area of soft tissue density but no definite mass lesion. Roentgen diagnosis: Intraductal process. Excisional biopsy was performed after localization of the lesion by means of a mammogram and injecting the suspected site with methylene-blue and urografin. The suspect microcalcifications of varying size, concentrated in groups were contained in the specimen. The figure above demonstrates these calcifications magnified 3 ×.
Histological diagnosis: Fibrocystic mastopathy with definite tendency towards proliferation. Sclerosing adenosis. Focal epithelial proliferation with some apocrine metaplasia. Foci of numerous microcalcifications within atrophic acini and dilated lactiferous ductules. Two foci of lobular carcinoma in situ. Microcalcifications were observed in neighboring acini but not within the carcinoma in situ. No evidence of invasive carcinoma.

Fig. **37**.4 Mammography revealed mammary dysplasia with some coarse structuring in a 43-year-old woman. A small group of microcalcifications was observed. The local area magnified 3 × shown in this figure reveals the varying density and shape of the calcifications. Roentgen diagnosis: Intraductal process. Histological diagnosis: Multicentric lobular carcinoma in situ.

in situ precedes that of invasive carcinoma by about 10 years.

Predisposing factors are not certain. Such factors as irregular menstrual periods, marriage, number of children and menopause in relation to this tumor may be chance associations (FARROW 1968).

Risk of Malignant Degeneration and Therapy

The significance of the discovery of a lobular carcinoma in situ is made clear from the results of treatment. "Simple mastectomy results in a zero recurrence rate". It is doubtful whether local excision alone is sufficient. In a study by

McDIVITT of 40 patients who underwent local excision of a lobular carcinoma in situ diagnosed between 1941 and 1952, a malignancy was found in the same breast in 35% of cases after a year follow-up and more than 50% after 23 years. CITOLER and DERBOLOWSKI (1971) from the Pathological Institute of the University of Bonn, between the years 1961 and 1967, discovered and followed clinically 14 cases of lobular carcinoma in situ found within a total of 4,770 histological preparations of breast tissue. In these cases there was no further operative or radiation therapy following the excisional biopsy. Examination of these patients four to ten years later revealed the development of breast carcinoma in the same breast in two patients. According to this study the malignancy risk is lower than in the report by McDIVITT.

Although these figures indicate an increased risk of carcinoma among these patients one must note that the excisional biopsies in such cases were confined to a very small localized area. It is therefore recommended that when focal (not multilocular) carcinoma in situ is found a more

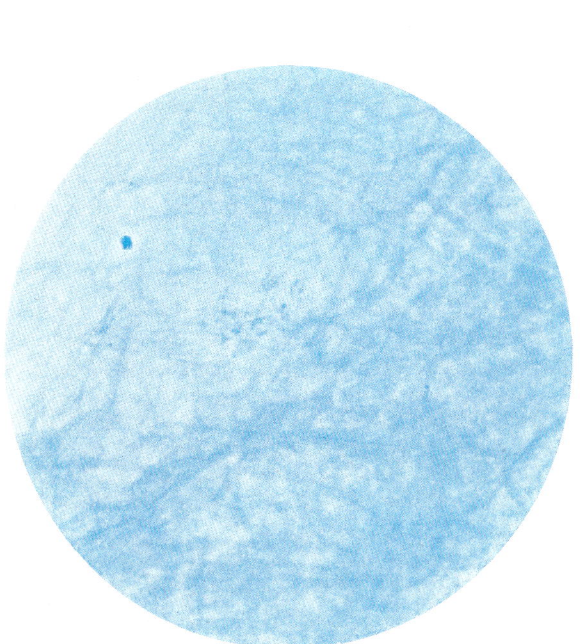

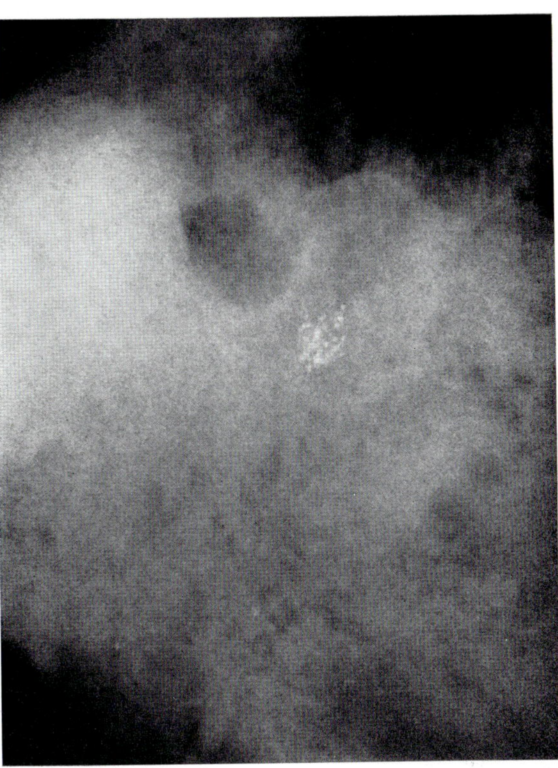

Fig. **37**.5   Xeromammogram (enlarged 2×): Numerous clustered microcalcifications in the periphery of the parenchyma (not present two years before). Roentgen diagnosis: Pathological intraductal process whose benignancy is not certain. Biopsy is recommended. Histological diagnosis: Lobular carcinoma in situ (type A).

Fig. **37**.6a   Mammogram (local area) reveals numerous, isolated microcalcifications in a 47-year-old woman. Additionally a group of irregularly formed microcalcifications as often seen in carcinoma is observed in an area of increased density measuring approximately 1 cm in diameter.

extensive regional extirpation should be performed instead of a disfiguring mastectomy. Furthermore, tests should be undertaken to determine whether it is not possible to undertake a complete removal of the entire remaining breast parenchyma, leaving the skin, with substitution of an indwelling breast prosthesis made from silastic or a fat-skin-plastic. These thoughts are based on the hope that by attaining early diagnosis of a breast tumor in the preinvasive stage one might spare the patient the disfiguring operation of mastectomy which is one of the primary aims of early diagnosis.

The transition of this tumor into invasive carcinoma occurs over a period of many months

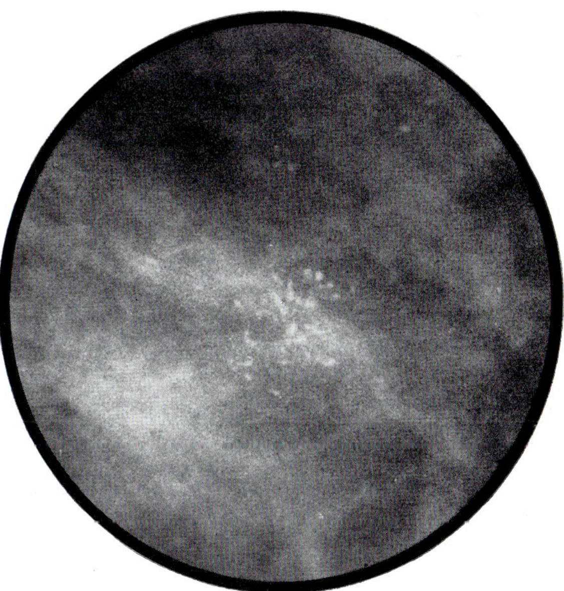

Fig. **37**.6b Mammogram of excisional biopsy, magnified 2×.
Histological diagnosis: Lobular carcinoma in situ.

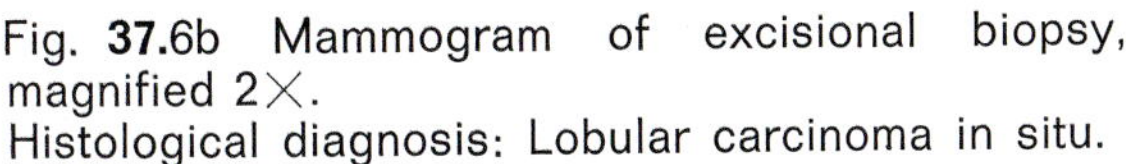

to years (GODWIN 1952; CUTLER 1952). The prognosis after the invasive stage has been attained is no different than with other breast carcinomas.

Clinical Findings

There are no typical clinical symptoms that will indicate lobular carcinoma in situ. One report of over 109 cases from the Memorial Cancer Hospital of New York, indicated that in four patients the clinical findings raised the suspicion of carcinoma (HUTTER et al 1969). Clinically the indication for biopsy generally depends on abnormal palpatory findings which are of concern to the patient or to the examining physician.

Roentgenology

There is no certain correlation between mammographic findings and the histological substrate of lobular carcinoma in situ. Despite this, in 46% of the published cases from the Memorial Hospital there were sufficient mammographic findings to indicate a biopsy. In our observations of 28 cases (LANYI et al 1972), 18 biopsies were performed on the basis of mammographic suspicion of an intraductal process or of malignant changes. This, in and of itself, indicates progress, insofar as in previous years this diagnosis was purely an accidental one made on histological examination.

There are specific microcalcifications which when seen cause us to urge excisional biopsy of the suspected lesion. The eventual histological findings have proved to represent intraductal proliferation, sclerosing adenosis, papillomatosis, a predominantly intraductal growing carcinoma, or lobular carcinoma in situ. It is not yet clear whether these microcalcifications are produced by the lobular carcinoma in situ itself or whether the two processes have an increased tendency to occur together. In support of the latter possibility it has been noted by HAAGENSEN that adenosis, in which condition we have seen similar microcalcifications, occurs in a greater than normal frequency in the vicinity of lobular carcinoma. Because of our increasing experience over the last several years we have urged excisional biopsy on the basis of microcalcifications with the following characteristics:

1) Numerous singular, round, moderately dense, plump calcifications as typically found in sclerosing adenosis demand close examination. In the case of such calcifications, whether they are localized to one section of the breast or are distributed diffusely in one breast or both breasts, if one discovers an additional small group of closely crowded, tiny microcalcifications, this portion of the breast particularly must be excised for histological examination. Biopsy is also recommended for such microcalcifications which have newly arisen since previous mammograms. This finding among our cases of lobular carcinoma in situ was the most frequent sign of a pathological intraductal process.

In such cases it is a remarkable fact, that with identical or very similar mammographic findings the histological section will reveal a lobular carcinoma in situ at one time or a type of mammary dysplasia at another (fig. 37.2a to d).

2) In other cases the calcifications found in the mammogram within an area of increased breast density are so sparse or poorly visible that they can only be found in over-exposed films using appropriate magnification techniques. These calcifications resemble those of any type of mammary dysplasia in their density as well as overall structures but they are crowded closer together or are within a group (fig. 37.3, 37.4, 37.5).

3) In another type of case a group of microcalcifications may be seen which are very dense, irregular in size and form and have the typical appearance of those associated with intraductal breast carcinoma (fig. 37.6a and b).

When such calcifications are observed in the mammogram there should be a suspicion of carcinoma. It is unclear why such "typically carcinomatous" calcifications are not restricted to invasive carcinoma but are also found in the preinvasive in situ type. One must assume a relationship because of the frequent agreement of roentgen and histological findings. There probably is some disturbance of the histochemical balance with subsequent precipitation of calcium salts somehow produced by a carcinoma or carcinoma in situ. The microcalcifications may lie in the periphery and not completely within the confines of the tumor or they may

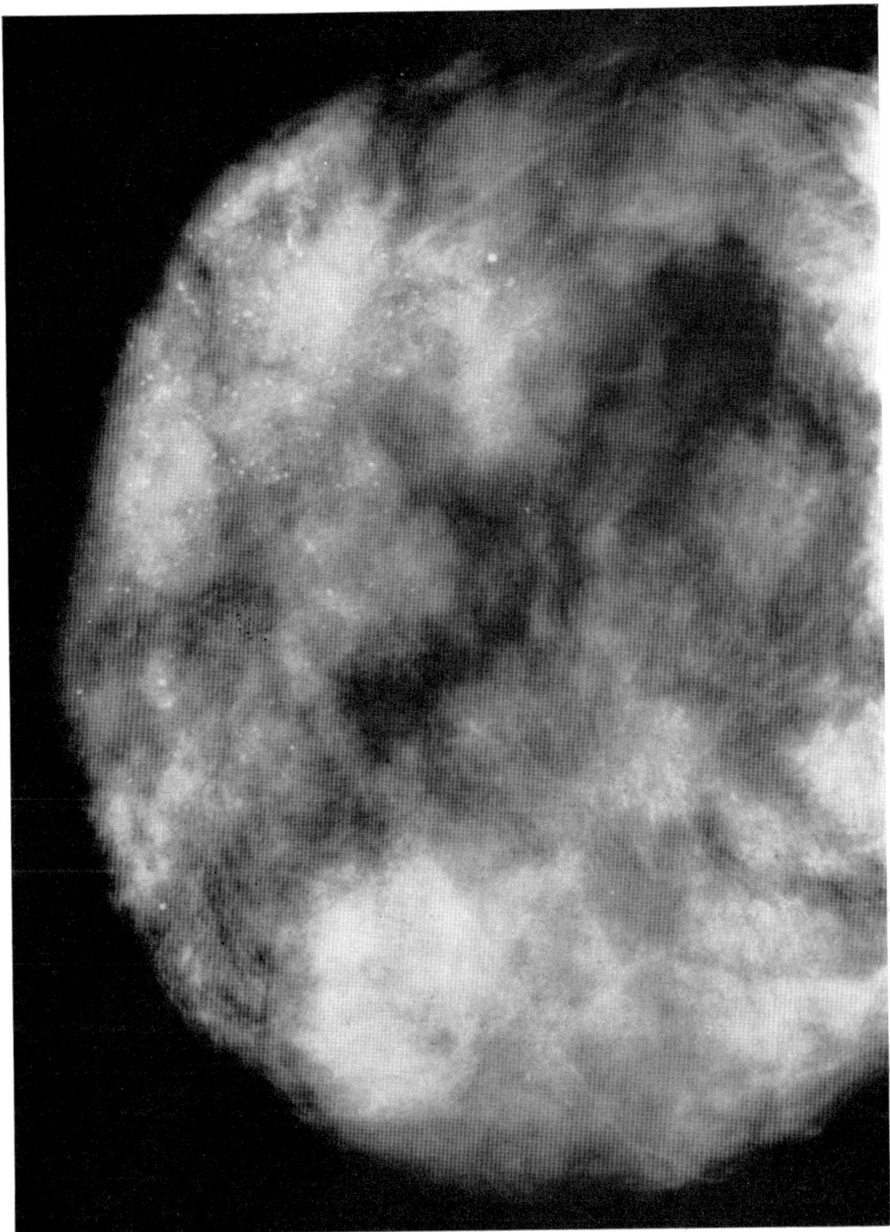

Fig. **37**.7   Diffuse mammary dysplasia of the right breast progressing over a period of 1 year. In the upper outerquadrant there are numerous, mostly coarse but also some very fine calcifications. The differential diagnosis here consists of sclerosing adenosis and a diffuse intraductal carcinoma (observations of Lendvai-Viragh, Porz/Cologne).

appear in fatty tissue where there is no definite evidence of tumor infiltration (SNYDER 1966; GERSHON-COHEN 1970; HUTTER et al 1969).

In the event of widespread multicentric lobular carcinoma one may find numerous, coarse calcifications. The roentgen image may resemble sclerosing adenosis or a diffuse intraductal carcinoma (fig. 37.7).

Mammography is making it possible for us not only to detect infiltrating carcinoma before there are clinical manifestations but also to discover lobular carcinoma in situ which is the preinvasive stage of carcinoma. It cannot be expected that with a macroscopic method of examination such as mammography one can reach a high degree of diagnostic accuracy in a disease which is, even today, still difficult to diagnose microscopically. Mammography will not be effective in diagnosing all cases of carcinoma in situ for this is not its responsibility. But it is a significant step forward that mammographic findings, leading to carefully localized excisional biopsy, may in addition to exhibiting extremely complex forms of mammary dysplasia, in many cases lead to the discovery of lobular carcinoma in situ.

Chapter 38

Lobular Infiltrating Carcinoma

Definition and Pathology

Infiltrating lobular carcinoma presumably does not originate as a primary tumor but evolves from lobular carcinoma in situ. It is relatively rare (MILLER and KAY: 1.5% of all breast cancers over a period of five years; BORDEN and GERSHON-COHEN: less than 1%). Lobular carcinoma is not a separate histological entity (STEWART). Typically it consists of a lobular tumor which in some cases may be diffusely infiltrating or in others may occur as scattered clumps of tumor cells.

Lobular carcinoma when widespread may resemble scirrhus carcinoma, but it can also resemble carcinoma simplex. HAAGENSEN once called this tumor "small cell carcinoma". Axillary lymph node metastases from this cancer may resemble lymphsarcoma histologically and sometimes result in a misdiagnosis in the cases in which the primary breast carcinoma is not discovered.

Clinical Findings

Lobular carcinoma is most frequent in the upper outer quadrant. This location, however, is not obligatory.

In some cases, which have recently evolved from a carcinoma in situ, there may be no clinical symptoms. Advanced lobular carcinoma results in the typical clinical signs and symptoms of breast cancer. One may palpate definite, lobular lumps or more widespread firm masses. Nipple retraction and skin fixation occur.

Roentgenology

Early lobular carcinoma may be detected in the mammogram as a so-called occult carcinoma. This is generally recognized in the fatty involutional breast as a small, irregular mass with poorly defined borders and delicate stellate extensions from its margin or in association with the "tail of the comet" sign. There is thus a resemblance to

scirrhus ductal carcinoma (fig. 38.1). In other cases the infiltrating lobular carcinoma may have a predominantly smooth contour, resembling medullary carcinoma (fig. 38.2a and b). Lobular carcinoma because of its basic lobular structure is easily overlooked in the dense fibroadenomatous breast or in the breast retaining a major portion of parenchymal tissue. In such cases this tumor may be recognized only by secondary signs of malignancy, the latter often detected only by comparison with views of the other breast.

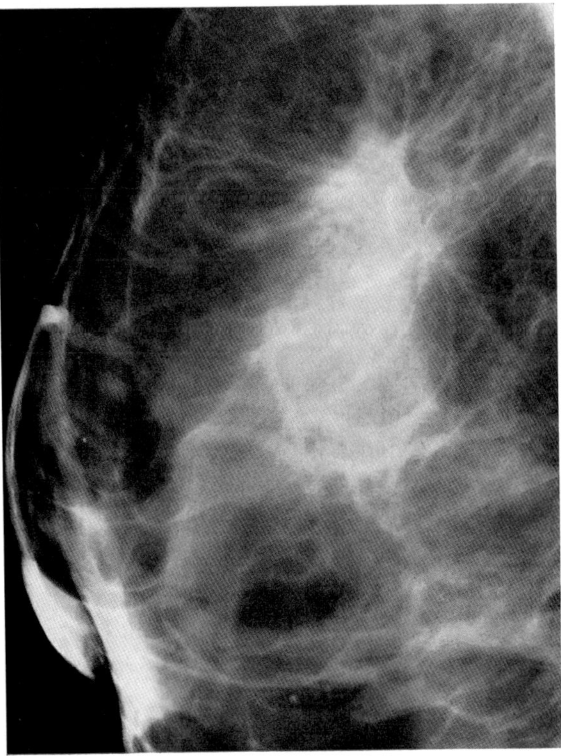

Fig. **38**.1 A circumscribed mass about 10 mm in diameter with irregular borders and containing occasional central calcifications.
Roentgen diagnosis: Suspicious for scirrhus carcinoma. Histological diagnosis: Diffuse lobular carcinoma, partly scirrhus. Lobular carcinoma in situ was also found.

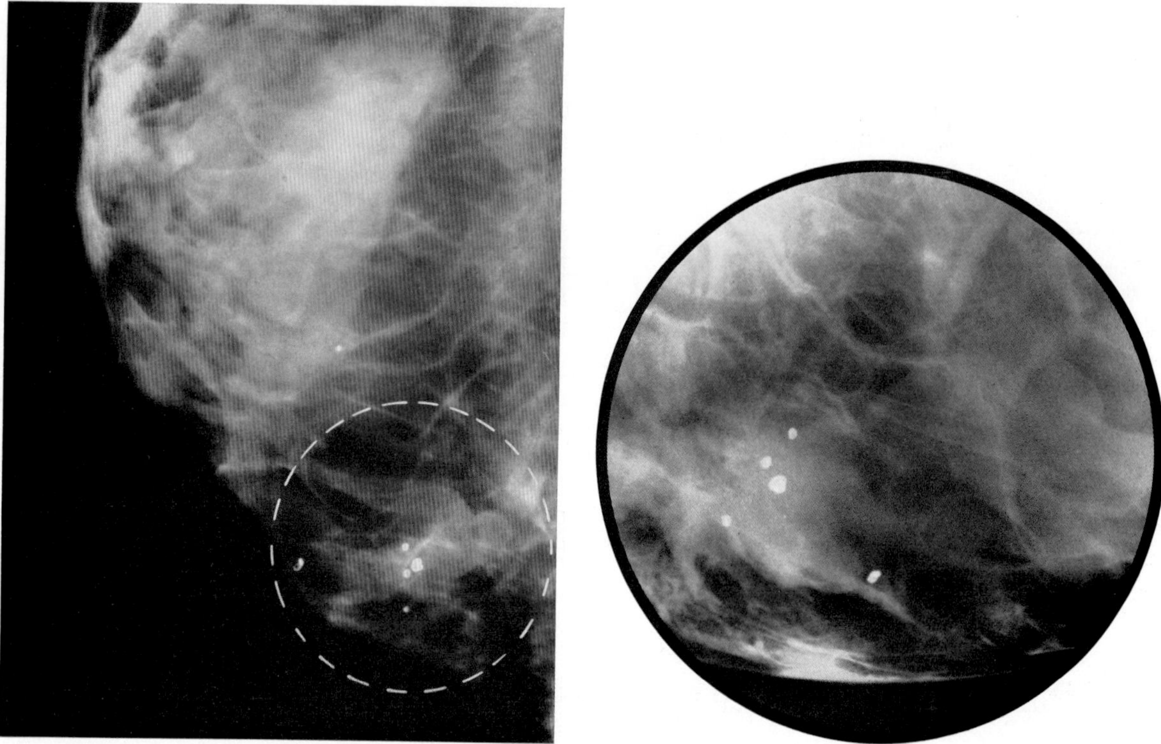

Fig. **38**.2a   Fig. **38**.2b

Fig. **38**.2 a, b   Painful but freely movable thickening beneath the nipple which is seen in the roentgeno-gram (a) as a rounded, fairly smoothly marginated density. Multiple areas of liponecrotic cysts. (b) Local area magnified 2 X. Roentgen diagnosis: Suspicious for malignancy.

Chapter 39

Sarcoma

Definition and Pathology

Mesenchymal malignancy of the breast is rare and it constitutes approximately 1% of malignant tumors of the breast. Sarcoma represents a greater proportion of the tumors of the breast in the male, 5.5%, than of the malignancies of the breast in the female (PETRACIC et al 1970). Sarcoma must be differentiated from the rare malignant variant of cystosarcoma phylloides, the latter tumor containing some epithelial elements. In addition to the more differentiated forms, fibro-, hemangio-, and liposarcoma as

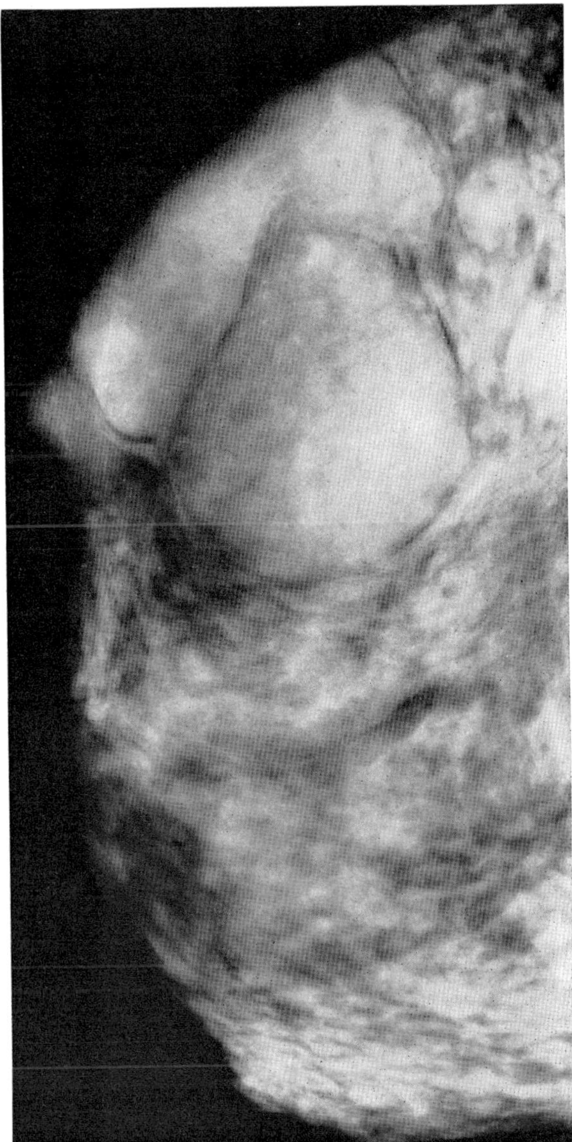

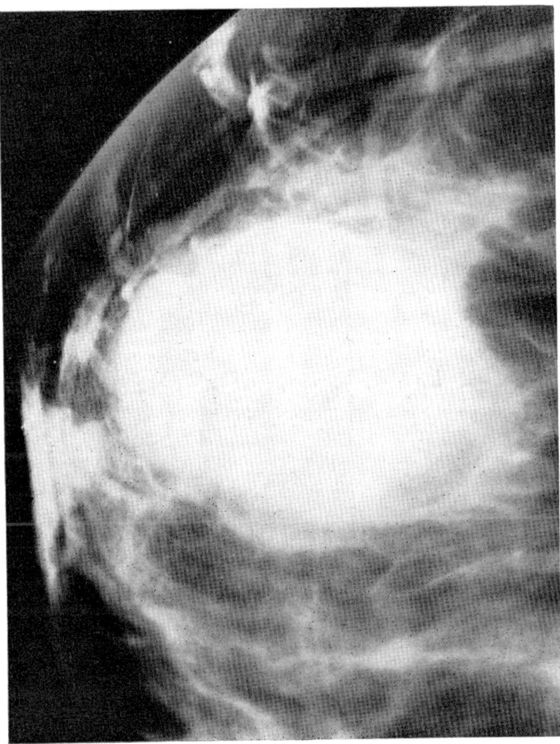

Fig. **39**.2 Clinical findings: Large, rapidly growing breast mass. No skin fixation. Patient being treated for lymphosarcoma. Roentgen findings: Rounded, slightly lobulated mass with some sharply marginated borders but also some ill-defined margins. Aspiration cytology: Numerous immature lymphoblasts: Lymphosarcoma. (Radiological Institute, University of Cologne, Women's Clinic, Professor Friedmann / Dr. Lanckohr).

Fig. **39**.1 Spindle cell sarcoma, rapidly growing. Mammogram: Sharply marginated lobular tumor mass. Occasional areas with microcalcifications. Displacement of the normal parenchyma by the rapidly growing tumor (Hüppe, Munich).

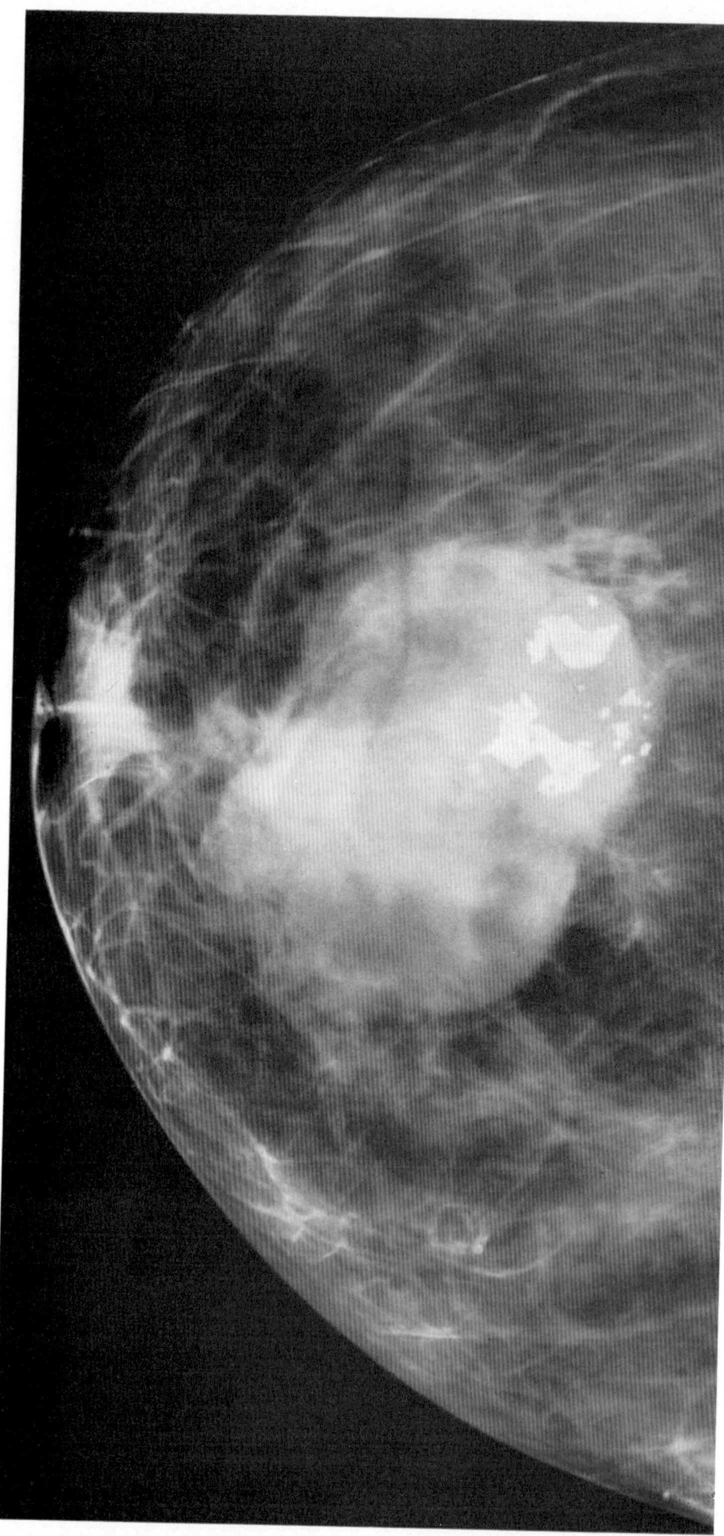

Fig. **39**.3 Polymorphocellular sarcoma with spindle cells and membranous bone forming components. Mammogram: Unusually large lobular mass with very smooth contours and coarse eccentric calcifications (Menges, Canton Hospital, Zürich).

well as the lymphoma and reticulum cell sarcomas, there are also anaplastic sarcomas, spindle, round, and pleomorphic sarcomas. Cartilage and bone formation have been observed in such tumors (SMITH and TAYLOR 1969). In addition to these there is the true breast sarcoma with a variable cytological appearance. This type of sarcoma is classified as "stromal sarcoma". Most likely the tumor consists, at least in part, of an undifferentiated liposarcoma which presents a very colorful histological picture.

Sarcomas may be relatively wellcircumscribed (for example, fibrosarcoma) or the borders may be ill-defined (for example, stromal sarcoma). Metastasis is primarily by way of the blood stream, however, OTT et al (1961) have indicated a 30% incidence of axillary lymph node involvement. This indicates an unfavorable prognosis (SINNER 1961). Angiosarcoma has a particularly poor prognosis. The prognosis is better with a highly differentiated fibrosarcoma or liposarcoma.

It is important to note that a medullary carcinoma associated with a rich proliferation of lymphoid stroma, particularly when associated with lymph node metastases, may very closely resemble lymphoreticular sarcoma. Therefore the diagnosis of the latter sort of breast sarcoma can only be made with careful and extensive histological examination.

To be complete one must also mention lymphoangiosarcoma of the shoulder and arm (STEWART-TREVES Syndrome, 1948) which may be associated with chronic edema of the arm following surgery or radiation therapy for breast carcinoma.

Clinical Findings

The tumor occurs most commonly between 45 and 55 years of age. Sarcomas never arise before puberty.

Rapid growth is characteristic of sarcomas. If a patient with a particularly large breast tumor indicates that growth occurred over a very short period of time, one should think of sarcoma.

It is important to note, however, that so-called cystosarcoma phylloides also may grow very rapidly.

At palpation a sarcoma is recognized as a large frequently mobile mass, not fixed to the skin. The nipple is also neither fixed nor retracted.

Large sarcomas may ulcerate. Fibrosarcoma is firm, somewhat nodular and not particularly

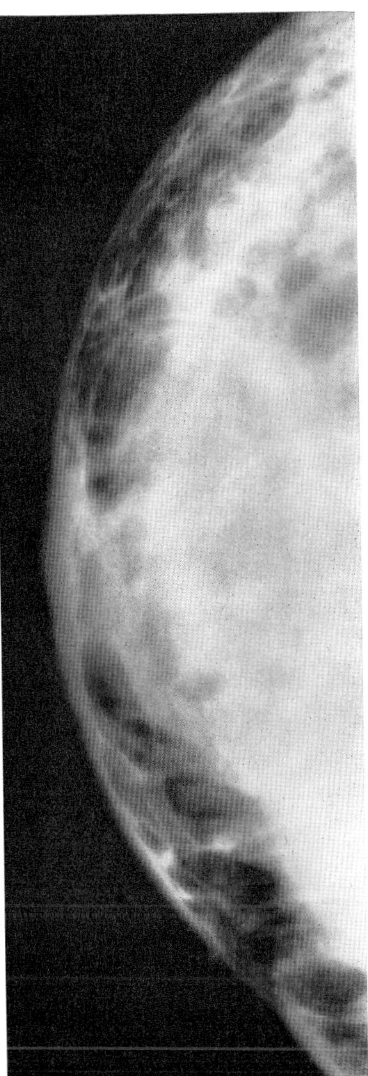

Fig. **39**.4   Fibroliposarcoma. Rapidly growing tumor first in the left then in the right breast of a 35-year-old woman. Massive enlargement and hardening of the breast with thickened erythematous skin. Excisional biopsy 4 weeks before: Fibrosis. Mammogram: Diffuse infiltration of the entire breast. Reticular infiltration of the subcutaneous fatty layer. Infiltrative thickening of the skin (Albring, Gelsenkirchen).

large. Lymphosarcomas and pleomorphic sarcomas are large, soft or spongy.

Opinions on adequate therapy vary. DA SILVA NETO (1970), on the basis of his observations of 22 cases, feels that simple mastectomy is sufficient. OTT et al (1961) because of their reported 30% incidence of axillary lymph node metastases advocate radical surgery. This view is shared by the Tübinger Surgical Clinic (PETRACIC et al

15*

1970) with the additional suggestion of "en bloc removal" of axillary lymph nodes followed by postoperative radiation. In our experience only lymphosarcoma and reticulum cell sarcoma have any radiation sensitivity whereas undifferentiated sarcomas are practically radioresistant. A radiation dose of 5,000 to 6,000 rads (cobalt[60]) to the axilla should not be exceeded. Such a dose is sufficient for radiosensitive sarcomas and a higher dose has no effect on radioresistant tumors.

Roentgenology

Differentiated sarcoma presents in the mammogram as large, round or lobular masses with sharp borders, occasionally surrounded by a sort of capsule (fig. 39.1, 39.2). The breast parenchyma is displaced by the rapidly growing expanding sarcoma. Bone formation or calcification may be seen within the tumor in the roentgenogram (fig. 39.3). One should consider sarcoma in any large breast mass containing coarse or bizarre calcium deposits similar to those found in fibroadenoma. On the whole extremely large, rapidly growing solid breast masses represent either sarcoma, giant fibroadenoma (cystosarcoma phylloides) or occasionally a large medullary carcinoma. Widespread carcinoma otherwise cannot be differentiated in the roentgenogram (fig. 39.4) from other diffuse infiltrating disease or edema of the breast.

Chapter 40

Lymphoma

Definition and Clinical Findings

It is rare that Hodgkin's disease manifests itself first in the breast.

The first description of lymphoma of the breast was by KÜCKENS (1928). There is a nodular and a diffuse form. The clinical picture of the nodular form may resemble breast carcinoma very closely, especially if there is involvement of the ipsilateral axillary lymph nodes. In the case of diffuse infiltrative breast lymphoma, as a rule, there is a rapid increase in size of the breast with edema and red discoloration of the overlying skin giving the appearance of a mastitis or inflammatory carcinoma (McGREGOR 1960; KUSHNER 1969; RANDALL and SPALDING 1945). Microscopic examination is necessary in this case to diagnose lymphoma.

It is more common to see breast involvement in advanced cases of Hodgkin's disease. Usually this diagnosis is not difficult although one must remember that primary carcinoma of the breast also may occur in a patient with lymphoma. However we ourselves have never seen or heard of a report of such a case.

Roentgenology

The nodular form of lymphoma of the breast is seen in the mammogram as a round or lobular relatively smooth mass described by ZWICKER and THELEN (1972) (fig. 40.1). It is difficult to differentiate the nodular form of lymphoma from medullary carcinoma. Lymphoma generally is not associated with microcalcifications or desmoplastic response; however, these signs are not obligatory with carcinoma either. The need to differentiate roentgenologically between nodular lymphoma of the breast, fibroadenoma and medullary carcinoma is infrequent and if so only possible when one is well informed about the general condition of the patient.

The same is true for the infiltrative form of Hodgkin's disease of the breast. BUTTENBERG

and WERNER (1962) described such a case which included a dense but nonhomogeneous retromammary infiltrative mass with irregular borders and unsharp contours 4 to 5 cm in diameter. In the diffuse form the entire breast may be permaeted by the neoplasm (fig. 40.2). The subcutaneous fatty tissue is permeated by linear and reticular structures and the overlying skin is thickened in a homogeneous or laminar fashion (WITTEN 1969). The diffuse form of breast lymphoma cannot be differentiated with any degree of certainty in the mammogram from diffuse or inflammatory carcinoma, obstructive lymphatic edema (KUSHNER 1969) or diffuse

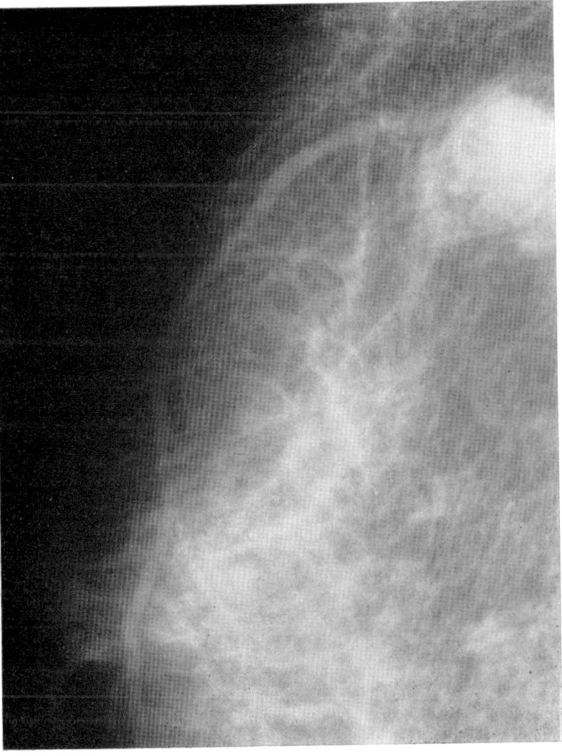

Fig. **40**.1 Nodular forms of breast lymphoma. In the upper half a relatively sharply marginated nodular mass. Dilated veins. (Zwicker and Thelen, University Radiological Clinic of Bonn).

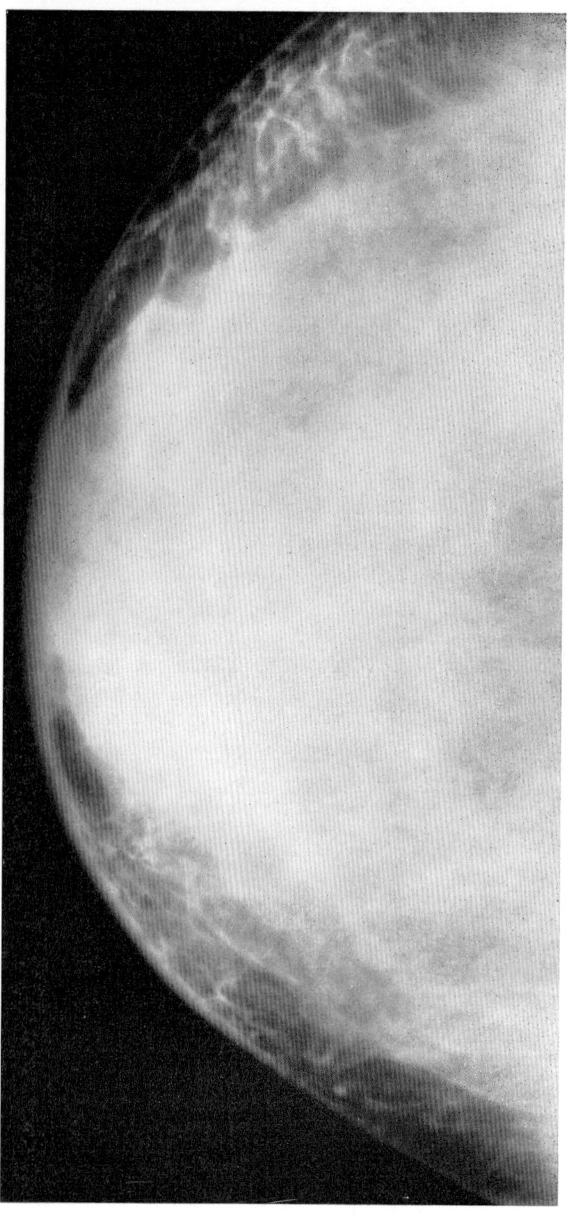

Fig. **40**.2 Diffuse form of breast lymphoma. Increased density of the entire breast with reticular infiltration of the subcutaneous fatty tissue. There is infiltration of the skin.

mastitis (HAAGENSEN 1971). Only familiarity with the underlying disease of the patient allows a reasonable differential diagnosis.

It is important to utilize all available clinical information in order to arrive at a differentiation between diffuse lymphoma of the breast and secondary obstructive lymphatic edema producing the same appearance, since staging and therapy of the disease depend on this. If local radiation therapy to the involved axillary lymph nodes results in regression of the breast changes a secondary obstructive lymphatic edema is assumed as the cause for the breast abnormality. If doubt still exists only excisional biopsy and histological examination of the breast tissue will permit a certain diagnosis.

Chapter 41

Leukemia

The breast tissue may be involved in acute as well as chronic leukemia with leukemic infiltrates. The first description of breast involvement in acute lymphocytic leukemia was by McWilliams and Hanes (1912).

In chronic lymphocytic leukemia intramammary lymph nodes may be involved. The most common breast involvement in this disease, however, is secondary generalized obstructive lymphatic edema of the breast because of involved enlarged axillary lymph nodes.

Clinical Findings

In leukemic infiltration of the breast there is a diffuse erythema of the skin which at clinical examination resembles an inflammatory process, an abcess or an inflammatory breast carcinoma. However, when the leukemic infiltration of the breast is bilateral, as it frequently is, and especially when there is knowledge regarding the basic hematological disorder of the patient, the differential diagnosis is not difficult.

Nodular leukemic infiltrates of the breast resemble carcinoma. These are most likely to occur in chronic myelogenous leukemia (Pascoe 1970).

Roentgenology

There are few reports concerning the mammographic findings in leukemic involvement of the breast.

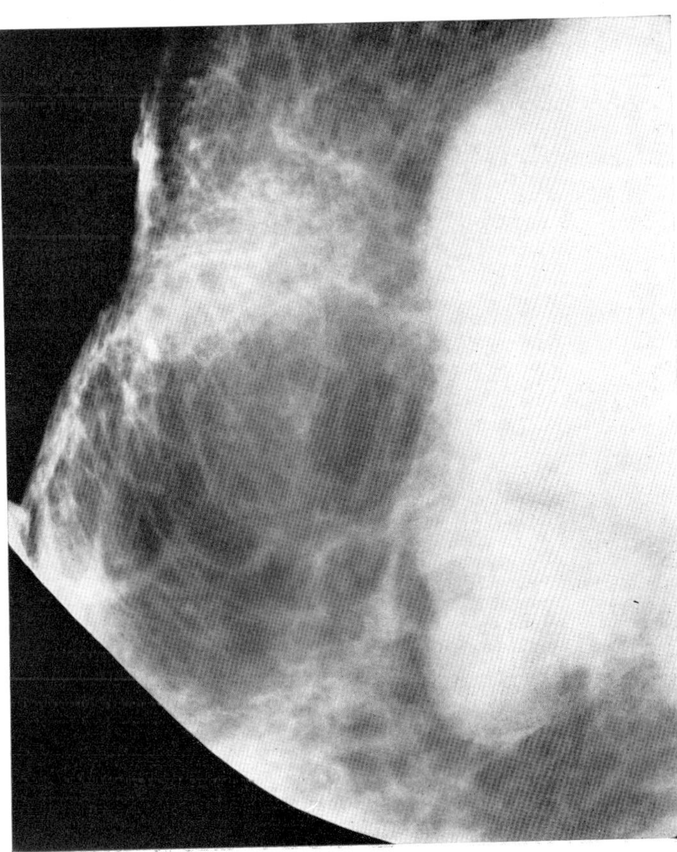

Fig. **41**.1 Giant lymph nodes in lymphocytic leukemia. The skin thickening and subcutaneous fibrosis in the upper half of the breast is the result of excisional biopsy.

Two cases have been reported by KENNEDY et al (1970). In diffuse leukemic breast infiltration the mammogram reveals a reticular infiltration with increased density of the entire breast parenchyma and of the subcutaneous fatty layer. The skin is normal or may be thickened in a scaly fashion. In acute leukemia one may find the above changes occurring in both breasts. Clinically the skin is deeply erythematous. However, it must be remembered that similar mammographic findings may be seen in chronic lymphadenosis occurring on one or both sides as a result of obstructive lymphedema. Clinically the two may be differentiated. If enlarged axillary lymph nodes are noted in the mammogram without pathological changes in the breast itself one should consider lymphoreticulosis (fig. 41.1). Adequate radiation therapy results in regression of the leukemic breast infiltrations as well as the lymphedema secondary to lymph node enlargement. A second form of leukemic breast involvement consists of nodular densities with irregular contours in the mammogram. Without knowledge of the underlying clinical condition these changes cannot be differentiated from the various forms of mammary dysplasia or breast carcinoma.

A further condition which provides problems in differential diagnosis is diffuse spontaneous hematoma which may accompany leukemia because of the associated hemorrhagic diathesis, but may also accompany breast carcinoma.

Diseases of the Male Breast

Chapter 42

Gynecomastia

Definition and Pathology

Gynecomastia consists of a benign enlargement of the male breast secondary to hyperplasia of the lactiferous ducts as well as connective tissue. Development of parenchymal tissue is very rare occurring only after long-term therapy with female hormone preparations or in hormonally active tumors.

Microscopically one finds proliferation of lactiferous ducts and connective tissue. Frequently proliferation of a fibrous stroma predominates, similar to the fibrous type of mammary dysplasia. In the older man a marked proliferation of fatty tissue may accompany the stromal development. Numerous fine papillary extensions off the ductal epithelium indicate a proliferative state. Epithelial metaplasia also occurs. If the intraductal papillary epithelial proliferation predominates it is described as proliferative gynecomastia. Whether this condition, which may be considered similar to the proliferative state of mammary dysplasia, indicates a greater risk of carcinomatous development is questionable but certainly it cannot be excluded (HAAGENSEN). Gynecomastia is most frequently observed in puberty ("puberty hypertrophy") or between the ages of 50 to 70 years ("senescent hypertrophy"). Endocrine disturbances are felt to be the cause. Unilateral gynecomastia is not rare and does not mitigate against a central, hormonal, metabolic, or iatrogenic etiology. Recently mammographic findings have indicated that such patients also show proliferative changes of the lactiferous ducts on the contralateral side; however, this is so minimal that it is not clinically detectable.

The exact etiology of pubertal gynecomastia is not known. The assumption that an alteration of the androgen/estrogen relationship with dominance of the estrogen effect is the cause is enlightening but has not been proved. JULL and DOSSETT (1964) as well as DECOURT et al (1962) were unable to demonstrate increased amounts of estradiol, estrogen or estriol in the urine. Against the theory of estrogen as the etiology of pubertal gynecomastia is the fact that treatment of these patients with testosterone results in an increase rather than decrease of the gynecomastia. It is more likely that a relationship exists between gynecomastia and the anterior lobe of the pituitary gland, because in hypophysectomized animals one is unable to produce gynecomastia either with the administration of estrogen or androgen (LEVY et al 1965). An increased production of gonadotropin may be involved in producing gynecomastia. Prolactin and pituitary hormone may also play a role in the development of pubertal gynecomastia (FREILINGER et al 1971; PAULSEN 1968).

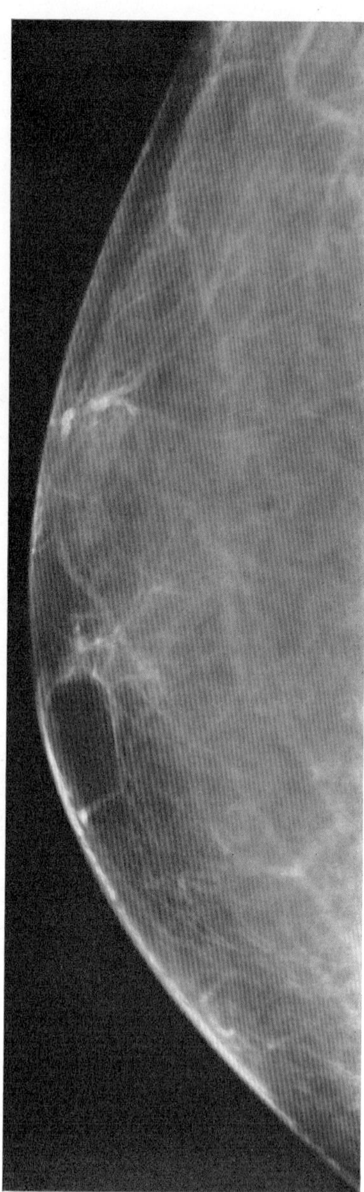

Fig. **42**.1a Delicate strands of connective tissue behind the nipple.

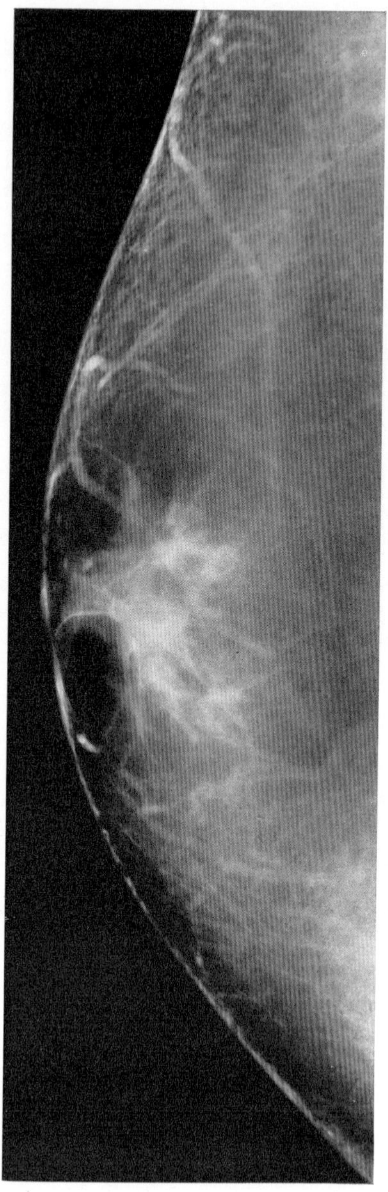

Fig. **42**.1b Ten months later there is coarsening of the strands and increased tissue density in the subareolar region: Fibrotic gynecomastia.

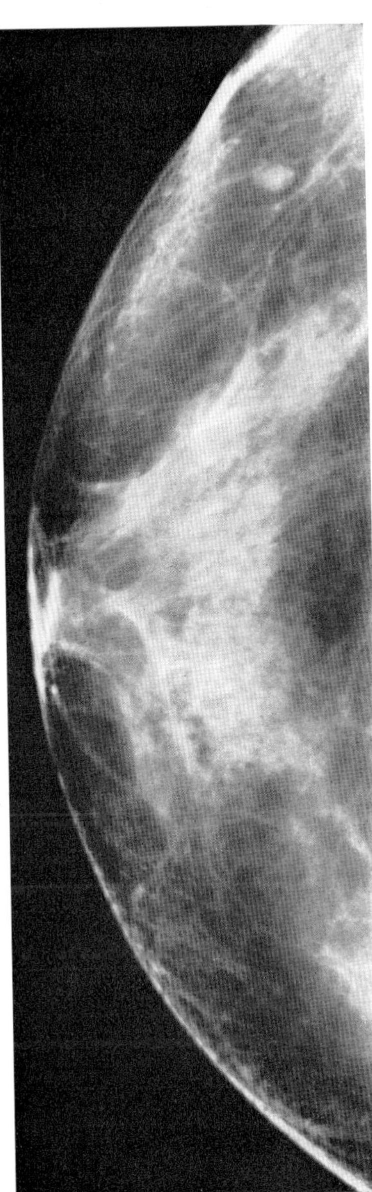

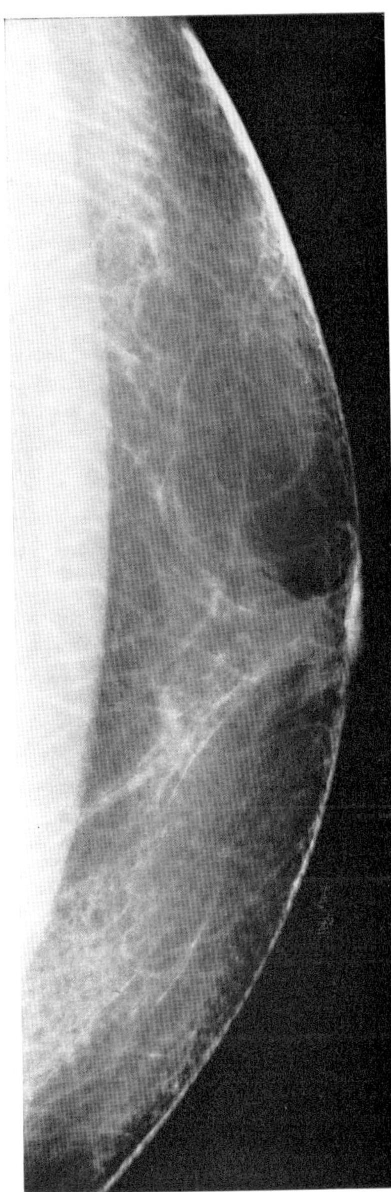

Fig. **42**.2a Clinical unilateral gynecomastia in a 63-year-old man. The roentgenogram reveals thickened radiating structures resulting in an extensive triangular subareolar increase in tissue density.

Fig. **42**.2b The contralateral breast was clinically normal. The roentgenogram, however, also reveals minimal gynecosmastia on this side.

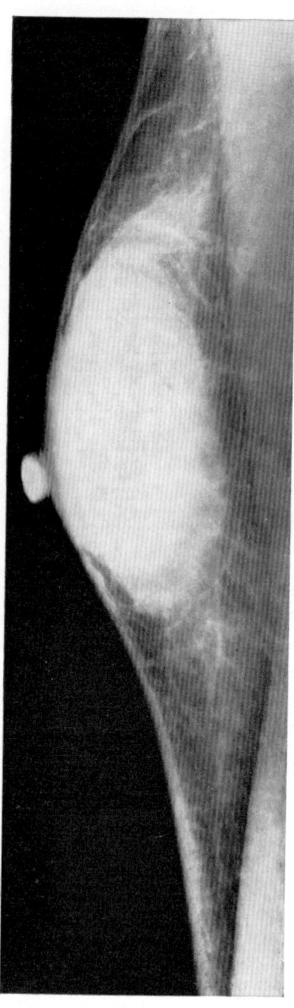

Fig. **42**.3 Gynecomastia with a large nodular subareolar soft tissue density in a 46-year-old man.

Gynecomastia has also been observed in malformations of the urogenital tract (for example, cryptorchism, hypospadias), Klinefelter's syndrome (XXY) and Reifenstein's syndrome, choriocarcinoma (malignant testicular teratoma with chorionic differentiation), testicular atrophy (posttraumatic, hydro- and varicocele), carcinoma of the adrenal cortex, chronic liver disease (cirrhosis) as well as in dystrophy ("gynecomastia of prisoners of war").

Drug-induced etiologies for gynecomastia include estrogen (treatment for prostatic carcinoma) as well as androgen therapy. The doses resulting in gynecomastia vary with the individual patient. Apparently even the absorption of hormones in the meat from animals treated with estrogens is sufficient to cause gynecomastia.

Further drugs which may result in gynecomastia in adults are phenothiazine, reserpine, methyldopa (this probably has its effect by way of the pituitary gland), digitalis, spironolactone.

Clinical Findings

Clinically one palpates a subareolar sharply-bordered, firm, rounded and movable mass with a diameter of 2 to 4 cm, or a more diffuse, soft, less well-defined fullness of varying size.

Gynecomastia of puberty is usually reversible and spontaneously regresses within a period of several months. In 25% of cases, however, it may remain over a period of two years, but rarely longer. Only rarely is surgical therapy indicated (FREILINGER et al 1971).

A careful history should be obtained in each patient with pubertal gynecomastia to rule out other etiologies. If there is no evidence in this direction one can reassure the parents and the patient and follow the patient at one or two monthly intervals. Today mammography is an essential part of the examination.

Gynecomastia of older patients ("virile climactic") also resolves spontaneously in most cases.

Fatty enlargement of the breast in a man without subareolar palpable parenchymal or connective tissue proliferations is not gynecomastia.

Roentgenology

There must be a proliferation of lactiferous ducts before gynecomastia may be objectively diagnosed by mammography.

In the normal adult male there is no increased density in the subareolar region. Any nodular or branching subareolar density is therefore abnormal even in the absence of clinical detectable gynecomastia.

In agreement with the histological appearance, the following mammographic types of gynecomastia may be differentiated (LISZKA et al 1968):

1) Fibrous gynecomastia is the most common form. In the mammogram one sees brushlike, subareolar radiating linear densities of varying extent (fig. **42**.1a and b). Such subareolar densities frequently have a triangular configuration.

In advanced "unilateral" gynecomastia one frequently sees smaller branching subareolar densities in the opposite "normal" breast (fig. 42.2a and b).

2) Large nodular gynecomastia (fig. 42.3) appear as a dense, almost homegeneous mass with round or oval contours (gynecomastia vera). This consists not only of proliferation of lactiferous ducts but also acinar proliferation.

3) Secretory gynecomastia is generally caused by hormonal therapy with androgens. Galactography is indicated in order to differentiate between simple secretory gynecomastia (fig. 42.4), ductal ectasia, and papillomatosis.

4) Pseudogynecomastia (adipose breast) is seen in generalized obesity. In the mammogram there is absence of lactiferous duct proliferation or increased tissue density. The only findings consist of an accumulation of fatty tissue.

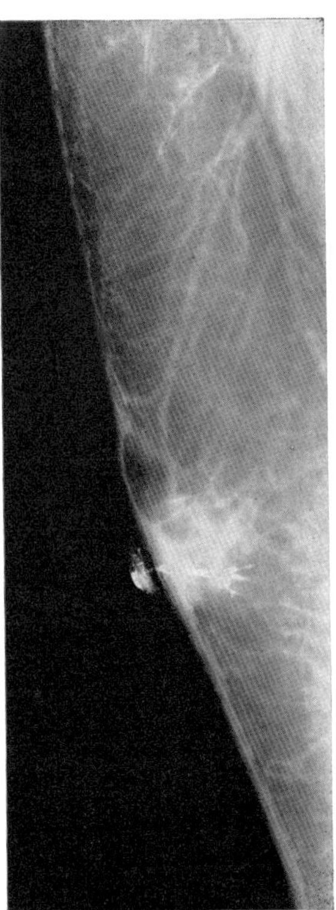

Fig. **42**.4 Gynecomastia with nipple discharge in a 36-year-old man. Ductography reveals a short branching duct.

Chapter 43

Fibromas and Cysts

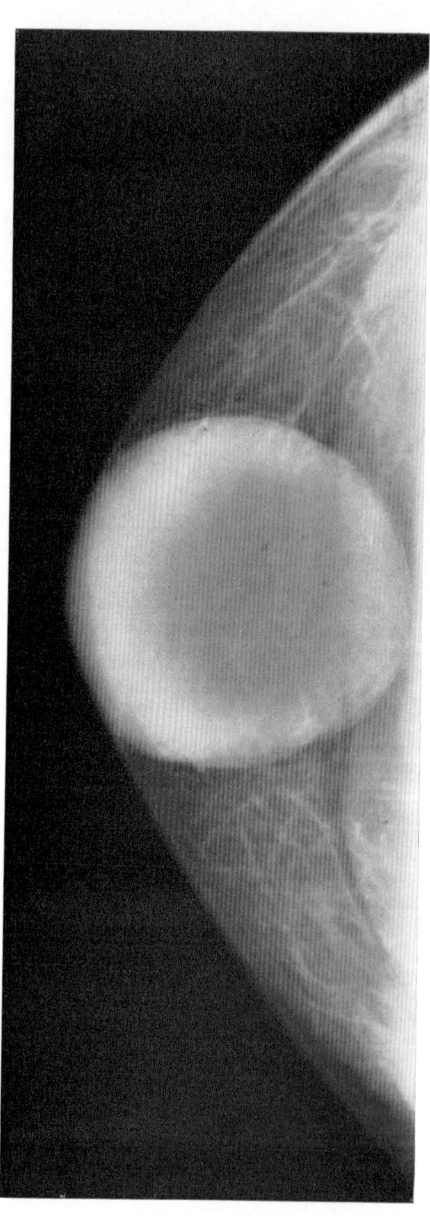

Fibromas and cysts of the male breast are no different macroscopically from those seen in the female breast.

In the mammogram there are found homogeneous, dense, round or oval structures with smooth and sharply demarcated borders. The differentiation between a cyst (fig. 43.1) and a fibroma is only possible with aspiration and pneumocystography.

Fig. **43**.1 Epithelial cyst in a 27-year-old man. The lesion has been present and enlarging gradually for 1½ years. On palpation a soft mass bulging beneath the areola was noted. Mammogram: Homogeneous round soft tissue mass with smooth borders.
Histology: Cyst surroundet by flat epithelium.

Chapter 44

Male Breast Carcinoma

Incidence, Pathology, Clinical Findings

Carcinoma of the male breast is rare. It constitutes 1% of all breast carcinomas (HAAGENSEN). Between 1960 and 1970 we have given radiation therapy to 19 male patients with carcinoma compared to 1,560 female patients, an incidence of 1.2%.

Clinically carcinoma of the male breast may be palpated as a firm or hard, poorly marginated, and somewhat fixed mass which generally occurs eccentrically in relation to the nipple. In advanced stages there may be ulceration. Frequently, even in the case of small carcinomatous masses, metastases to the axillary lymph nodes have developed.

Microscopically carcinoma of the breast in the male assumes the same forms as in the female. There is a tendency towards greater degree of differentiation. Paget's carcinoma may occasionally be seen in the male breast. The 10-year survival rate following radical mastectomy is 35—50% (HAAGENSEN).

McDIVITT, STEWART and BERG are very critical of the notion that carcinoma of the male breast arises as a result of hormonal therapy of prostatic carcinoma. According to their view the possibility of intramammary metastases from prostatic carcinoma with secondary invasion of the lactiferous ducts may occur and therby give the impression of a primary breast carcinoma.

Roentgenology

The appearance in the mammogram of carcinoma of the male breast is identical to that of carcinoma in the female.

Occasionally there may be diagnostic difficulty with stellate or radial streaky subareolar thickening of ductal tissues as found in fibrous gynecomastia. This process, however, is always symmetrically distributed beneath the areola and nipple whereas carcinoma is invariably eccentric in location (fig. 44.1).

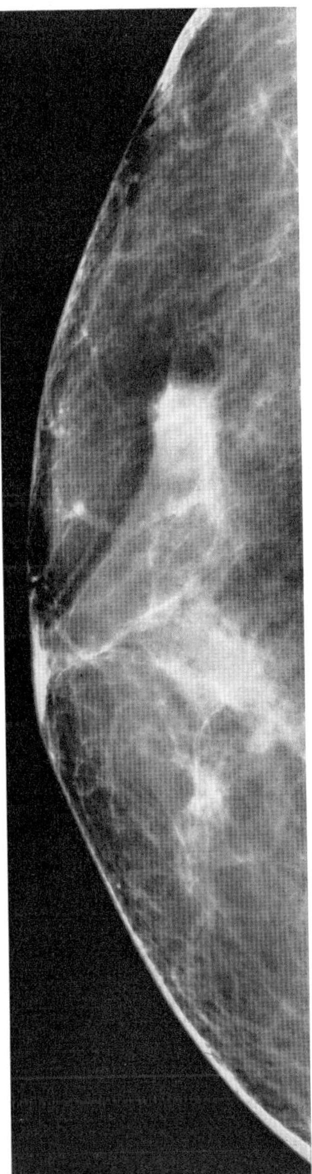

Fig. **44**.1   Small scirrhus carcinoma in a 65-year-old man.

The Breast Following Surgery and Radiation Therapy

Postsurgical changes may create problems in the roentgen examination of the breast. These are important not only as to their cause but also because of their frequency. In our case material, for example, 38% of the patients had postbiopsy scars and 5% had scars resulting from incision and drainage of mastitis. Cosmetic surgical scars are less frequent.

The evaluation and definition of any pathological process in the anatomically intact breast is difficult enough. In the surgically deformed breast the problems of differential diagnosis are much greater. It is especially difficult to differentiate a postincisional intramammary fibrosis with skin thickening from the similar changes produced by a scirrhus carcinoma. Accurate history, palpation and inspection are as important in mammographic evaluation of the post-operative breast as in any other roentgen examination. Clinically doubtful findings are frequently resolved by mammography. It is unusually difficult clinically to evaluate the character of a palpable mass beneath a surgical scar. Roentgen examination in such cases also demands great experience in order to differentiate between postsurgical changes which result in skin thickening, increase in subcutaneous tissue density, and even microcalcifications all of which resemble carcinoma.

Naturally there are borderline cases in which neither clinical nor roentgen findings are clear enough to avoid repeat biopsy.

The effects of radiation therapy of breast carcinoma are accurately determined by mammography. Regression of the tumor, or radiation resistance with recurrence or spread may be accurately detected by roentgen examination making mammography indispensable, the decisive examination to document the effectiveness of radiation therapy on a breast carcinoma.

Chapter 45

The Breast Following Incision and Biopsy

Scars and Parenchymal Defects

Incision for mastitis as well as biopsy results in scarring and thickening of the skin and reticular or linear nodules in the subcutaneous tissues, in the region of the surgery. Fewer diagnostic problems, however, are noted following incision and drainage for mastitis than with excisional biopsy. Incision and drainage does not result in deformity of breast parenchyma; it does occur in excisional biopsy because of the removal of tissue. The primary finding in the parenchyma may be a nodular increase in density. Incision and drainage scars do not result in microcalcification of the incisional scars or the development of oil cysts. If the incision for mastitis occurred many years ago then the residual findings are fairly sparse since the skin thickening gradually regresses and there is reorganization of the parenchyma as well.

Excisional biopsy scars are recognized on the tangential roentgenogram as an area of skin

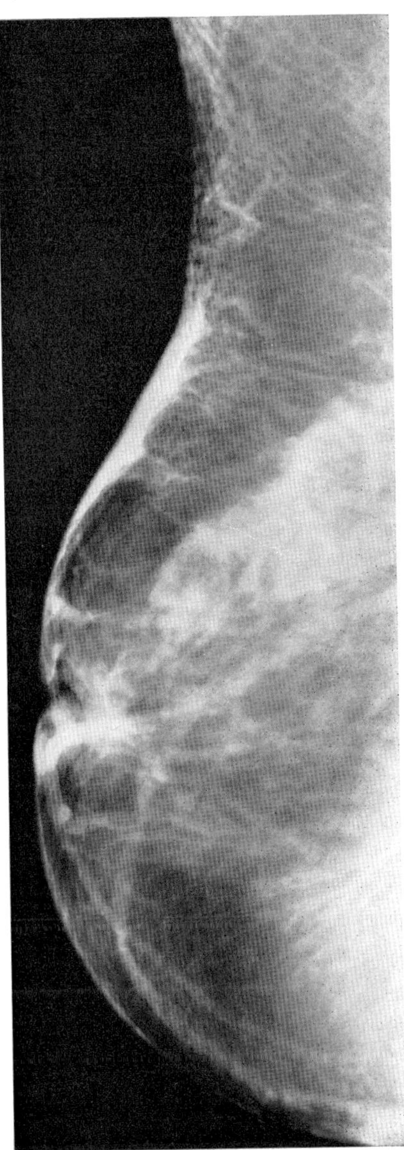

Fig. **45**.1a   Scar 4 weeks after excisional biopsy. Thickening of the skin in the region of the scar. Delicate linear and reticular connective tissue proliferation subcutaneously.

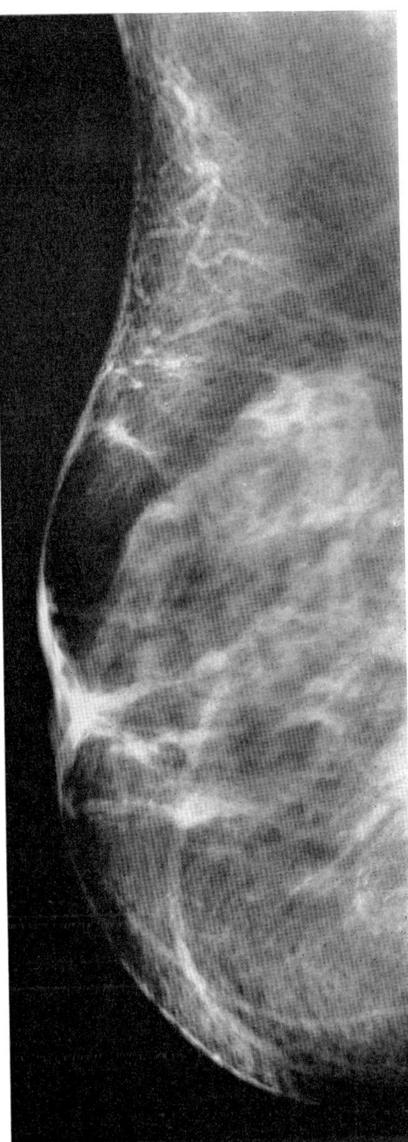

Fig. **45**.1b   Six months after excisional biopsy the skin thickening has regressed. Some small connective tissue strands, however, remain in the subcutaneous fatty layer.

thickening. Beneath this thickened skin the subcutaneous fatty tissue is permeated with fine linear strands of fibrous tissue which may assume a netlike pattern. These scars regress with time and become smaller and more focal (fig. 45.1a and b). There may be increased skin thickening and subcutaneous fibrosis if there were postoperative complications such as infection and inflammation. The more extensive the biopsy, particularly in cases of multiple simultaneous biopsies, the more extensive are the changes

noted within the breast parenchyma and fatty tissue (fig. 45.2). Thus there may be a diffuse reticular permeation by fibrous tissue of the subcutaneous as well as intramammary fat and the breast parenchyma with extensive overlying skin thickening which, without prior knowledge of surgical manipulation, may be interpreted in the mammogram as a diffuse breast malignancy. The same error may be made by the mammographer when there has been surgical removal of a large group of axillary lymph nodes and subsequent

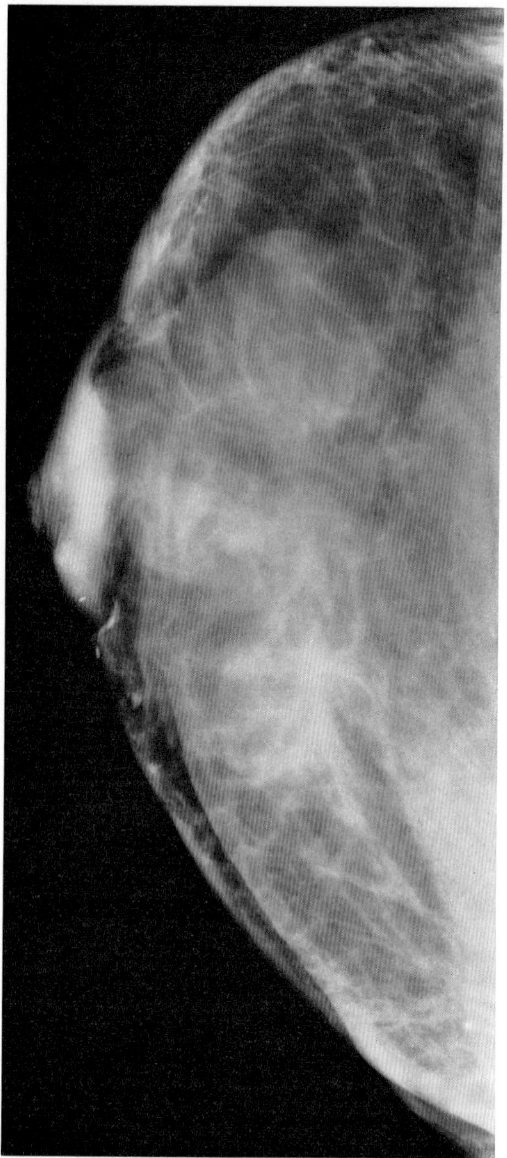

Fig. **45**.2 Diffuse reticular connective tissue proliferation in the subcutaneous fatty layer and
throughout the whole breast after repeated extensive excisional biopsy. Skin thickening secondary
to scar formation and inflammatory postoperative
complications. In the absence of the history this
could be confused with diffuse carcinoma or
mastitis.

Fig. **45**.3 Mammogram after excision of lateral
breast parenchyma. A small parenchymal rest persists in the subareolar area.

lymphatic block has occurred resulting in diffuse
edema of the breast. Surgical parenchymal defects
are not a diagnostic problem mammographically
when a section of the breast parenchyma has
been completely removed. The parenchymal mass
is then smaller and appears "amputated" (fig.
45.3).

If excisional biopsy of the central portion of the
breast parenchyma has been performed, the
subsequent fibrotic reaction of this focus and the
surrounding parenchyma results in a stellate
intramammary scar which is very difficult to
differentiate mammographically from scirrhus—
carcinoma (fig. 45.4). This problem is compound-

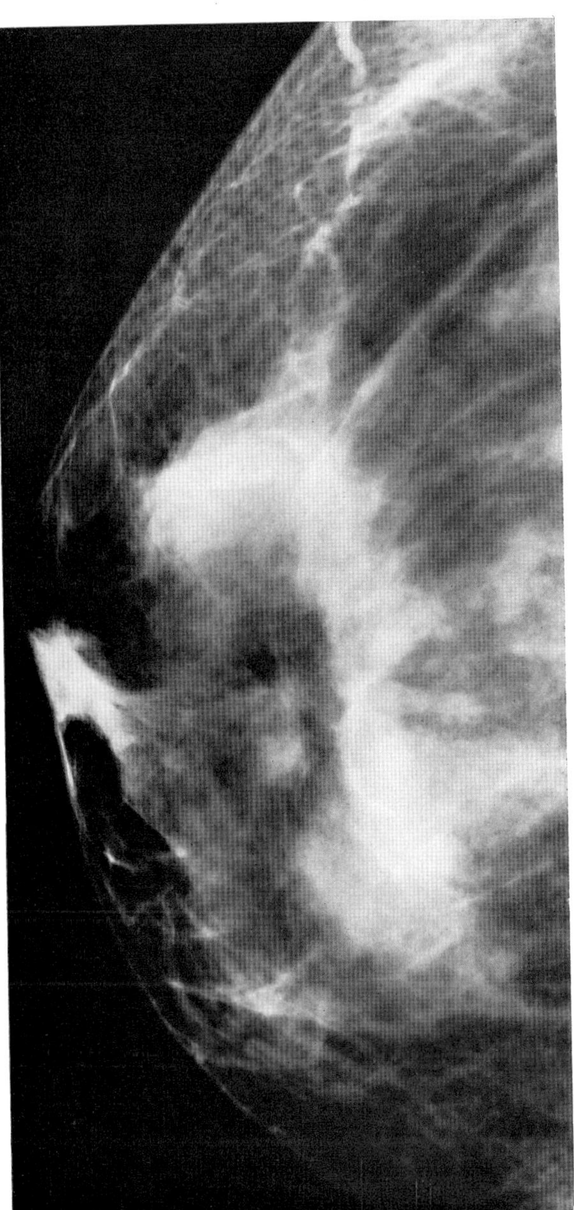

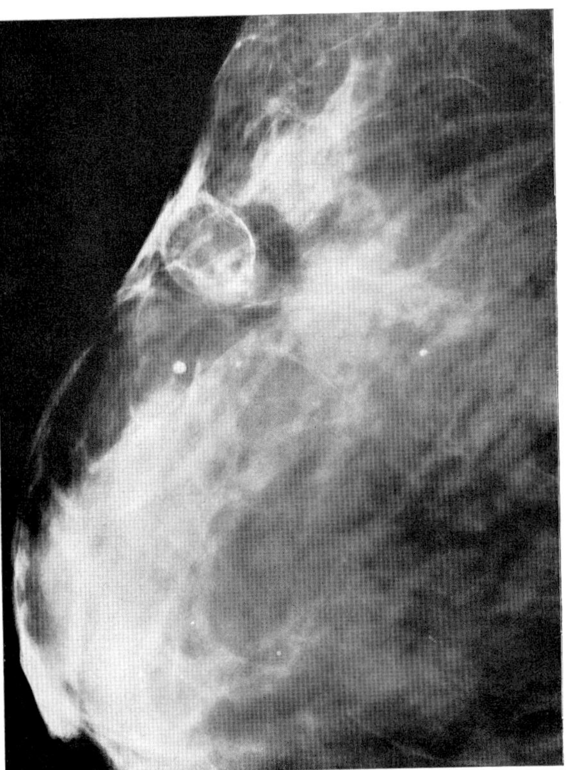

Fig. **45**.5 Typical oil cysts in a surgical scar clinically palpable as spherical lumps. Near by are two cystlike calcifications (liponecrosis microcystica calcificans, Leborgne).

Fig. **45**.4 Rounded defect in the center of the breast parenchyma with central, stellate connective tissue fibrosis following excisional biopsy. In the absence of the clinical history this may be misconstrued as scirrhus carcinoma.

ed when nipple retraction results as part of the postoperative fibrosis or when microcalcifications form within the parenchymal scar. Further problems occur when, as a result of excisional biopsy, the breast parenchyma is divided into two sections and when one of those sections is left more or less intact. This may appear at palpation as a nodular mass and on the roentgeno-

gram gives the impression of an isolated area of increased density within the breast. This creates even more concern when dysplastic changes occur in this tissue or when it remains as a residual parenchyma while the other portions of the breast involute in later years. In such cases it is helpful to have prior knowledge of the exact localization of the excisional biopsy. In doubtful cases biopsy of the questionable tissue must be performed. Simple follow-up examinations of such lesions are only justifiable when no suspicion of malignancy exists clinically or roentgenologically.

Calcifications

Calcification in postoperative scars is not infrequent. Since they may indicate malignancy and because on palpation the findings beneath a scar also frequently raise similar suspicions, it is important to become very familiar with the appearance of such postoperative calcifications. The calcifications of a postexcisional biopsy scar

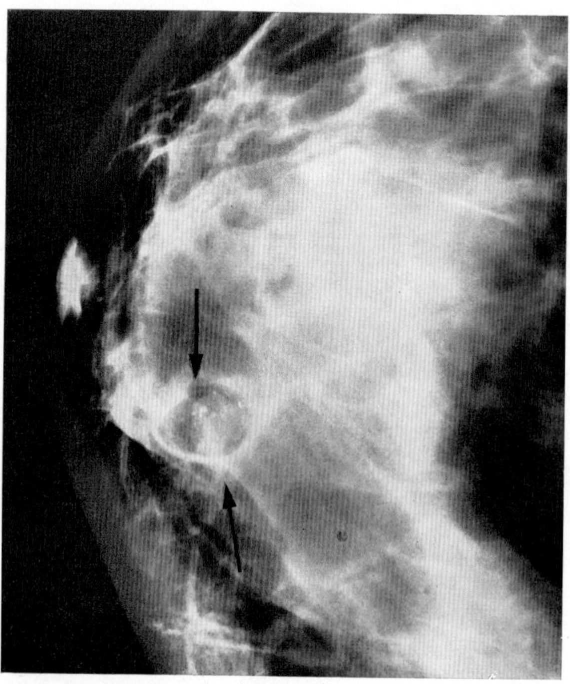

Fig. **45**.6   Punctate calcifications within the confines of an oil cyst.

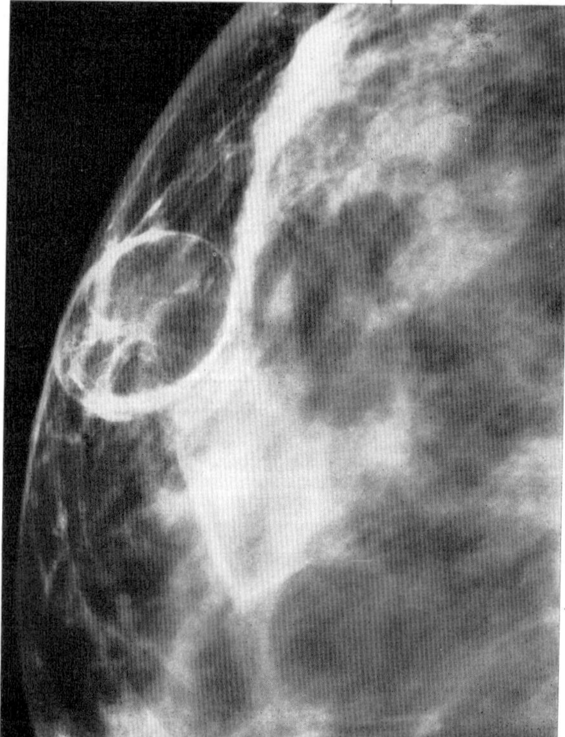

Fig. **45**.7   Mammogram following compression injury to the breast. Ringlike lesion in the subcutaneous area is seen, corresponding to palpatory findings. The inner portion of the ring is radiolucent and aspiration revealed oily contents.

are mostly within the subcutaneous fatty tissue, whereas calcifications of malignant disease do not occur in this area. Additionally postoperative calcifications are few and singular (see fig. 49.21). They frequently have a peculiar linear or bubbly configuration which is often characteristic enough to allow their identification. It is more difficult when these microcalcifications lie deeper within the breast and then resemble more closely the calcium of carcinoma.

If microcalcifications appear as a group in the region of the operative scar one must then proceed as one would for microcalcifications associated with carcinoma. Only accurate excisional biopsy and careful histological examination of the suspicious lesion will allow an accurate differential diagnosis. It is not uncommon to see small areas of fat necrosis in postoperative scars. These result in small bubbly or cystlike calcifications.

They are found most frequently in the region of a scar and thus verify the theory of LEBORGNE, who was the first to recognize this cystlike calcification as a sign of fat necrosis (see fig. 45.5).

Oil Cysts

Of particular interest is the appearance of so-called "oil cysts" in postoperative scars. We have seen this not only in scars following excisional biopsy and cosmetic surgery but also in crushing trauma to the breast. In the mammogram one sees a delicate ringlike shadow the center of which has the same density as the fat tissue of the breast (fig. 45.5, 45.6, 45.7). It has been assumed that this appearance indicates that the content of such lesions must be firm or liquid fat. We have shown this hypothesis to be true by puncture and aspiration. A clear oily liquid is aspirated. We have performed chemical and physical analysis of the oily content of the cyst. Analysis (LEUPOLD) of the material resulted in a total lipoid content of 210 mg% which consisted almost completely of neutral fat, the exact determination of which resulted in 195 mg%. Traces of other lipoids such as cholesterol and phosphatine were found. Lipoid electrophoresis verified the above findings. We are essentially then dealing with pure triglyceride or perhaps chylomicrons with minimal protein content, and thus the designation of "oil cysts" is entirely correct.

Histologically the oil cyst is lined by a single-layered epithelium. The fat content can be verified on the Sudan stain. We explain the formation of such oil cysts in excisional biopsy scars as a result of ischemia of fatty tissue following the surgery with subsequent fat necrosis and coalescence of fatty contents around which a connective tissue capsule is formed.

The size and shape of such oil cysts varies ranging from 4 to 10 mm in diameter. An exceptional oil cyst may have a longitudinal or oval configuration. These atypical configurations probably result from the shape of the surrounding fibrosis and are seen only in relatively recent scars. As the scar and surrounding fibrotic reaction matures the oil cysts invariably evolve into their later rounded form.

Since oil cysts may suggest a firm or solid mass on palpation, excision is often performed because of the clinical findings. The roentgen appearance of oil cysts, however, is so characteristic that any other cause of a mass in the breast can be easily excluded and excision avoided.

If the contents of an oil cyst are not completely liquid, particularly when a few microcalcifications are associated, the lesion can resemble a solid intracystic mass (fig. 45.6). In such a case excisional biopsy and histological examination is indicated to rule out malignancy.

The wall of an oil cyst rarely may calcify. LEBORGNE has named this liponecrosis macrocystica calcificans.

Foreign Bodies in the Breast

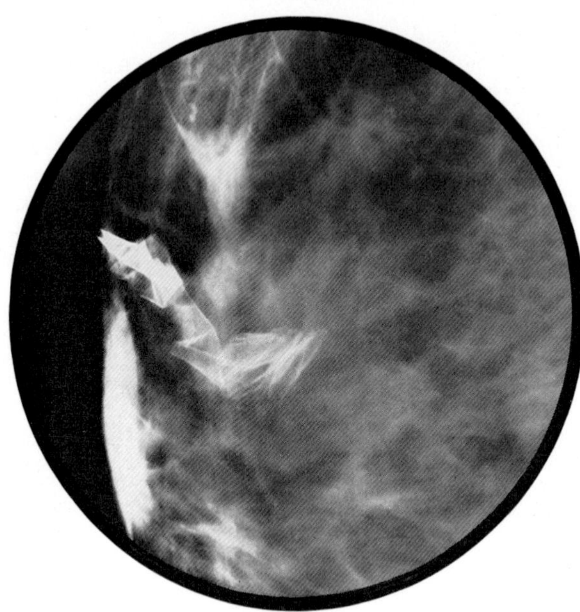

Fig. **46**.1 Retained gauze following excisional biopsy.

Foreign bodies in the breast most commonly are surgical materials inadvertently left behind during the operation. Gauze (fig. **46**.1), drainage tubes (fig. **46**.2), pieces of rubber, fractured surgical needles (fig. **46**.3) have been found. Suture material is only recognizable in the roentgenogram when it is metallic or when it becomes calcified (fig. **46**.4).

Noniatrogenic foreign bodies of the breast are rare. The most common are sewing needles which may have been introduced into the breast accidentally or purposely; the latter may be seen in women prisoners or psychologically disturbed patients.

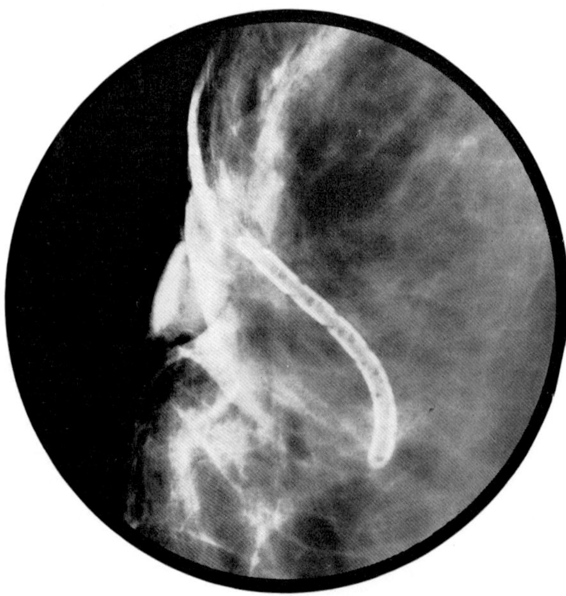

Fig. **46**.2 Retained drain following excisional biopsy.

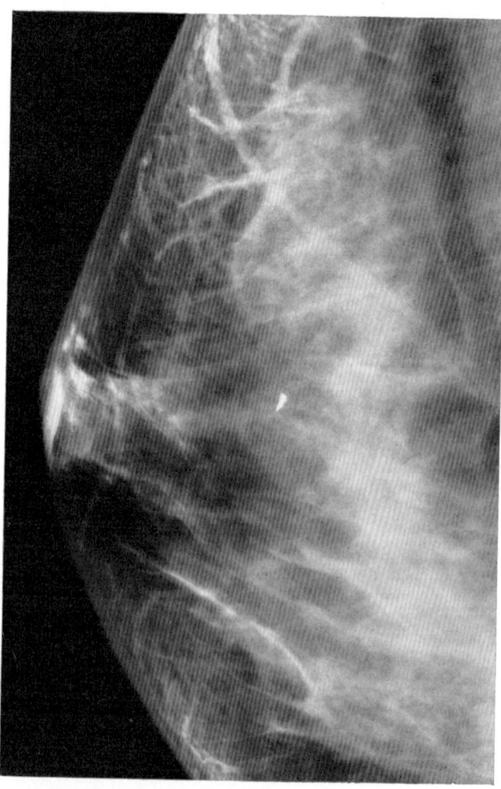

Fig. **46**.3 Fragment of surgical needle.

The diagnostic problem posed by an intra-mammary foreign body is not to mistake the fibrosis surrounding the foreign body for a tumor when the breast is palpated. The identification of radio-opaque foreign bodies is readily accomplished with a roentgenogram. For this reason mammography is obligatory before any other further investigation of a postsurgical positive palpatory finding. Foreign bodies need not always be removed. "Secretory disease" in a breast containing a foreign body does not necessarily mean they are related. Care should be taken not to miss a carcinoma developing in the vicinity of a foreign body in the breast.

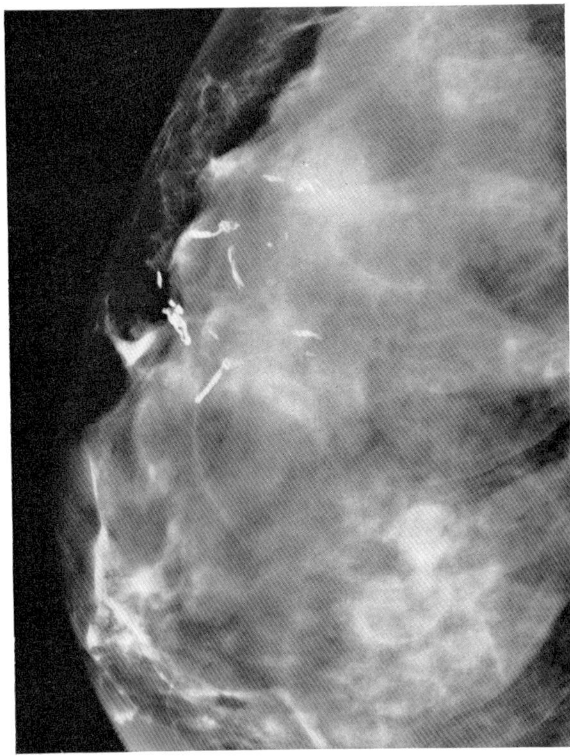

Fig. **46**.4   Calcified suture material, following excisional biopsy.

Chapter 47

Plastic Surgery of the Breast

Knowledge of the most common methods of plastic surgery of the breast is necessary in order to correctly assess a mammogram of a patient who has undergone such an operation. In problematic cases the operative report should be considered.

Surgical Elevation of the Papilla

This is recognized at inspection of the breast by a circular row of sutures surrounding the areola associated with a short linear row of sutures extending in a crosslike fashion into each quadrant of the breast (fig. 47.1). This correction is performed for congenitally retracted nipple which may cause difficulties in lactation and impede proper hygiene of the area. In the mammogram there are no structural changes within the breast. In the vicinity of the skin incisions, however, one can expect scars and individual, fine microcalcifications. The sub-areolar area may be somewhat enlarged or broadened.

Reduction Mammoplasty

Reduction mammoplasty of a unilateral or bilaterally enlarged breast is generally performed by extensive excision of tissue from the upper hemisphere (LEXER, BERSON and others) or through partial amputation of the upper portion of the breast (GOHRBANDT-LODGE). The operative approach resembles that of an extensive excisional biopsy in accordance with the need to reduce the size of the breast.

The classical type of incision in a reduction mammoplasty is depicted in fig. 47.2. A curvilinear incision at the base of the breast is performed with a vertical incision extending to the areola and encircling it.

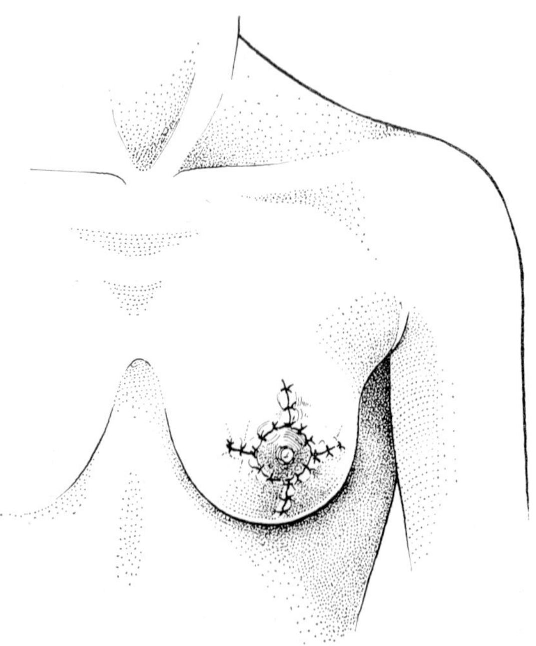

Fig. **47**.1 The breast after corrective surgery for retracted nipple.

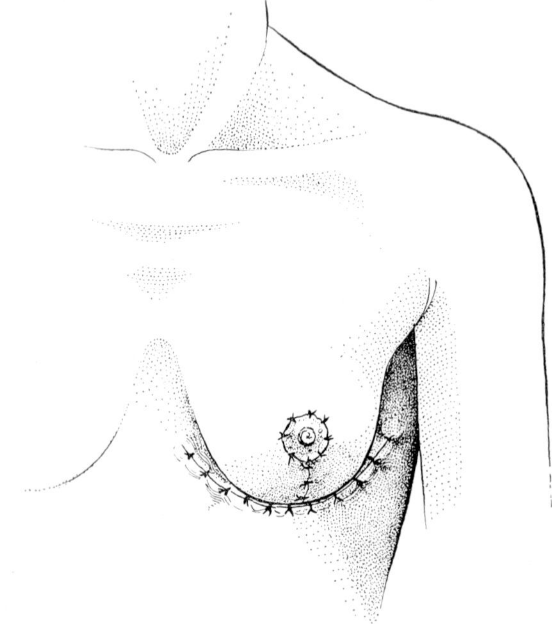

Fig. **47**.2 The breast following surgery for reduction mammoplasty.

In the mammogram one notes large defects in the parenchyma and its displacement into atypical locations.

Within the region of the surgical scar calcifications may occur which can produce difficulty in differentiation from those found in intraductal carcinoma. The absence of signs of infiltration mitigates against carcinoma. One must give careful consideration to the palpatory findings, in the final diagnosis.

Augmentation Mammoplasty

In order to reconstruct the breast either uni- or bilaterally because of hypoplasia or following mastectomy one may use autologous tissue or synthetics. Autologous material is generally taken from the fat rich tissues of the buttocks or from the anterior abdominal wall directly inferior to the breast (fig. 47.3). This adipose tissue is positioned into the breast by way of an inferior curvilinear incision. Such fatty implants are recognized in the mammogram by their radiolucent character. Most have a rounded shape (fig. 47.4a). A disadvantage of fatty implants is their tendency to shrink later and eventually to undergo dissolution. In such an event one may see isolated rests of the original fat implant and numerous coarse calcifications (fig. 47.4b). Such calcifications may also be seen in an otherwise intact implant (fig. 47.5). It is of particular significance when such calcifications occur in the periphery of the transplant within the displaced breast parenchyma. Roentgenologically it is then difficult to decide whether these calcific deposits and accompanying increased tissue density result from the transplant or could be part of an adjacent developing tumor. Clinically, recognition of carcinoma in such patients is also difficult because transplants normally present a nodular surface on palpation.

A second method of augmentation mammoplasty is by the use of synthetics. Earlier attempts were made using Ivalon sponges which were shaped to the desired size and form of the breast and then introduced into the fascial planes of the breast (fig. 47.6). In the mammogram the Ivalon sponges are very dense. More recently use has been made of plastic prostheses made of silicone (for example, silastic mammary prosthesis*). Silicone prostheses are available in various sizes.

---

* Dow Corning Company, USA

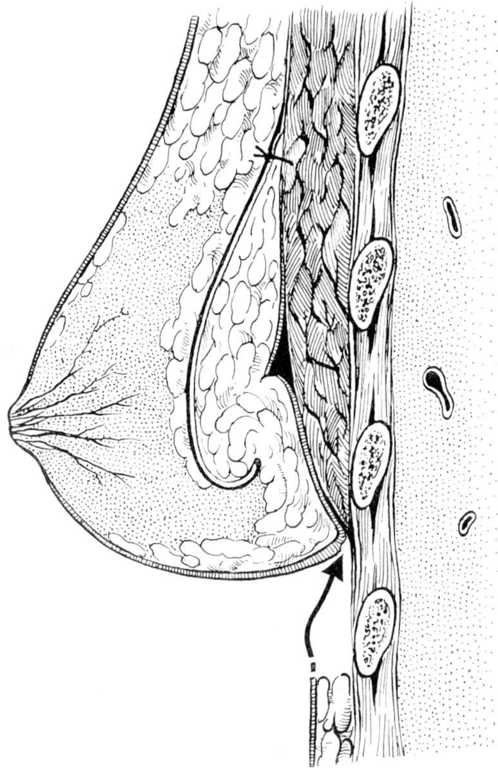

Fig. **47**.3 Augmentation mammoplasty using homologous fat. The fat tissue is attached to the thoracic wall at the level of the inframammary fold and then implanted beneath the fascial base of the breast.

In the mammogram such silastic prostheses are homogeneously dense. They produce various deformities within the breast which on palpation feel like ridges and masses thus creating serious diagnostic problems (fig. 47.7). The breast tissue is displaced by these plastic materials and surrounds the prosthesis as a narrow band.

Incidence of Carcinoma in the Postsurgical Breast

A causal relationship between carcinoma and preceding breast surgery has been considered in isolated cases but has not yet been proved in a general sense. Scar carcinomas are exceedingly rare. BUCHWALD et al (1970) who have investigated this problem have so far discovered four cases.

It is hardly likely that a carcinoma would arise from autologous adipose material used as an implant. The use of synthetic materials in augmentation mammoplasty always raises the heretofore unsettled question regarding the

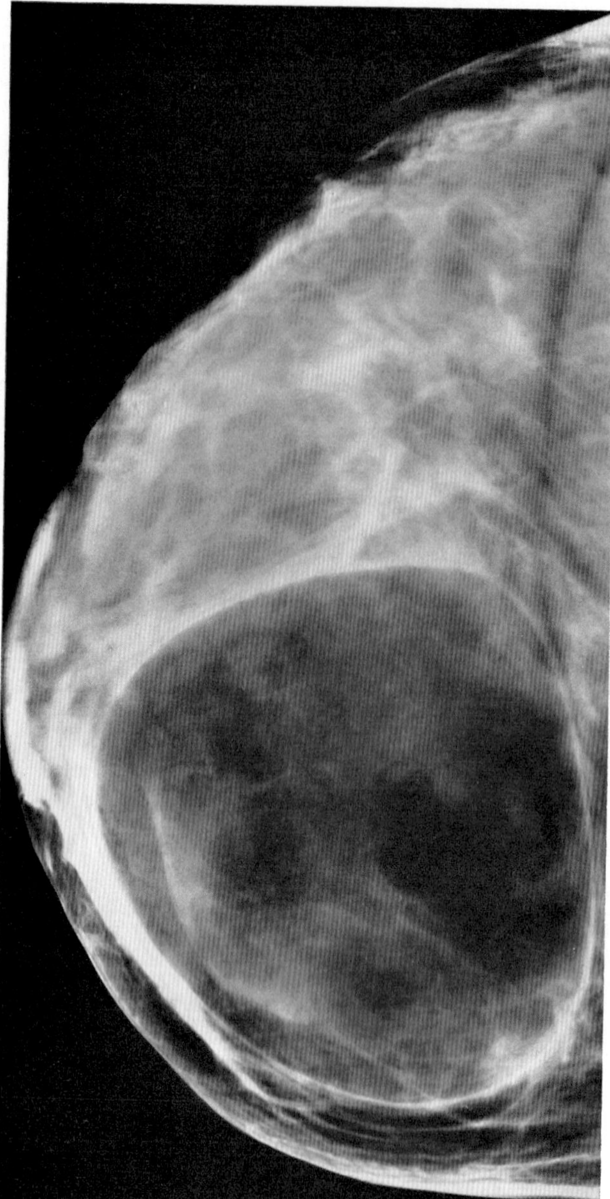

Fig. **47.4a**   Lipomatous implant following augmentation mammoplasty.

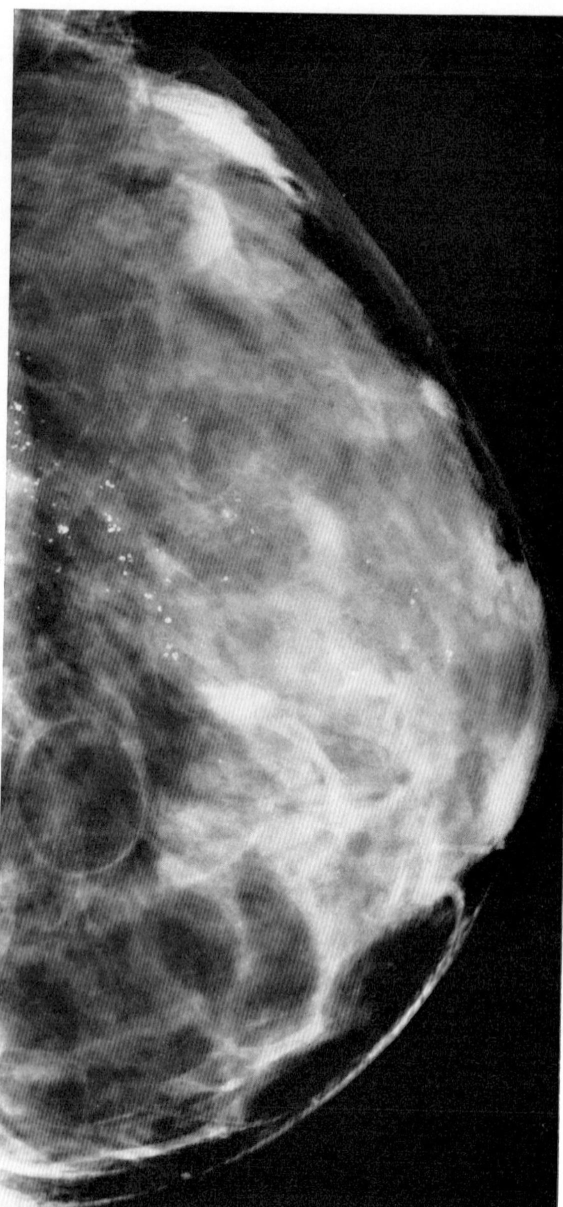

Fig. **47.4b**   The implant in the remaining breast has disrupted. Only a small section approximately 2 cm in diameter remains. There are numerous calcifications secondary to scarring.

possibility of carcinogenesis. Definite carcinogenesis with such synthetic materials in the breast has not yet been proved. The new elastic silicone prosthesis has a very smooth surface which would hardly result in irritation of the overlying breast parenchyma. Plastic surgeons have many years' experience with such prosthetic material and to date there are no grounds for any suspicions about its use.

One case of the development of carcinoma adjacent to a breast prosthesis was reported by BUCHWALD (1970).

In recent years there have been increasing efforts to achieve nondisfiguring therapy for breast carcinoma. Subcutaneous mastectomy leaving the skin, nipple and subcutaneous fat inctact followed by reconstruction of the breast using prosthesis, is a method now being pursued. It is

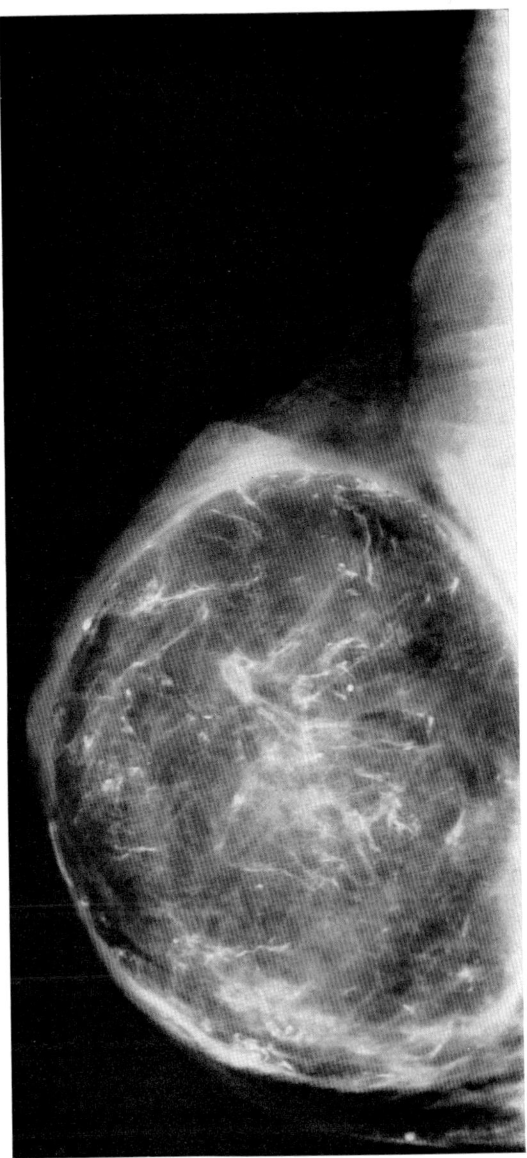

Fig. **47**.5 Lipomatous implant with numerous linear calcifications.

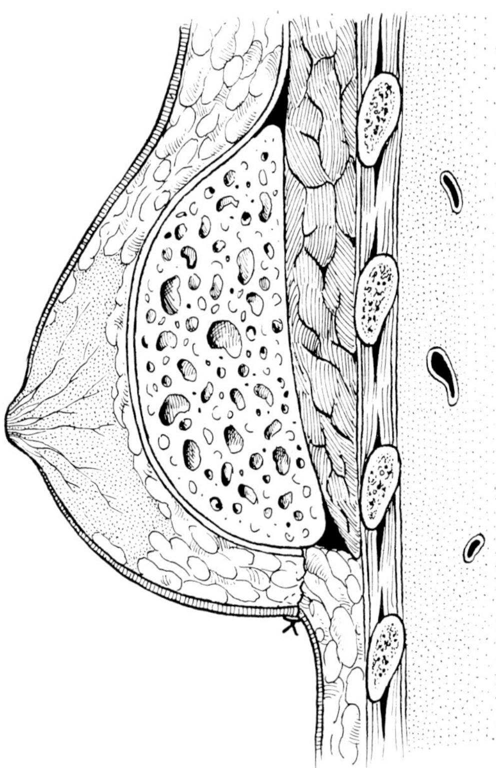

Fig. **47**.6 Schematic drawing of Ivalon sponge prosthesis.

important for the roentgenologist to be familiar with such postoperative findings because a prosthetic silicone device in the breast presents as a soft tissue density in the chest film and may suggest an intrathoracic tumor (fig. 47.8). Roentgen examination in two projections and examination with an intense light source will avoid such an error. A similar shadow may be produced by a glycerin prosthesis worn within the brassiere of women following mastectomy. If inadvertently a chest examination is performed on a patient without prior removal of brassiere

and prosthesis one will see a large round density with a horizontal fluid level. At first this might be considered to be an air-fluid level within the thorax or possibly a hiatal hernia. Inquiry and examination of the patient will clear up this situation.

Breast prostheses made of silicone have a density of approximately 1.4 grams per cubic centimeter and contain enough silicone to have a radiographic density which is 14 times greater than that of water or soft tissue. In the usual radiographic technique and particularly with mammographic technique this results in essentially homogeneously dense shadows. The HEYER-SCHULTE breast prosthesis is radiolucent and thus does not interfere with mammographic examinations.

Silicone prostheses will interfere with radiation therapy using conventional radiation because of significant radiation absorption. This absorption difference between silicone prostheses and soft tissues is diminished during gamma radiation therapy using Cobalt-60. However, the absorption differential again increases when ultra-hard

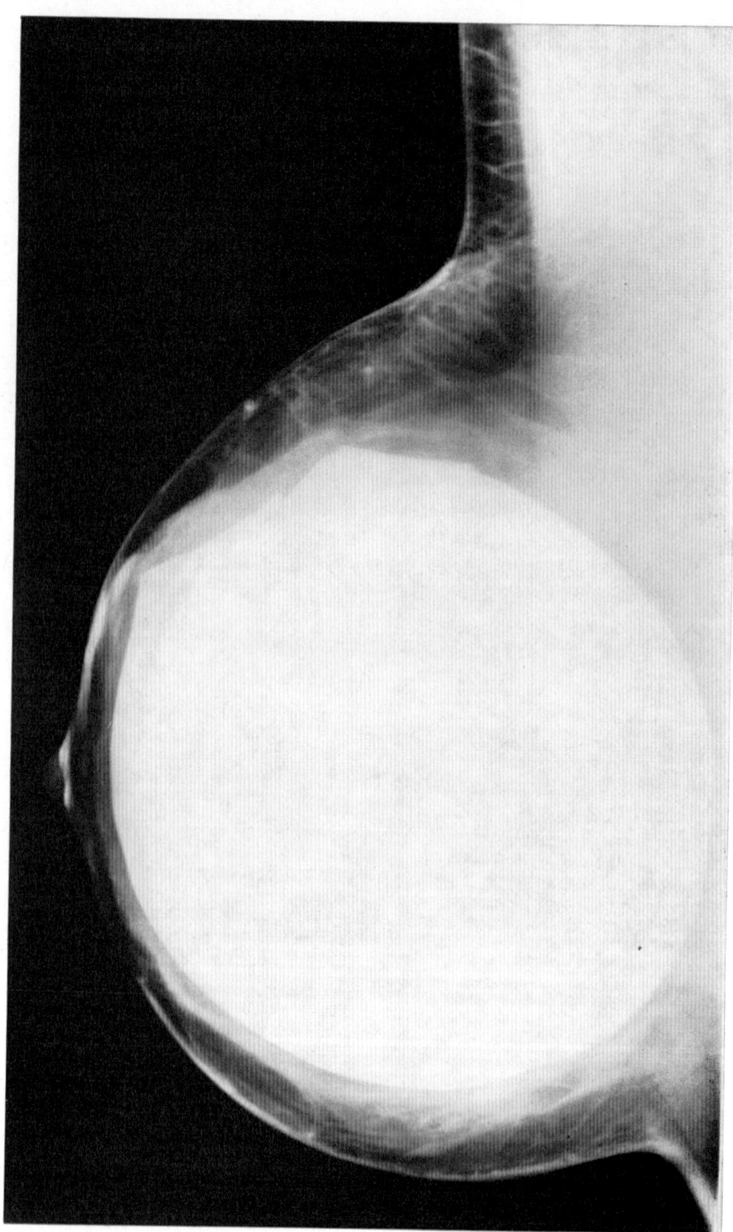

Fig. **47**.7   The posterior border of the Silastic prosthesis which should be resting against the thoracic wall has tilted anteriorly and was palpated clinically as a nodular mass. The mammogram revels the true state of affairs.

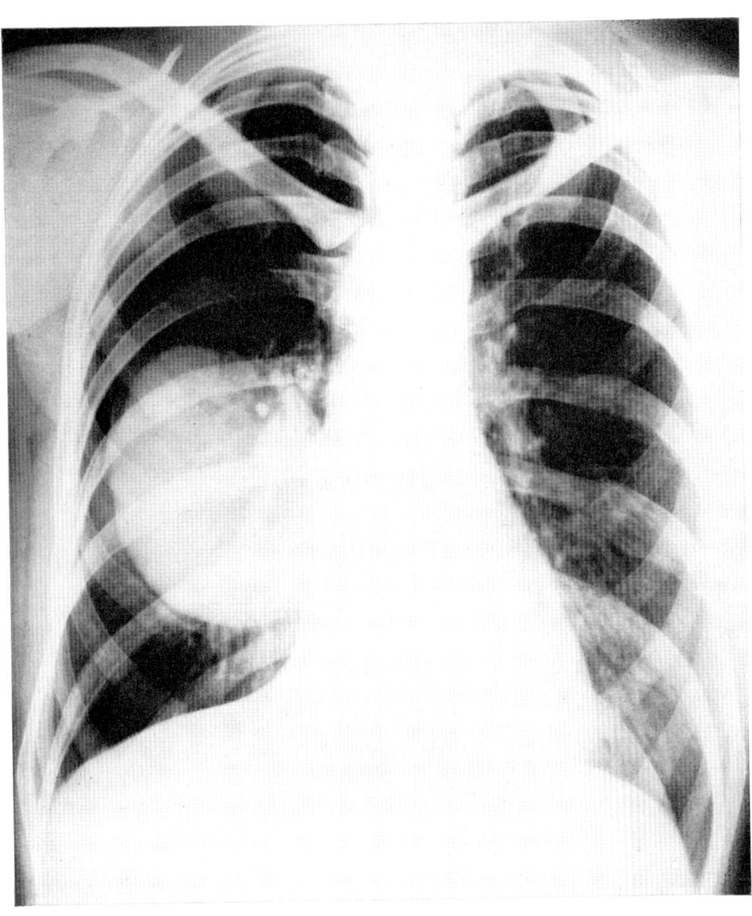

Fig. **47**.8   Silastic prosthesis following right-sided mastectomy which
mimics an intrathoracic process

Bremsstrahlung, for example, radiation with the 42 MeV Betatron. In the latter therapy, however, the penetration is much greater and thus the prosthesis will interfere only minimally in the delivered radiation dosage. The absorption in the silastic material and soft tissues is about equal with radiation therapy using an electron beam in the range of 10 to 25 MeV. The result is that in electron beam radiotherapy, a silastic prosthesis will not produce a lack of homogeneity. As a result patients with silastic breast implants may undergo radiation therapy using Cobalt-60, ultra-hard x-rays and fast electron beams without the prosthesis having a noticeable effect on dose distribution. When conventional x-rays are used for radiation therapy one must expect significant differences in dose distribution depending on the size of the prosthesis so that this method of radiation therapy cannot be used in such patients.

Alterations of the silicone prosthesis secondary to radiation-induced chemical changes need not be expected with the dose used for radiation therapy.

Chapter 48

The Breast after Radiation Therapy

In earlier days the assessment of therapeutic effects of radiation therapy could only be done by clinical examination. With mammography we are in the position today to document accurately the effect of radiotherapy in the same fashion as roentgen examination can assess the effects of treatment of fractures or diseases such as pneumonia, ulcers, etc. We are indebted in this respect to French investigators who have accurately recorded the roentgen changes in a breast carcinoma treated by radiation therapy (GROS 1963).

At the present time the nondisfiguring treatment of breast carcinoma is again achieving popularity thus lending new importance to mammographically controlled radiation therapy. The most important phenomena are regression of the tumor, dissolution of tumor calcification and connective tissue response.

1) At first the tumor mass loses its contour, secondary to exudative processes, but decreases in size and may eventually disappear (fig. 48.1a and b). The latter is particularly true for medullary carcinoma and carcinoma simplex, whereas in scirrhus carcinoma there may occasionally only be a decrease in size and not complete disappearance of the tumor. It is noteworthy that with scirrhus carcinoma, even though there may be complete regression of the central tumor mass, the fibrotic portion with the radiating extension of connective tissue may remain unchanged (fig. 48.2b).

2) After the onset of radiation therapy microcalcifications may in some cases become more easily definable as the density of the tumor diminishes, but they may also be less easily seen if there is much edema. Later on, the microcalcifications disappear in part or completely (fig. 48.2a and b). This is most astounding because one is more inclined to expect an increase in calcium deposition with radiation therapy as a result of tumor necrosis rather than the actual disappearance of the microcalcifications.

Perhaps this observation will eventually yield greater knowledge about the tumor biology of breast carcinoma.

3) In the earlier stages radiation changes in the connective tissue of the breast and skin consist of an exudative, edematous reaction, followed by indurational fibrosis. Therefore, following radiation therapy and depending on the dose, the skin becomes thickened, the subcutaneous fatty tissue is interrupted by a reticular fibrotic proliferation and the connective tissue septa of the breast as a rule also are thickened (fig. 48.1b).

At the site of the tumor mass a stellate, streaky fibrotic reaction occurs which gradually shrinks down as time goes on. Breast carcinoma, depending on its radiation sensitivity, may regress more or less completely. The mammogram provides an objective evaluation of the effectiveness of radiation therapy in achieving the desired tumor regression and serves as a basis for decisions regarding any further therapeutics. It is to be emphasized, however, that mammography reflects only the macroscopic picture of the effects of radiation therapy and gives no information about the microscopic situation or the vitality of the tumor tissue. Although one can assume extensive destruction of cancer cells when macroscopically there appears complete regression of the tumor mass, nevertheless, the persistence of an occasional complex of viable tumor cells cannot be ruled out. Follow-up examinations at first, every three months, then every six months and later on at yearly intervals are necessary.

It should be mentioned that mammography may also be utilized to verify correct placement of radium needles and radioactive gold seeds within breast tumors. Additionally this mode of examination may be used to follow effectiveness of therapy in reducing the size of axillary lymph nodes involved with breast carcinoma, or systemic disorders such as leukemia and Hodgkin's disease.

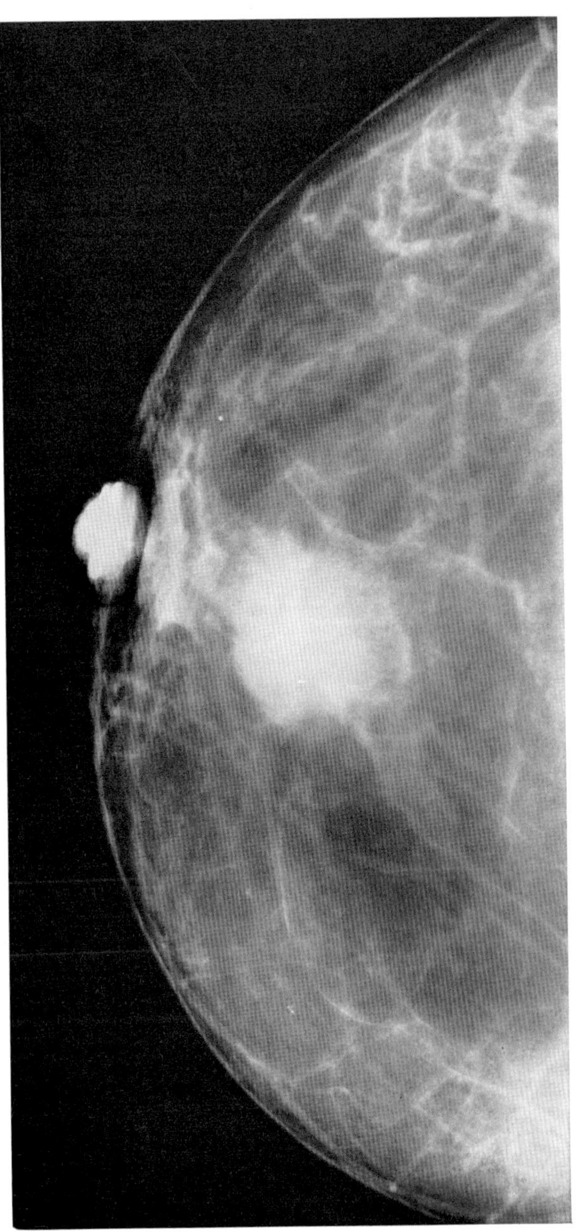

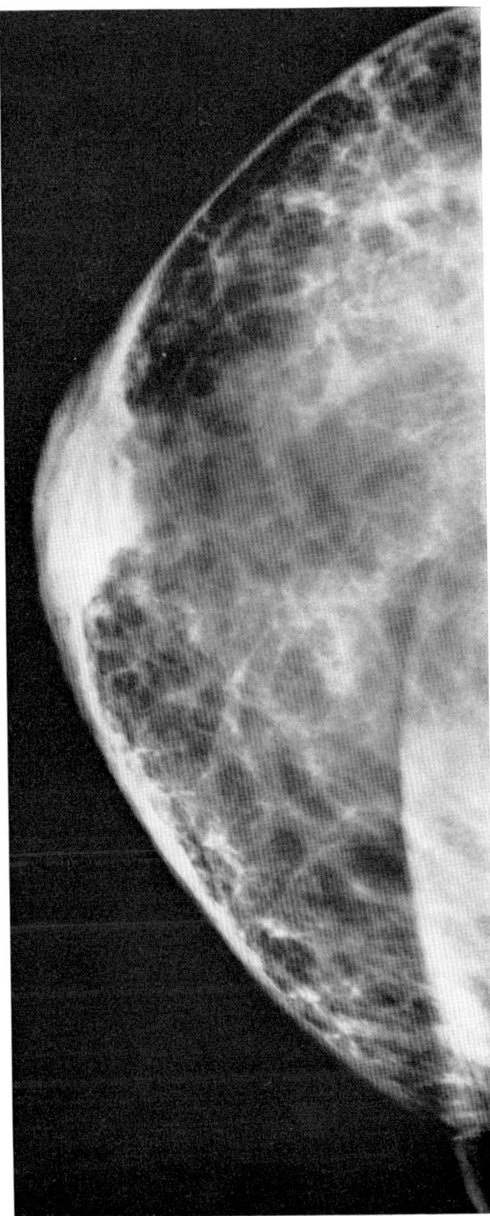

Fig. **48**.1a Typical subareolar carcinoma simplex with fine, stellate infiltrations.

Fig. **48**.1b The same case 2 months later following cobalt therapy (6,000 rads). The tumor mass has disappeared completely and the entire breast is diminished in size. Areola and skin of the breast are thickened. Connective tissue trabeculae are thickened. There is reticular connective tissue proliferation within the fatty tissue. The entire picture resembles lymphatic carcinomatosis and may easily be mistaken for this in the roentgenogram. Only the clinical history allows the correct diagnosis: Postradiation breast.

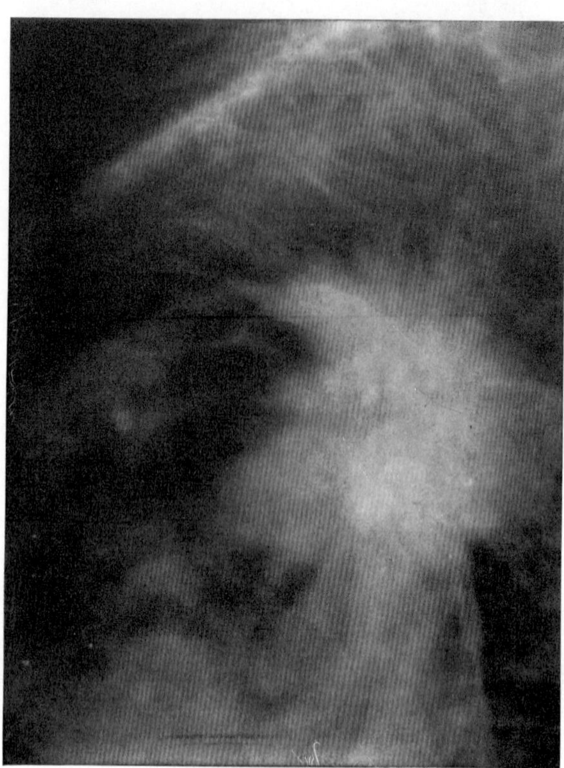

Fig. **48**.2a   Typical scirrhus carcinoma with microcalcifications (magnification 2×).

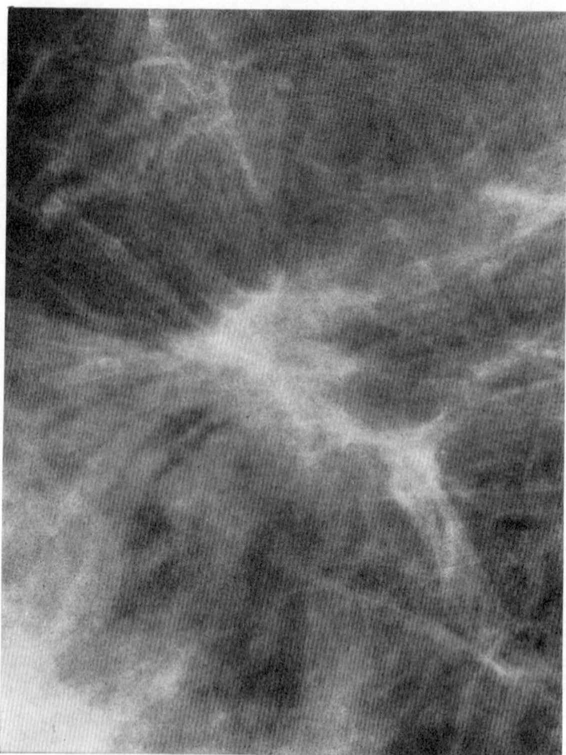

Fig. **48**.2b   The same case 2 months later following cobalt therapy (4,500 rads tumor dose). There is complete regression of the central tumor mass but the fibrotic component remains. No microcalcifications are recognizable.

Roentgen Findings in the Differential Diagnosis of Breast Diseases

The radiologist confronted with roentgen signs, by analysis and synthesis of the roentgen image, formulates a pathological/anatomical concept leading to a clinical diagnosis. There have been earlier attempts to organize the roentgen differential diagnosis of diseases of the breast (among others KÜBLER 1955; GERSHON-COHEN et al 1966; PRAGER and HASERT 1969; BUCHWALD et al 1970; REHM et al 1970). In all these accounts, however, the clinical aspects or pathological/ anatomical disease concepts remained predominant. In our opinion the radiologist after careful evaluation of each roentgen finding and making a judgment regarding its meaning and significance should be able to use this as a basis for a diagnosis. Although repeated emphasis is given to the importance of history and clinical findings, the following chapters will deal primarily with the radiographic findings in mammography and their significance.

Chapter 49

Differential Diagnosis of Breast Calcifications

Coarse Calcifications

The differential diagnosis of coarse calcification is based on two groups of pathological entities: fibroadenoma and carcinoma. The coarse calcifications of fibroadenoma are so characteristic in their bizarre form, their division into several centers of calcification and their slow increase in size over a period of prolonged observation that the diagnosis of fibroadenoma may be made with a high degree of certainty on the basis of these special mammographic signs (fig. 49.1).

Coarse calcifications present a problem when they arise in a carcinoma, which is uncommon. This type of carcinoma is predominantly carcinoma simplex which in the mammogram has a nodular contour and when it contains such calcifications may resemble a fibroadenoma to the unwary mammographer (fig. 49.2). The configuration of the calcifications does not allow a differential diagnosis since the calcium deposits within the tumor mass result from tumor necrosis and appear coarse, bizarre, fragmented and dense as they do when they arise from degeneration of a fibroadenoma. The difference between the two, therefore, is not to be found in the calcifications but rather in the configuration of the soft tissue mass. A fibroadenoma is nodular, rounded but always has a sharp smooth contour. A carcinoma will have some margins which are poorly defined, cometlike connective tissue extensions, or spiculations of connective tissue in the periphery of

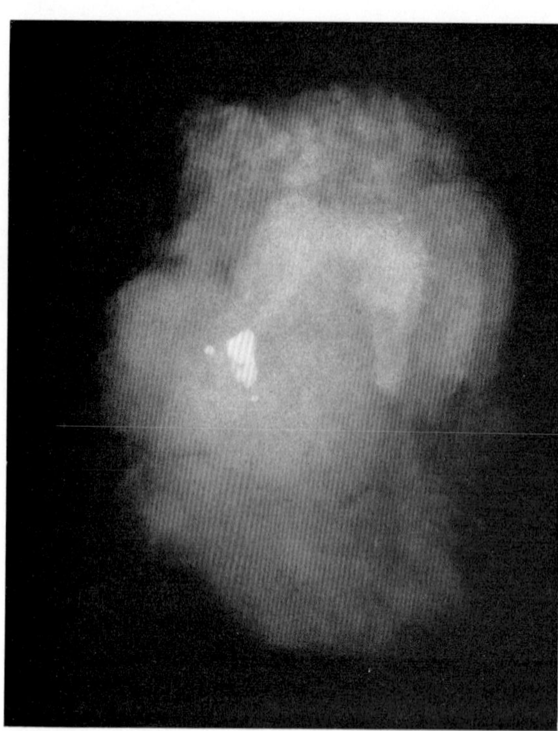

Fig. **49**.1   Fibroadenoma (roentgenogram of the surgical specimen, magnified 3×): Coarse calcification with two small foci of rounded calcific deposits.

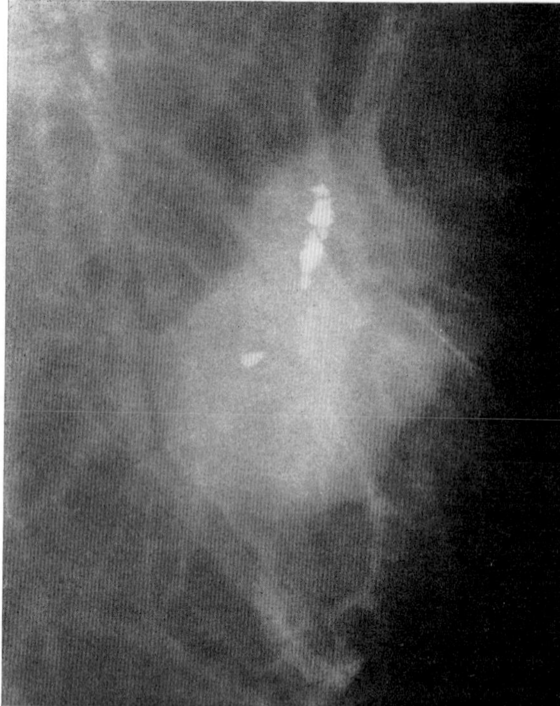

Fig. **49**.2   Carcinoma simplex (mammogram magnified 2×): Irregular, somewhat fragmented calcifications. Lobular mass with broad and cometlike tumor extensions.

the tumor mass. Caution is advised, however, because medullary carcinoma and colloid carcinoma may have relatively smooth margins. If the slightest degree of uncertainty exists and particularly if there is a difference between size estimation at palpation and that at mammography, biopsy is indicated.

Ringlike Calcifications

Ringlike calcifications always indicate benign changes. They never occur within a carcinoma; however, they may be present incidentally in the periphery of a carcinoma.

Ringlike, cystlike or occasionally spherical calcifications imply deposition of calcium within the wall of a round or rounded pathological process (cyst, fibroadenoma, fat necrosis, oil cyst) or

within rounded anatomical structures (chronically inflamed, thickened lactiferous ducts, dilated sebaceous glands of the skin); they may also result from external artifacts (fig. 49.3), such as zinc-containing medication applied to the nipple, or sequestered in a fistulous opening, et cetera.

Rounded, circular or curvilinear calcifications are found within the walls of cysts or in the periphery of fibroadenomas (fig. 49.4). One cannot differentiate between the two in the mammogram.

Cystlike or spherical calcifications (fig. **49**.5) are found in liponecrosis microcystica calcificans (Leborgne), which is frequently focal, but may be multiple in the same or in both breasts. Characteristically this lesion is within the subcutaneous fatty tissue, occasionally lies within

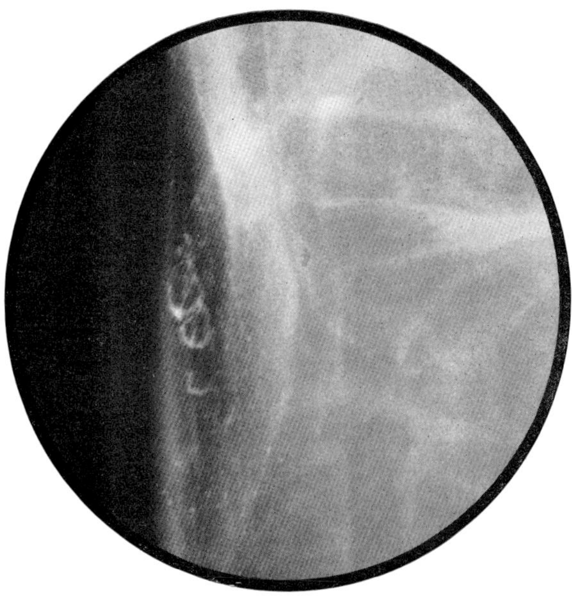

Fig. **49**.3 Residual medication (zinc containing compound) and ulcer following resection of the nipple. (Mammogram, magnified 3 ×.)

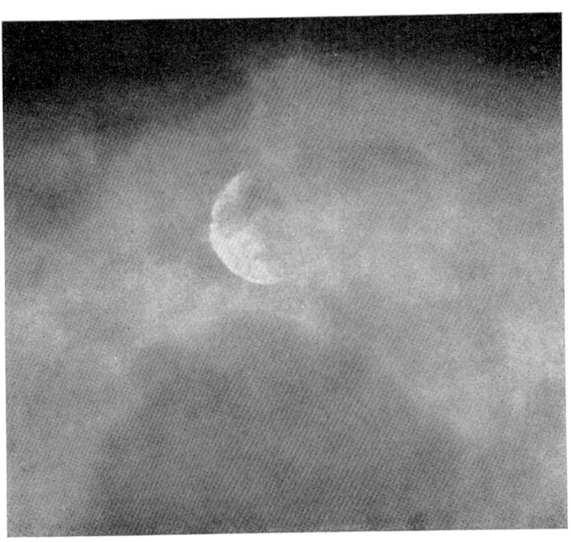

Fig. **49**.4 Semilunar calcification of a cyst wall or a fibroadenoma. (Mammogram, magnified 3×.)

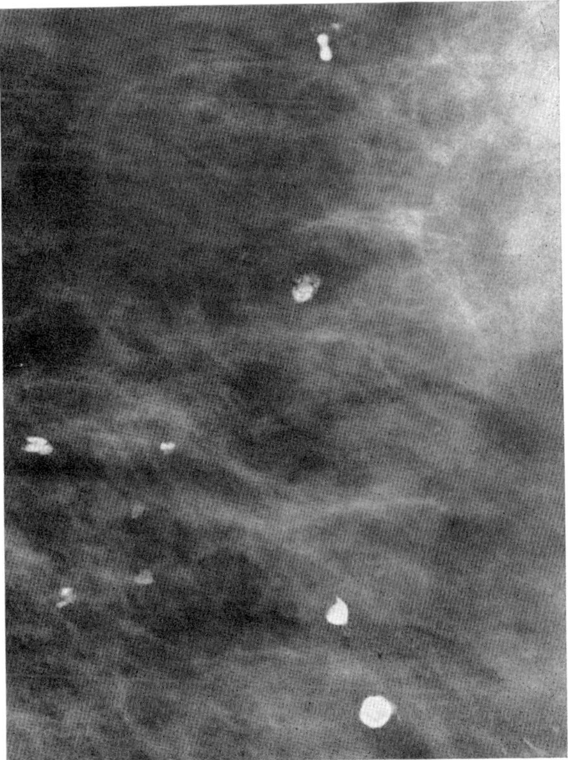

Fig. **49**.5 Calcified fat necrosis. (Mammogram, magnified 2 ×.) Small spheres, a few millimeters in diameter, within fatty tissue without surrounding fibrosis but partially or completely calcified.

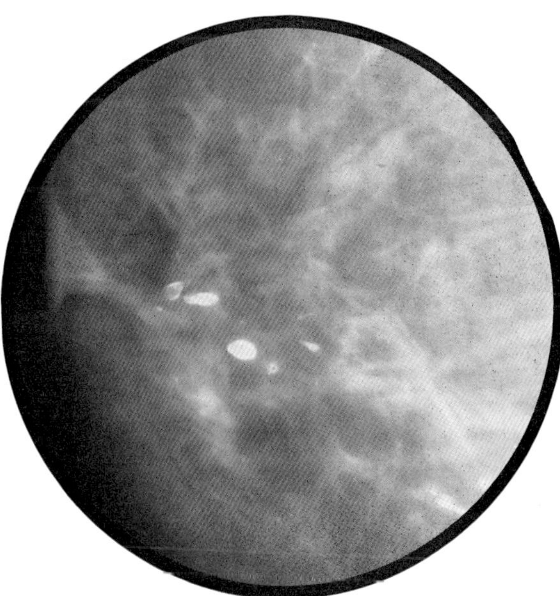

Fig. **49**.6 Plasma cell mastitis. (Mammogram magnified 2 ×.) Typical ring-shaped and oval calcifications oriented in the radiating pattern of lactiferous ducts behind the nipple, with surrounding fibrosis.

17*

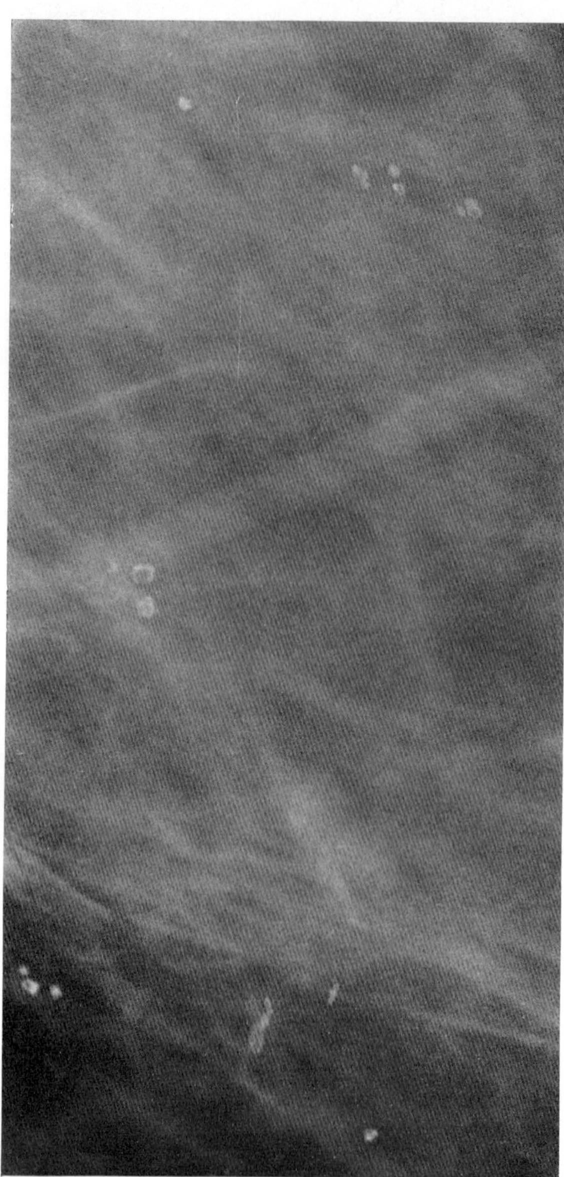

Fig. **49**.7a   Calcified sebaceous glands of the skin (mammogram, magnified 3×): Ringlike, slightly irregular calcifications 2 to 3 mm in diameter.

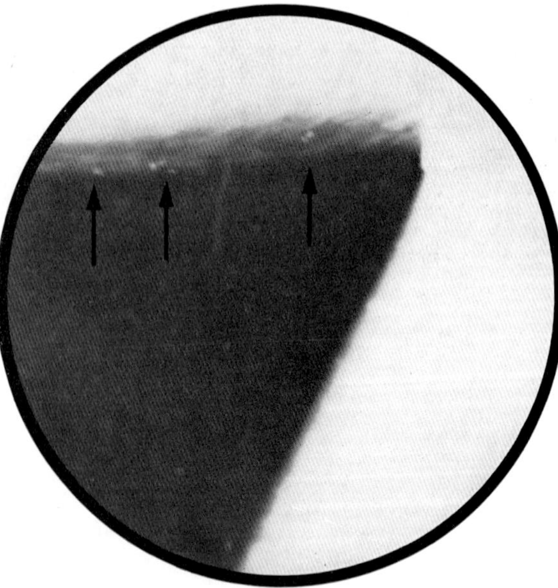

Fig. **49**.7b   Tangential view of the skin: The calcifications are seen to be within the skin.

the body of the breast, but invariably is free of surrounding fibrotic reaction. The lesion is found particularly in older women, occasionally in the vicinity of a carcinoma. Within the cystlike or ringlike calcifications there are occasionally further punctate flecks of calcium suggesting a buttonlike appearance. The calcifications of fat necrosis also may have a dumbbell shape. Those lesions previously described as phleboliths are in fact the spherical calcifications of fat necrosis. Calcifications within the walls of oil cysts are to be found when surgery has been done and a scar remains. The central portions of oil cysts are radiolucent.

Oval or thickened linear, multiple calcifications, radially distributed in a retroareolar location, are so characteristic for plasma cell mastitis that it is easily diagnosed (fig. **49**.6). This is occasionally accompanied by a singular or multiple linear or even V-shaped calcification of the inspissated secretion. Active fibrosis is invariably found in the surrounding tissues.

Calcification of dilated sebaceous glands in the skin (fig. **49**.7a) resemble the calcifications of fat necrosis, but they are smaller, crenated and are to be found within the skin. The latter location can only be verified by tangential views (fig. **49**.7b). If this sort of calcification is projected over the breast parenchyma it resembles the smaller calcifications of fat necrosis or the calcification of plasma cell mastitis. Multiple cystlike calcifications the size of peas or slightly larger may be found in both breasts with Pfeiffer-Weber-Christiansen disease (panniculitis disseminata).

Linear Calcifications

Linear calcifications occur in normal anatomical structures of the breast. Such calcifications are found in the walls of arteries and reflect the course and caliber of the vessels. They appear as two parallel lines of calcium, easily recognized as to their nature. Calcifications of the walls of veins does not occur; neither do phleboliths. Calcifications of lactiferous ducts appear as solid densities ranging from a few millimeters to centimeters in length. Linear calcifications may also occur in the walls of lactiferous ducts but are then generally shorter and frequently associated with ring-shaped or oval calcifications. Such intraductal and periductal calcifications occur within inspissated secretions and in a fibrotic thickened

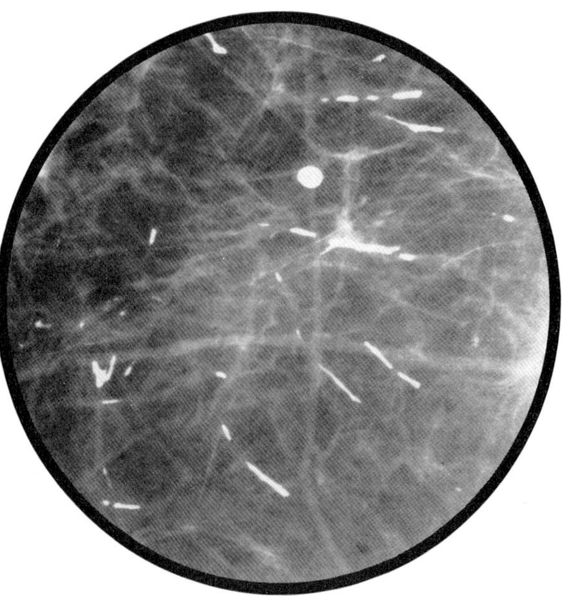

Fig. **49**.8 Plasma cell mastitis (mammogram, magnified 2×): Linear calcifications of lactiferous ducts. A single completely calcified focus of fat necrosis is evident.

duct wall, particularly in "secretory disease" and plasma cell mastitis (fig. 49.8). A direct relationship to carcinoma does not occur although such linear calcifications are occasionally found in the vicinity of a carcinoma.

Microcalcifications Occurring in Groups

The differential diagnosis of microcalcification is the most difficult problem for the mammographer. The earlier concept that microcalcifications distributed in groups are pathognomonic for carcinoma needs to be corrected in light of recent knowledge of comparative roentgenology and histology. Improved mammographic technique, evolved over the last several years, has been paramount in deciding on the significance of microcalcifications and has permitted the detection of such calcium deposits at a much earlier stage than previously possible. Pathologists have also made progress in learning more about the significance of breast calcification. But in spite of all this there still is no certain understanding about the etiology, histochemical relationships, actual localization within tissues and etiological relationship with the basic breast disease. The general uncertainty regarding the significance of microcalcifications is increased by the fact that there is occasionally lack of support of the

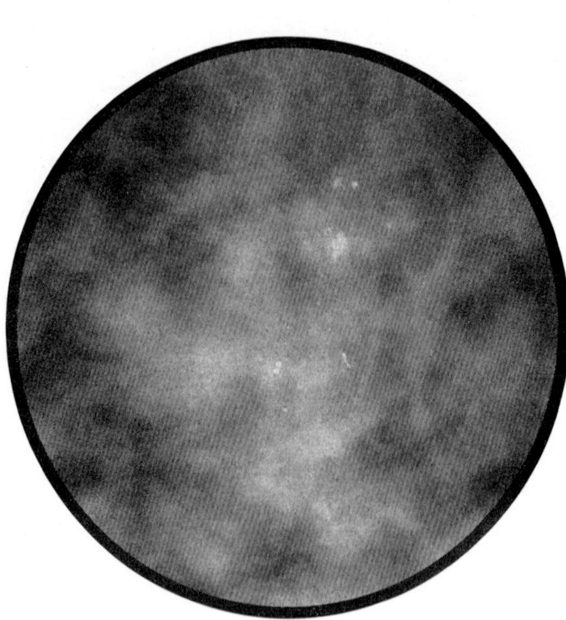

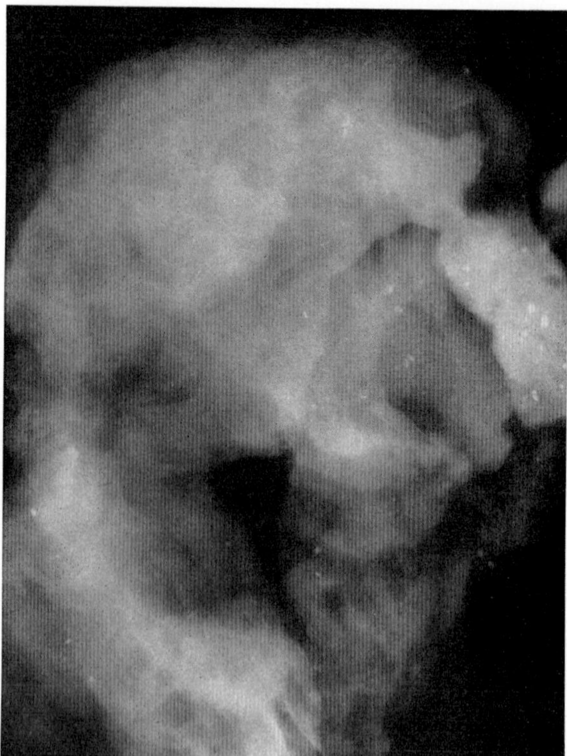

Fig. **49**.9   Mammogram, magnified 3×. Amorphous, irregular, not particularly dense microcalcifications of varying size gathered into a group. There is surrounding fibrosis.
Roentgen diagnosis: Pathological intraductal process.
Clinical findings: No palpable nodule. Excisional biopsy was performed.
Histology: Fibrocystic disease. Some local inflammatory changes with calcification.

Fig. **49**.10   Roentgenogram of the surgical specimen, enlarged 2×. Granular microcalcifications of varying size, some round or oval, some distributed in groups. The density of these calcifications is not very great. No bizarre forms are seen.
Roentgen diagnosis: Pathological intraductal process, probably benign.
Clinical findings: Palpatory findings indicate fibrocystic disease.
Histology: Fibrocystic disease with areas of myoepithelial proliferation. Periductal fibrosis, stasis of secretions and siderophagic activity around lactiferous ducts. No evidence of malignancy.

original suspicion by the eventual histological diagnosis. There is always a question as to whether the tiny area which appears suspicious in the mammogram is in fact the same as that examined by the pathologist. Through the use of photographic enlargement techniques we are able today to more closely examine and learn the form, structure and density of such microcalcifications allowing a greater differentiation in regard to the various processes which cause their formation.

Calcifications localized in groups that are not within the confines of a nodule but instead appear within breast parenchyma or in an area of minimal connective tissue proliferation are most

likely intraductal calcifications. It is our experience, however, that it is as difficult to differentiate between a benign mammary dysplasia and a proliferating pathological process of the breast as it is to differentiate between a lobular carcinoma in situ and an intraductal carcinoma (fig. 49.9 to 49.20). In the following discussion we will describe the typical calcifications of various processes with the warning, however, to be extremely cautious about permitting the roentgen differentiation to dictate therapy of the breast disorder.

Nevertheless, it is the significant contribution of mammography to allow discovery, localization and excision of malignant breast disease, espe-

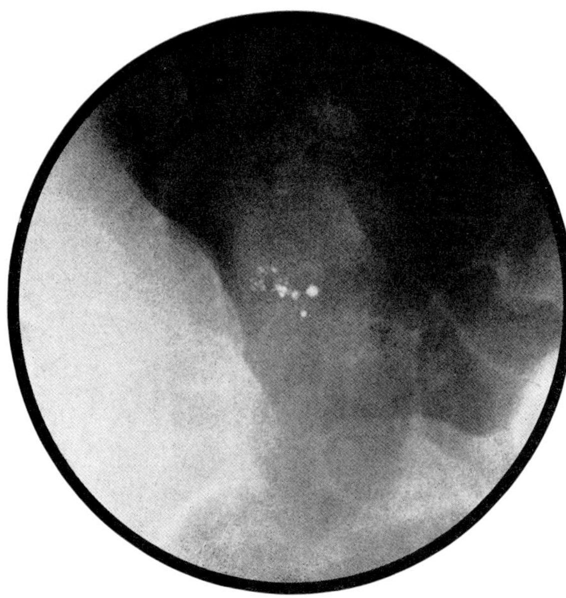

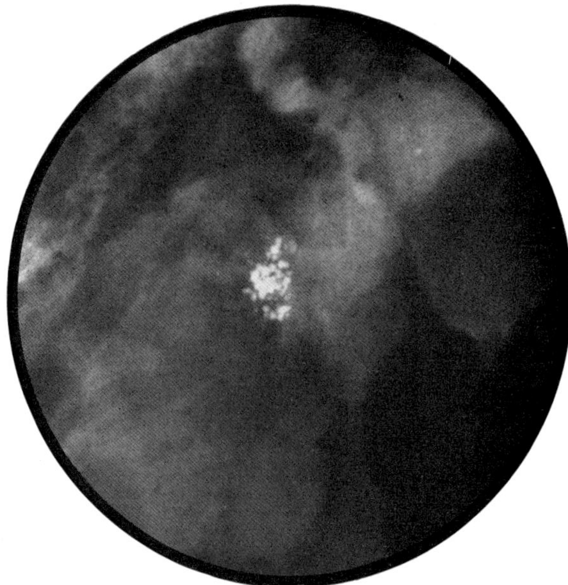

Fig. **49**.11 Roentgenogram of the surgical specimen, magnified 3×. Coarse and fine rounded calcifications distributed in a group within a nodular mass. Roentgen diagnosis: Pathological intraductal process.
Clinical findings: Palpatory findings indicate fibrocystic disease.
Histology: Fibrocystic disease with foci of calcified sclerosing adenosis and myoepithelial proliferation.

Fig. **49**.12 Roentgenogram of the surgical specimen, magnified 2×. Numerous microcalcifications of varying size and shape distributed closely within a group. The calcifications are very dense, some are rounded, others have a crystalline appearance. Roentgen diagnosis: Pathological intraductal process.
Histology: Intraductal epithelial proliferation with some atypical epithelial cells.

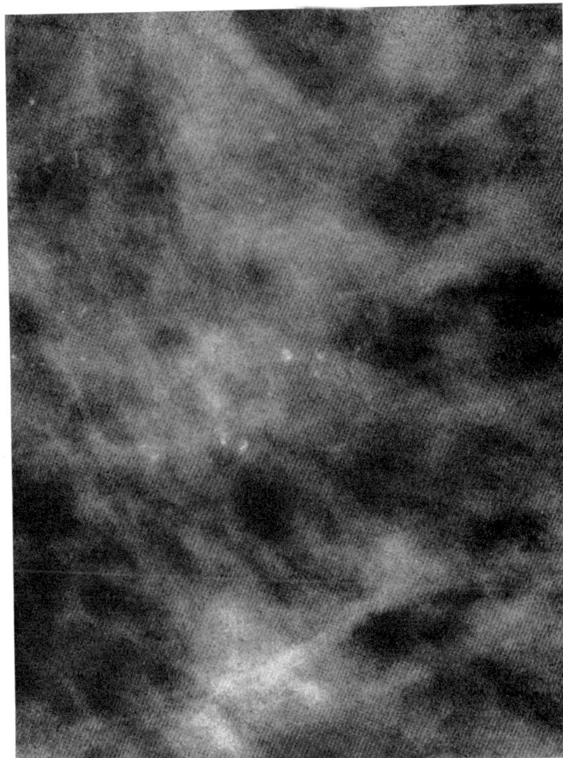

Fig. **49**.13 Mammogram, magnified 3×. Amorphous microcalcifications of varying size distributed in groups. Density of the microcalcification is minimal. Surrounding soft tissues do not appear to be exceptionally dense. Roentgen diagnosis: Pathological intraductal process.
Clinical findings: Normal breast.
Histology: Proliferative fibrocystic disease. Marked epithelial proliferation with complete filling of milk ducts. Papillomatosis. Occasional foci of calcifications in areas of apocrine metaplasia. Follow-up examination recommended!

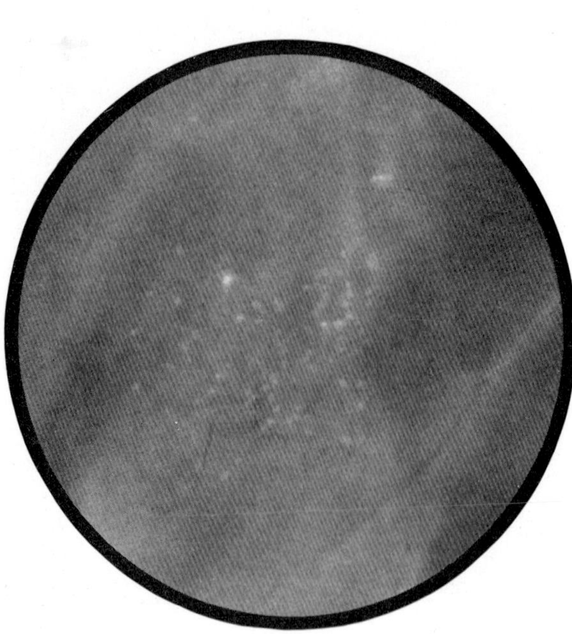

Fig. **49**.14   Mammogram, magnified 5×. Numerous amorphous microcalcifications of varying size and density.
Roentgen diagnosis: Pathological intraductal process. Benignancy is not certain.
Clinical findings: No clinical symptoms. Palpatory findings indicate fibrocystic disease. Excisional biopsy was performed.
Histology: Fibrocystic disease with atypical intraductal epithelial proliferation.

Fig. **49**.15   Mammogram, magnified 3×. Numerous microcalcifications some distributed singularly, others in groups. Irregular and even some bizarre forms. Density of the calcifications is not great.
Roentgen diagnosis: Pathological intraductal process suspicious for malignancy.
Clinical findings: Normal breast.
Histology: Extensive sclerosing adenosis and intraductal carcinoma.

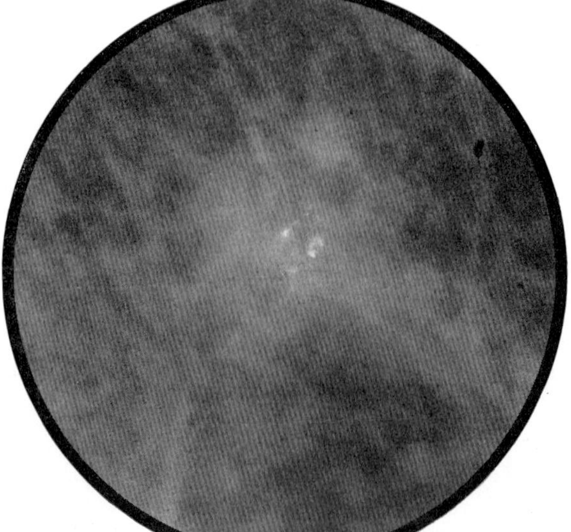

Fig. **49**.16   Mammogram, magnified 3×. Sparse microcalcifications which are very small and of varying form and density. The calcifications are localized within soft tissue of increased density.
Roentgen diagnosis: Pathological intraductal process suspicious for malignancy.
Clinical findings: Routine breast examination, normal. Mastectomy on the other side for carcinoma 3 years before.
Histology: Invasive ductal carcinoma. The diameter of the primary tumor was 1 cm. Lymph node metastases were demonstrated.

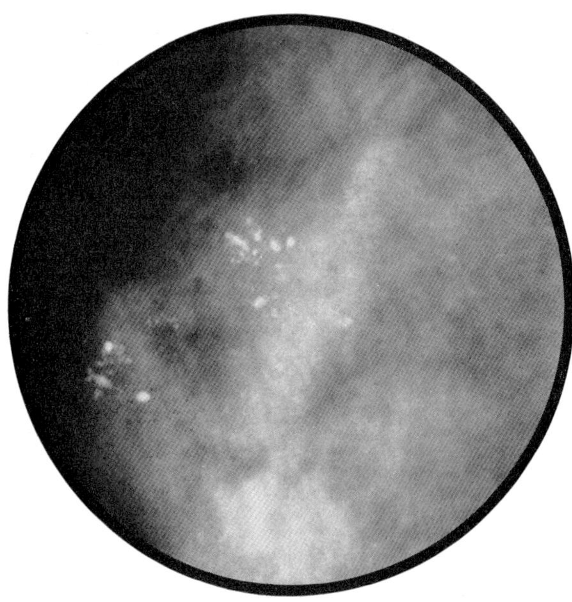

Fig. **49**.17   Mammogram, magnified 3×. Numerous microcalcifications of varying shape and size, very dense, appearing fragmented and distributed in two groups. Between these groups are even tinier calcifications, barely visible.
Roentgen diagnosis: Intraductal carcinoma.
Clinical findings: Palpable mass.
Histology: Intraductal carcinoma.

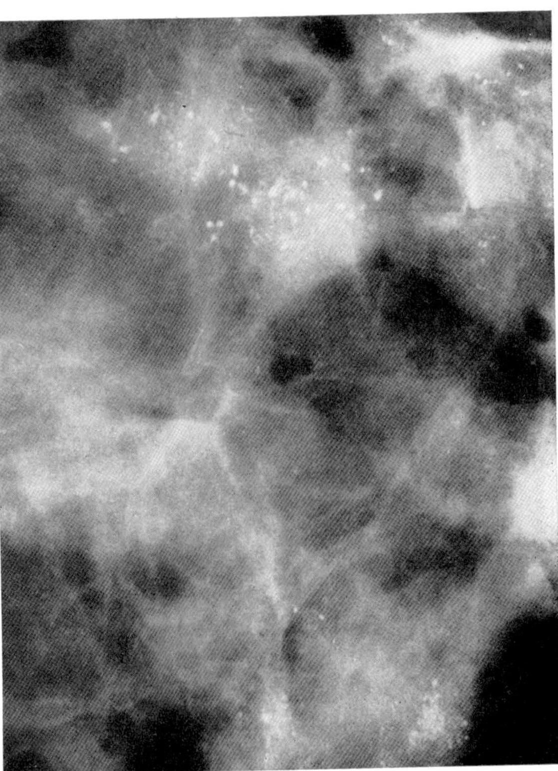

Fig. **49**.18   Roentgenogram of the surgical specimen, magnified 3×. Numerous small and larger groups of closely positioned microcalcifications of varying size, shape and density resembling "scattered salt". There are amorphous, bizarre and fragmented pieces of calcium.
Roentgen diagnosis: Intraductal carcinoma.
Clinical findings: Family history of breast carcinoma. Breast examination in this patient was normal.
Histology: Invasive intraductal carcinoma.

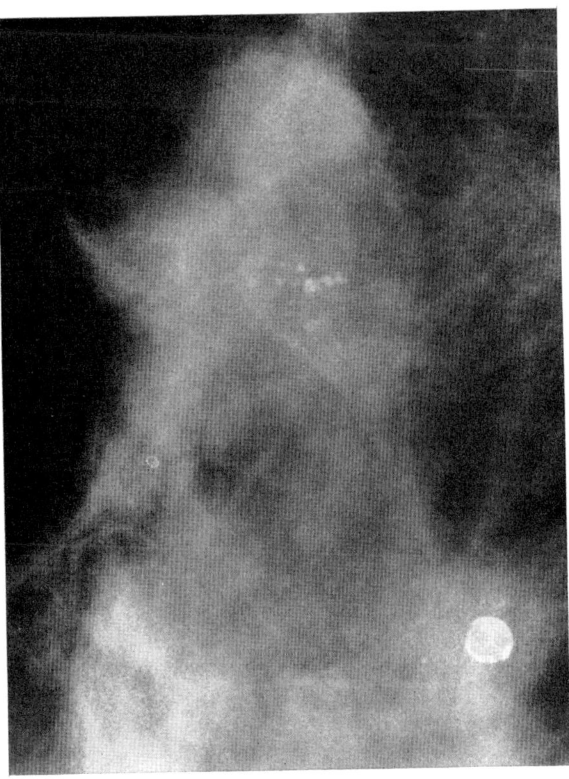

Fig. **49**.19   Mammogram, magnified 3×. Sparse microcalcifications of varying form and size. Slight increased soft tissue density in the area. The calcifications are within a nodular soft tissue mass with some linear extension into surrounding tissue. Calcified fat necrosis is seen in the vicinity.
Roentgen diagnosis: Carcinoma.
Clinical findings: A nodule was palpated.
Histology: Breast carcinoma with apocrine and scirrhus characteristics.

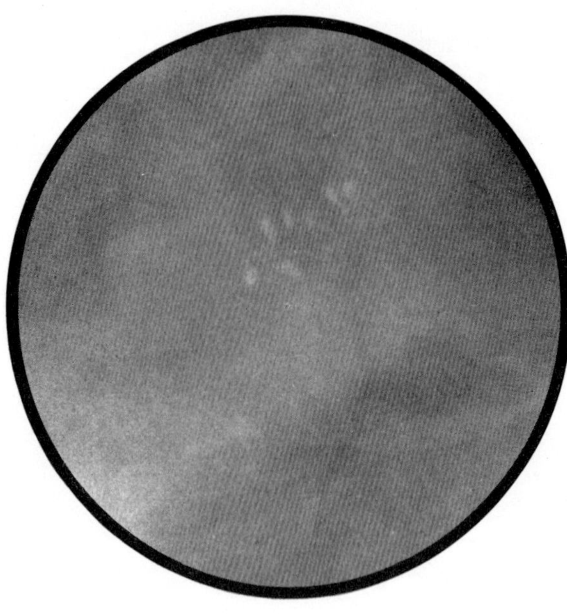

Fig. **49**.20   Mammogram, magnified 5×. A group of amorphous microcalcifications of low density. Roentgen diagnosis: Suspicion for malignancy. Histology: Lobular carcinoma in situ.

cially with the aid of the diagnosis of microcalcifications, long before there are clinical manifestations of the disorder. With mammographically localized excision, intra- and postoperative mammographic examination of the specimen, and careful subsequent histological examination, this method of diagnosis should reach a state in which carcinoma in situ will be discovered frequently.

Histological examination following excisional biopsy because of clustered microcalcifications in 212 patients indicates the statistical probability of various breast diseases which may be expected:

| Benign Alterations |

Mammary dysplasia *without* atypical proliferation	78	
Fibroadenoma	7	44%
Papilloma (solitary)	8	
Mammary dysplasia *with* atypical proliferation	61	29%

| Lobular and ductal carcinoma in situ |

	32	15%

| Carcinoma |

Intraductal growth	9	
Invasive growth	17	12%

(Citoler, Gawlich, Lanyi, Tismer and Zippel [1975], Women's Clinic and Radiological Institute of the University of Cologne and Roentgen Institute of AOK Cologne.)

This problematic situation does not include the grouped microcalcifications found in surgical scars (fig. **49**.21), fibroadenomas (fig. **49**.22, **49**.23a and b, **49**.24), cysts (fig. **49**.25a—c), and in the walls of arteries (fig. **49**.26a and b). The history, clinical findings and demonstration of benign nodules (aspiration and cytological examination) will support the roentgen diagnosis in these cases. It is particularly important to be aware of and not to misinterpret film artifacts (dust on the film surface, water bubbles in the developer, fingerprints on the film, metal debris in the tube head, radiation absorbing medications on the skin). Such errors are avoided by demonstrating the suspected calcification in two different projections to be *within* the breast, thus localizing it and determining in which type of tissue it occurs. Microcalcifications are frequently seen only with over exposures and often can be detected only in coned-down compression films. Microcalcifications may be considered typical of carcinoma when they have the following characteristics:

1) delicate, varying in size, crystallike in appearance, bizarre and fragmented;
2) varying density;

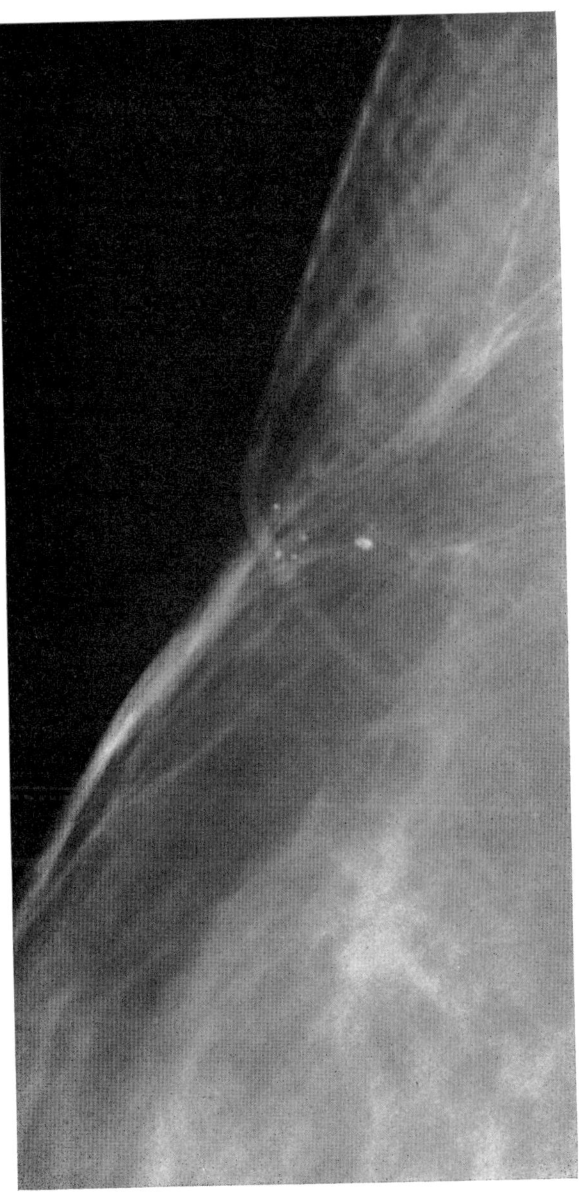

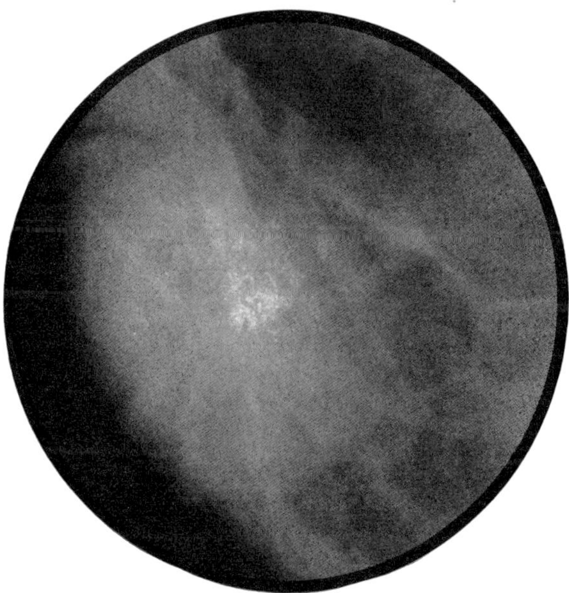

Fig. **49**.21   Punctate microcalcifications of varying size, quite dense within the confines of a scar. Roentgen diagnosis: Calcifications within excisional biopsy scar. Follow-up examination is recommended. No change in repeat examination after 6 months.

Fig. **49**.22   Mammogram, magnified 3×. Numerous tiny closely grouped microcalcifications within an oval superficial mass with relatively sharp margins. No evidence of infiltration.
Roentgen diagnosis: Fibroadenoma? Suspicion of malignant degeneration.
Clinical findings: Smooth, rounded, freely movable subcutaneous mass in a 26-year-old woman.
Histology: Fibroadenoma without evidence of malignancy.

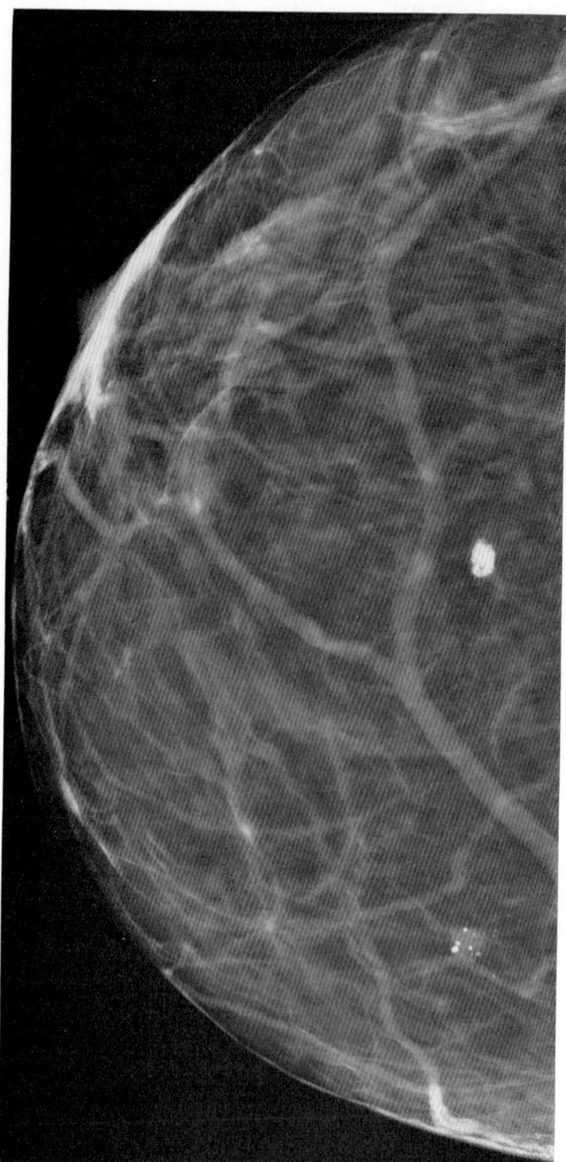

Fig. **49**.23a Mammogram. Soft tissue nodule about 5 mm in diameter with several punctate calcifications. Additionally there is a nearly completely calcified soft tissue nodule in the vicinity.

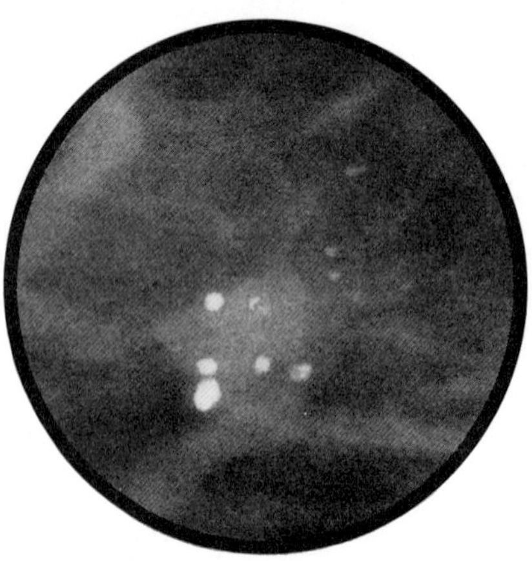

Fig. **49**.23b Local area magnified 3×. Punctate, rounded, very dense calcifications within and at the periphery of the soft tissue nodule.
Roentgen diagnosis: Incomplete and complete calcifications of two small fibroadenomas.

3) localized into a group or gathered together in a well-circumscribed tissue density or scattered diffusely throughout the entire breast.
Such calcifications are found in intraductal carcinoma as well as within the extensions of an invasive breast carcinoma. There are variations, however, on this classical description of carcinomatous microcalcifications so that occasionally one can only indicate an "intraductal process" and must withhold further diagnostic differentiation.

Diffusely Distributed Microcalcifications

In the differential diagnosis one must decide between those microcalcifications that, for the most part, lie close together in a parenchymal area or occupy part of the parenchyma, and solitary calcifications distributed over the entire breast. Furthermore it is important to describe whether only a segment of parenchyma contains such calcifications and whether the distribution

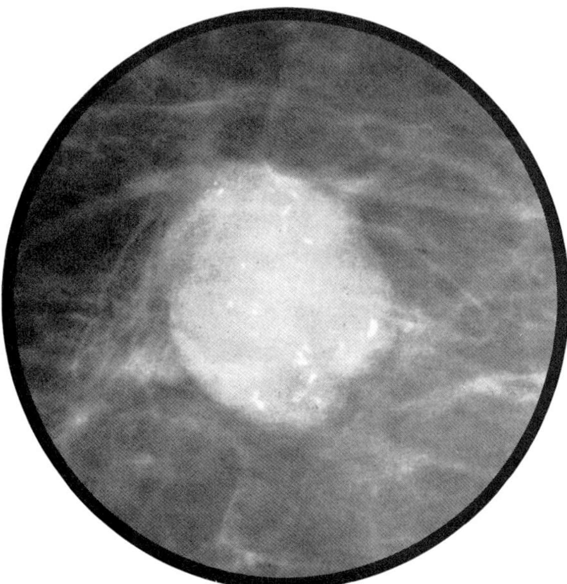

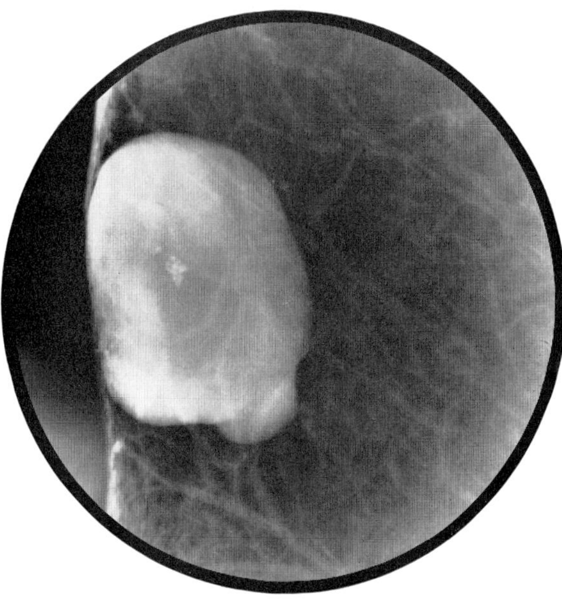

Fig. **49**.24 Mass with relatively sharp borders, somewhat lobulated with a "tail of the comet" extension at one point. Within the mass there are numerous, irregular, amorphous and very dense calcifications of varying size.
Roentgen diagnosis: Fibroadenoma with beginning calcific degeneration. Excisional biopsy recommended to rule out medullary carcinoma.
Clinical findings: Large breast, no mass palpated.
Histology: Fibroadenoma with calcification.

Fig. **49**.25a Coned-down roentgenogram. Minimally lobulated but smoothly bordered oval mass, containing punctate calcifications within a single group.

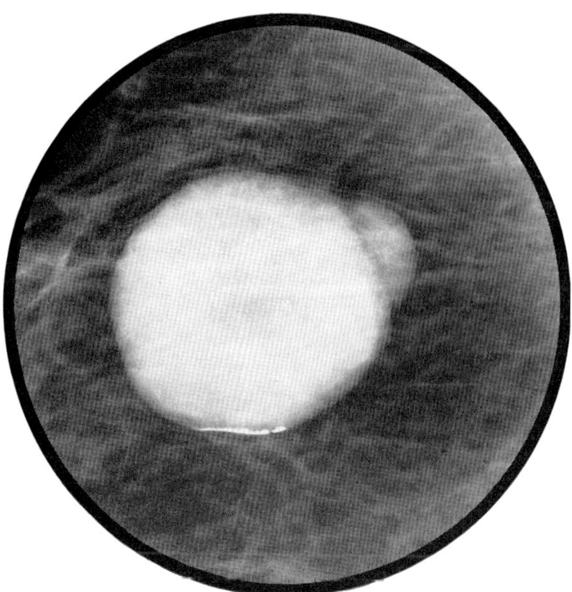

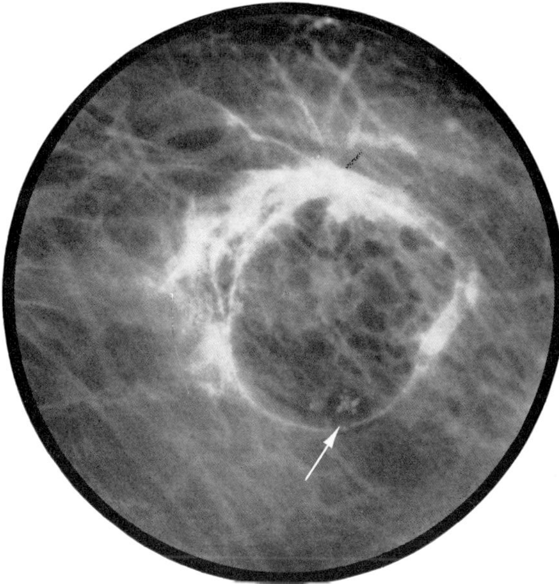

Fig. **49**.25b Roentgenogram in the opposite projection. The calcifications lie along the margin of the mass and are linear.

Fig. **49**.25c Pneumocystogram. The microcalcifications are demonstrated to be within the cyst wall (arrow): Benign calcification of cyst wall.

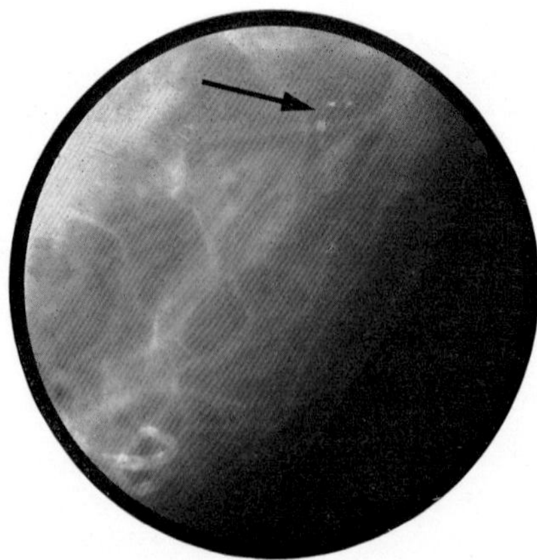

Fig. **49**.26a   Mammogram. Punctate subareolar calcifications (arrow). Arterial calcification in the periphery.

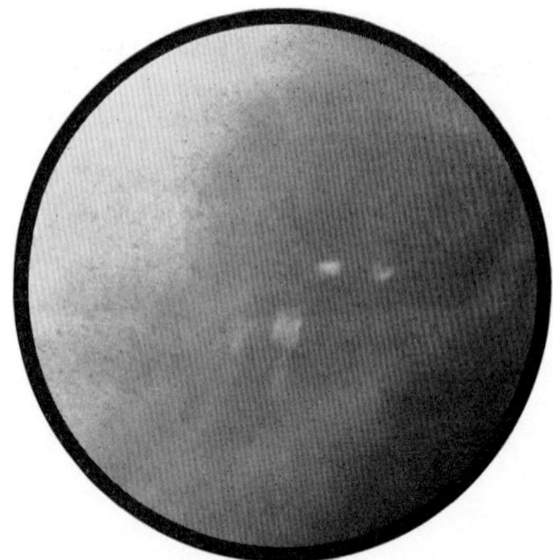

Fig. **49**.26b   Magnified 3×. Punctate calcifications within an arterial wall.

is equal throughout or whether in part the calcifications are localized into groups. Further yet one must analyse whether the calcifications are rounded, of low density and somewhat ill-defined or whether they are crystallike, very dense and possess very sharp contours.

If such diffusely distributed calcifications are seen as solitary calcific deposits in *both* breasts, are not very dense, appear rounded and have a diameter approximately 0.5 mm or more, then it is most likely that this represents sclerosing adenosis or another form of fibrous mammary dysplasia (fig. 49.27, 49.28).

If the above criteria (bilaterality, diffuse distribution in the entire breast) are not present and particularly if the calcifications are small (0.1 to 0.2 mm), are not rounded but instead are crystallike, fragmented and very dense then one should think of a malignant intraductal process (fig. 49.29, 49.30). The latter conclusion is particularly justified when some of the calcifications are localized into groups and there is a corresponding palpatory finding in this area or other clinical suspicion of malignancy. Suspicion must be particularly great when such calcifications are very numerous and are unilateral (fig. 49.31, 49.32, 49.33, 49.34). Theoretically it is no doubt possible that a bilateral comedocarcinoma can exist although we have never seen such a case. Follow-up examinations are of some help in the

final decision; however, this is only justified when there is not the slightest trace of suspicion of malignancy both clinically and roentgenologically. If this is not the case excisional biopsy must be performed and a definite histological diagnosis made. This is also indicated even in a benign-appearing fibrous dysplasia in order to clear up any doubts regarding a possible tendency of the process to proliferate. It is always a problem, particularly in diffusely distributed calcifications without palpatory findings, whether to accept without doubt the result of the histological findings on excisional biopsy, because one is never exactly sure if the removed tissue specimen is truly representative of the pathological changes of the entire breast. Therefore all patients with such mammographic changes belong in a special risk group who should be followed with mammography in spite of histologically verified mammary dysplasia. Examination every year is essentially too long an interval for we have seen numerous cases in which a carcinoma developed within a period of 6 or 7 months and resulted in lymph node metastases even though clinical and roentgen findings beforehand were not suspicious of malignancy. On the other hand, it is hard to justify roentgen examination at 6 months intervals because of the risk of radiation damage. In the isolated case a suitable compromise in regard to these factors must be made.

Fig. **49**.27 Mammogram, magnified 3×. Numerous, minimally dense and somewhat ill-defined flecks of calcium distributed throughout the entire parenchyma of the left and right breast in a uniform fashion. The picture resembles that of the "milky way". Roentgen diagnosis: Diffuse fibrocystic disease of both breasts, probably of the fibrous type. Clinical findings: Nodularity of breast parenchyma bilaterally but slightly increased on the left.
Histology: Fibrocystic disease, fibrous type with minimal inflammatory changes and microcalcifications.

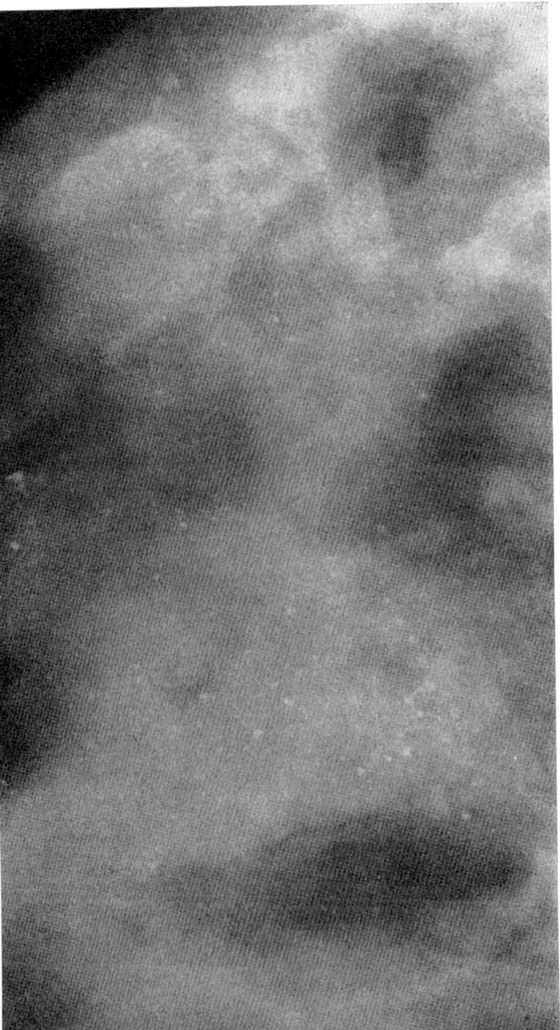

Fig. **49**.28 Mammogram, magnified 3×. Numerous evenly distributed calcifications are seen in the upper outer quadrant of the right breast with an area of increased soft tissue density suggesting mammary dysplasia.
Roentgen diagnosis: Mammary dysplasia with intraductal process.
Clinical findings: Nodular mammary dysplasia. No dominant mass palpated. The breast examination was routine since there were no clinical symptoms.
Histology: Peculiar type of sclerosing adenosis with myoepithelial and papillary proliferation. There is insufficient experience with this atypical type of sclerosing adenosis to warrant surgical therapy.
The histological findings in this case indicate how difficult it is even for the experienced histologist to categorize pathological processes which are only identifiable in the mammogram.

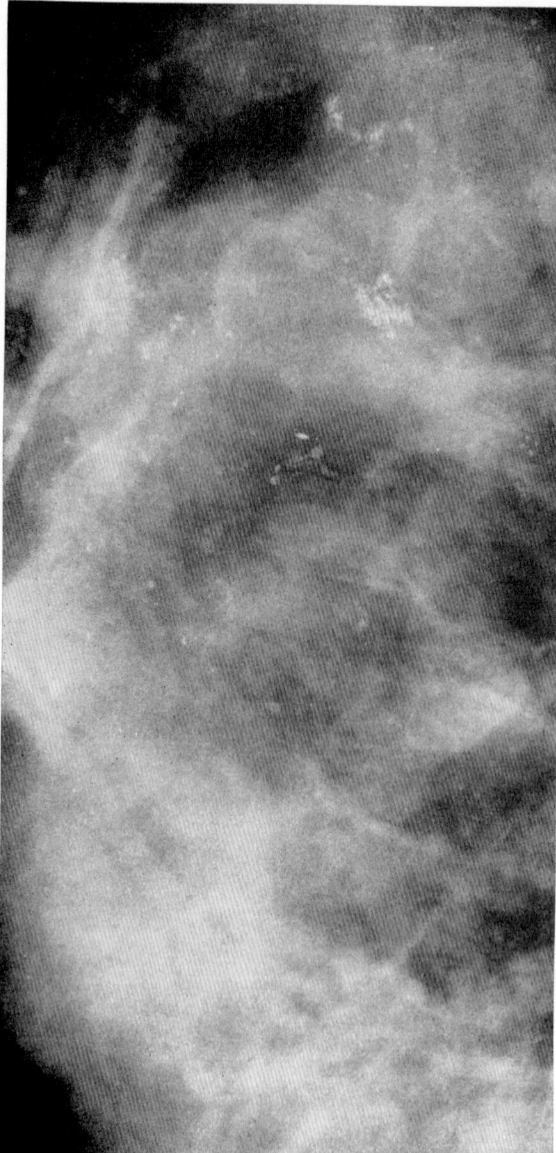

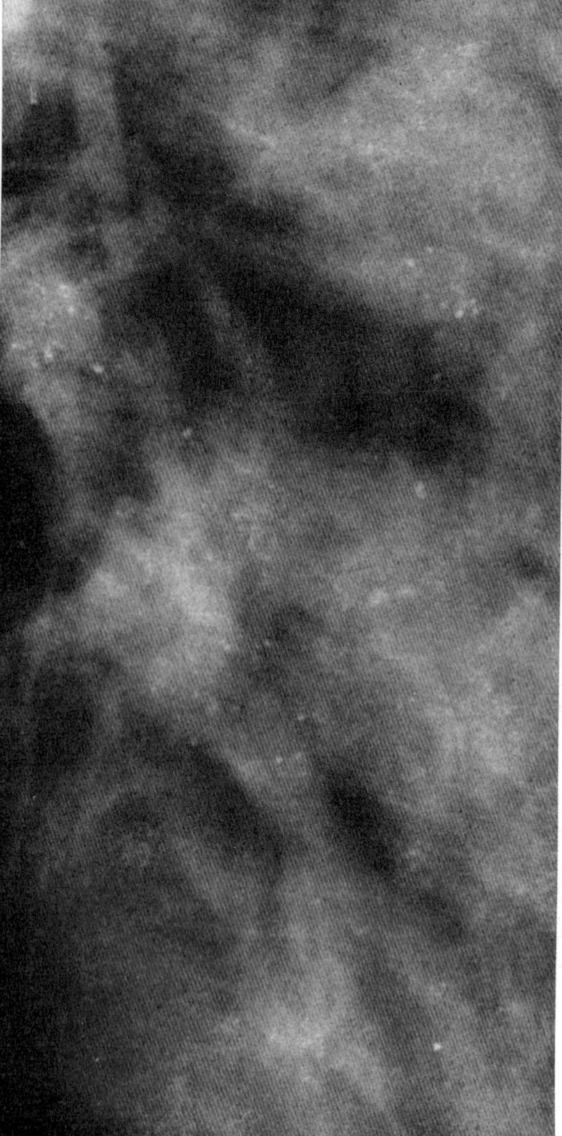

Fig. **49**.29   Mammogram, magnified 2×. Microcalcifications scattered throughout the entire breast evenly and in groups, and most numerous in the subareolar region. The calcifications are rounded, somewhat ill-defined but of about the same density. A few calcifications appear more dense than others, are localized into groups and have a fragmented appearance.
Roentgen diagnosis: Intraductal process. The calcifications localized into groups may indicate carcinoma and for these excisional biopsy for histological examination is recommended.
Clinical findings: Minimal milky nipple discharge.
Cytology: Negative.
Histology: Fibrocystic disease, papillary and cystic form, with intraductal epithelial proliferation. No evidence of carcinoma.

Fig. **49**.30   Mammogram, magnified 4 ×. Diffusely distributed, tiny microcalcifications with are somewhat ill-defined and of varying density. The differences in density of the calcification makes roentgen classification difficult. This may represent malignant degeneration of an intraductal process. It was elected to follow this patient conservatively because there were no significant palpatory findings in the breast and a single puncture revealed a negative cytology. Additionally there had been four excisional biopsies in the other breast. Three years later a second excisional biopsy was performed.
Histology: Fibrocystic disease. Signs of secretory stasis. No evidence of malignancy.

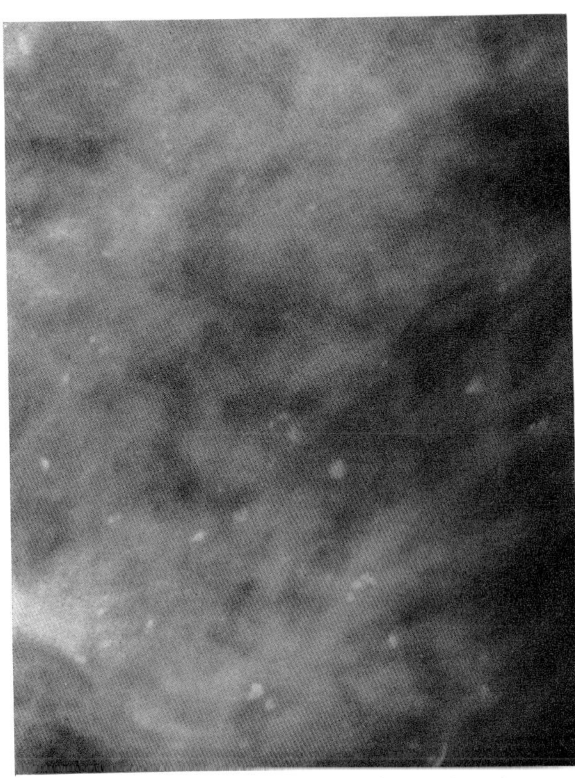

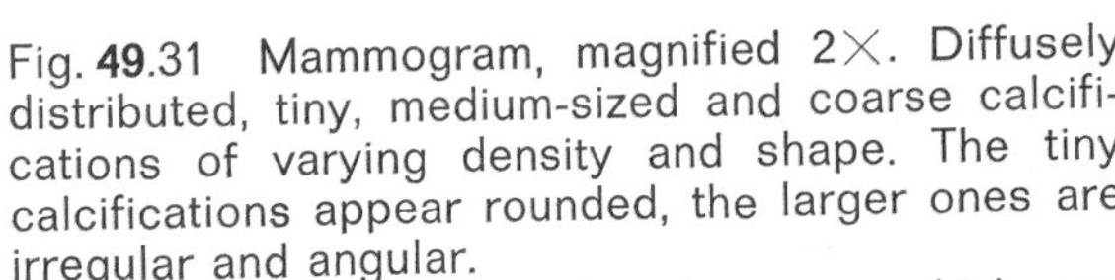

Fig. **49**.31 Mammogram, magnified 2×. Diffusely distributed, tiny, medium-sized and coarse calcifications of varying density and shape. The tiny calcifications appear rounded, the larger ones are irregular and angular.
Roentgen diagnosis: Intraductal process which may indicate malignancy.
Clinical findings: Pain, circumscribed induration beneath the areola.
Histology: Intraductal, necrotic carcinoma in situ associated with extensive periductal inflammatory fibrosis.

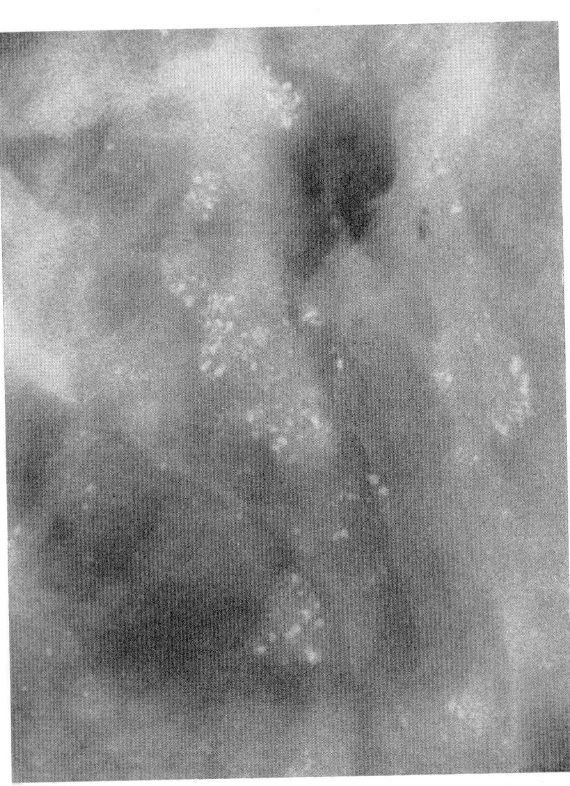

Fig. **49**.32 Roentgenogram of the surgical specimen, magnified 3×. Diffuse calcifications, many of which are in groups, of varying size and shape but quite dense.
Roentgen diagnosis: Suspect intraductal carcinoma. Recommend wide excisional biopsy.
Clinical findings: No palpable mass.
Histology: Intraductal carcinoma.

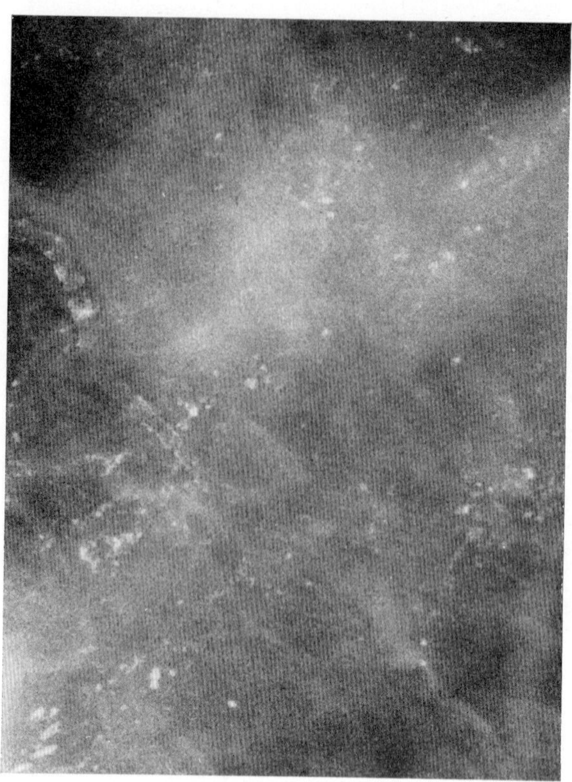

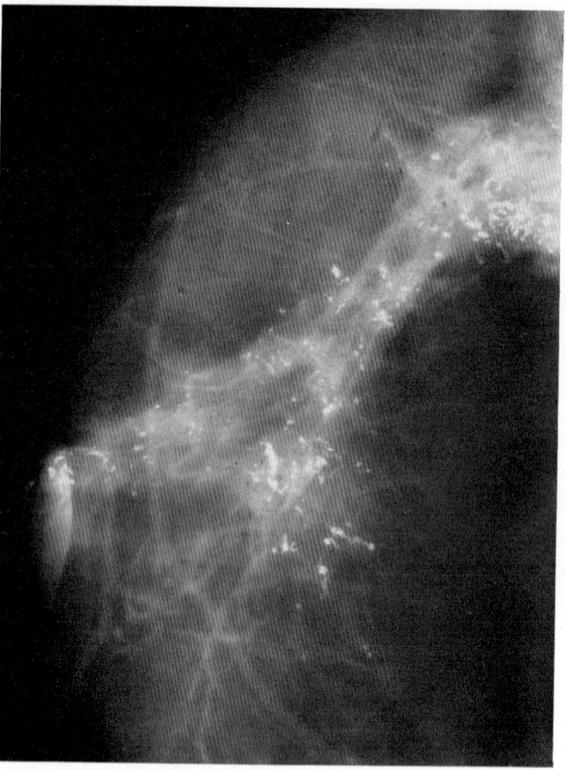

Fig. **49**.33 Mammogram, magnified 3×. Diffuse microcalcifications varying in size, quite dense, some of which are distributed into groups. A calcified vessel is identified.
Roentgen diagnosis: Definite intraductal carcinoma.
Clinical findings: Family hstory of breast carcinoma. A dominant mass is not palpated.
Histology: Intraductal carcinoma.

Fig. **49**.34 Mammogram. Very dense, irregularly shaped microcalcifications of varying size distributed within the course of a lactiferous duct extending from a soft tissue mass to the nipple. There is associated fibrosis.
Roentgen diagnosis: Because there is eczema of the nipple this appearance is consistent with Paget's carcinoma.
Histology: Paget's carcinoma of the areola and nipple. Intraductal carcinoma.

In order to simplify the differential diagnosis as to the etiology of various calcifications found in the mammogram, we have tabulated the usual pathological processes associated with some common calcifications. The table contains diseases not included in this chapter but which have been discussed in prededing chapters.

Differential Diagnosis of Breast Calcifications

Coarse:
Fibroadenoma
Carcinoma with central necrosis

Semicircular and circular shape:
Cysts
Fibroadenoma
Liponecrosis microcystica calcificans
Panniculitis nodularis nonsuppurativa febrilis
(Pfeiffer-Weber-Christian)
Oil cysts
Plasma cell mastitis
Calcified sebaceous glands

Linear:
Arteriosclerosis
Plasma cell mastitis
Lactiferous duct carcinoma

Microcalcifications localized into groups:
Lactiferous duct carcinoma
Proliferative mastopathy (epithelial hyperplasia,
intraductal papillomatosis)
Fibrosing mammary dysplasia
Sclerosing adenosis
Lobular carcinoma in situ
Scar calcification
Beginning calcification within a fibroadenoma
and cyst
Beginning calcifications in arteries

Diffuse scattered microcalcifications:
Sclerosing adenosis
Lactiferous duct carcinoma
Multicentric lobular carcinoma in situ
Epithelial proliferation in mammary dysplasia
Fibrosing mammary dysplasia

In addition to the above all calcifications may represent artifacts.

18*

Chapter 50

Differential Diagnosis of Round Masses in the Breast

A round mass in the breast may be produced by many anatomical or pathological conditions. Although the differential diagnosis of a round mass in the breast is a daily problem, there have been few publications on the subject: GERSHON-COHEN and SCHORR (1969), PRAGER and HASERT (1969), REHM et al (1970).

The preliminary requirement for the appearance of a round shadow is a body having the density of water or soft tissue. It is not possible to make any decision as to the substrate of a shadow in the roentgenogram on the basis of its density, although a few authors claim to be able to do this. The maximum radiodensity of soft tissue components of the breast are essentially the same as water. Greater density is only possible if there is an intermixing of iron (hemosiderosis) or calcium. A lesser density results if there is a mixture of fat or oil. The differential diagnosis of a round shadow in the mammogram is based on its form, size and borders, the surrounding tissue reaction and the clinical history.

The *form* of a round shadow gives no certain clue as to the nature of the lesion. Only a longitudinal or lobulated configuration has any importance in differential diagnosis and raises the possibility of a multiloculated cyst, fibroadenoma, subcutaneous neurofibroma, giant fibroadenoma, hemangioma, intraductal papilloma, lymph node, sarcoma or atypical carcinoma.

A completely round density verified in two different projections includes many possibilities of differential diagnosis (see page 288).

The *size* of a rounded density also gives only limited information. Very large round shadows may indicate cysts, giant fibroadenomas, medullary carcinoma and sarcoma, whereas medium-sized and small round densities have no particular differential diagnostic significance.

A *smooth contour*, however, suggests a benign expansile process (cyst or fibroadenoma), but this sign must not be relied upon absolutely.

Likewise, poorly defined borders of a mass, although predominantly found in carcinoma, do not always definitely indicate that the lesion is malignant. One must adhere to the clinically approved rule that every definable nodule which is definitely palpable should be removed. The following are exceptions to this rule:

1) The uncomplicated cyst, emptied by aspiration and demonstrating a smooth inner border on pneumocystography, the aspirate of which is normal on histological examination and in which mammography after three months indicates regression of the cyst.

2) The fibroadenoma of the young girl which is verified by puncture with cytological examination. Excision of the tumor may be excluded providing careful follow-up is obtained.

3) The small or medium-size fibroadenoma of the older woman, the diagnosis of which is quite certain on the basis of its typical mammographic signs (smooth contours and typical coarse calcifications). Excision may be excluded on the basis of the age of the patient providing that careful follow-up is obtained.

4) The unilateral nodular parenchymal proliferation developing in a girl at the beginning of puberty which often simulates an isolated breast nodule. Removal of this results in permanent disfigurement.

5) Palpatory findings that simulate breast nodules but which on mammography or other diagnostic methods turn out not to be solid masses but instead lipomas, inflammatory processes, hematomas, postoperative changes or changes following tetanus vaccination, et cetera. There do not require excision but careful observation.

In the following mammograms we will show some of the problems of the differential diagnosis of breast masses and indicate the considerations needed for correct differential diagnosis: (Numerous representative cases follow).

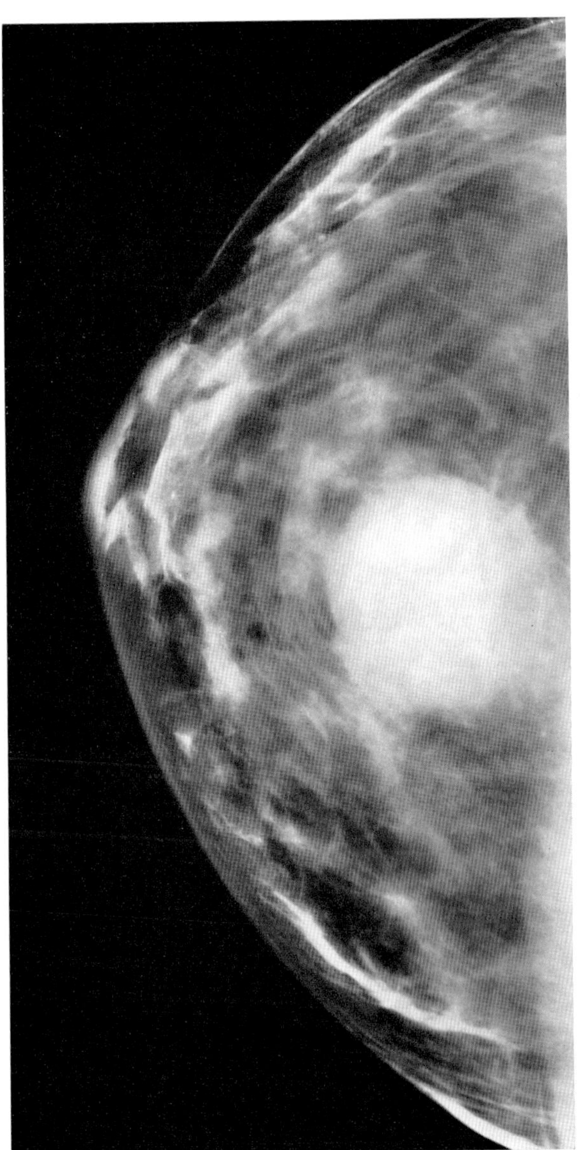

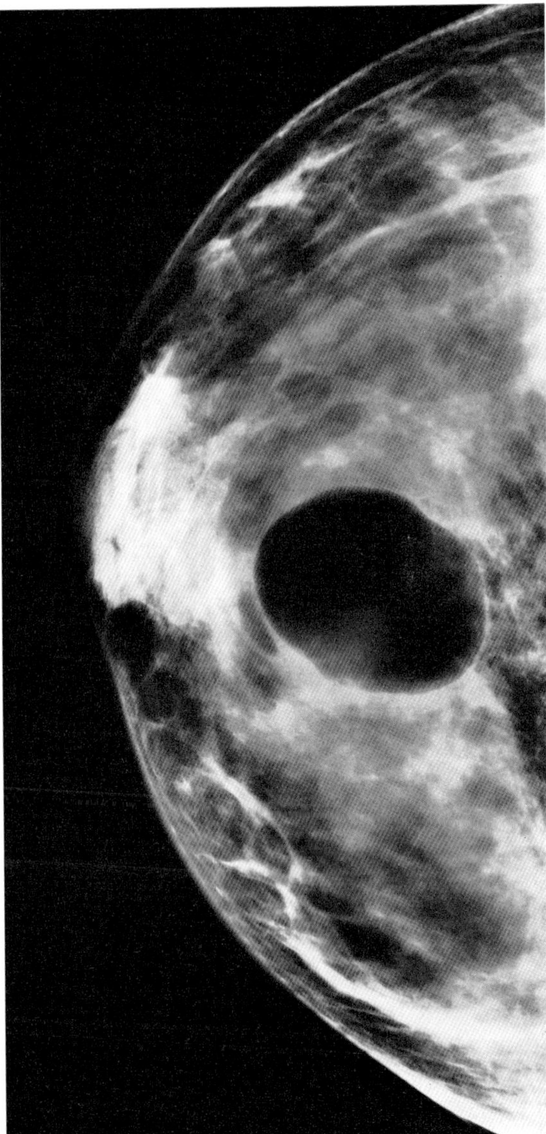

Fig. **50**.1a Smoothly marginated oval mass with minimal lobulation.
Clinical findings: Smooth freely movable mass corresponding in size to the lesion noted on the roentgenogram.
Differential diagnosis: Clinically or roentgenologically one cannot differentiate this lesion from fibroadenoma, medullary carcinoma, cyst, intracystic carcinoma or papilloma.
Aspiration: Yellow-green aspirate.

Fig. **50**.1b Pneumocystogram: Smoothly marginated inner wall. No soft tissue masses. Cytology: Occasional histiocyte, otherwise negative. Course: Complete regression on follow-up examination 3 months later.
Note: Aspiration, pneumocystography, cytology, and follow-up examination are necessary for final diagnosis.

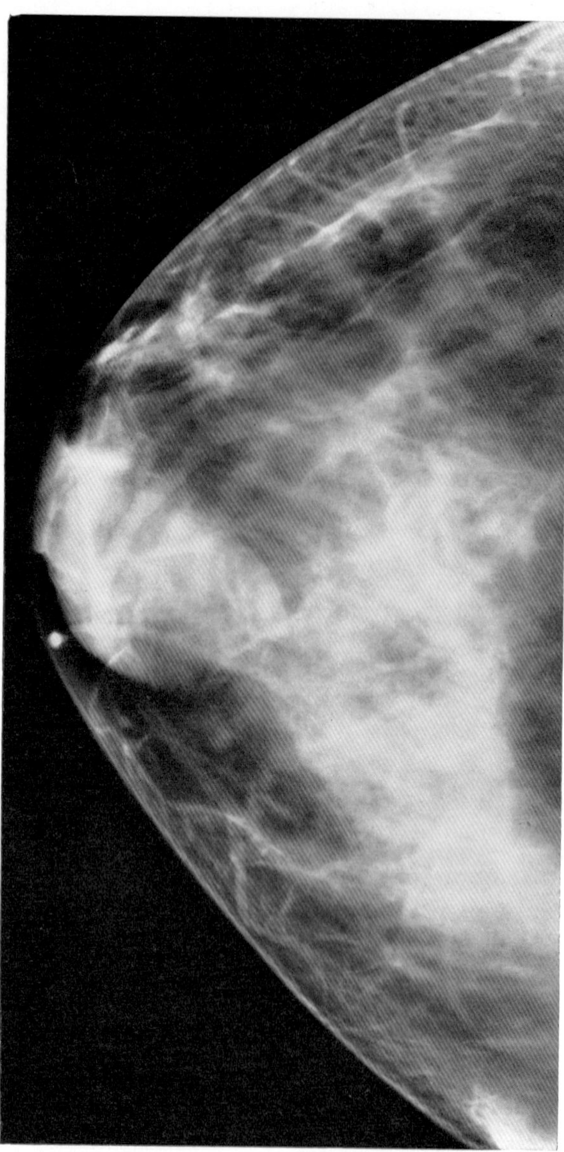

Fig. **50**.2 Subareolar smoothly marginated oval mass. No sign of malignancy. (The dilated vein was present in the other breast as well.)
Clinical findings: Sharply defined subareolar mass.
Differential diagnosis: The subareolar location and oval shape of a mass in a 30-year-old woman suggests fibroadenoma. A cyst or intracystic papilloma cannot be ruled out. Carcinoma is unlikely. Aspiration: Solid material. Cytology: Fibroadenoma.
Note: Aspiration determines the final diagnosis.

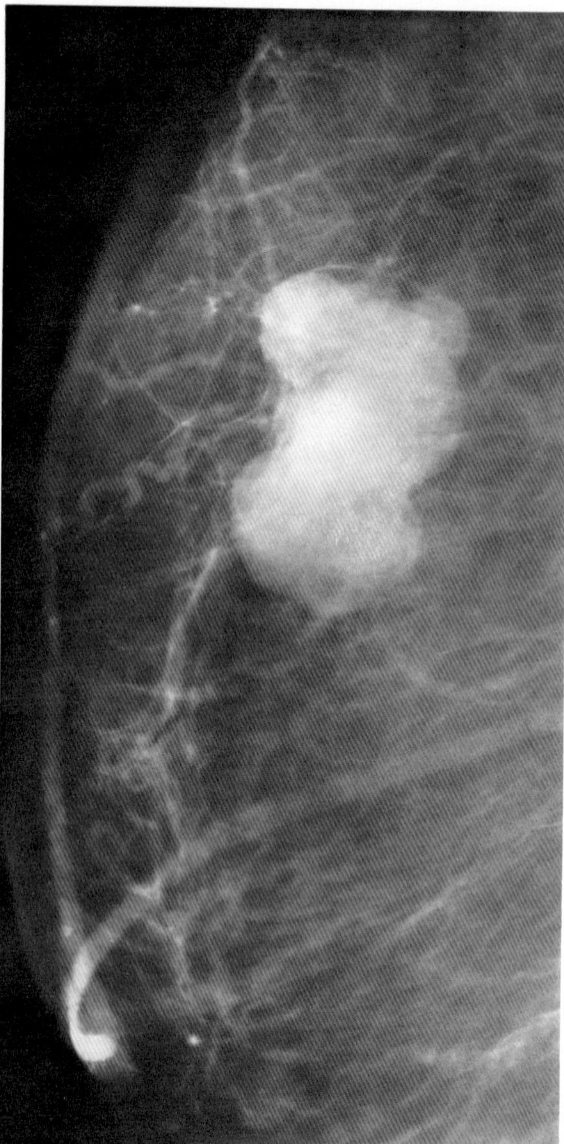

Fig. **50**.3   Lobular mass with sharp margins.
Clinical findings: Easily definable, movable, firm nodule. No skin or nipple abnormality.
Differential diagnosis: This includes lobular fibroadenoma, loculated cyst, solid or medullary carcinoma. Of significance is the demonstration of a tortuous, dilated corkscrew vein between the tumor nodule and the skin.   This suggests carcinoma.
Histology: Invasive intraductal carcinoma.
Note: The dilated tortuous vein suggested the correct diagnosis.

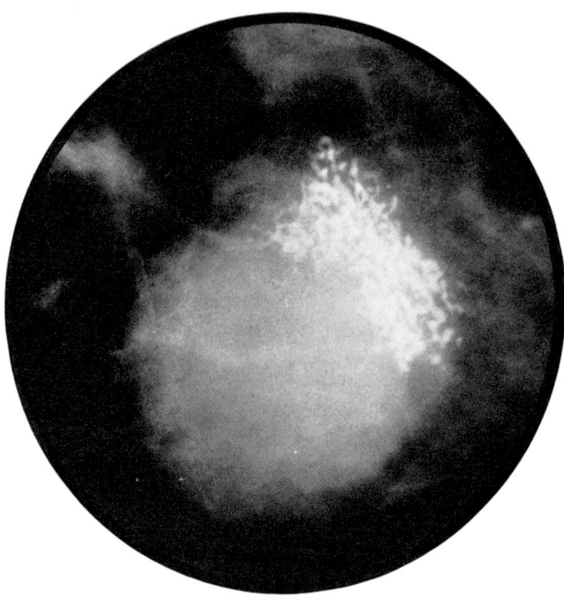

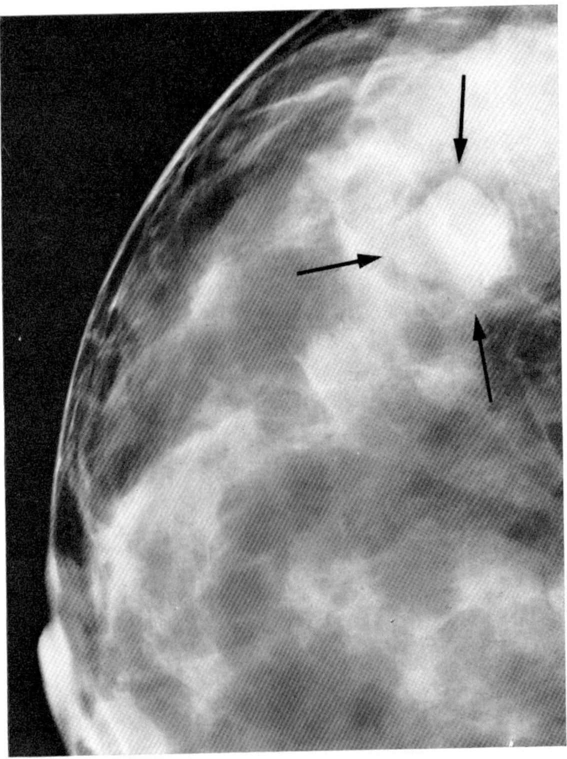

Fig. **50**.5a

Fig. **50**.4 Rounded mass with relatively smooth border.
Clinical findings: Well-defined, somewhat hard but freely movable mass. Size corresponded to that in the roentgenogram. Fibroadenoma was suspected.
Differential diagnosis: In the roentgenogram within the confines of the mass there are numerous, closely grouped very dense microcalcifications of irregular and sometimes bizarre shape. These calcifications are so typical of carcinoma that there need be no doubt of the diagnosis.
Histology: Intraductal carcinoma with medullary components.
Note: Typical microcalcifications are diagnostic.

Fig. **50**.5a Smoothly marginated, somewhat lobulated mass surrounded by a fatty margin and contained within dense parenchyma. A corresponding mass was not clinically palpable. Because of this puncture and aspiration would have been difficult and were not performed.Under the assumption that this represents a fibroadenoma, follow-up examination is indicated to verify benignancy of this process.

Fig. **50**.5b Follow-up examination 7 months later: The mass has increased in size. It is again not palpable so that puncture and aspiration are not possible. Although the increase in size can occur with a cyst or fibroadenoma, carcinoma can no longer be ruled out. Excisional biopsy is unavoidable.
Histology: Poorly differentiated carcinoma.
Note: Enlargement of a mass on follow-up examination is always suggestive of carcinoma.

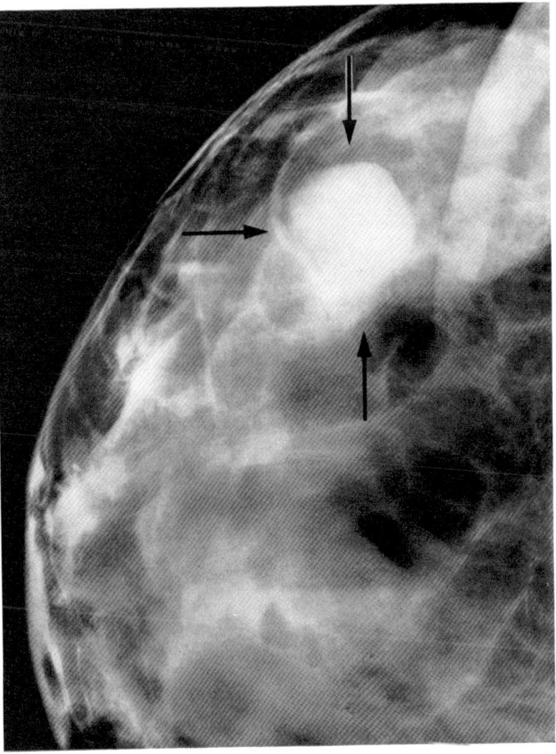

Fig. **50**.5b

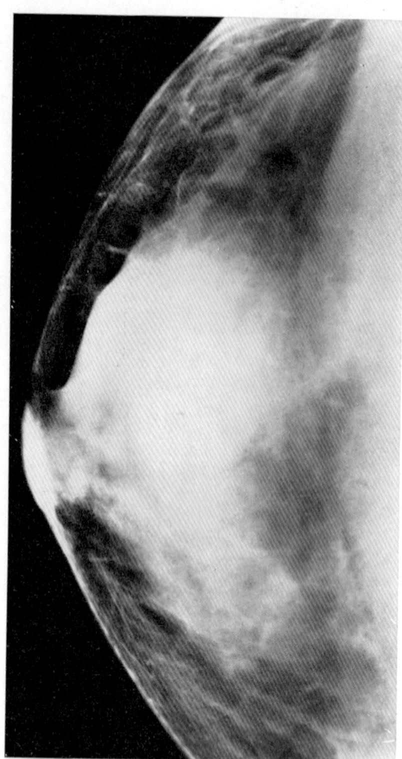

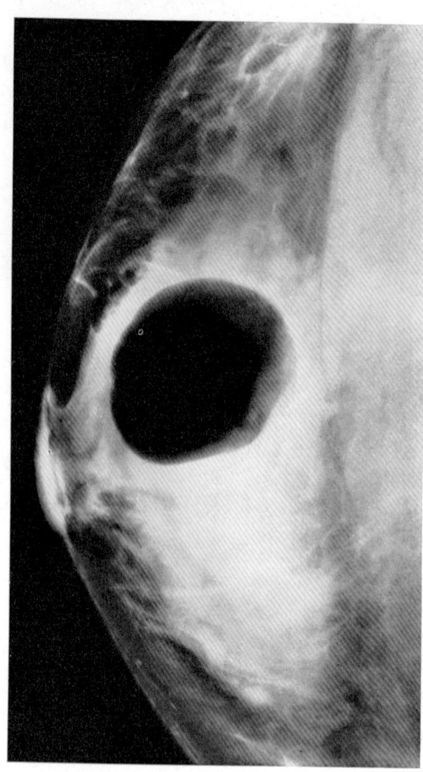

Fig. **50**.6a   Poorly defined subareolar mass without sharp margins differentiating it from breast parenchyma. Clinical findings: Tense subareolar mass, freely movable, painful.
Differential diagnosis: In the mammogram neither microcalcifications, increased vascularity nor desmoplastic response are visible; however, because of the ill-defined margins this cannot be considered a cyst or fibroadenoma with any degree of certainty. Further work-up with aspiration or excisional biopsy is indicated. Aspiration: 5 cc straw-colored fluid.

Fig. **50**.6b   Pneumocystogram: Loculated cyst with smooth margins.
Cytology: Occasional foam cells.
Course: The cyst regressed within 3 months.
Note: In any mass with poorly defined borders the diagnosis must be made by aspiration, cytology or histology. Simple observation of the lesion is incorrect management.

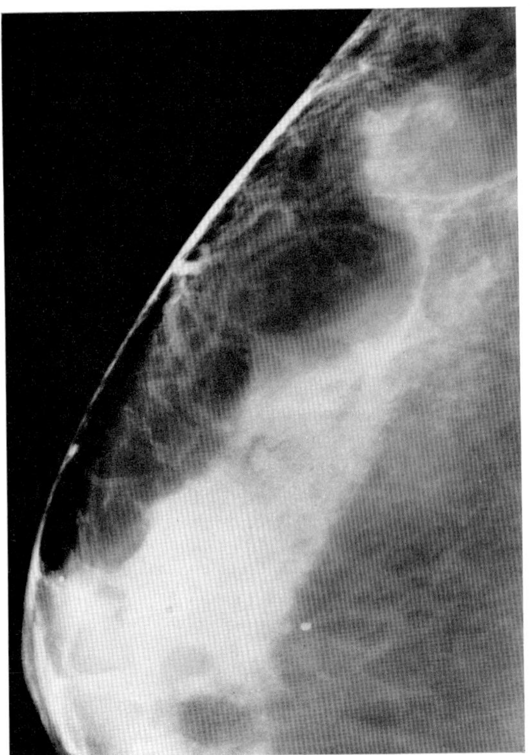

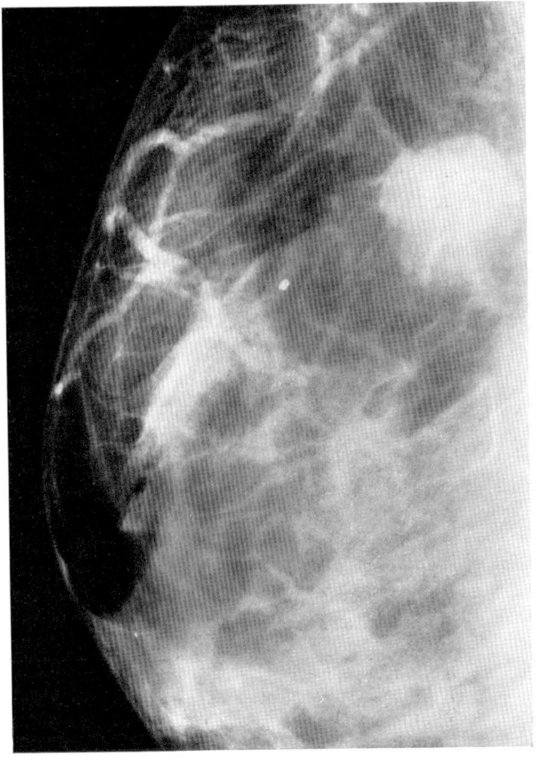

Fig. **50**.7a   Mass with poorly defined borders situated within the subcutaneous fatty layer peripheral to the breast parenchyma.
Clinical findings: Irregular, somewhat fixed nodule which on palpation was felt to be larger than its size in the roentgenogram. Contralateral mastectomy had been performed in the past for breast carcinoma.
Differential diagnosis: The poor definition and occasional umbilication of the borders of the mass as well as the curvilinear connections to the parenchyma are signs suspicious of carcinoma.

Fig. **50**.7b   The configuration of this mass in the other projection indicates definite signs of carcinoma. This diagnosis is supported by the fact that the patient belonged to a high risk group. Histology: Poorly differentiated solid breast carcinoma.
Note: Poorly defined and umbilicated borders and size discrepancy between palpatory and roentgen findings as well as the history indicate the correct diagnosis of carcinoma.

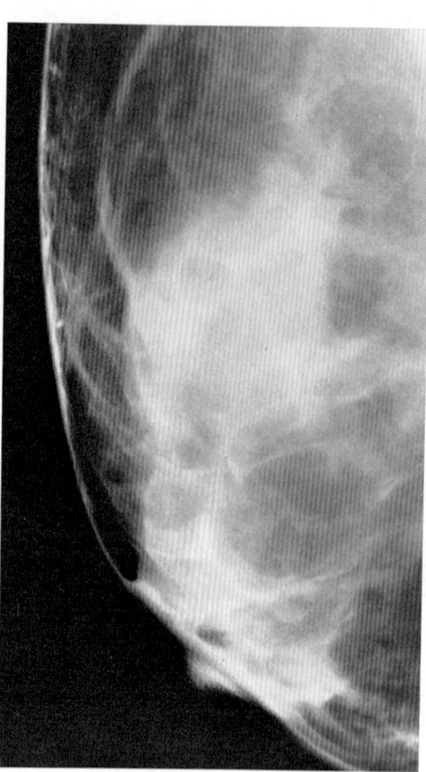

Fig. **50**.8 Large primarily smoothly marginated mass in the lateral aspect of the breast parenchyma. At some points there is ill-defined extension into neighboring tissue. Curvilinear densities extend from the mass towards the axilla.
Clinical findings: Recent history of erythematous skin changes and development of a painful mass with fever.
Differential diagnosis: The differentation here includes abscess, inflamed cyst and inflammatory carcinoma. The absence of increased vascularity and typical microcalcifications mitigate against carcinoma. With inflammatory skin changes aspiration is contraindicated. Surgery must be performed for final diagnosis. This turned out to be an abscess.
Note: Masses and inflammatory changes not associated with gestation are always suspicious for carcinoma. Mammographic differentiation between abscess, infected cyst and carcinoma is difficult.

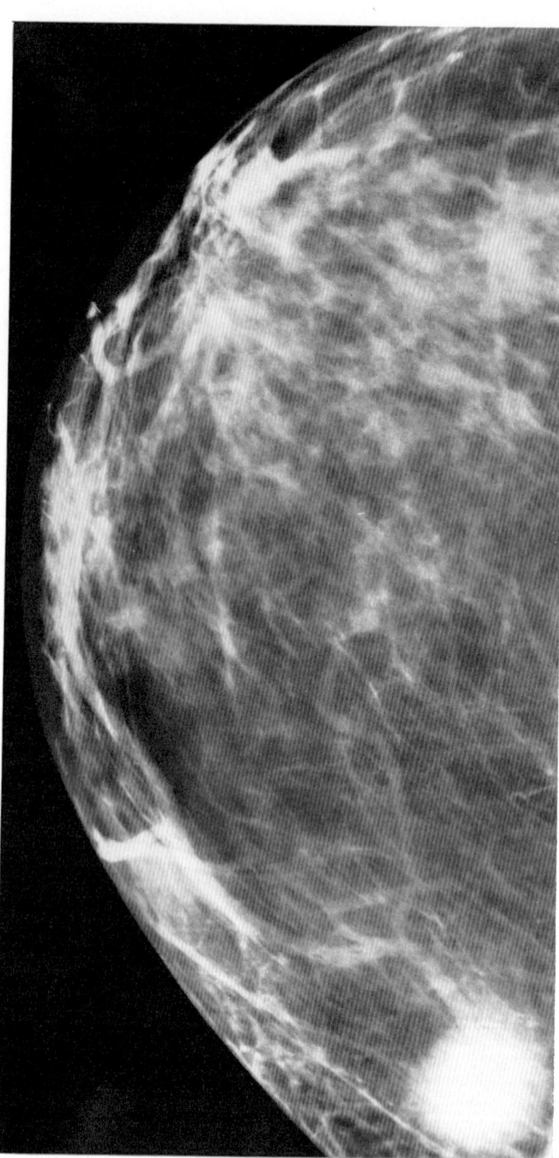

Fig. **50**.9 Ill-defined, poorly marginated mass beneath the skin in the inferior half of the breast.
Clinical findings: Typical furuncle.
Differential diagnosis: There are no mammographic signs characteristic for this lesion.
Note: Clinical findings led to the correct diagnosis.

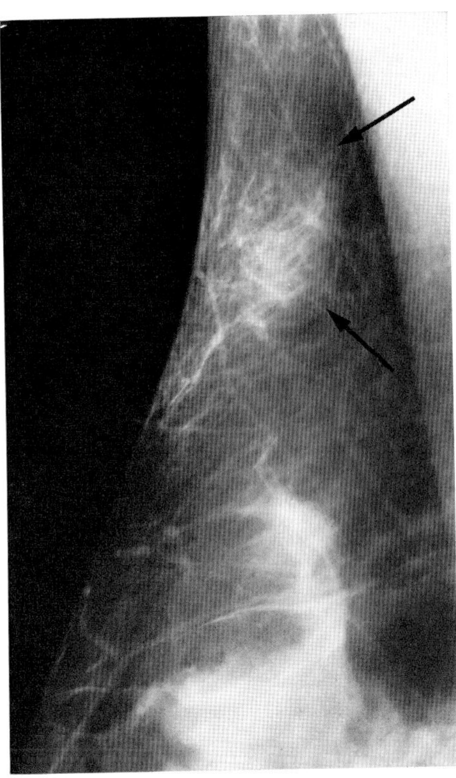

Fig. **50**.10 Minimal soft tissue density within the sucutaneous fatty layer at the base of the breast, beyond the breast parenchyma.
Clinical findings: Fairly firm, painful mass about 1 cm in size. No skin fixation. Closer inquiry revealed that a few weeks before, tetanus vaccination had been performed in this location.
Note: History established the diagnosis.

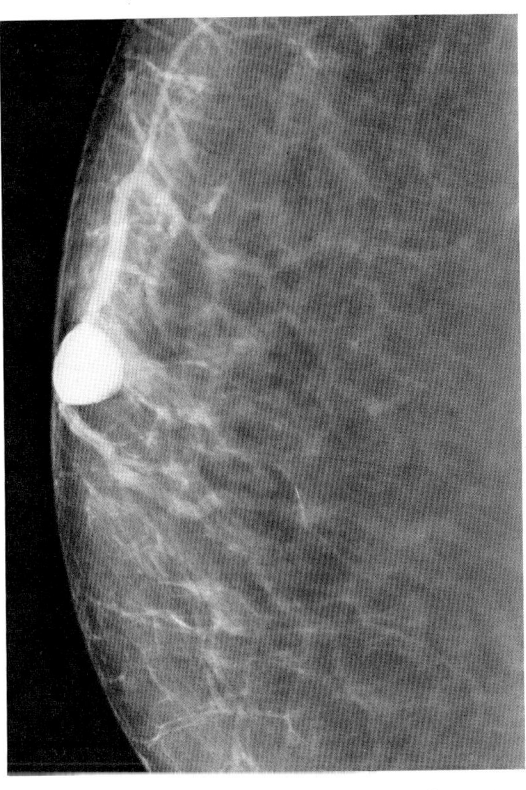

Fig. **50**.11 Sharply marginated mass about 1 cm in diameter beneath the skin in the center of the breast.
Clinical findings: No palpable nodule.
Differential diagnosis: The absence of palpatory findings called attention to the absence of the nipple shadow in the mammogram. This results from a failure of proper positioning of the breast resulting in projection of the nipple end—on, to produce the unusual shadow.
Note: Correct positioning is particularly important in evaluation of lesions or findings in the area of the nipple and areola.

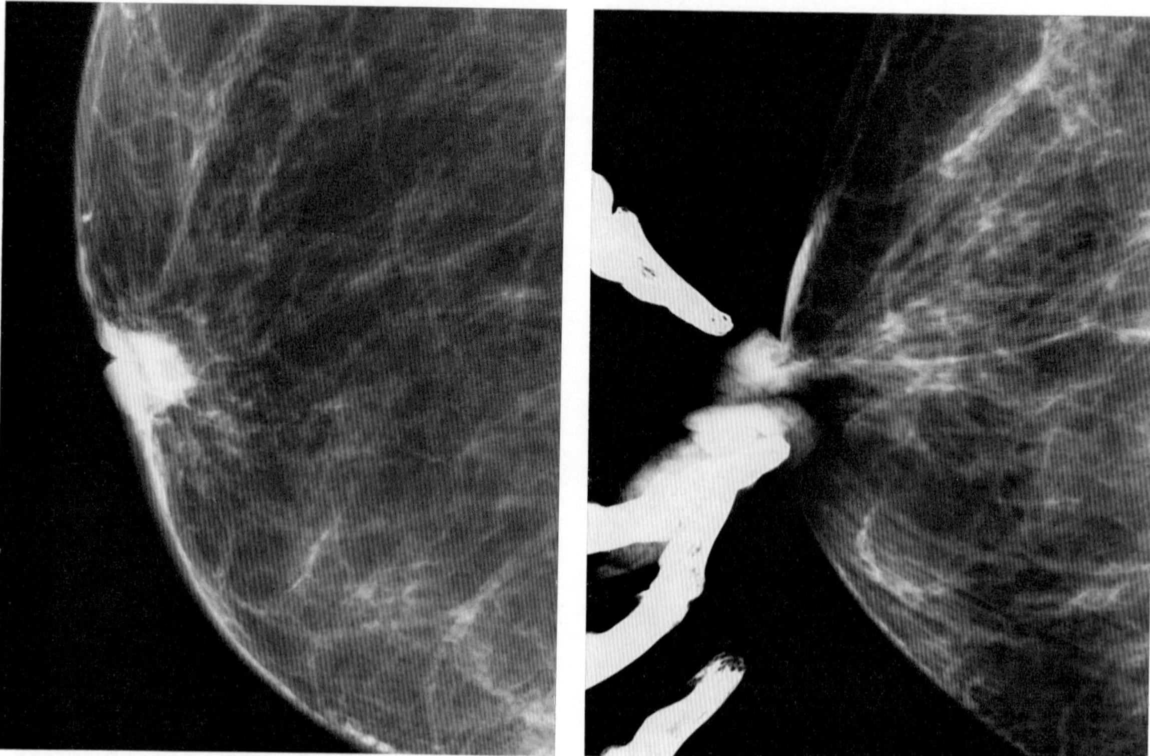

Fig. **50**.12, a, b   Rounded density consisting of retracted nipple. Clinical findings: Congenitally retracted nipple which could be pulled forward manually (b).
Note: Mammogram performed when the nipple is pulled forward reveals no abnormality of the breast.

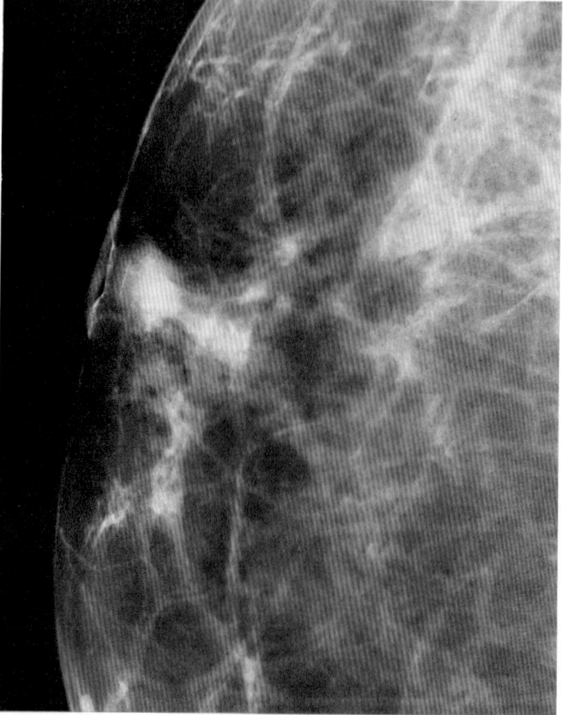

Fig. **50**.13   Subareolar round soft tissue density associated with flattened nipple.
Clinical findings: Recent nipple retraction with palpable subareolar firmness.
Differential diagnosis: Radiating linear densities are seen to extend from the subareolar soft tissue density deeply into the breast. A small focus of calcification is seen within the mass. This suggests a pathological intraductal process. In association with recently developed nipple retraction these subareolar changes are suspicious of carcinoma and indicate the need for histological examination.
Histology: Adenocarcinoma.
Note: When linear extensions and calcifications are seen in association with a mass further diagnostic workup is indicated.

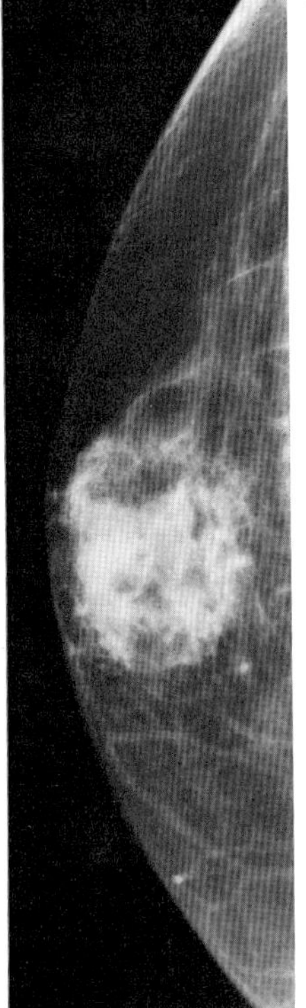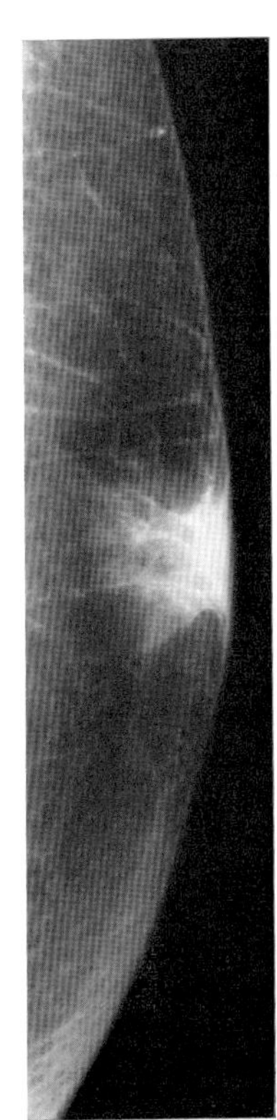

Fig. **50**.14a   Right breast of a 10-year-old girl with rounded soft tissue density about 2 cm in diameter.
Fig. **50**.14b   Left breast of this patient demonstrating subareolar parenchyma about 1 cm in size.
Clinical findings: Palpable and painful lump in the right breast. Is surgery indicated?
Differential diagnosis: There is no evidence of smooth round or homogenous mass density within the immature breast tissue. This represents asymmetrically developing breast parenchyma.
Note: Parenchyma development of the breast in children during puberty frequently mimics a mass. Mammography clarifies the situation.

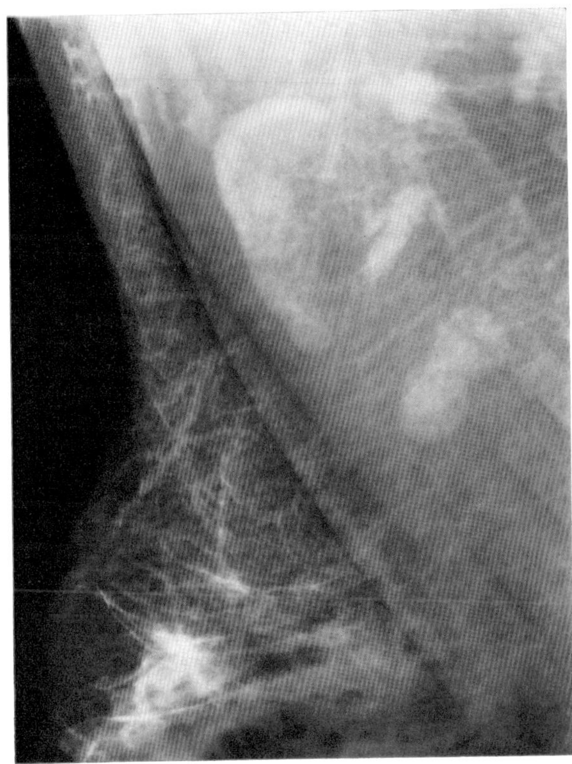

Fig. **50**.15   Two closely positioned soft tissue masses associated with smaller masses and a large semilunar density are observed in the anterior axillary fold.
Clinical findings: Palpable lymph nodes.
Differential diagnosis: Lymph nodes the size of beans normally occur in the anterior axillary fold. The central radiolucency in the largest lymph node indicates fat infiltration.
Note: The small lymph nodes are not suspicious for metastases. Clinical follow-up examination, however, is recommended.

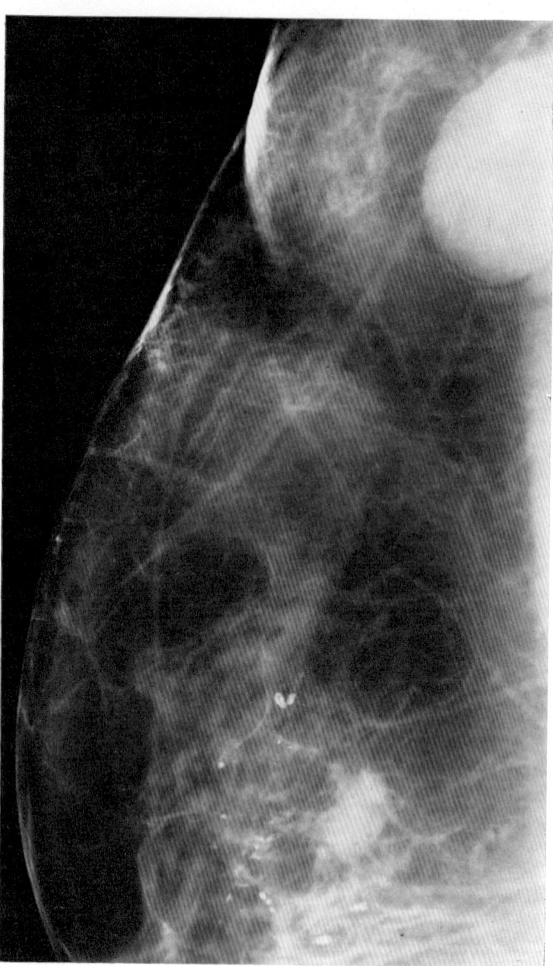

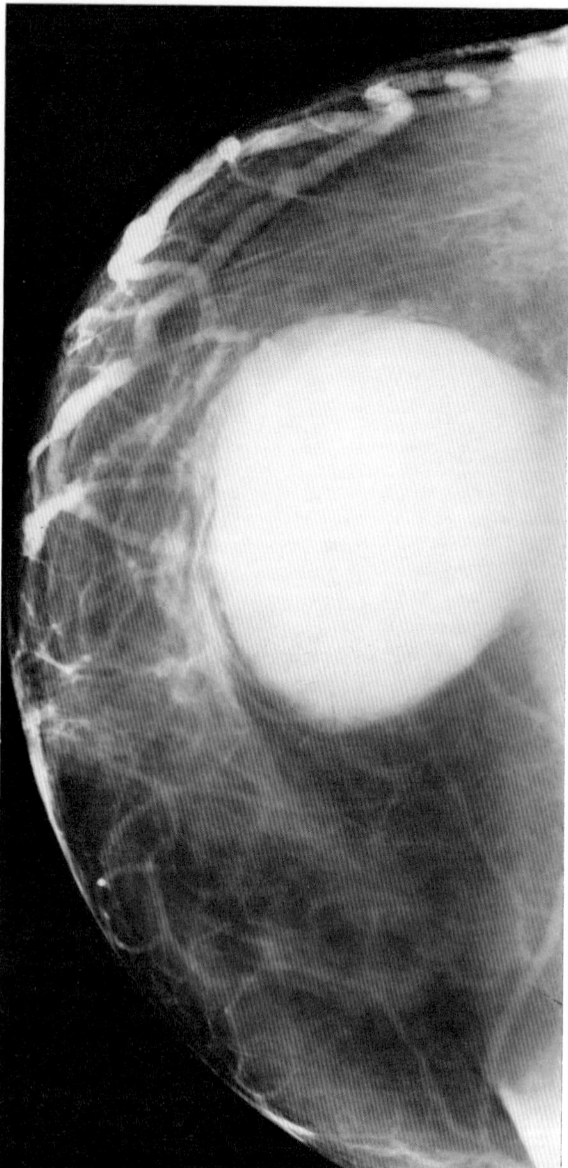

Fig. **50**.16   Walnut-sized mass with smooth borders beneath the anterior axillary fold.
Clinical findings: Enlarged lymph nodes. No abnormal palpatory findings in the breast.
Differential diagnosis: In this location the lymph node is abnormally enlarged. This may represent systemic disease as well as lymph node metastases. The mammogram, however, reveals an occult intraductal carcinoma within the lateral parenchyma containing small intraductal calcifications and a spiculated border.
Note: Dense lymph nodes within the axilla larger than a bean are generally pathological. Smooth borders do not rule out metastatic disease.

Fig. **50**.17   Large smoothly bordered mass displacing surrounding tissues. There is an obvious dilated and tortuous vein seen between the mass and the skin. This represents a metastasis from a hypernephroma.
Note: Differential diagnosis between this metastatic lesion and that of a cyst, fibroadenoma or even a large medullary carcinoma was possible with the help of the clinical history (pulmonary metastases had been observed on the chest film). (Radiological Clinic University of Goettingen, Prof. Gregl.)

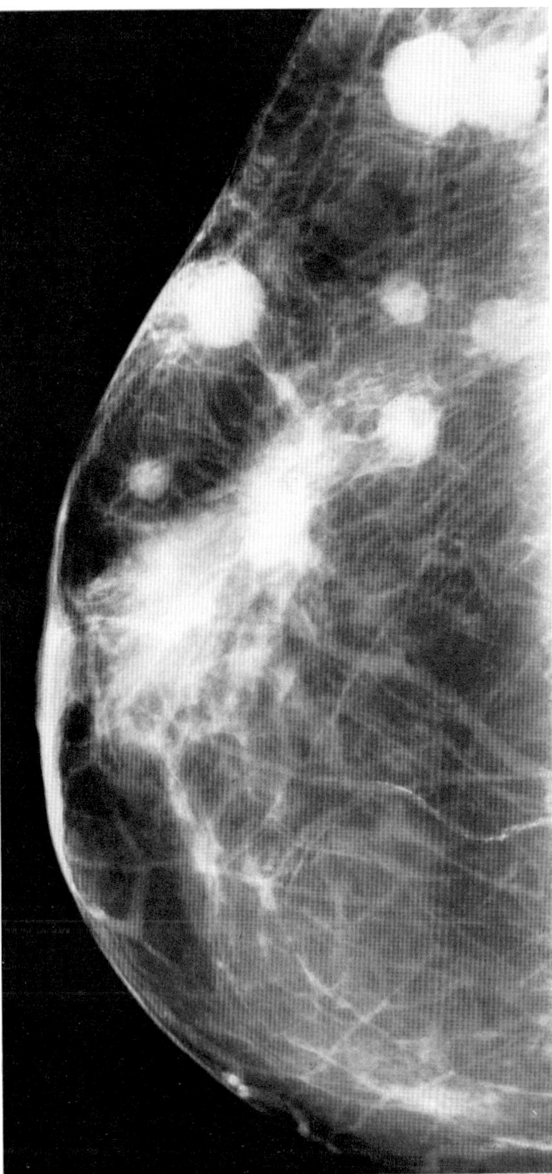

Fig. **50**.18 Smoothly marginated masses distributed unevenly in an involuted breast. Closer examination allows classification of these nodules into
three groups all of different sizes.
Clinical findings: Previous contralateral mastectomy.
Differential diagnosis: Multiple cysts? Multiple fibroadenomas? Cysts of fibrocystic disease and
multiple fibroadenomas are always of different
sizes since they arise at different points in time.
This mammogram, however, reveals that the larger
nodules are approximately the same in size. The
same is true of the smaller group. This is strong
indication of metastases from a primary breast carcinoma. This was verified histologically.
Note: History and uniformity of the nodules led to
the correct diagnosis.

To make the differential diagnosis of round shadows in the mammogram easier we have compiled the following table of some of the more common pathological entities causing this change.

Included in this table are entities discussed in the previous chapters.

The following pathological entities manifest themselves as round shadows in the mammogram:

Differential Diagnosis of Round Shadows

1) Cyst
2) Intracystic papilloma (benign or malignant)
3) Fibroadenoma
4) Giant fibroadenoma
5) Hyalinized fibroadenoma without associated reactive fibrosis
6) Intraductal papilloma
7) Hemangioma
8) Fibroadenolipoma
9) Subcutaneous neurofibroma
10) Various types of carcinoma (medullary carcinoma, gelatinous carcinoma, papillary carcinoma, carcinoma simplex)
11) Carcinoma metastasis
12) Sarcoma
13) Sarcoma metastasis
14) Nodular form of lymphoma
15) Abscess
16) Skin furuncle
17) Tetanus vaccination
18) Nodular form of tuberculosis
19) Hematoma
20) Lymph node metastasis
21) Atheroma, comedo
22) Skin wart
23) Neurofibromatosis.

Normal structures that may appear as round shadows in the mammogram are as follows:

24) Early developing parenchyma of the pubertal girl
25) Circumscribed normal breast parenchyma
26) Retracted nipple or a nipple not seen tangentially in the roentgenogram
27) Orthograde projection of a vein (vein seen end on)
28) Normal lymph node.

Chapter 51

Differential Diagnosis of Stellate Shaped Structures in the Breast

The differential diagnosis of stellate densities in the mammogram consists of differentiating scirrhus carcinoma from acute or chronic inflammations, the fibrosing type of mammary dysplasia, sclerosing adenosis and fibrosis following infection, surgery or trauma. To be differentiated from all these pathological processes are the stellate densities created by summation shadows.

Scirrhus carcinoma may only be diagnosed with reasonable certainty if there is a central tumor mass from which radiate stellate connective tissue extensions. Typical microcalcifications, increased vascularity, skin changes, retraction of the nipple and suspicious palpatory findings are further supportive signs of carcinoma. These signs and symptoms, however, are not definite and each case must be individually considered before the diagnosis is made. Only the uninitiated will find it easy to make the diagnosis of scirrhus carcinoma simply on the basis of a stellate shaped density. On the other hand, every stellate shaped structure within the confines of the breast, no matter how discrete, must be carefully examined because it may prove to be a scirrhus carcinoma. In the final interpretation of a stellate shaped density in the mammogram clinical findings and history must be taken carefully into account. Subsequent illustrations will show stellate densities in the roentgenogram all of which are very similar to one another; however, some are scirrhus carcinoma and others are benign fibrotic conditions. In these cases the definite diagnostic differentiation cannot be made (fig. 51.1, 51.2, 51.3a and b).

Furthermore two cases are presented here in which there are very similar stellate densities both of which contain central microcalcifications; however, each case represents a different disease (fig. 51.4a and b; 51.5a and b).

Fig. 51.6 and 51.7 illustrate stellate densities resulting from scar formation following surgery. As a comparison we present a retro-areolar scirrhus carcinoma which developed in the course of numerous inflammatory afflictions of the breast (fig. 51.8).

The postoperative breast is particularly difficult for the radiologist in making a decision as to whether a palpable tissue density represents a surgical scar or a carcinoma. On his judgement depends the correct or incorrect indication for excisional biopsy.

Follow-up mammograms are occasionally diagnostic; however, this type of management can only be done for a limited period of time.

Hyalinized fibroadenomas bear a strong resemblance to scirrhus carcinoma because this benign tumor consists of a central mass which as the result of hyaline degeneration shrinks down and becomes surrounded with radiating fibrous bands (fig. 51.9). Macroscopically, the appearance of this benign tumor is as difficult to differentiate from scirrhus carcinoma as in the roentgenogram or on clinical examination. One must be acquainted with these potential errors in order to prevent mastectomy on the basis of clinical and roentgen impressions of scirrhus carcinoma without the absolutely necessary histological verification. Fortunately hyalinized fibroadenoma which resembles scirrhus carcinoma is extremely rare, thus diminishing the chance of mistaking it for a malignancy.

Clinical signs as they are found in scirrhus carcinoma are not always reliable when applied to the differential diagnosis of stellate lesions in the mammogram. The clinical findings must not be over-weighted in importance when significant roentgen signs are absent. Circumscribed skin retraction occurs not only in scirrhus carcinoma but also as a result of traumatic scar formation with organizing hematoma (fig. 51.10).

In reaching a judgment on stellate shaped densities in the roentgenogram, projections at opposite angles, as well as coned-down compression views are very important. If the lesion is not reproducible on two 90° projections at right angles to each other, then one is dealing with a summation effect of normal tissue structures. However, one must be very careful in coming to this conclusion and guard against making errors as to localization. Such artificial stellate densities are shown in fig. 51.11a, b and 51.12a, b in conjunction with a radiating retromammary parenchymal rest (fig. 51.13).

More remote causes of stellate structures in the breast are tuberculosis, actinomycosis and fistula formation. These disorders are very rare and are of little importance in the differential diagnosis. In uncertain cases, mammographically guided biopsies must be instituted for final diagnosis.

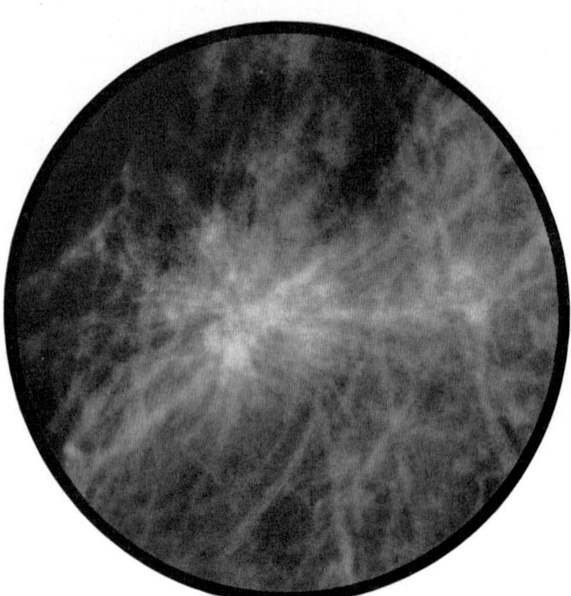

Fig. **51**.1   Stellate soft tissue density with a central discrete nodule. No palpatory findings. Scirrhus carcinoma of the contralateral breast was demonstrated clinically and roentgenologically.
Histology: Bilateral scirrhus carcinoma.
Note: The existence of a carcinoma in the other breast was significantly important in arriving at the mammographic diagnosis in spite of the absence of clinical findings.

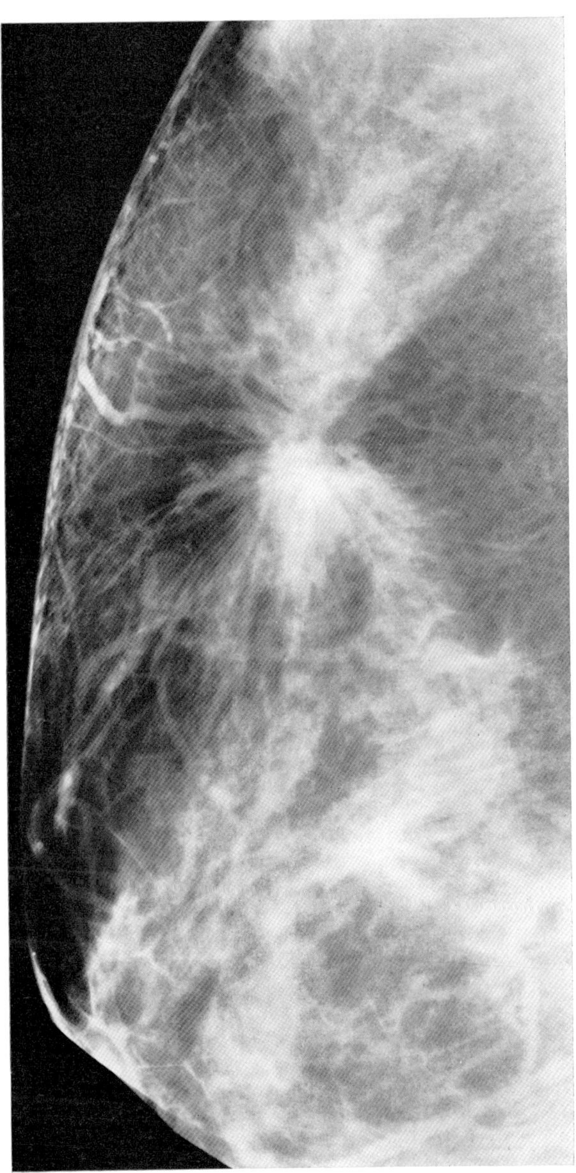

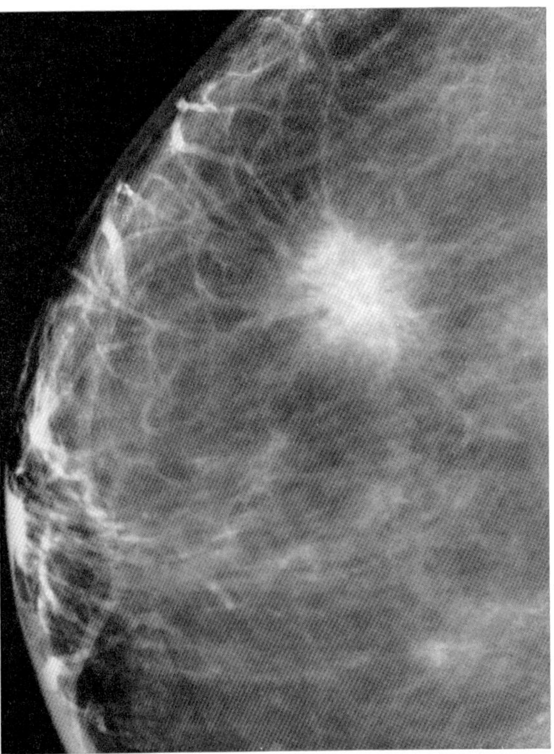

Fig. **51**.3a   Mass, 1 cm in diameter, with ill-defined spiculated margins easily demonstrated in two projections at right angles. A central mass of greater density is not seen. Skin infiltration is not demonstrated roentgenologically or clinically. No microcalcifications. Vascular pattern is normal. Excisional biopsy was undertaken with the presumptive diagnosis of fibrocystic disease. Intraoperative roentgenogram of the biopsy specimen to verify localization (Fig. 51.3b) reveals the mass and a single central microcalcification. Histology: Fibrous mastopathy. Examination of serial sections failed to reveal evidence of scirrhus carcinoma.
Note: The presumptive diagnosis of fibrous mastopathy is supported by the absence of a central nodular tumor mass as well as other signs of carcinoma. However, excisional biopsy of such lesions is still indicated.

Fig. **51**.2   Stellate soft tissue density with far-reaching linear extensions but relative sparing of a section of the breast dorsally. A central mass is absent. However, a tortuous vein extending from the center of the abnormal tissue to the skin suggests scirrhus carcinoma. On the basis of this suspicion excisional biopsy was performed even in the absence of palpatory findings.

Histology:Fibrous mastopathy.
Because of the discrepancy between roentgenological and histological findings the biopsy specimen was examined very carefully in order to avoid overlooking a tiny central scirrhus carcinoma. Reexamination, however, failed to reveal tumor.

Note: Supporting the diagnosis of fibrocystic disease is the fact that because of special circumstances this patient did not come to excisional biopsy until 9 months following the mammographic examination. During this time no roentgen changes had been observed, nor were there clinical symptoms to suggest scirrhus carcinoma.

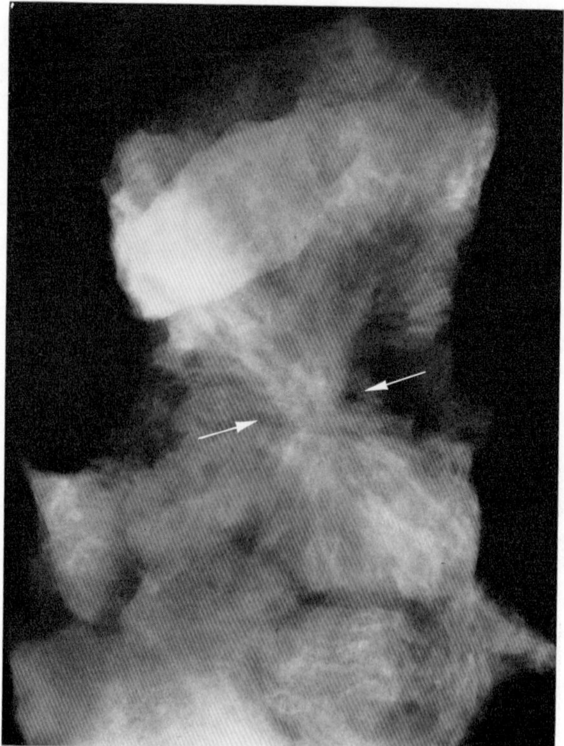

Fig. **51**.3b

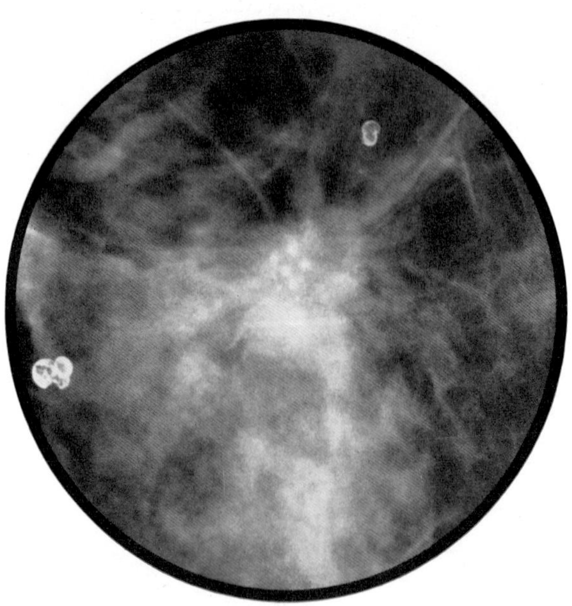

Fig. **51**.4b

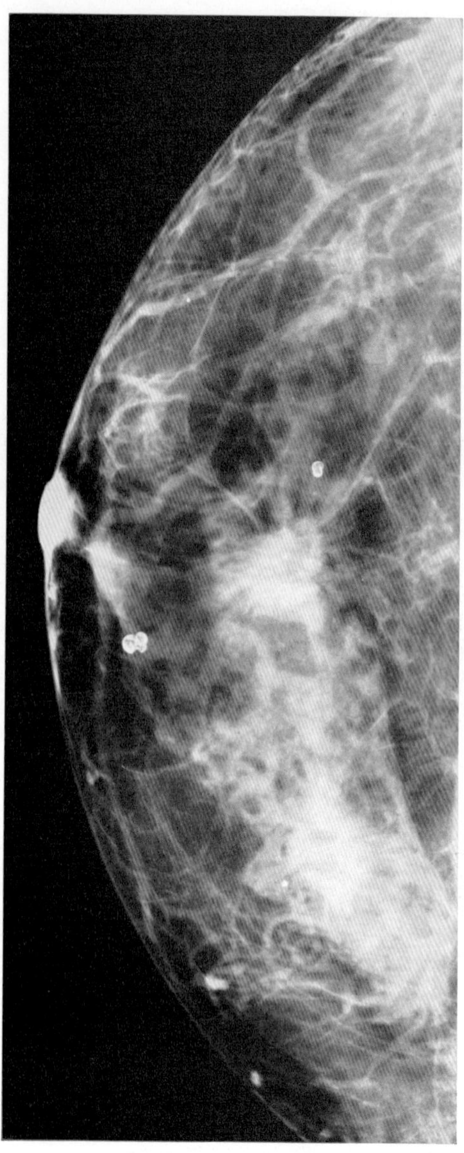

Fig. **51**.4a   Stellate soft tissue density with a central, somewhat nodular mass, containing microcalcifications. Increased vascularity. Two foci of calcified fat necrosis are observed.

Fig. **51**.4b   Local area magnified 2× to show lesion. Clinical findings: No palpable mass. Excisional biopsy was undertaken because of the suspicion of occult scirrhus carcinoma.

Histology: Scirrhus carcinoma.

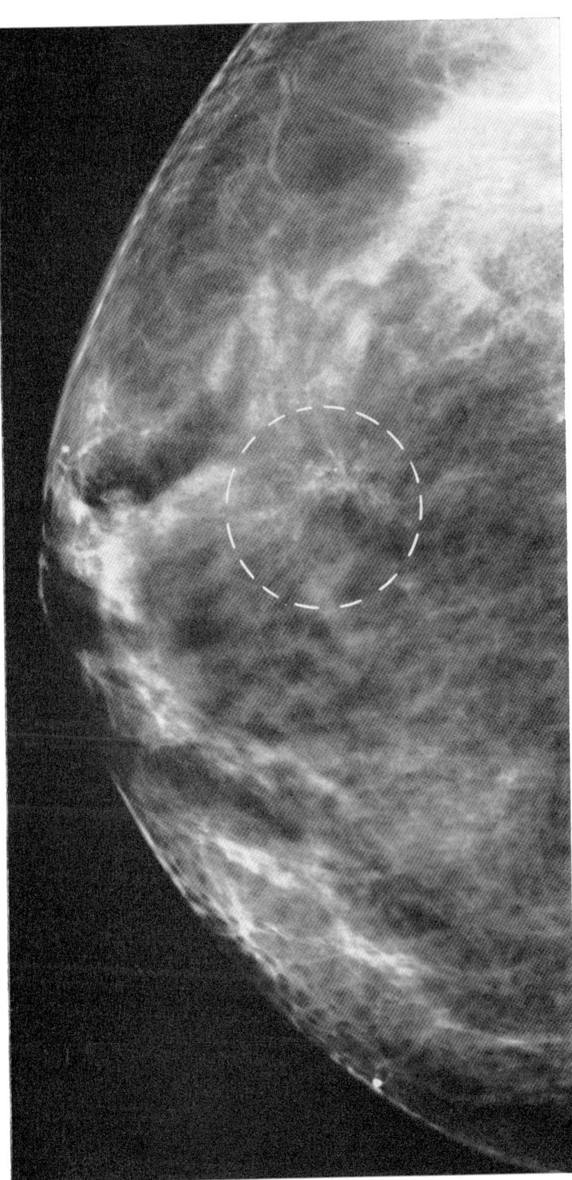

Fig. **51**.5a

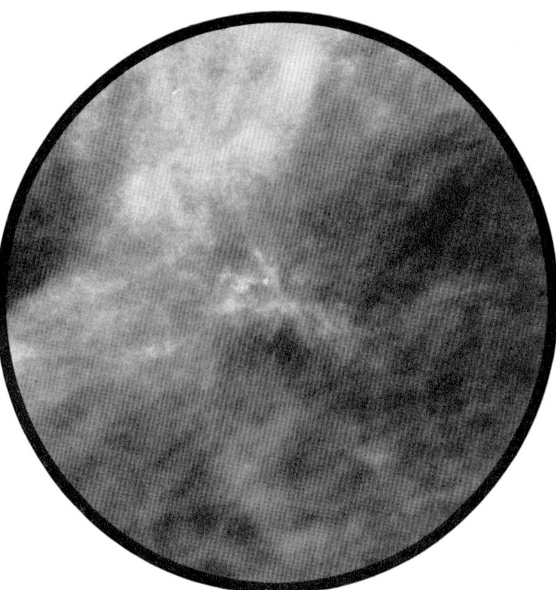

Fig. **51**.5b

Fig. **51**.5a Delicate stellate pattern containing microcalcifications resembling those of Fig 51.4a and b. A central tumor mass is not visible, and this is verified in Fig. 51.5b, local area magnified 2 ✕.
Clinical findings: Normal.
Excisional biopsy was performed to differentiate fibrous changes from scirrhus carcinoma.
Histology: Fibrous mastopathy.
Note: A positive differentiation between stellate soft tissue lesions, as illustrated in Figs.51.4 and 51.5, is not possible in the mammogram. In such lesions the task of mammography is accurate localization for excisional biopsy rather than differential diagnosis.

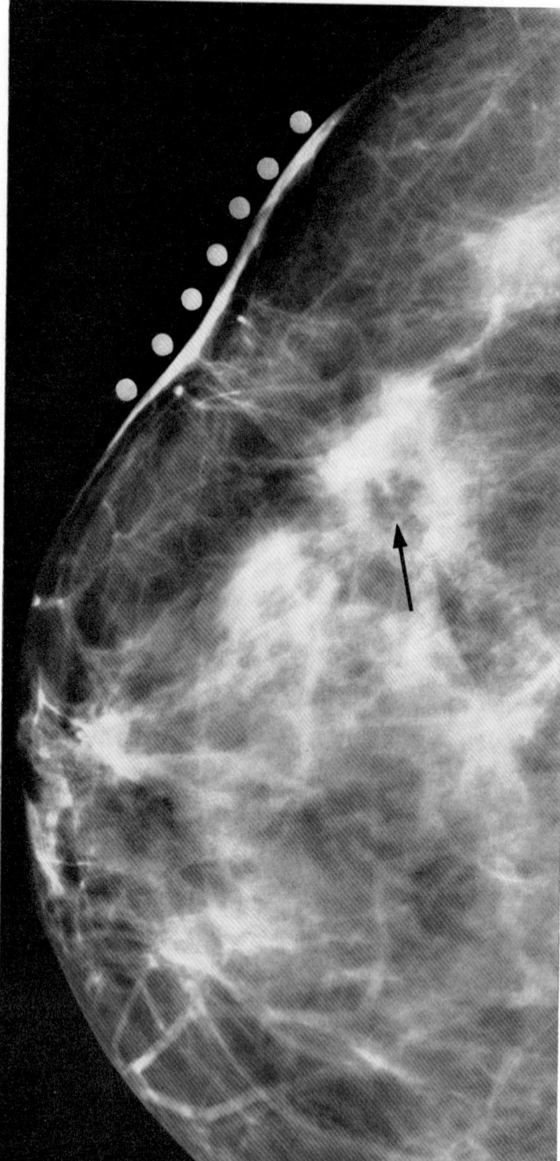

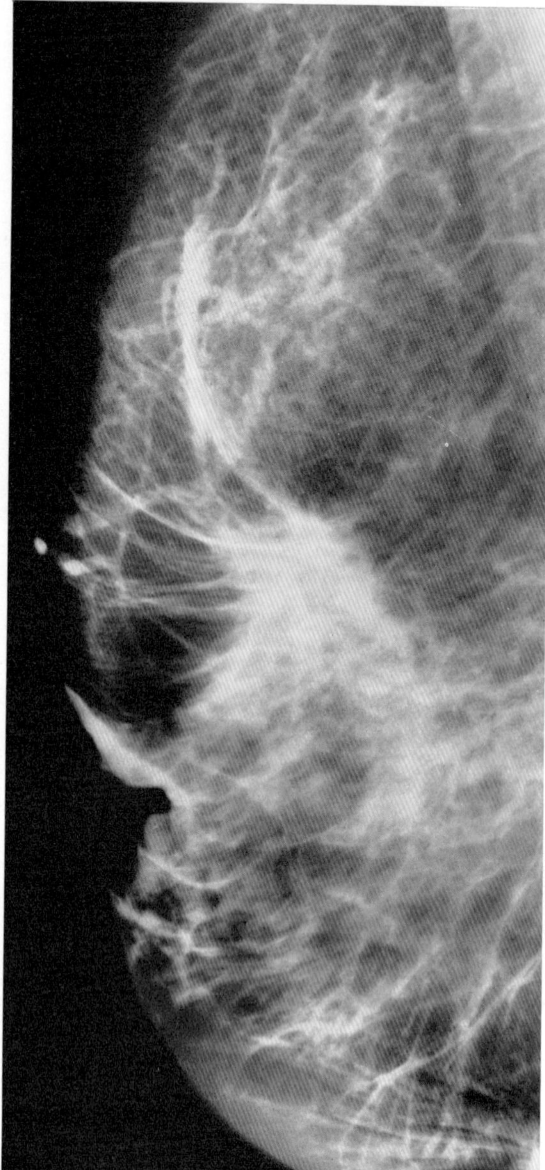

Fig. **51**.6   Coarse stellate density in the periphery of the breast parenchyma (arrow) with thickened subcutaneous septa and local skin thickening. Roentgenologically this is compatible with scirrhus carcinoma infiltrating into the skin. Clinical history indicates that there had been a previous excisional biopsy. The next step in the examination is to verify whether the existing scar corresponds to the area of skin thickening in the mammogram. Spot mammography as recommended by Gershon-Cohen should be performed. The scar may be localized with lead markers and a tangential projection performed. This case represents a scar and local fibrotic changes secondary to excisional biopsy.

Note: Precise knowledge of clinical history and careful roentgen examination is necessary for accurate diagnosis in patients with questionable postoperative findings. Even in these cases follow-up examination is necessary.

Fig. **51**.7   Stellate soft tissue lesion with radiating linear extensions to the subcutaneous tissue paralleling Cooper's ligaments. These are some extensions into the parenchyma and also to the posterior surface of the retracted and thickened nipple and areola. Roentgenologically this is consistent with scirrhus carcinoma. Clinical history indicates repeated incision and drainage for puerperal mastitis 36 years before. There has been no change in the degree of nipple retraction since that time. This then is a case of scarring and deeper fibrotic changes after mastitis and surgical drainage.

Note: Correct diagnosis could only be made by accurate knowledge of the clinical history.

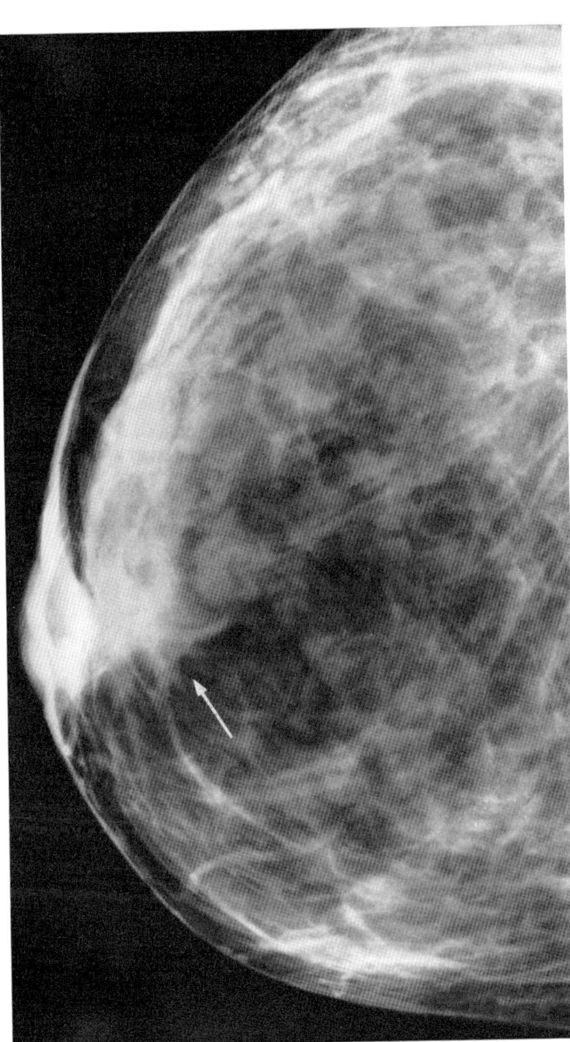

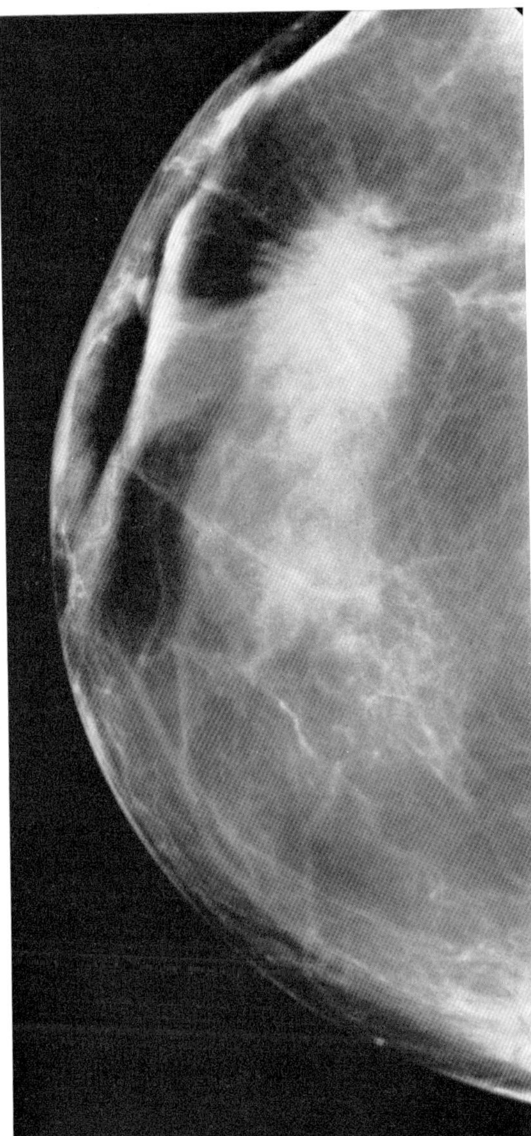

Fig. **51**.8 Subareolar soft tissue mass with ill-defined contours and stellate marginal extensions (arrow). Thickening of the subareolar tissues and lactiferous ducts. Clinical history indicates repeated inflammations of the nipple and areola. The nipple although it appears normal is fixed. A firmness is palpable in the subareolar region. The differential diagnosis includes scirrhus carcinoma versus fibrotic changes following mastitis. Excisional biopsy is indicated for clarification.
Histology: Infiltrating adenocarcinoma with solid and scirrhus components.
Note: In this case the mammographic suspicion of malignancy was the prime consideration resulting in excisional biopsy. Whenever there are suspicious roentgen findings excisional biopsy is recommended even if the clinical history suggests a post-operative or postinflammatory process.

Fig. **51**.9 Subareolar tumor mass with numerous tumor extensions to the periphery. Skin thickening and retraction of the nipple accompany the other signs.
Clinical and roentgen impression: Carcinoma.
Histology: Hyalinized fibroadenoma.
Note: There are no reliable roentgen signs to accurately differentiate between scirrhus carcinoma and hyalinized fibroadenoma.

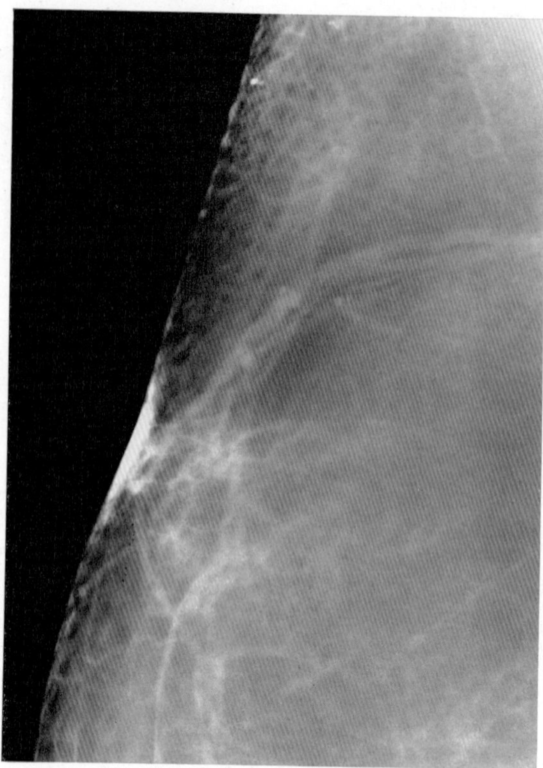

Fig. **51.**10   Focal skin thickening with somewhat atypical subcutaneous fibrosis. Clinical examination indicated plateauing of the skin.
Patient referred for mammography because of this skin fixation and the clinical suspicion of possible carcinoma. A definite tumor mass was not palpable. On the basis of benign mammographic findings the differential diagnosis was changed from previous suspicion of carcinoma to posttraumatic fibrosis since closer questioning indicated a breast hematoma following an auto accident 3 months before.
Note: Clinical history, benign mammograms and complete disappearance of this fibrosis on follow-up examinations resulted in the final correct diagnosis. However, plateau formation of the skin is always suspicious.

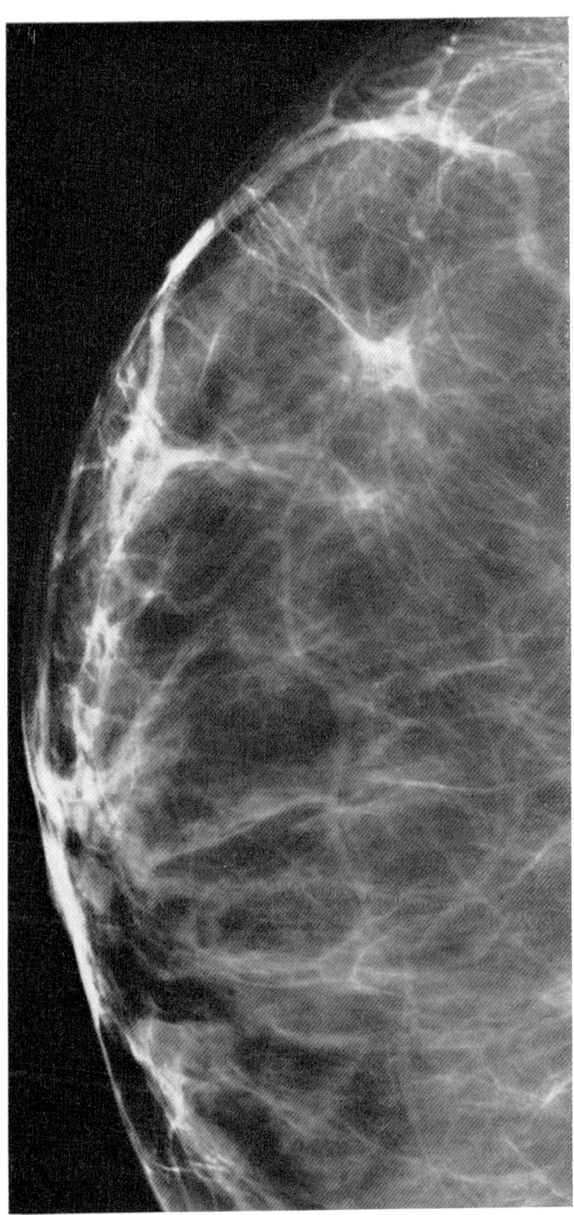

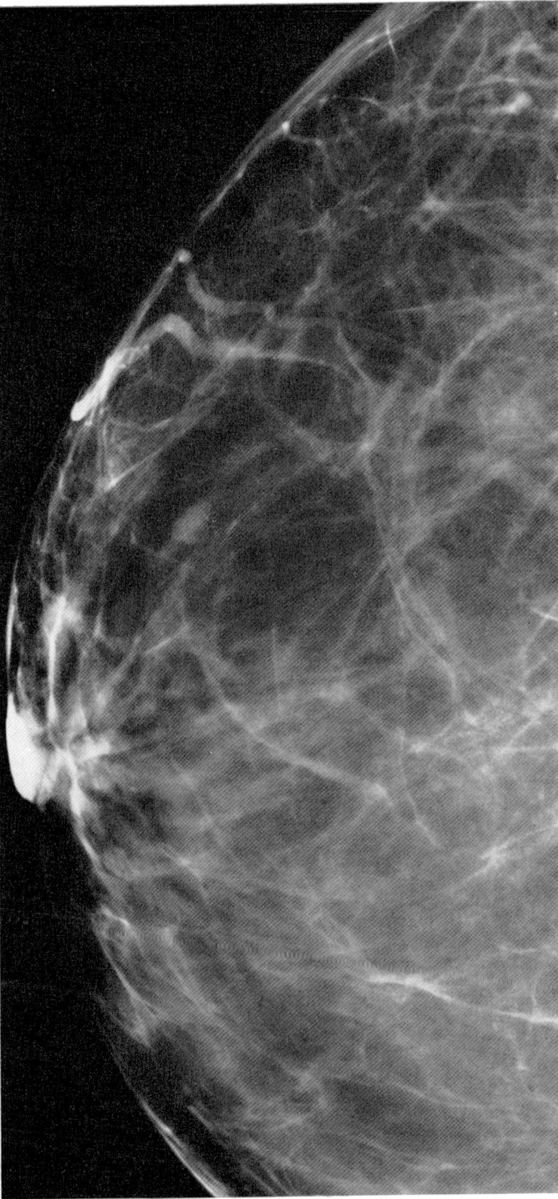

Fig. **51**.11a　The lateral mammogram reveals a stellate soft tissue density with widespread extensions.

Fig. **51**.11b　The craniocaudal view reveals an involutional breast with normal connective tissue septa and vascular structures. The stellate soft tissue density on the lateral view represented a summation shadow.
Note: A carcinoma should be seen in both right angled projections.

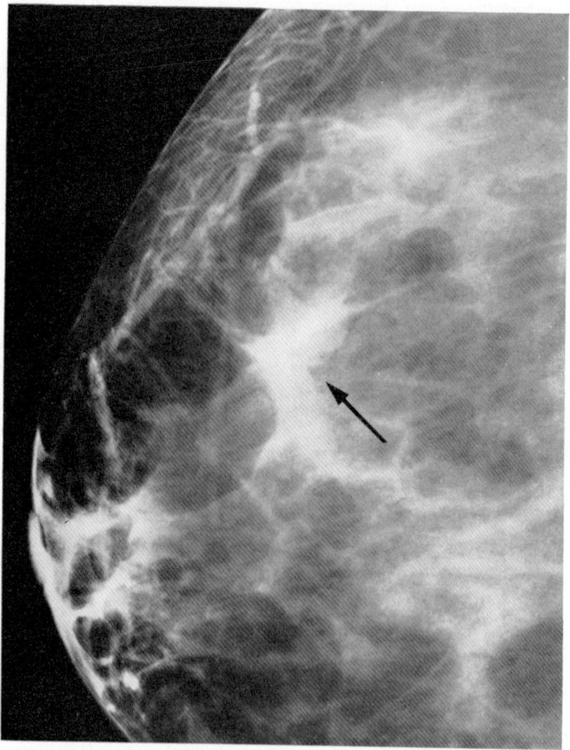

Fig. **51**.12a   In the craniocaudad projection there appears to be a thickened area of parenchyma with somewhat stellate borders just lateral to the region of the nipple (arrow).

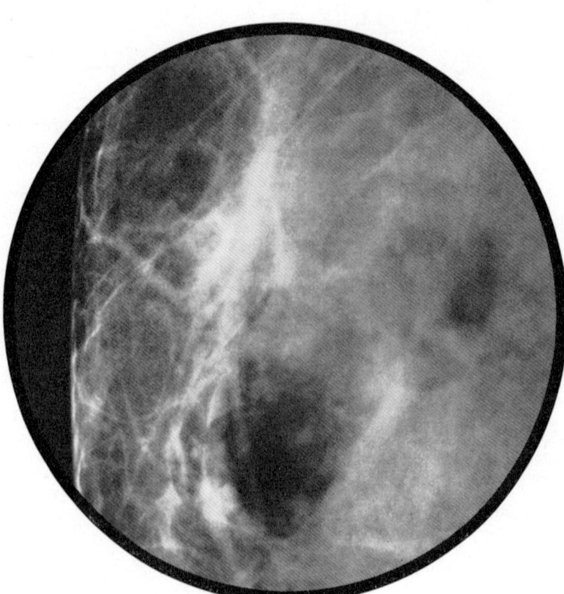

Fig. **51**.12b   Compression view of this area reveals normal parenchyma and no stellate mass. The finding in the craniocaudad examination represented a summation shadow.

Note: In evaluating a stellate shaped density, the compression mammogram with a smaller tube head is very important. This will either support or negate the original diagnostic suspicion.

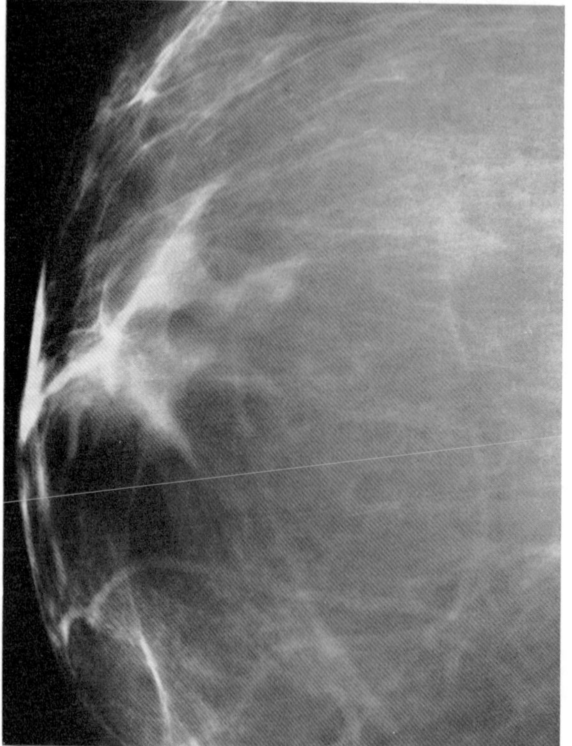

Fig. **51**.13   Subareolar stellate soft tissue density in an involutional breast. This represented a subareolar parenchymal rest.

Note: The differentiation of such a finding from a subareolar scirrhus carcinoma can only be accomplished by the use of compression, mammograms with manual pulling on the nipple. This is especially true if the clinical findings are negative (also see fig. 51.8).

In order to make the differential diagnosis of stellate shaped densities in the mammogram easier the following table of pathological and other etiologies causing this kind of pattern is provided.

Entities described in previous chapters are included in this table.

Stellate shaped irregular densities in the mammogram of the female breast may represent the following pathological entities:

Differential Diagnosis of Stellate Shaped Densities

1) Scirrhus carcinoma and carcinoma simplex with scirrhus components
2) Sclerosing adenosis
3) Hyalinized fibroadenoma with fibrosis
4) Hyalinized fibroadenoma
5) Circumscribed fibrosing mammary dysplasia
6) Acute mastitis
7) Sclerosing form of tuberculosis
8) Actinomycosis
9) Fistula formation
10) Subareolar fibrosis secondary to plasma cell mastitis (secretory disease)
11) Healed fat necrosis with associated fibrosis
12) Scars following incision and drainage or excisional biopsy
13) Scars following trauma
14) Scars following inflammation
15) Summation shadows.

Chapter 52

Differential Diagnosis of Diffuse Density of the Breast

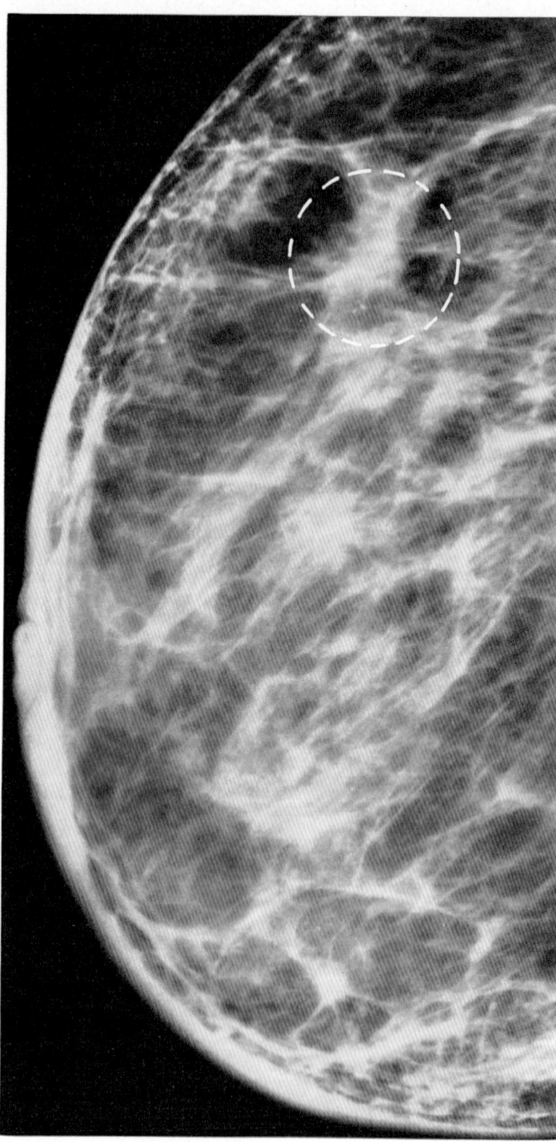

Fig. **52**.1   Diffuse reticular infiltration of the subcutaneous tissues and of the entire mass of this involutional breast in a 75-year-old woman. There is skin thickening between the region of the nipple and the inframammary fold.
Differential diagnosis: Lymphangitis carcinomatosa? Lymphatic block? Extensive acute mastitis? Fibroliposarcoma?
Note: The diagnosis of carcinoma was made on the basis of a localized soft tissue density containing microcalcifications typical for carcinoma in the upper half of the breast.

In the differential diagnosis of diffuse increased density of the breast one must decide whether this density is restricted to the body of the breast and that the skin thickness and subcutaneous fatty layer are normal or that it is the result of thickening of the skin and reticular proliferation of the subcuteneous connective tissues. Whenever such diffuse changes are encountered one must perform an overexposed mammogram to rule out a mass or microcalcifications which might be obscured by the diffuse increased density of the breast.

If one is dealing with a diffuse reticular connective tissue proliferation in the subcutaneous tissues or a diffuse overlying skin thickening of the breast one cannot decide from the mammogram whether this process is the result of carcinomatous infiltration, ordinary infection and inflammation, a diffuse hematoma, or breast edema secondary to cardiac failure or lymphatic obstruction. The ill-defined and blurred posterior margin of the overlying skin as well as the ill-defined blending of thickened skin into areas of normal thickness, although typical for mastitis, may also occur in carcinoma.

The diffuse reticular permeation of the subcutaneous fatty layer by a carcinoma is also very difficult to differentiate from edema as well as from a hematoma.

The clinical signs as well as the roentgen findings are not decisive since erythema of the skin may be found in mastitis as well as inflammatory carcinoma. Skin edema in the form of "peau d'orange" may be found in carcinoma as well as local edema secondary to lymphatic obstruction in the axillary nodes secondary to Hodgkin's disease or leukemia, and also in cardiac anasarca. Retraction of the nipple in diffuse skin edema may occur in carcinoma as well as in all other causes of breast edema.

We will show cases in which the differential diagnosis of the underlying cause of the roentgen findings is problematic. Only careful analysis of all the roentgen changes considered with the clinical signs, historical data and course of the disease will lead to the correct diagnosis.

In certain rare cases of diffuse breast disease the differential diagnosis given here is limited because these cases are not part of our own experience or observation. For example, the *diffuse* form of tuberculosis we only know from the literature (LEBORGNE) since we have not seen such a case. The history indicated the presence of pulmonary or extrapulmonary tuberculosis; however, this was not obligatory. The mammographic picture resembles that of diffuse carcinoma. It also resembles ordinary mastitis. A specific roentgen diagnosis is impossible. The disease however is rare.

The manifestations of acute lymphocytic leukemia of the breast are extremely rare. Since the first description by McWILLIAMS (1912) a total of 7 cases have been reported, one of which was a 15-year-old girl (KENNEDY et al 1970) with bilateral involvement.

In these cases, roentgenologically, there was diffuse infiltration of the breast. Clinical examination revealed tense enlarged breasts with ecchymosis. Following adequate therapy the clinical and roentgen findings disappeared within a period of four days. The correct diagnosis can only be made taking into account the history, clinical and laboratory data.

Leiomyomatosis consists of an essentially benign neoplasm of smooth muscle (erector pili muscles, muscle tissue associated with sweat glands, tunica media of blood vessels, smooth muscle fibers of the nipple). We mention leimyomatosis as the cause of diffuse breast density only for completeness. MISGELT et al reported a case in the fall of 1970 which mammographically resembled that of carcinomatous lymphangitis without evidence of tumor or microcalcification. Histologically the diagnosis was leiomyomatosis.

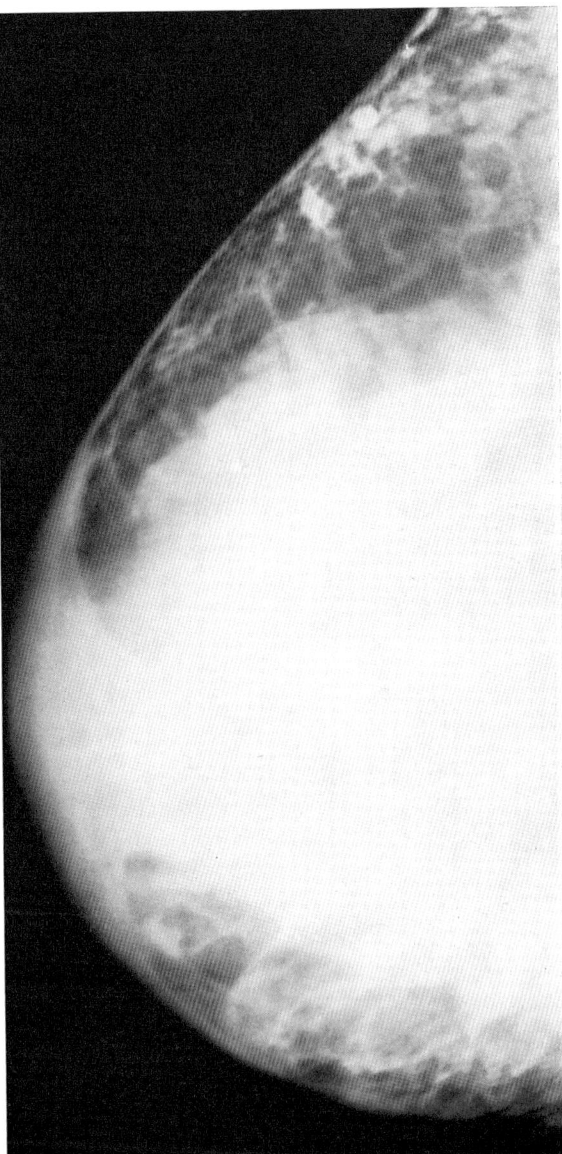

Fig. **52**.2 Diffuse increased density of the breast with a nodular mass in the upper half and a reticular infiltration in the lower half. There is infiltration of the subcutaneous fatty layer and diffuse skin thickening in this 65-year-old woman. The nodular mass suggests diffuse carcinoma.
Histology: Carcinoma.
Note: The diagnosis of inflammatory disease of the breast should not be the first consideration in the absence of recent gestation or lactation. This basic principle applies to local as well as diffuse breast disease.

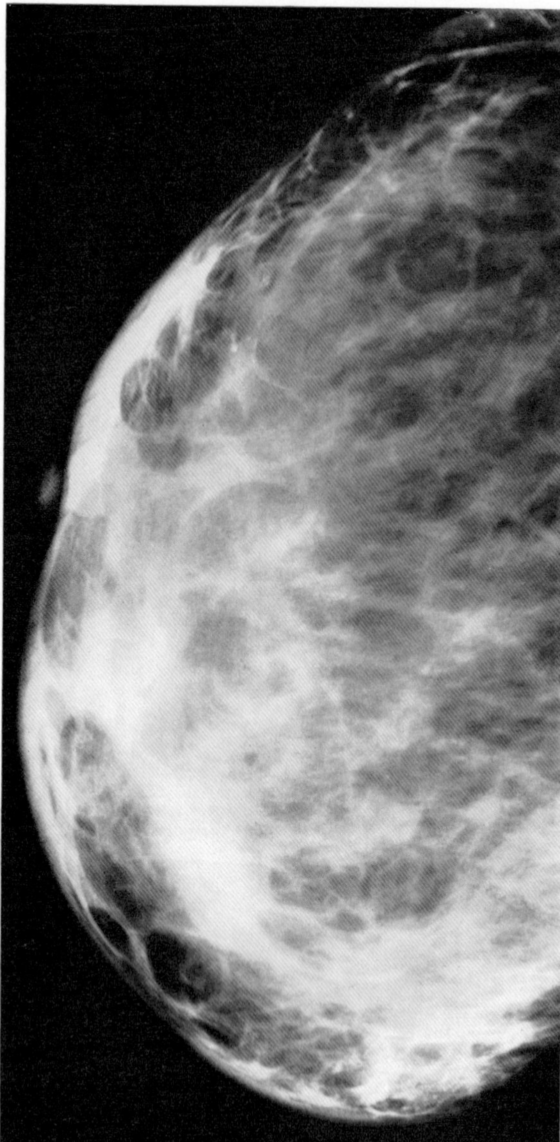

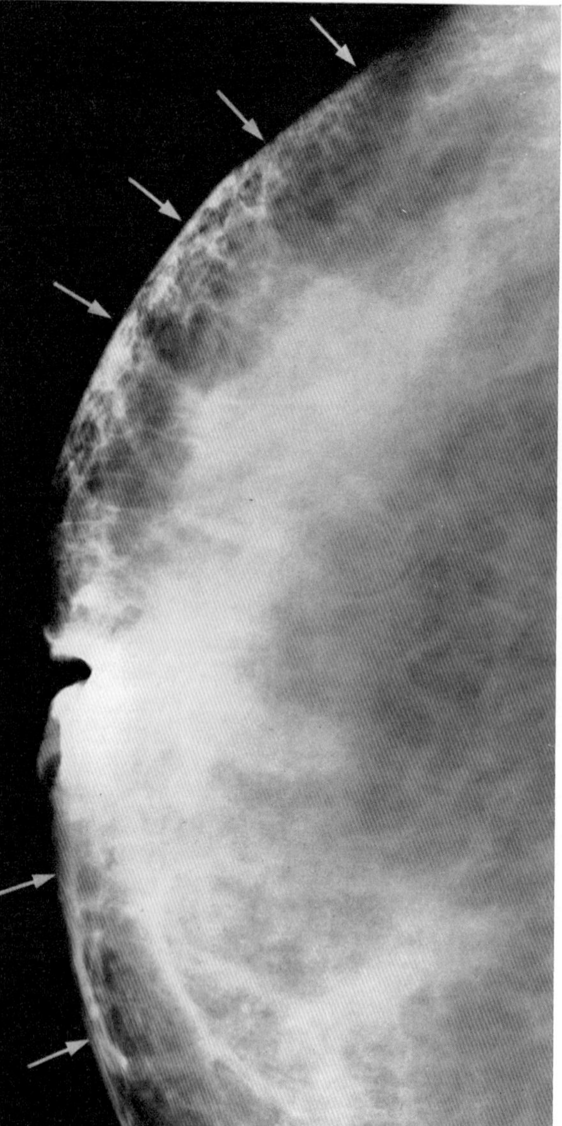

Fig. **52**.3 Diffuse coarsely reticular infiltration of the entire breast including the subcutaneous fatty layer, associated with generalized skin thickening in a 45-year-old woman. In addition to a unilaterally firm breast with diffuse skin edema (peau d'orange) a group of matted hard lymph nodes was palpated in the axilla.

Important in the diagnosis is the knowledge that the patient has a histologically verified lymphoma. Following radiation therapy to the axillary lymph nodes, the edematous changes of the breast disappeared. The breast abnormality represented lymphedema rather than direct lymphomatous involvement of the breast.

Note: In this case the differential diagnosis is based on clinical history and physical examination.

Fig. **52**.4 Diffuse infiltration of the breast with reticular infiltration of the subcutaneous fatty layer in the lateral half of the breast (4 arrows) with normal subcutaneous fatty layer medially (2 arrows). There is nipple retraction.

Clinical history indicates recent incision and drainage of an abscess just to the left of the areola. There is widespread mastitis in the lateral half of the breast. It is this process which has caused the subcutaneous infiltration and the skin thickening in the lateral half of the breast, as seen in the roentgenogram.

Note: In any case of mastitis not associated with recent pregnancy and lactation, carcinoma can only be ruled out by biopsy and histological investigation, and follow-up mammographic and clinical examinations.

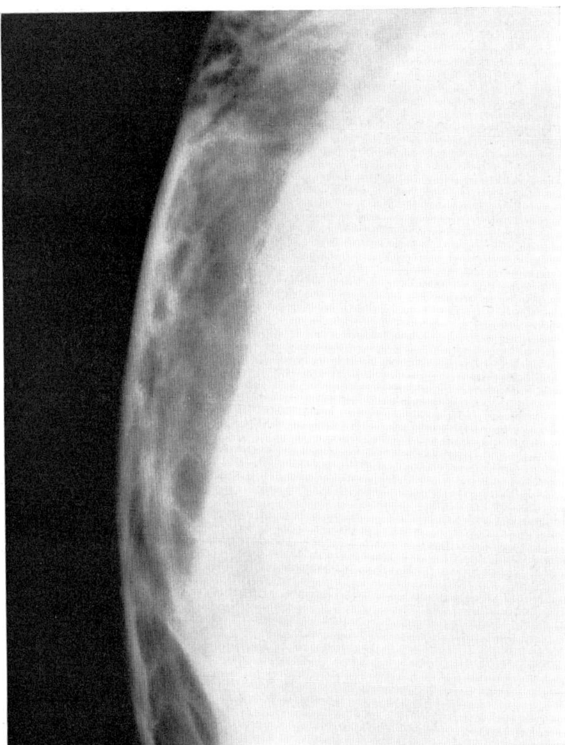

Fig. **52**.5a   Thickening of the skin, edematous appearance of the subcutaneous tissues. As a result there is shown a ground-glass, somewhat reticular blurring of the subcutaneous fat layer.
Clinical impression: Typical hematoma following auto accident. Follow-up mammogram 6 weeks after definite regression of clinical findings reveals a normal breast (Fig. 52.5b). Skin and subcutaneous tissues are unremarkable.
Note: History and clinical examination led to the correct diagnosis.
In any hematoma of the breast, however, carcinoma must be considered because a tumor eroding blood vessels may result in spontaneous breast hematoma.

Fig. **52**.5a

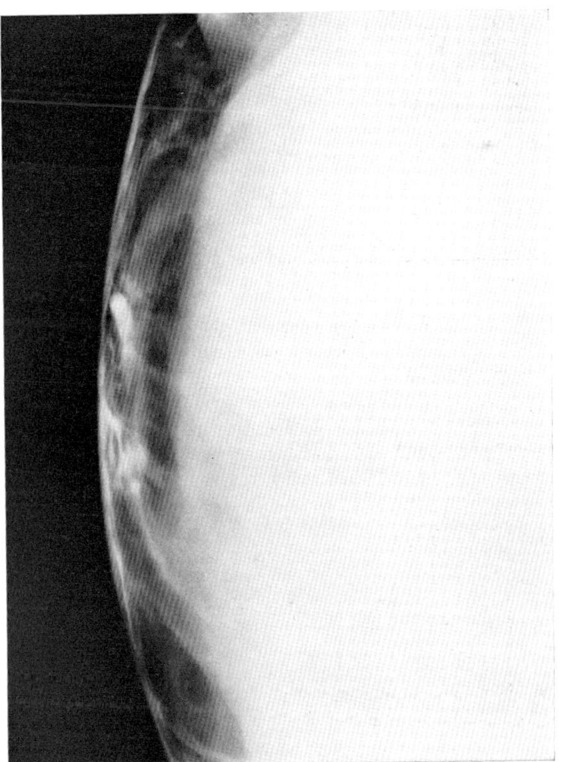

Fig. **52**.5b

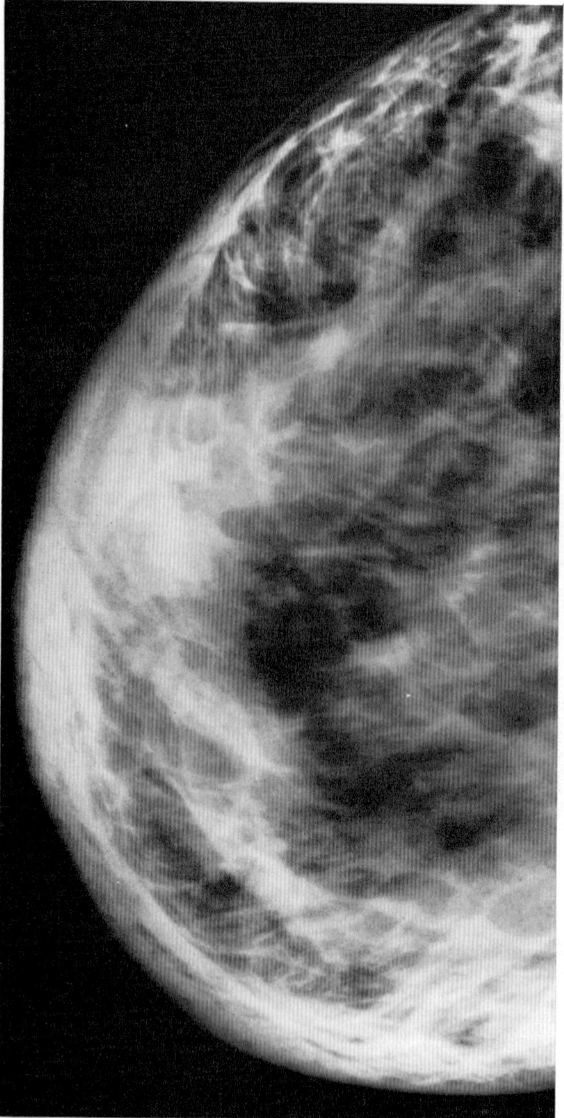

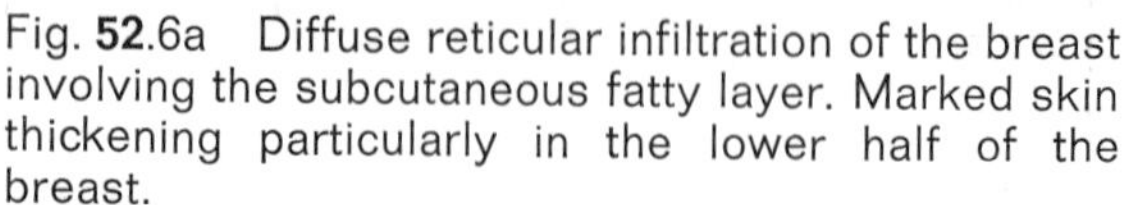

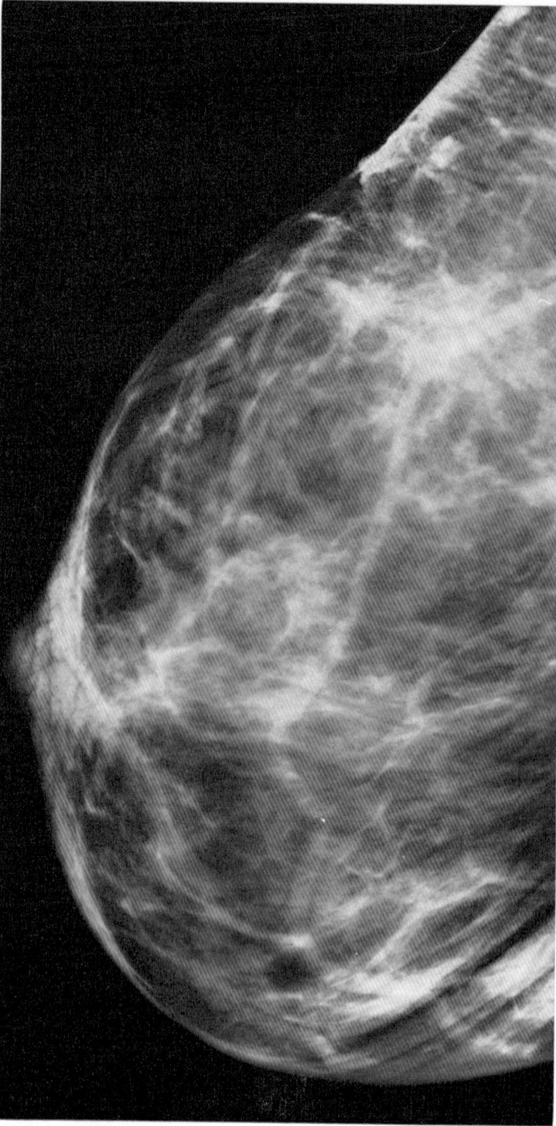

Fig. **52**.6a   Diffuse reticular infiltration of the breast involving the subcutaneous fatty layer. Marked skin thickening particularly in the lower half of the breast.
The same findings were noted in the other breast suggesting a bilateral diffuse carcinoma.
Clinically there was bilateral skin thickening with peau d'orange. Furthermore, heart failure with hepatomegaly and severe bilateral dependent edema was observed. Differential diagnosis now leans toward bilateral breast edema secondary to congestive heart failure.

Fig. **52**.6b   Following treatment of congestive heart failure and resolution of edema, mammography 8 days later reveals bilaterally normal breasts.
Note: In the event of bilateral breast edema a cardial origin should be considered.

In order to make the differential diagnosis of diffuse increased density of the breast easier we have compiled the following table of frequently occurring pathological entities which may produce this appearance. Some of the entities in the table have been discussed in previous chapters.

The following pathological entities may manifest as diffuse density of the breast in the roentgenogram:

Differential Diagnosis of Diffuse Breast Changes

1) Diffuse carcinoma
2) Hodgkin's disease
3) Lymphatic obstruction
4) Cardiac edema
5) Leukemia
6) Extensive acute mastitis
7) Diffuse form of tuberculosis
8) Status post multiple excisional biopsies
9) Status after radiation therapy
10) Exceptionally large hematoma
11) Giant fibroadenoma
12) Fibroliposarcoma
13) Silicone prosthesis
14) Advanced mammary dysplasia
15) Leiomyomatosis.

Early Detection of Breast Carcinoma

The incidence of breast carcinoma is increasing in almost all countries. In spite of this the mortality has remained unchanged in the last 30 to 50 years (SHIMKIN 1967). The improved prognosis is primarily a function of earlier diagnosis and treatment whereas other factors (histological nature of the tumor, host resistance) play a secondary role. The various methods of therapy differ little among one another in achieved results.

"Early diagnosis" may be considered as that stage when the diameter of the tumor is less than 2 cm (stage T-1) and the regional lymph nodes are histologically free of metastases. The 10-year survival rate in the absence of axillary lymph node involvement is 70—90% and with lymph node involvement 29—33% according to EGAN (1969) and GILBERTSEN (1966).

According to FARROW (1970) the discovery of a noninvasive carcinoma constitutes the "earliest" diagnosis. The "earliest" and "early diagnosis" of breast carcinoma may be achieved through the use of the following three diagnostic methods according to FARROW (1968):

1) broad clinical indications for excisional biopsy and extensive excisional biopsy;
2) serial sectioning of the entire excised preparation;
3) mammography.

We shall not deal with the first two modes of diagnosis but concern ourselves primarily with the role of roentgen diagnostic methods in the detection of clinically occult breast carcinoma and also deal with serial and survey examinations using mammography.

Chapter 53

Clinically Occult Breast Carcinoma

Breast carcinoma is considered occult when it is not detectable with the usual clinical methods of examination. There are "occult early carcinomas' without metastases and "occult late carcinomas" with metastases; in the latter case the primary tumor of the breast is not diagnosable clinically. A carcinoma may be clinically occult when:

1) the tumor is too small to be palpable;
2) the tumor is small in relation to a large breast, or the tumor is deep within the breast;
3) there is no change in consistency between the tumor and the surrounding tissues because the carcinoma is soft, is growing primarily intraductally, or is located within an area of fibrous dysplasia or mastitis.

An occult breast carcinoma is discovered by survey or prophylactic examinations or by accident.

Included in this category are occult late carcinomas which are discovered during the search

Table 53.1

Author	Total number of examinations	Serial examinations	Occult total	Occult by serial examinations	Axillary metastases in occult carcinoma	Microcalcification as the only sign of occult carcinoma	Remarks
Asch (1963)	500	—	4	—	—	—	
Doane and Williams (1963)	108	—	1	—	—	—	
Egan (1964)	3818	—	85	—	27	—	10% of all carcinomas are occult.
Friedman et al (1966)	2022	—	7	—	—	—	
Gershon-Cohen et al (1967)	—	about 22 000 on 1120 women	20	20	—	6(?)	Serial examinations at half year intervals for ten years.
Gros (1960)	—	—	60	—	—	—	
Lanyi and Littmann (1970)	2550	1450	13	4	6	6	
Lee et al (1963)	1035	603	11	3	—	—	
Lindell and Boyle (1961)	206	—	4	—	—	—	
Picard and Desprez-Curley 1958)	2500	—	35	—	—	—	In 11 cases of palpable carcinoma one contralateral occult carcinoma.
Rogers, Powell and Egan (1966)	6311	—	21	—	—	—	5% of all carcinomas were occult. 58 biopsies performed on the basis of roentgenological indications.
Scherer and Seifert (1968)	—	1080	5	5	—	—	Published material and personal communication.
Stevens (1966 and 1967)	—	3943	6	6	—	—	Published material and personal communication.
Strax et al (1967)	—	20 211	21	21	4 (19%)	—	Of 21 occult carcinomas, 18 are clinically negative, three cases uncertain.
Tortora et al (1967)	—	2000	4	4	—	—	
Witten (1967)	35 000	5014	132	8	—	—	Published material and personal communication. Among 57 carcinomas not discovered by serial examination 19% had axillary metastases. In eight occult carcinomas discovered by serial examination, no metastases.
Wolfe (1965 and 1967)	20 000	4000	16	16	2	2	Published material and personal communication.

for a primary tumor on the basis of demonstrated metastases. To our knowledge the first work on roentgen diagnosis of occult breast carcinoma was published by GERSHON-COHEN et al in 1956. According to our search of the literature (table 53.1) 445 clinically occult breast carcinomas have been discovered with the help of mammography up to the year 1970. This number, however, in no way reflects the actual situation because through personal communications we have recorded more than 200 cases of occult breast carcinoma discovered in this fashion, none of which were published. The number of roentgenologically discovered breast carcinomas builds up as experience increases. We have ourselves been able to find more than 50 clinically occult breast carcinomas between 1969 and 1971.

There are few reports in the literature as to any numerical relationship between occult late carcinoma and occult early carcinoma. According to a study by LANYI and LITTMANN (1970) of 179 cases in which the status of metastases was known there were 50 cases with demonstrable metastases in the axillary lymph nodes. According to this data approximately 75% of occult breast carcinomas belong in the early group and approximately 25% of cases fall into the category of late carcinoma.

Some of these occult breast carcinomas diagnosed with the help of mammography were in the "in situ" stage.

The roentgen signs of occult breast carcinoma are the same as those for the nonoccult variety. The characteristic microcalcifications are the predominant finding and about 40% of occult carcinomas were discovered solely on the basis of microcalcifications (LANYI and LITTMANN 1970). In other cases the suspicion of occult carcinoma was engendered by small stellate or round densities or, much more rarely, by unilateral subareolar lactiferous duct ectasia, or increased vascularity. In the breast with hemorrhagic discharge ductography (GROS and BURG 1957) resulted in the diagnosis of small, nonpalpable intraductal carcinoma.

Naturally not every clinically negative but roentgenologically suspect case will result in the histological diagnosis of breast carcinoma. According to URBAN (1960) one may count on a histologically verified roentgen diagnosis of occult breast carcinomas in approximately 50% of cases; according to GRIESBACH (1969) as well

as LANYI and LITTMANN (1970) the figure is approximately 33% of cases while GERSHON-COHEN et al (1958) report the figure as only 20% of cases. Frequently histological examination will reveal intraductal epithelial proliferation with cellular atypia of varying grades which is considered a precancerous stage (GALLAGER and MARTIN 1969), making the roentgen suspicion of occult carcinoma in such cases actually correct.

Of course there are not only clinically occult but also *roentgenologically occult* breast carcinomas which are only discovered later on in a follow-up examination. In this regard the words of INGLEBY and GERSHON-COHEN are appropriate:

"It is incorrect to insist that every 'clinically occult' tumor may be diagnosed roentgenologically . . . . . ., but we should not forget that months or years may pass before a preclinical tumor achieves the stage at which it can be detected by physical methods. If the radiologist missed the chance at an early cure, his only consolation is that at the time when he was confronted with the problem no one else was able to make the diagnosis either."

There are three groups of tumors that fall into the roentgenologically false negative diagnostic category:

1) Carcinomas which were not recognized in the roentgenogram. This involves primarily the interpretation of a medullary carcinoma as a fibroadenoma or cyst (puncture, aspiration and cytological examination were not performed!), interpretation of microcalcification of a carcinoma as the calcification of sclerosing adenosis, and the interpretation of carcinomatous connective tissue changes as mammary dysplasia.

2) Carcinomas which were missed because of incomplete roentgen examination. Such misdiagnoses are based on errors in technique; for example, underpenetrated mammograms or incomplete representation of the breast in the mammogram, or failure to include areas with positive clinical findings in the mammogram.

3) Carcinomas which, in spite of optimal mammographic technique and examination, cannot be diagnosed in the mammogram. The latter category consists primarily of intraductal duct carcinoma which because of the absence of tumor necrosis failed to exhibit

microcalcifications. If such carcinomas occur in a portion of the breast which is dense because it is rich in parenchyma or are associated with an area of increased tissue density secondary to mammary dysplasia they are not recognizable in the roentgenogram. These tumors may be extensive and even invasive. As long as nodular or scirrhus changes are absent the tumor cannot be recognized in the mammogram. This latter category is a natural shortcoming of mammography as a method of diagnosis, whereas the preceding two categories of false negative diagnosis indicate a fault of the mammographer and/or the technique of mammography.

Preparation for Biopsy and Histological Examination of Occult Breast Carcinoma

The axiom that any suspicious change in the breast warrants histological examination is true not only for the clinician but also for the mammographer. However, there are still cases where histological examination of an occult carcinoma, diagnosed in the roentgenogram, was not undertaken because biopsy was refused by the patient, the referring physician and the surgeon. Therefore some preparation of the patient, the referring physician and the surgeon is necessary to obtain permission for biopsy.

The patient is usually willing to permit biopsy when the occult carcinoma is symptomatic as with pain or swelling of lymph nodes. She is also so inclined if one breast has already been removed, if there is cancer phobia or if someone in the family or in the neighborhood has had a breast carcinoma. It is extremely important to convince the referring physician about the need for biopsy. The patient is more inclined to agree to biopsy if her own physician shares this conviction.

A close working relationship with the surgeon is particularly important and in the best interest of the patient. The "skeptical surgeon" as described by GERSHON-COHEN et al can do significant damage to the patient either by advising against biopsy or failing to consult the mammographer prior to biopsy and thus missing the carcinoma at operation (LANYI 1967; LANYI et al 1968). It is therefore recommended that the biopsy be performed by a surgeon who is well informed concerning the value as well as the limits of mammography. The best result is obtained by teamwork between a surgeon and a roentgenologist who enjoy one another's confidence. Therefore, we should, with the consent of the supervising physician, always try to convince the patient to agree to that diagnostic procedure which is most likely to yield a correct diagnosis of occult carcinoma. We have found, as have BARKER et al (1969), that personal consultation with the surgeon is best on the day preceding surgery rather than the same day since at the time the patient is already premedicated and localization of the suspicious area interferes with the normal activities preceding surgery.

Geometric Localization

We have worked out the following procedure in localization (fig. 53.1 a—c):
1) the exact location of the suspicious area on the roentgenogram is located by coordinates on an X and Y axis;
2) the suspicious area is localized on the skin of the breast in relation to the nipple with non-washable ink (for example fuchsin);
3) the measurements of the above coordinates are transferred to the skin of the breast thus localizing the lesion precisely for the surgeon.

Geometric localization is not a very precise method of indicating what portion of the breast tissue is to be excised because of the changes in the position of the breast during surgery. Therefore, even with this method of localization, any excision of a nonpalpable process means removal of a large volume of tissue. Intraoperative specimen radiography is essential.

In the case of occult carcinoma located in a subareolar position the above method of localization is not necessary. All that is needed is to indicate the depth of the process in centimeters.

Needle Localization

Localization of an occult process by geometric methods may be made more precise by insertion of one or two needles. The position of the needles must be corrected and verified by repeat mammograms in both lateral and craniocaudal projections. The disadvantages of this method are:
1) pain;
2) problems with sterility of the tissues;
3) inadvertent displacement of the indwelling needle during mammograms for needle localization and during transport of the patient to the operating table or during surgery.

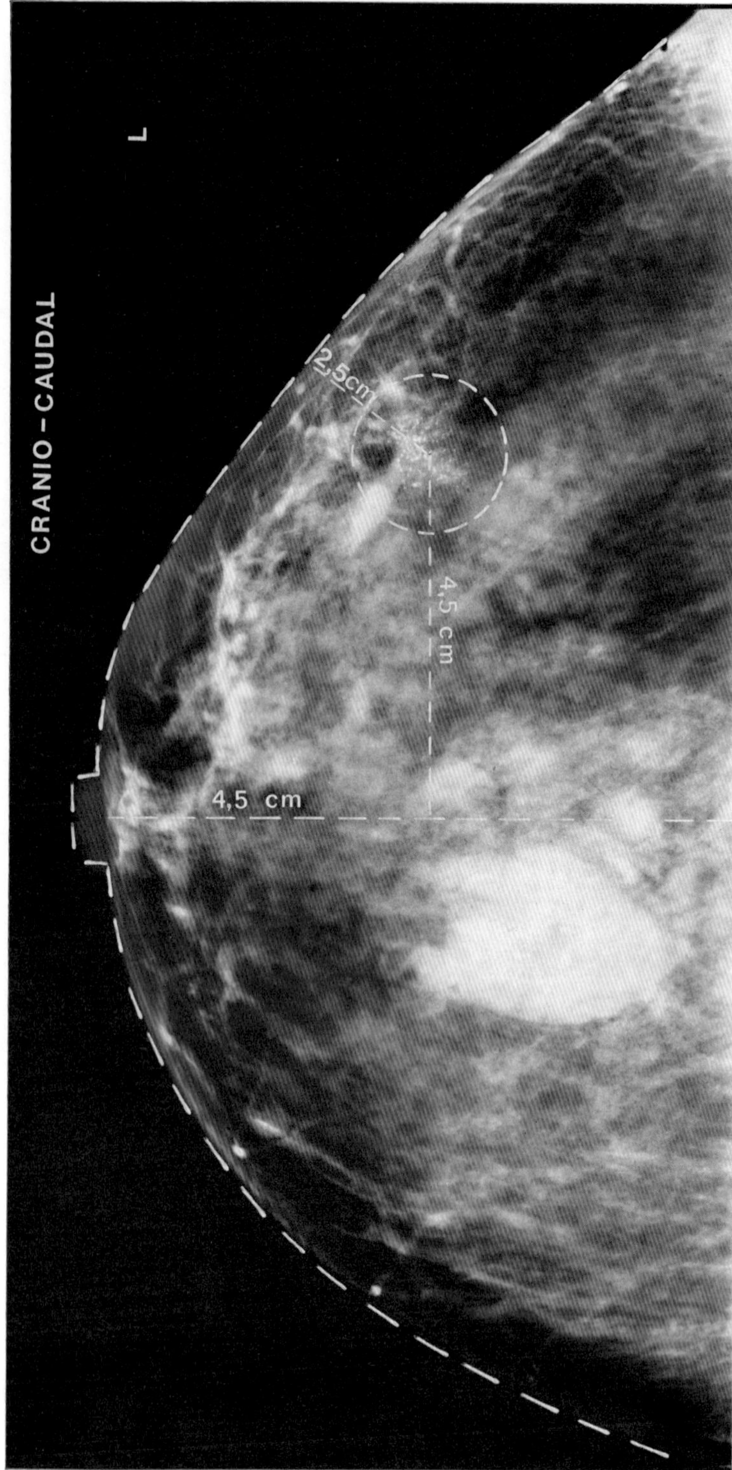

Fig. **53.**1a   Craniocaudal projection.

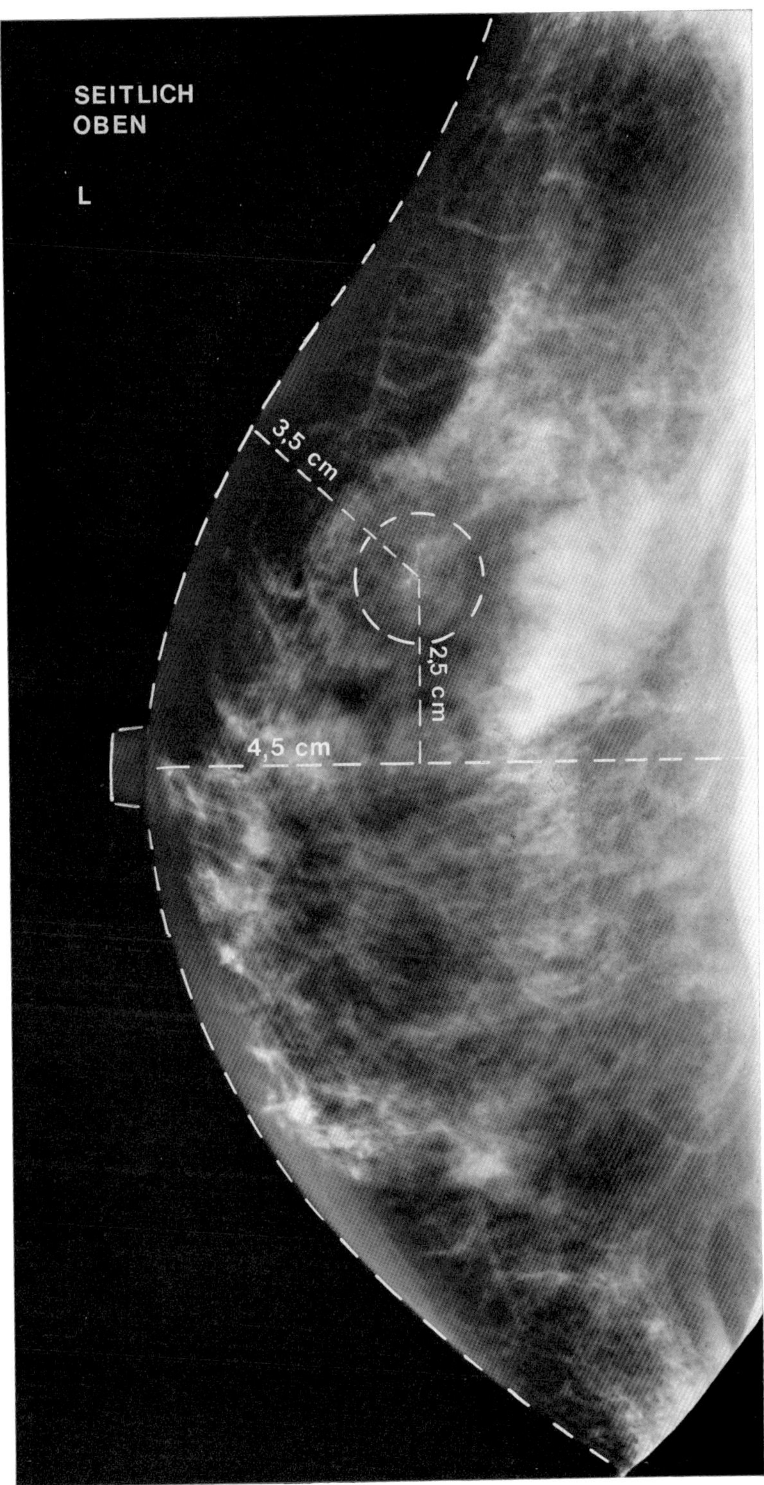

Fig. **53.**1 b.   Lateral projection.
The suspicious group of microcalcifications is localized in relation to the vertical and horizontal lines drawn on the breast and relative to the skin.

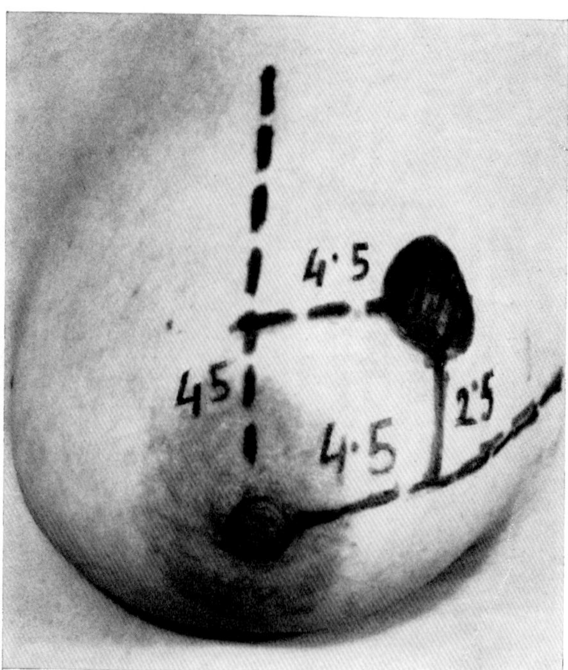

Fig. **53**.1c The measurements obtained on the mammogram are then transferred to the skin of the breast with indelible ink. The numbers indicate the depth of the lesion as noted on the roentgenogram, not the distance on the skin.

Contrast — Color Dye Localization

A reliable localization of a suspicious process may be obtained by injection of a mixture of radiographic contrast material and colored dye. Geometric localization is followed by intra-mammary localization by injection of a mixture of 0.4 cc of radiographic contrast material and 0.1 cc of colored dye. Any aqueous iodinated radiographic contrast material which is excreted by the kidneys is suitable. Concentration should be approximately 60—70%. Patent Blue or similar colored indicators are suitable for the colored dye. The amount of the mixture used for such localization should be kept to a minimum.

Follow-up mammograms in two projections at right angles will indicate whether the spot of contrast material is exactly within the region of the suspicious process (fig. 53.2a and b). If this is not the case, it is necessary to advise the surgeon as to the exact location of the suspicious lesion in relation to the dye collection. In order to prevent extensive diffusion of the colored dye within the breast it is recommended that no more than 30 minutes time interval occur between injection and surgery.

The surgeon orients the approach for biopsy according to the location of the dye deposit. In order to insure that the suspicious tissue has been removed intraoperative specimen radiography is essential (fig. 53.3a). Sectioning of a larger biopsy specimen into smaller portions and repeat specimen radiography lightens the task of the pathologist in localizing the tissue containing the suspected lesion (fig. 53.3b). Small carcinomas, even those *not* containing microcalcifications are reliably and rapidly excisable using this technique (fig. 53.4).

If the suspected lesion consists only of micro-calcifications, frozen section should not be performed.

If mammographic findings and histological results do not coincide and there is significant doubt that the cause of the variants is the result of examining the wrong biopsy section, a further examination must be performed and should include:

1) follow-up mammography of the patient and eventual repeat biopsy;
2) repeat specimen radiography of the paraffin blocks containing the tissue and eventual further sectioning.

Lactiferous Duct Localization

Localization of an occult lesion detected at ductography may also be performed through the use of a mixture of contrast material and colored dye (Patent Blue). The suspicious duct is injected with the mixture, and the correct localization verified by follow-up mammograms in cranio-caudad and lateral projections. The surgeon then explores and excises the stained duct.

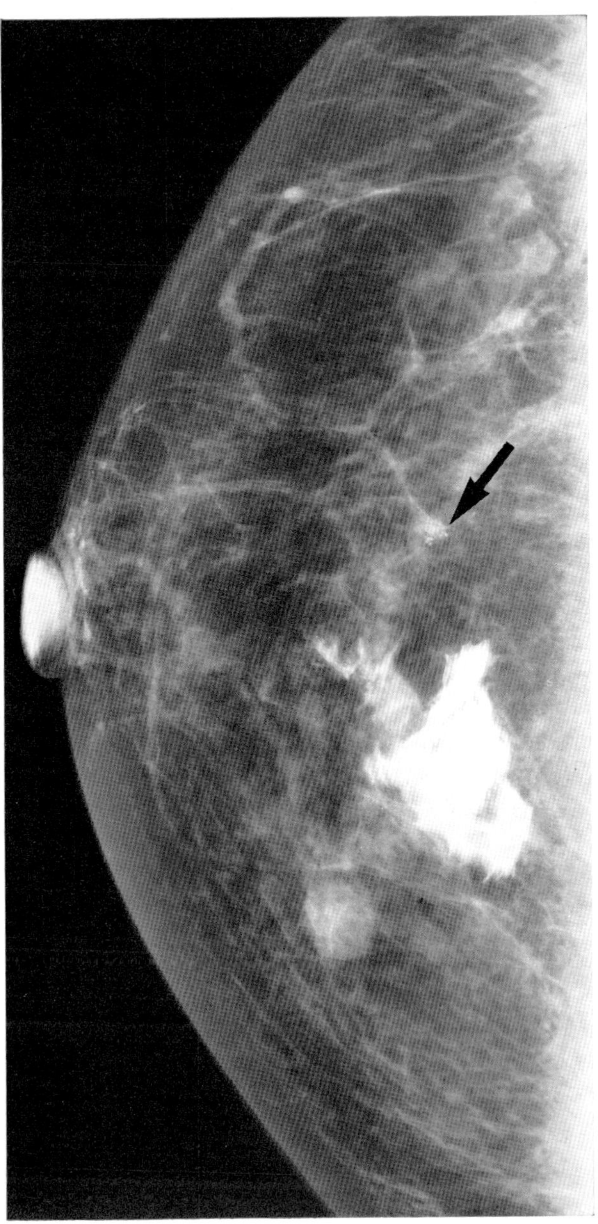

Fig. **53**.2a   Localization of a cluster of microcalcifications with contrast media — Patent-Blue — injection (lateral view).

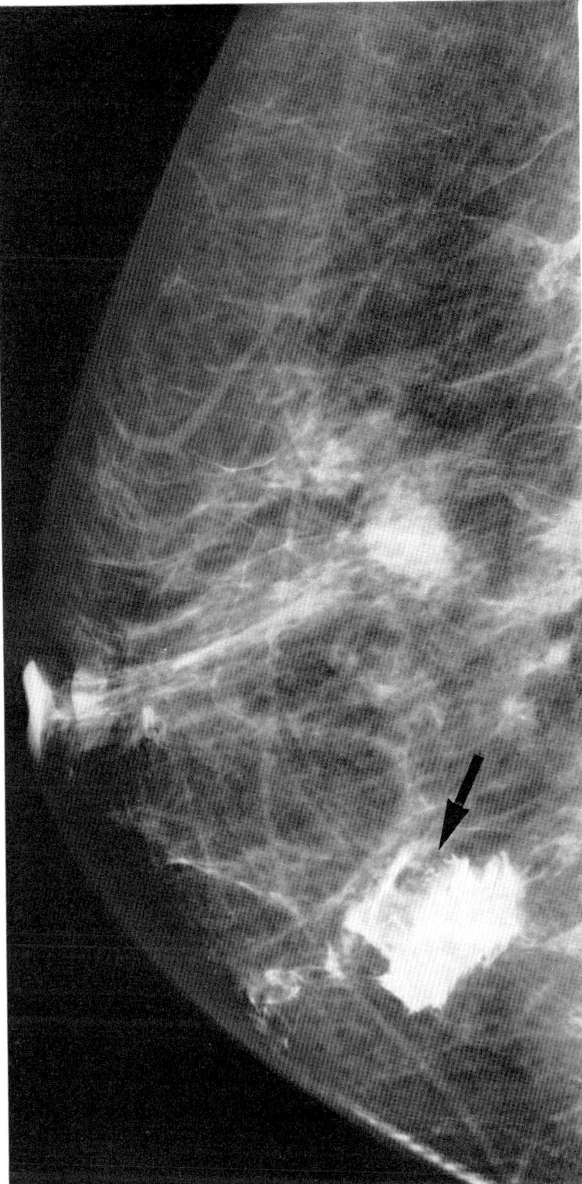

Fig. **53**.2b   The craniocaudad projection indicates that the contrast material was injected approximately 2 cm away from the cluster of microcalcifications. The deposit of dye facilitates easier open biopsy for the surgeon.

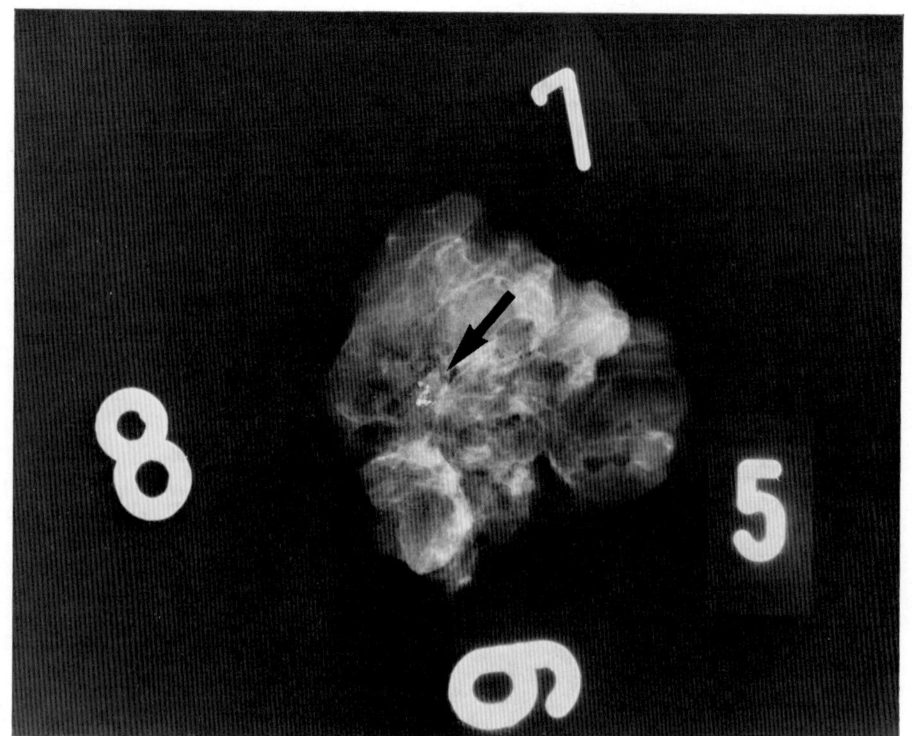

Fig. **53**.3a   Intraoperative mammographic examination of the biopsy material: The suspicious cluster of microcalcifications has been excised.

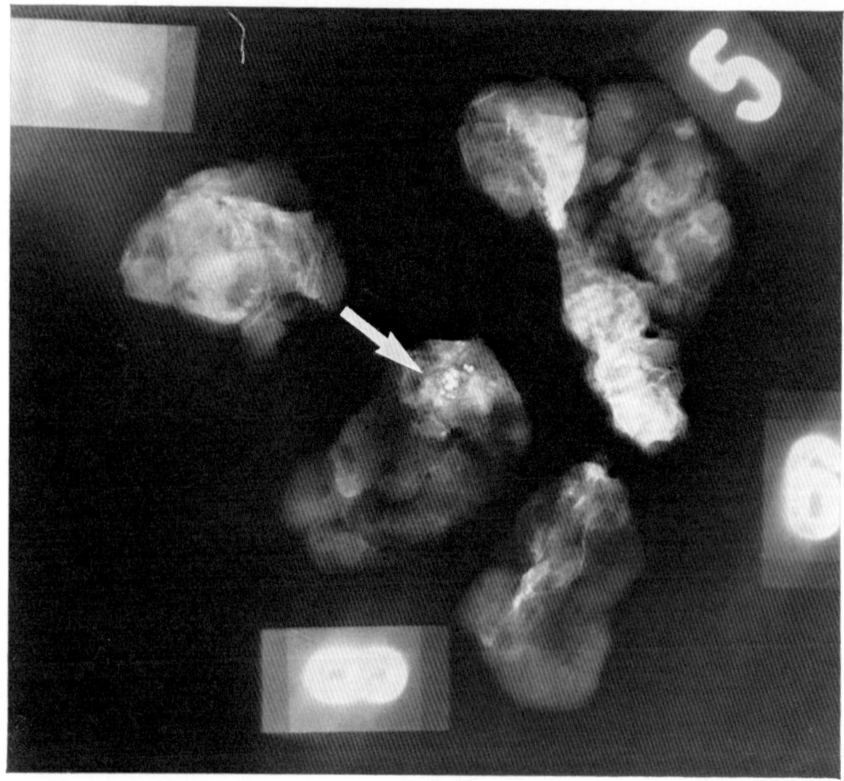

Fig. **53**.3b   Specimen radiography of the sectioned biopsy. This makes it easier for the pathologist to find and examine the suspicious microcalcifications. The individual biopsy sections are indicated by lead markers.

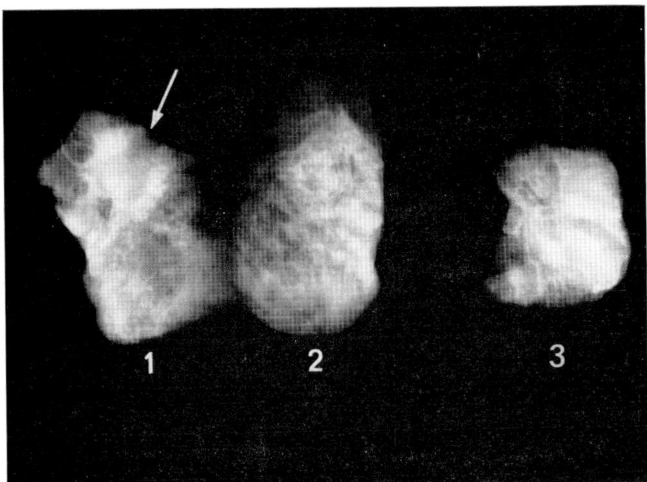

Fig. **53**.4   Roentgenogram of surgical specimens: Only after the third attempt was it possible to remove the specimen containing the occult carcinoma. The preparation demarcated with the numbers 2 and 3 were roentgenologically not suspicious. In the specimen marked with numeral 1 the tumor nodule was found (arrow).

Serial Examinations

In the majority of cases (90—95%) breast carcinoma is discovered by the patient herself (FARROW 1965; GERSHON-COHEN et al 1967). Sixty-five to ninety percent of carcinomas so discovered are already no longer in the Steinthal I stage (GERSHON-COHEN et al 1967; MANNHERZ and KUHWALD 1966). Among these patients there is an approximately 50% five-year survival following diagnosis. According to CUTLER (1966) periodic routine self-examination raises the incidence of discovery of carcinoma in earlier stages by about 4%. Although this is a small figure, one cannot dispute the value of self-examination. GILBERTSEN (1969) has reported on a 21-year-long observation (40,633 examinations) of 7,819 women who performed monthly self examination. Of the 66 carcinomas discovered in these patients, 25 were discovered by the patients themselves (38%). Of these ten carcinomas were already in Steinthal stage II.

Consequently the discovery of breast carcinoma must not be left to the patient or to chance but one must "organize" chance discovery for early diagnosis. The key to "organited chance discovery" is serial examination, namely:

1) clinical serial examination;
2) thermographic serial examination;
3) mammographic serial examination;
4) combined serial examination.

The value of *clinical serial examination* for the early detection of carcinoma is debatable. According to MCDONALD (1966) breast carcinomas discovered by clinical examinations should never be considered to be in an early stage. LEIS (1970) agrees and indicates that a palpable carcinoma even in the absence of lymph node metastases is never an early carcinoma. According to the experience of URBAN (1960) on the other hand, there is a five-year survival rate of 76% in patients with palpable carcinoma without lymph node metastases and 38.6% among those with lymph node metastases. BARNES et al (1968) in their clinical serial examination of 654 symptom-free women found 16 with breast changes. Among these five turned out to be carcinomas, one of which had lymph node metastases. Among 41 cases of breast carcinoma discovered during clinical serial examinations by GILBERTSEN (1969), eight patients demonstrated regional lymph node metastases. Clinical serial examination therefore increases the percentage of early diagnosis when carefully performed by an experienced examiner. However, it is inadequate as the only serial examination method.

The use of *thermography* as a method of serial examination, that is, in women without breast complaints, is much discussed in the current literature. The accuracy of this method is supposed to be 84—98% (GERSHON-COHEN and HERMEL 1969; HABERMANN 1968; NOTTER and MELANDER 1968; AARTS 1969). Many authors use thermography as an adjunct to mammography in order to increase the accuracy of the latter method of diagnosis (VAILLANT 1970).

HOFFMAN (1967) reports good results with 1,924 women. He found 24 histologically verified carcinomas of which 91.6% were correctly detected by thermography. Of these 24 carcinomas 16.7% were in an early stage. HOFFMAN therefore pleads for the use of thermography even though he has a 20% false positive diagnosis rate. HITCHCOCK et al (1968) by combining clinical and thermographic serial examination were only able to find one carcinoma among 2,523 women. Three carcinomas were missed. These authors also complained about the large group of false positive cases (13%).

Further criticism is offered by NATHAN et al (1972). They report on 346 patients examined with thermography. In 115 patients (59%) with localized hot spots no histological evidence of disease was found. The thermogram in these cases was falsely positive. In a further group of

Table 54.1

Author	Number of examinations	Number of carcinomas	Clinically occult	Lymph node metastases	Remarks
Dowdy et al (1970)	1735	17 (0.98%)	3	10	Combined serial examination. One bilateral carcinoma, four false negative cases.
Gershon-Cohen et al (1967)	22000	36 (0.163%)	20	11	Serial examinations at six months intervals of the same 1120 patients. Bilateral carcinoma in three cases.
Griesbach (1969)	25209	31 (0.12%)	12	12	Combined serial examinations. Among a total of 54 carcinomas 23 were roentgenologically occult.
Irvine and James (1969)	912	—	—	—	Combined serial examinations. No carcinoma detected clinically or roentgenologically.
Lanyi et al (1970)	1450	6 (0.41%)	4	1	Combined serial examination.
Rasmussen (1967)	1450	12 (0.83%)	8	—	Personal communication.
Scherer and Seifert (1968)	1080	8 (0.74%)	5	2	Combined serial examinations. 62 patients were symptomatic.
Stevens and Weigen (1969)	4706	14 (0.29%)	12	1	Annual combined serial examinations of the same 1223 patients. Six occult carcinomas were palpable at repeat examinations.
Strax et al (1967)	20211	31 (0.155%)	18	12	Combined serial examinations. See also: Shapiro et al (1966).
Tortora et al (1967)	2000	7 (0.35%)	4	1	—
Witten and Thurber (1964)	5014	8 (0.15%)	8	—	—
Wolfe (1965)	3891	16 (0.41%)	16	2	—
Total	89658	186 (0.2%)	110 (59%)	52 (27.9%)	—

164 patients with normal thermograms seven had carcinoma. The thermogram was normal 21% of the time in women with known breast carcinoma but registered an increased heat signal in 50% of healthy women.

As a method of serial examination, a 13—20% false positive rate is not tolerable. The missed carcinomas in the series reported by Hitchcock add further to this conclusion. Leis (1970) also expresses doubts about the value of thermography for the reason that small breast carcinomas often show no thermographic changes whatsoever. A final conclusion, however, cannot yet be made. The value of thermography as a method of serial examination will be decided after further comparative studies. We have our doubts.

Serial examination with *mammography* has been previously recommended by Gershon-Cohen et al (1956). These authors performed serial examinations of their patients at six months' intervals and have reported their results after five years (1961) and ten years (1967), and these are summarized in table 54.1. Mammographic serial examinations were performed in the United States by Dowdy et al (1970), Griesbach and Eads (1966), Griesbach (1969), Shapiro et al (1966), Strax et al (1967), (Shapiro and Strax are members of the same group of workers), Stevens and Weigen (1966), Stevens (1967), Witten and Thurber (1964), and Wolfe (1965). European publications on this method have been produced by Rasmussen (1967), Irvine and James (1969), Lanyi (1967), Lanyi et al (1970), Scherer and Seifert (1968), Tortora et al (1967). As stated above the results reported by most of these authors are summarized in table 54.1. This tabulation shows that among a total of almost 90,000 mammographic serial examinations 186 (0.2%) carcinomas were discovered. 60% of these carcinomas were occult and in 28% lymph node metastases were demonstrated.

The use of mammography as a method of serial examination in spite of the good results provides *numerous problems*. Witten summarizes some of these:

1) The accuracy of mammographic serial examination is low in premenopausal patients because the dense structure of the breast parenchyma may obscure carcinoma.

2) Mammographic serial examination demands a very considerable financial, technical, and personnel investment so that wide application is probably not feasible.

3) There is no statistical evidence so far that the mortality of patients in whom a breast carcinoma is found by serial examination is any less than if the examination had not taken place.

We *do not agree* with most of these considerations.

1) The accuracy of serial examination is obviously directly related to morbidity. In countries with low morbidity of breast carcinoma the accuracy of clinical as well as mammographic serial examination is lower than in countries with a higher incidence of breast carcinoma. The first objective and the great significance of mammographic serial examination is the early detection of clinically occult breast carcinomas. Even though the number of breast carcinomas so discovered according to table 4.1 represents only 0.2% of all examinations, the discovery of these clinically occult carcinomas still justifies serial roentgen examination. Without mammography these tumors would be treated later and therefore with a poorer prognosis. A further point in favor of mammographic serial examination is that in those breast carcinomas detected only 28% had lymph node metastases whereas the average incidence of metastases among clinically palpable breast carcinomas is 55—65% (GERSHON-COHEN et al 1967).

No doubt there are roentgenologically occult but clinically detectable carcinomas (STRAX et al 1967). This, however, does not miltate against mammography but rather indicates the need for combined serial examinations.

2) To solve these problems many recommendations have been made:

(a) Serial mammography should be restricted to high risk patients (see page 319): BYRNE et al (1968), DUNN (1969), HAYDEN (1969), LEWISON (1969), STEVENS and WEIGEN (1969), WYNDER (1969), and MAASS (1971).

(b) A combination of mammographic serial examination with gynecological serial examination has been recommended (DOWDY et al 1970). By restriction of mammographic examination only to clinically suspect cases, according to our statistics in table 54.1, only 76 carcinomas instead of 186 would have been found.

Aside from restricting the examination as described above there have been other suggestions to expedite this method of examination and also to decrease the expense:

The use of the Odelca camera for mammography has been recommended by STRAX (1965). However, the experience of LANYI (1970) in this regard in sot supportive.

The mechanization of diagnosis by the use of computers has been recommended by WINSBERG et al (1967) but so far has found no support.

The use of nonphysicians as specially trained personnel to conduct the examination has been recommended by DOWDY et al (1969). ALCORN and O'DONELL (1969) have had the only experience with this method to date.

3) GERSHON-COHEN et al (1967) report a 45% 5-year survival in patients whose breast carcinoma was not discovered by serial examinations compared to a 90% 5-year survival in those patients whose breast carcinoma was found by mammography. This report concerns only 33 cases and cannot be considered the final answer on this issue.

The extensive number of examinations conducted by SHAPIRO, STRAX and VENET (1971) produced the following results:

Among 31,000 women who underwent regular careful mammographic and clinical examinations for six years, 31 died of breast cancer. In the control group in which there was no regular examinations, 52 patients died of breast cancer. The difference is significant.

In our opinion it is absurd to forego the use of serial examination, which has been shown to increase the number of early diagnoses and therefore to improve the prognosis, because of its great expense or cost in personnel. This objection should be dismissed until cheaper methods which are equally effective become available.

Groups with Special Risk	Risk Factor
1) Patients with a family history of breast carcinoma	2 or more
2) With previous carcinoma of the other breast	8—10
3) With a long history of estrogen treatment	Unknown
4) Postmenopausal patients with vaginal smear revealing hormonal grade 3—4	Unknown
5) Patients with advanced mammary dysplasia	2
6) With proliferative complicated mammary dysplasia as revealed by biopsy	Approximately 2
7) With numerous mammographically demonstrated breast calcifications	Unknown
8) Patients with large breasts	Uncertainty of the clinical examination
9) Nulligravidae who have never lactated	1.5 to 2.3 (?)
10) Patients of advanced age	Increasing risk.

Results

Chapter 55

Statistics

The first statistics about the accuracy of mammographic diagnosis, originally published by WARREN (1930), are only of historical value. As summarized in table 55.1 the accuracy ranges from 46 to 98.8%. This variation is explainable by the differences in the evaluations, particularly as regards the inclusion of the diagnosis labeled as "suspicious". If the latter type of diagnosis were correct in terms of the final diagnosis then the accuracy rate will be high but if the "suspicion of carcinoma" is counted as a misdiagnosis then the statistical results will be poor. Additionally one must recall that over the years the technique of mammography has been improved and it is really not possible to compare previous statistics with those of today. Furthermore today ductography, pneumocystography, cytology, and thermography are used as adjuncts to mammographic diagnosis, making an isolated value judgment by roentgen examination really only of academic interest.

Much more important it seems to us is an evaluation of the causes of misdiagnoses. The blame for failing to diagnose a breast carcinoma may rest on the mammographer, the surgeon or the pathologist. We will concern ourselves only with the causes of radiological misdiagnosis. GERSHON-COHEN et al list technically inadequate roentgenograms, dense breast parenchyma or failure to recognize a significant roentgen sign as the primary causes of radiological misdiagnosis.

According to EGAN, false positive diagnoses are more frequent in sclerosing adenosis, infected cysts and abscesses of the breast. FRIEDMAN considers the diagnostic accuracy of mammography to be proportional to the age of the patient correlating approximately to the progressively decreasing density of the parenchyma with increasing age.

WOLFE (1966) lists dense and small breasts, and failure to recognize the significance of calcifications as the main causes of his diagnostic errors. Our views on the causes of diagnostic errors were explained in Chapter 53. These agree with the experience of GERSHON-COHEN and the other authors listed above.

Table 55.1

Author	Total number	Number of histological examinations			Accuracy of mammographic diagnosis (percent)		
		total	malignant	benign	total	malignant	benign
Asch (1963)	500	259	84	175	90.0	86.0	84.0
Buttenberg and Werner (1962)	860	158	—	—	96.1	91.9	99.8
Clark et al (1965)	1580	1580	475	1105	87.1	79.0	90.0
Dormann and Labusch (1958)	157	157	—	—	86.6	88.9	80.0
Egan (1964)	3818	1217	728	489	94.6	97.1	91.0
Friedman et al (1966)	2022	776	233	543	72.8	68.0	75.0
Gershon-Cohen et al (1954) (1960)	210 1500	210 536	47 —	163 —	94.7 98.0	85.0	97.0
Hessler and Gershon-Cohen (1965)	213	215	58	157	88.8	91.4	98.1
Kaufmann (1969)	—	619	259	360	56.5	61.0	53.3
Kremens (1958)	1000	372	124	248	62.6	98.8	97.9
Lanyi et al (1966)	440	140	—	—	77.0	—	—
Lohbeck and Frischbier (1969)	—	525	194	331	—	88.0	79.0
De Luca and Wentworth (1966)	5000	700	175	525	—	85.2	—
Martinelli et al (1969)	300	186	23	163	87.1	86.3	—
Muntean (1961)	488	168	79	89	90.0	92.4	92.1
Picard and Desprez-Curley (1958)	2500	569	430	139	82.2	86.4	67.6
Philipp et al (1964)	50	50	20	30	48.0	50.0	46.0
Rogers et al (1966)	3379	1270	411	859	80—88	70—88	76—96
Samuel and Young (1964)	450	245	—	—	82.4	—	—
Skinner (1963)	294	174	53	121	90.0	92.5	90.0
Warren (1930)	—	—	—	—	85.0	—	—
Weinstein and Endlich (1966)	13	13	—	13	92.0	—	92.0
Wolfe (1964)	2000	759	161	598	89.0	92.0	88.0

SUPPLEMENT

Thermography

Thermography is a method using a heat-sensing device, for the graphic recording of the natural emission of infrared radiation from the human body. It does not produce any ionizing radiation, is noninvasive, completely harmless, quickly and easily performed and readily interpreted.

LAWSON in 1956 observed circumscribed areas of increased temperatures on the skin of the breast in patients with breast carcinoma. These temperature changes were used to develop a new diagnostic method over the subsequent years. The recording of skin temperature in its simplest application can be performed with a contact thermometer, such as the Heimann bolometer (BUCHWALD). In the meanwhile technical advances have allowed the development of means for detecting and pictorially recording the temperature distribution of large portions of the body. These methods detect the heat radiated from the skin in the form of infrared emission. According to the law of Stefan-Boltzmann the heat radiated from a surface is directly proportional to the fourth power of its absolute temperature and the emissivity of the surfaces. Absolute temperature is measured according to the scale of K (Kelvin) and is derived by adding 273 to the centigrade temperature (for example, the body temperature of 37 C is 310 K). According to the law of Wien one may calculate the maximum wave length of the radiated heat spectrum according to the formula λmax T = 2898 in which the wave length is expressed in microns and the temperature is recorded according to the scale of Kelvin. For a skin temperature of 35° centigrade (308 K) the maximum emission is 9.4 microns which is in the deep infrared spectrum. Investigations by HARDY have shown that the skin in the infrared spectrum is similar to a "black body", thereby possessing a significant index of measurability.

Thermography

The detector of the thermographic apparatus (fig. 1) consists of an indium-antimony or a mercury-cadmium telluride crystal whose electrical resistance is altered by infrared rays (photoresistance; inner photoeffect). In order to reach the necessary sensitivity this crystal must be cooled with liquid nitrogen. Through the use of a system of rotating mirrors the detector scans areas of the body surface and transforms the heat radiation into electronic signals. These are displayed on the screen of a cathode ray tube

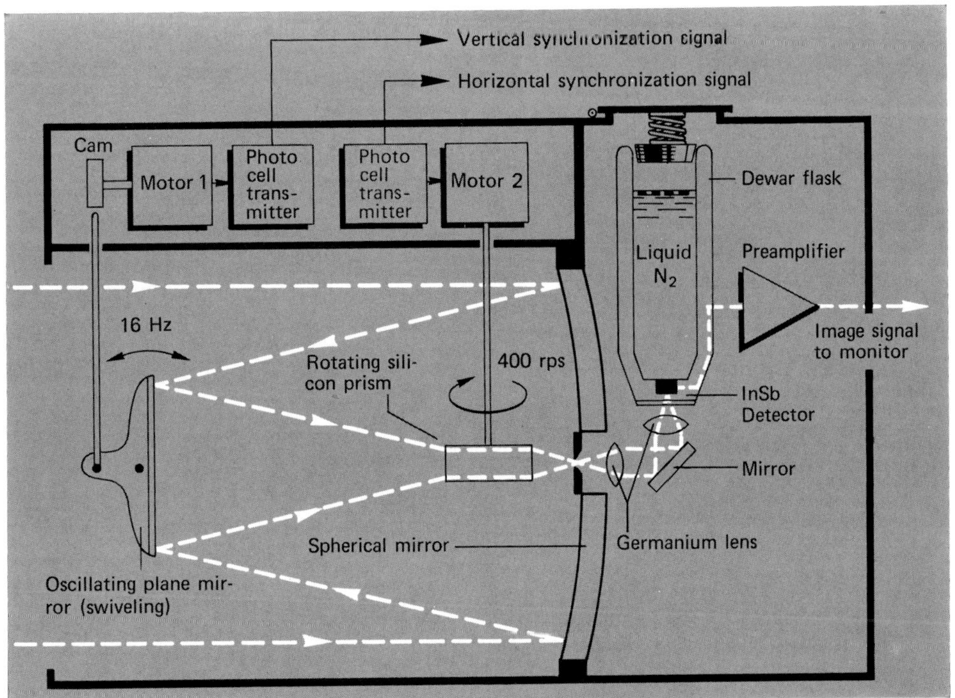

Fig. 1. Schematic diagram of the AGA camera unit.

similar to the method of television. The result is a black and white picture in which the warmest areas are white and the coldest black. This display may be photographed with polaroid film or by other photographic methods. Most units contain an electronic reversal mechanism allowing the choice of looking at "negative" or "positive" pictures. Furthermore many of these units contain a mechanism allowing dominant display of previously selected temperature ranges (isotherms). In some units a color display is also available. The table below summarizes some technical data of three of the most extensively used devices produced in Germany.

Method of Examination

Thermographic examination must be preceded by a cooling of the skin of the area to be examined. This may be performed by requiring the patient to sit for ten minutes in a room cooled to 68° to 70° F (or through the use of alcohol sprays and ventilator). The examination itself may require only an additional five minutes.

The use of a climatized room offers the advantage of a stable, controlled and repoducible environment for the examination. Normally, depending on variations in body contour, hair growth, the presence or absence of blood vessels in the vicinity of the area to be examined and the addition of numerous outside factors such as ventilation, which may influence the heat distribution, the pattern of warmth is more or less irregular. The infrared pattern emitted in particular regions of any individual body remains relatively constant.

The thermogram of the normal female breast will reveal irregularities in temperature distribution. Frequently there is an increased heat in both upper inner quadrants, the axillary portion of each breast and possibly that portion of the breast overlying the heart although the latter is doubtful. Superficial blood vessels produce an increased heat signal in the overlying skin. Hormonal stimulation (pregnancy, lactation, menses, ovulation) influence the heat pattern of the breast.

The heat pattern of the breast is determined primarily by the superficial vascularity. This is individually highly variable. Numerous attempts have been made to map out this vascularity in order to create a pattern for a normal thermogram (JONES 1968; HABERMAN 1968; LAPAYOWKER 1971; AMALRIC 1972: fig. 2; GROS 1972; PATIL 1972).

Diagnostic Signs

Thermography is not used to visualize disease but rather to record differences in heat emission. Contrary to earlier theories it is not differences in metabolism but differences in vascularity that is measured. Breast disease is therefore only recognizable on the thermogram when it involves an increase in vascularization.

Thermographic evaluation is made easier by comparing the differences in the temperature between the two breasts. There may be asymmetrical heat distribution in normal breasts and these are explained as a rule by the varying courses of the superficial veins. Such temperature differences, however, are not greater than 2 to 2.1° F. Numerous experiences have been reported in several symposia (New York 1963; Strassburg 1966; Leiden 1968; Toulouse 1972) setting some uniform guide lines which may be applied to interpretation of breast thermograms.

Mammary Dysplasia: Hypervascularity unilateral or bilateral, extensive or circumscribed. Temperature differences between corresponding locations is less than 2.7° F.

Mastitis: Hypervascularity of a circumscribed area indicating a "hot spot". Temperature

	AGA	Bofors	Rank
Image size	90 × 90 mm²	70 × 70 mm²	145 × 120 mm²
Image frequency	16/s	2/s	46/s
Film distance	0.95 m — ∞	0.2 m — ∞	0.25 m — ∞
Temperature range	—15° to +55°	—20° to +150°	0° to +200°

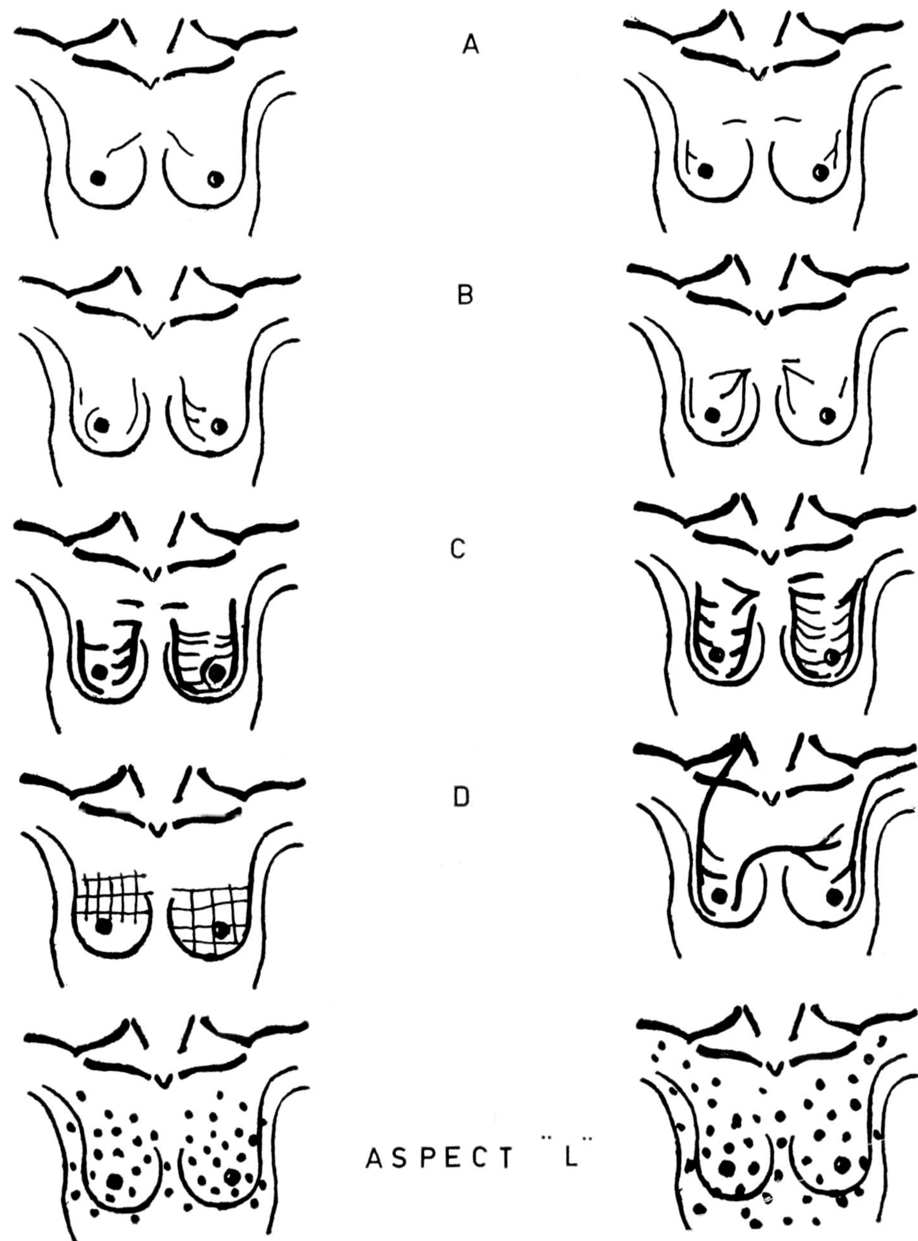

Fig. 2 Types of vascularization of the female breast according to Amalric (1972).
Type A: Avascular
Type B: Bilateral vascularization with 2 to 3 linear vessels; relatively symmetrical, witih demonstration of medial, lateral and periareolar vessels
Type C: Hypervascularity with normal vessels
Type D: Hypervascularity with atyplcal vessels
Configuration L: (leopard skin) spotted thermogram

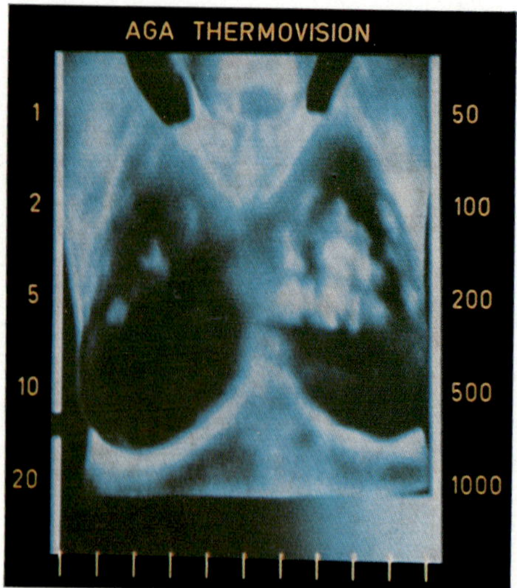

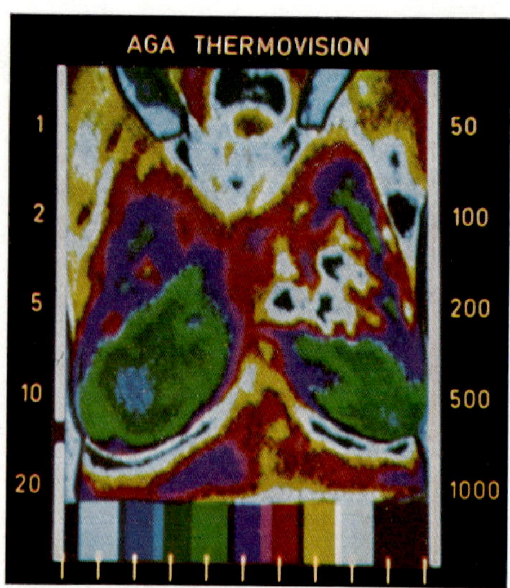

Fig. 3 a, b.   Ductal carcinoma of the left breast with solid and scirrhus components. Mammogram of the left breast revealed a mass about 1 cm in diameter above the areola with numerous tumor extensions from the margins.
Electrothermography: a) Black and white thermogram: Dark equals cool, light equals warm. There is a hot spot in the upper inner quadrant of the left breast. Temperature difference between this and the corresponding area of the right breast was greater than 2° centigrade. — b) Color thermogram of the same case: Fragmented warm spot in the upper inner quadrant of the left breast. Corresponding temperature difference with the right breast was 3° centigrade

difference 3.5° F or more, only if just under the skin.

Carcinoma: Circumscribed atypical hypervascularity must be just under the skin producing "hot spots" (fig. 3a and 3b). Temperature difference of the corresponding area 3.5° F or more. Warm areola and nipple.

It is not possible to differentiate inflammatory processes from carcinoma or dysplasia in the thermogram. The greatest problem in differential diagnosis, however, consists of separating carcinoma from normal variants and mammary dysplasia. The margin of error is great. In the occasional case when the pathological process is not associated with increased vascularity thermography will consistently fail to detect it. Scirrhus carcinoma, for this very reason, is occasionally not detectable in the thermogram (90% of all breast carcinoma is scirrhus)*. Furthermore it must be noted that the hyperthermic region may not be in the same location as the pathological process.

Thermography cannot be considered a substitute for clinical or mammographic examination but is an adjunct procedure. Its importance consists in supporting the clinical-mammographical diagnosis and in the rare discovery of a carcinoma not seen in the mammogram. Thermography plays an important role in supporting the differential diagnosis made by other types of breast examination.**

Plate Thermography

In recent years a further method of examination using the temperature pattern of the skin has been developed. FERGASON demonstrated in 1964 that "liquid" cholesterol crystals will undergo varying color changes within a narrow range of temperatures. By suitable selection of such crystals one can apply this characteristic of changing color within the range of skin temperatures. In the earliest attempts the substance was applied in liquid form and in numerous layers onto the skin where it solidified and a color

---

* This appears to contradict the experience in the U. S. The peripheral reaction induced by scirrhus carcinoma should, in fact, result in greater vascularity and thus more positive thermograms.

** Many investigators in the U.S.A. believe that thermography is only a screening procedure so that a positive result necessitates mammography but is not significant in itself. More recent studies have thrown grave doubt even on this aspect of thermography and at present the value of the method must still be established.

thermogram developed (SELAWRY 1966; GROS et al 1970; GRALL and TRICOIRE 1967). The heat diffusion along the borders made the picture relatively blurred and washed out.

Progress was made when the crystals were applied to a very thin foil which was brought into chemical contact with the skin. These foils are reusable for a long period of time. The color picture develops in seconds and may be photographed. Reports on the use of this technique are available from GROS et al (1970) and TRICOIRE et al (1970).

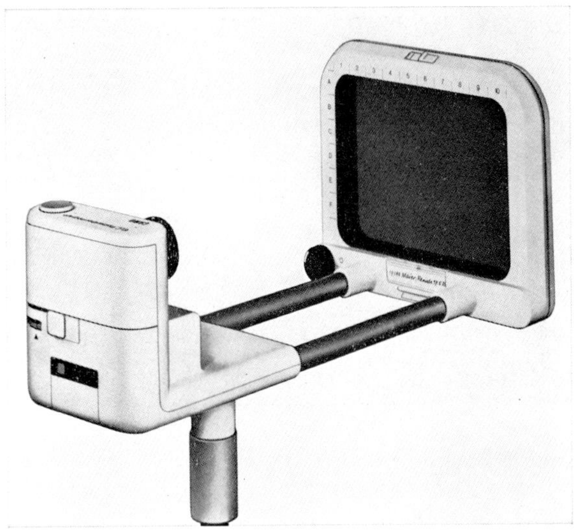

Fig. **4** Plate thermography after Tricoire. Arrangement for examination (Elco-Thermo-System).

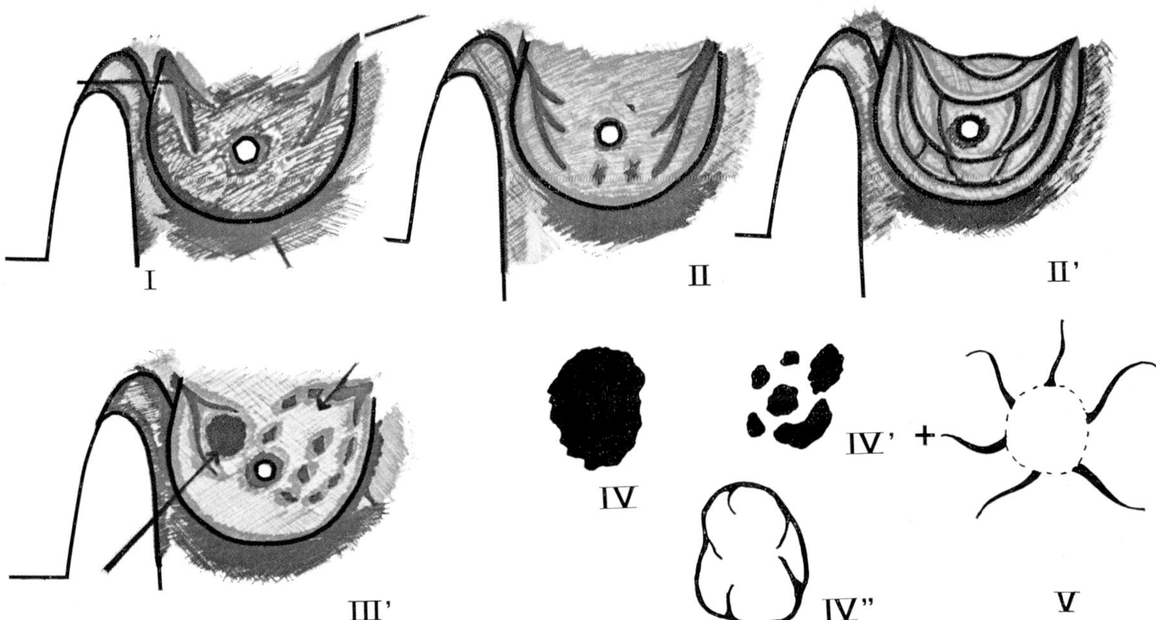

Fig. **5.** Sketches of normal and pathological findings using plate thermography, according to Tricoire (La Presse Medicale 1970).

I   No hormonal activity (prepubertal, senility)

II   Normal vascularity

II′   Hypervascularity (pregnancy, mastodynia, premenstrual syndrome)

III′ "Cold" spot in parenchyma (benign, palpable tumor)

IV′   Fragmented warm spot (malignant tumor)

IV″   Varying loops of vessels entering a tumor (malignant)

IV   Homogeneous warm spot (malignant tumor)

V   Stellate, converging vessels (malignant)

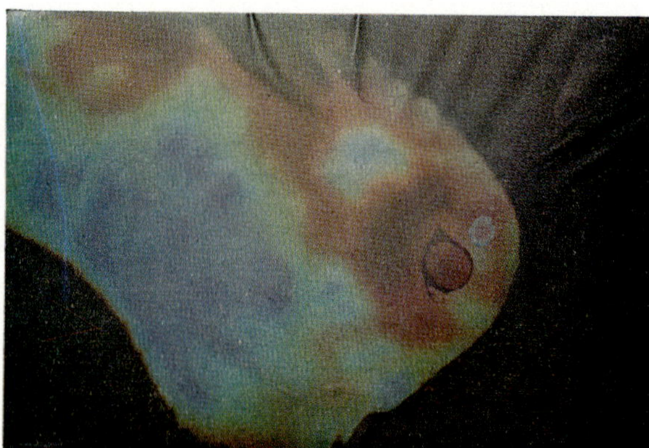

Fig. 6 Plate thermogram of a carcinoma in the outer portion of the right breast. Extensive pathological vascularity resulting in easily recognizable blue staining of these vessels. The cool portions of the breasts are brown. The nipple is also cool.

Method of Examination

Plate thermography (sheet thermography) according to TRICOIRE (fig. 4) may be used as a static type of examination by recording the existing warmth pattern of the skin of the breast or as a dynamic method of examination by recording the reappearance of vascular markings following cooling of the skin of the breast.

During examination using sheet thermography the skin is cooled by a fan or ventilator and the abnormal vascularity will impress as a persistent hot spot. Since the examination is very rapid, the cooling of the skin attained by having the patient remain in a climatized room, is not necessary.

Plate thermography, according to TRICOIRE, results in a relatively sharply demarcated pattern of color which is reproducible in a few seconds by reapplication of the plate onto the skin. This allows a quick determination whether the changes in temperature correspond to the clinical findings.

Plate thermography, because of its good resolution, reflects accurately any abnormal vascularity. The detection of a "hot spot" is a more generalized finding which is of secondary importance.

An overview of the characteristic abnormal vascular patterns and their significance as signs of carcinoma is seen in the schematic representation by TRICOIRE (fig. 5).

The resultant thermogram may be recorded with a camera and color film (fig. 6); however, the diagnosis is essentially made during the examination.

Plate or sheet thermography like electrothermography, is a method of diagnosis based on skin and vascular heat and therefore both have approximately the same accuracy and margin of error.

The apparatus consists of a thermographic plate, tripod, and camera (fig. 4) in contrast to the necessary electronic equipment for electrothermography. The operating costs consist essentially of the photographic film used for documentation.

We use plate thermography as a quick source of information and as an adjunct for differential diagnosis in addition to electrothermography, mammography and clinical examination.

Ultrasound Diagnosis of the Breast

The application of ultrasound to breast examination is based on the fact that ultrasound impulses reflect from the interfaces of intramammary masses, cysts and carcinomas. With the so-called B-mode one can record on an oscilloscopic screen all sound reflecting interfaces between different types of tissues within a portion of the body (ICHIKAWA et al 1966; MARI et al 1966; WAGAI et al 1965; HAYASHI et al 1962).

Several types of ultrasound units are available (Siemens Vidoson, Picker Lamniograph, Kretz Technik Combison). The advantage of this method is that it is harmless, thus allowing serial and control examinations. The disadvantage in comparison to mammography consists in its rather poor resolution. It is unlikely therefore, that small clinically occult carcinomas can be detected with this method. Publications on the method to date (DELAND 1970, and others) deal with ultrasonic demonstration of tumors that are already clinically detectable and therefore this does not constitute early detection. Ultrasound examination is being applied increasingly for the differential diagnosis of benign and malignant solid tumors as well as cysts.

However, thin needle aspiration and cytological examination are easy to perform and are more accurate.

Benign breast tumors reveal a regular border in the two dimensional ultrasonogram. Only a few echoes are detected within the confines of the tumor. In malignant tumors the borders appear irregular. The inner portion of the tumor mass will in most cases reflect a great number of echoes (DELAND 1970).

Attempts to apply ultrasound technique for examination of the female breast in the University of Cologne Women's Clinic have produced results which agree with those found in the literature. The ultrasonograms (figs. 7 to 9) supplied by SCHLENSKER from the University of Cologne Women's Clinic, 1972, demonstrate some normal and pathological breast findings.

Diaphanoscopy (Transillumination)

Diaphanoscopy is used primarily in the Gros Clinic in Strasbourg. This consists of transilluminating the breast with a strong light source (manufacturer: Ateliers St. Joseph, Molsheim, France) showing parenchymal and other non-homogeneous tissues as ill-defined shadows.

With considerable experience some differential diagnostic determinations are possible. GROS has high regard for this method as an adjunct to mammography (GROS 1951; GROS 1972).

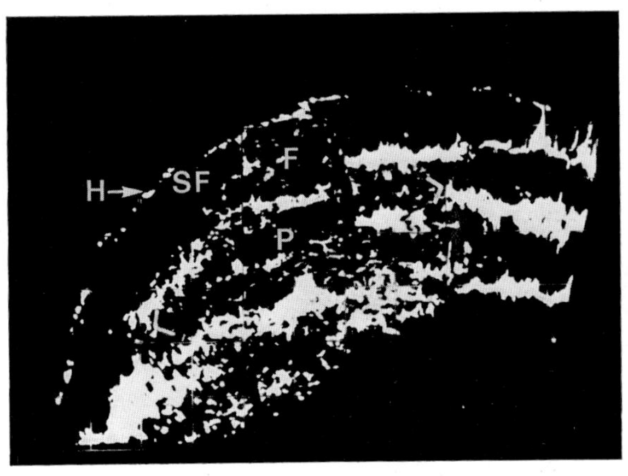

Fig. 7 Ultrasonogram of the right breast. Sonographic section 2 cm above the areola. Frequency is 4 MHz. One square in the sonogram is equivalent to 1 cm.
F = fibroadenoma, diameter is 2 cm
H = skin
SF = subcutaneous fatty tissue
P = breast parenchyma

Fig. 8 a to e Ultrasound examination of breast cyst

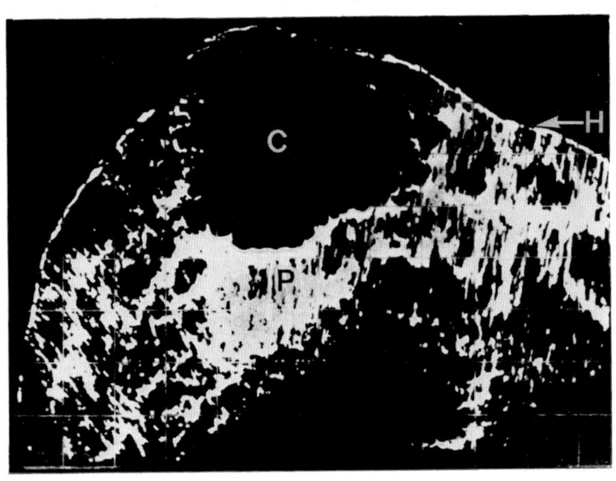

Fig. 8 a

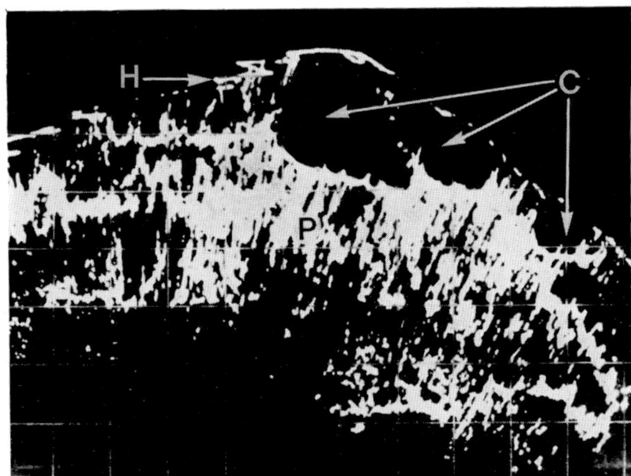

Fig. 8 b

Fig. 8 a, b **Ultrasonogram.** a = right, b = left. Transverse section along upper margin of areola. Frequency was 4 MHz. One square equals 1 cm. C = cyst, H = skin, P = breast parenchyma.

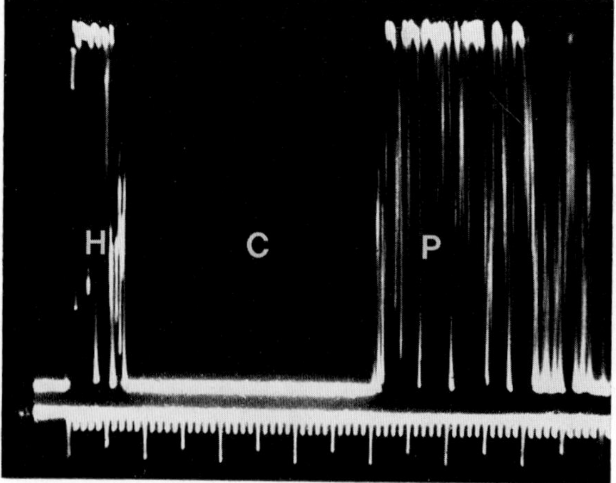

Fig. **8** c

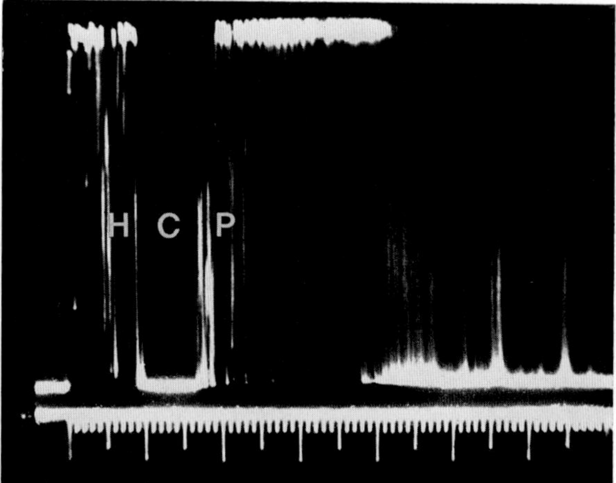

Fig. **8** d

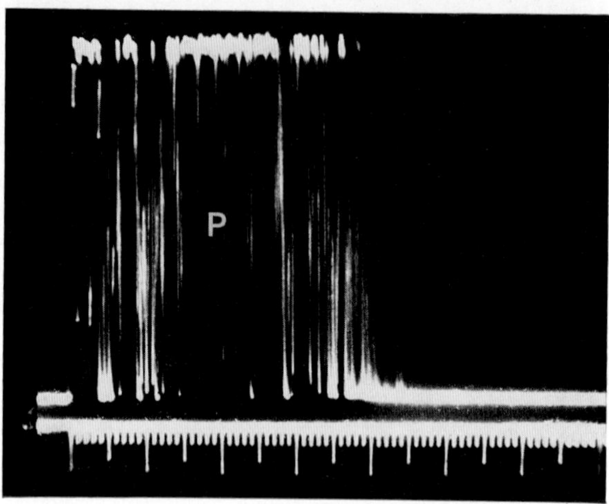

Fig. **8** e

Fig. **8c, d, e** A-mode ultrasonogram. Frequency was 4 MHz. One square equals 1 mm.
Fig. **8c** Demonstration of a large right-sided cyst as in fig. 8a.
Fig. **8d** Demonstration of a small cyst as in fig. 8b.
Fig. **8e** Breast tissue without cysts.

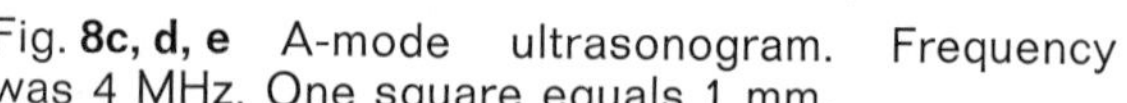

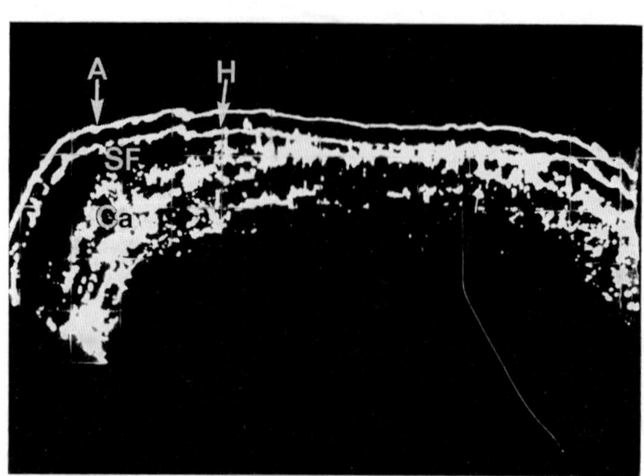

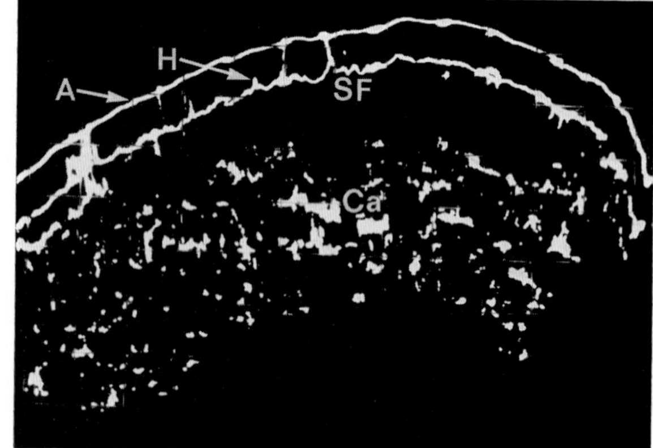

Fig. **9** a, b. **Extensive carcinoma of the right breast.** Ultrasonogram, Skin = H, subcutaneous fatty tissue; SF, carcinoma = Ca; contour A indicates the course of the probe. Frequency was 4 MHz.
Fig. **9** a. Cross-section performed through both breasts 3 cm above the areola. One square equals 2 cm.
Fig. **9** b. Cross-section through the right breast 1 cm beneath the areola. One square equals 1 cm.

References

AARTS, N. J. M.: The use of thermography in the detection of breast cancer. Medical Thermography. Karger, Basel 1969

ADAM, G., M. BARTEL: Beitrag zur Pathogenese, Klinik und Prognose des Riesenfibroadenoms der weiblichen Brustdrüse. Zbl. Chir. 94 (1969) 840

AGNEW, D. H.: The Principles and Practice of Surgery. Vol. III. Lippincott, Philadelphia, 1883

ALBRING, E.: Personal communication 1970

ALCORN, F. S., E. O'DONELL: The training of nonphysician personnel for use in a mammography program. Cancer (Philad.) 23 (1969) 879

AMALRIC, R., J. M. SPITALIER, J. LEVRAUD, C. ALTSCHULER: Classification des images thermovisuelles des carcinomes mammaires. Symposium des thérapeutiques non mutilantes des cancéreuses du sein. Strasbourg, June 1972

AMERSON, J. R.: Cystosarcoma phyllodes in adolescent females. A report of seven patients. Ann. Surg. 171 (1970) 849

ANACKER, H., A. GAUL, P. BERNETT: Die Arteriographie des Mammakarzinoms. Fortschr. Röntgenstr. 113 (1970) 448

ASCH, TH.: Mammography: A study of 580 patients. Amer. J. Roentgenol. 90 (1963) 366

ATKINS, H. J. B.: Mamillary fistula. Brit. med. J. 1955/II, 1473

AUFERMAUR, M.: Präkanzeröse Veränderungen der weiblichen Brustdrüse, mit besonderer Berücksichtigung der Zystenmamma. Schweiz. med. Wschr. 99 (1969) 1779

BACLESSE, F., A. WILLEMIN: Atlas of mammography. Librairie des Facultes, Paris 1967

BÄSSLER, R.: Das sogenannte lobuläre Karzinom der Mamma. Dtsch. med. Wschr. 94 (1969) 108;
Neuere Aspekte der normalen und pathologischen Feinstruktur der Mamma. Hippokrates 39 (1968) 327

BARALDI, A.: Roentgen-neumo-mastia. Rev. Cirurg. (B. Aires) 14 (1935) 321

BARKER, W. F., L. SPERLING, A. H. DOWDY, L. J. ZELDIS, W. P. LONGMIRE jr.: Management of nonpalpable breast carcinoma discovered by mammography. Ann. Surg. 170 (1969) 385

BARNES, S., W. H. C. BERRY, M. J. WILLIAMS, M. BAUM, W. D. MACKAY, C. T. HOWE, J. G. MURRAY: Mass screening for cancer of the breast. Lancet 1968/1, 1417

BATSON, O. V.: The role of the vertebral veins in metastatic processes. Amer. Int. Med. 16 (1942) 38

BERG, J. W., G. F. ROBBINS: A late look at the safety of aspiration biopsy. Cancer (Philad.) 15 (1962) 826

BERGER, S. M.: Inflammatory carcinoma of the breast. Amer. J. Roentgenol. 88 (1962) 1109

BERGER, S. M., B. M. CURCIO, J. GERSHON-COHEN, H. J. ISARD: Mammographic localization of unsuspected breast cancer. Amer. J. Roentgenol. 46 (1966) 1046

BERNDT, H., S. MARWITZ: Mastopathie und Mammokarzinom. Arch. Geschwulstforsch. 32 (1968) 137

BERSON, M. I.: Atlas of Plastic Surgery, 2nd edn. Grune & Stratton, New York 1963

BILLROTH, TH.: Die Krankheiten der Brustdrüsen. Enke, Stuttgart 1880

BJÖRN-HANSEN, R.: Contrast-mammography. Brit. J. Radiol. 38 (1965) 947

BJÖRN-HANSEN, R., K. TALLE: Diagnostic significance of secretion from the mammary papilla. T. norske Laegeforen. 87 (1966) 1979

BLOODGOOD, J. C.: The clinical picture of dilated ducts beneath the nipple frequently to be palpated as a doughy worm-like mass —
the varicocele tumors of the breast. Surg. Gynec. Obstet. 36 (1923) 486;
The blue-domed cyst in chronic cystic mastitis. J. Amer. med. Ass. 93 (1929) 1056;
Comedo carcinoma (or comedo-adenoma) of the female breast. Amer. J. Cancer 22 (1934) 842

BÖHMIG, R.: Mastopathia fibrosa cystica, ihre Epithelproliferationen und deren Beziehungen zum Karzinom. Ergebn. allg. Path. path. Anat. 25 (1964) 39

BOHRER, S. P.: Mammographie. Röntgenpraxis 18 (1965) 149

BORCHARDT, M., R. JAFFÈ: Zur Kenntnis der Zystenmamma. Beitr. klin. Chir. 155 (1932) 481

BOREADIS BORDEN, A. G., J. GERSHON-COHEN: Mammography of lobular carcinoma. Radiology 81 (1963) 17

BRASNIKOV, N. N.: Funktionelle und altersbedingte Besonderheiten im Röntgenbild der normalen und pathologisch veränderten Mamma. Radiol. diagn. (Berl.) 5 (1964) 459

BRAUN-FALCO, O.: Über strangförmige oberflächliche Phlebitiden (gleichzeitig ein Beitrag zur Kenntnis der Mondorschen Krankheit). Derm. Wschr. 127 (1953) 506

BREIT, A., W. LOY, W. HAUBOLD: Bildverstärkung auf fotografischem Weg: Ein Beitrag zur Behandlung des Mammakarzinoms. Strahlentherapie 117 (1962) 525

BRISSAUD, E.: Anatomie pathologique de la maladie kystique des mamelles. Arch. physiol. norm. et path. 3 (1884) 98

BRODIE, B. C.: Lectures Illustrative of Various Subjects in Pathology and Surgery. Longmans, London 1846

BUCHWALD, W.: Die Differentialdiagnose der voroperierten Brustdrüse in der Mammographie: Narbe — Narbenkarzinom. Fortschr. Röntgenstr. 105 (1966) 857,
Infrarotthermometrie in der Diagnostik von Brustdrüsenerkrankungen. Röntgen-Bl. 21 (1968) 60—64

BUCHWALD, W., R. HÜLSE, H. FASEL: Zur Differentialdiagnose des malignen Herdschattens in der Mammographie: Fortschr. Röntgenstr. 112 (1970) 369

BUTTENBERG, D., K. WERNER: Die Mammographie. Schattauer, Stuttgart 1962

BYRNE, R. N., W. FOX: J. GERSHON-COHEN, Periodic postoperative mammography. Int. Surg. 50 (1968) 415

CHARDOT, C., R. M. PARACHE, C. CHEVAL: Une forme remarquable des cancers du sein: le carcinoma «circonscrit» ou «médullaire». Ann. Méd. Nancy 91 (1970) 189

CHAVANNE, G., A. GREGOIRE: Diagnostic radiologique des tumeurs de la glande mammaire. Publication des Étudiants de la Faculté de Médicine de Louvain. July 1956

CHEATLE, G. L., M. CUTLER: Tumors of the Breast. Arnold, London 1931

CHELIUS, M. J.: Zit. nach: ADAM, BARTEL: Beitrag zur Pathogenese, Klinik und Prognose des Riesenfibroadenoms der weiblichen Brustdrüse. Zbl. Chir. 94 (1969) 840

CITOLER, P., S. DERBOLOWSKI: Stellt das lobuläre Carcinoma in situ der Mamma eine Rarität dar? Vortrag auf der Sitzung der Nordrhein-Westfälischen Pathologen am 4. 12. 1971 in Düsseldorf

CITOLER, P.: Pers. Mitt. 1972

CLAGETT, O. T., N. C. PLIMPTON, G. T. ROOT: Lesions of the breast; the relationship of benign lesions to carcinoma. Surgery 15 (1944) 413

CLARK, R. L., M. M. COPELAND, R. L. EGAN, H. S. GALLAGER, H. GELLER, J. P. LINDSAY, L. C. ROBBINS, E. C. WHITE: Reproducibility of the technic of mammography (EGAN) for cancer of the breast. Amer. J. Surg. 109 (1965) 127

CONSIGLIO, V., M. FILOTICO, L. CONSIGLIO: L'Infarto Della Ghiandola Mammaria Funzionante. Arch. ital. Chir. 93 (1967) 580

COOPER, A. P.: The Anatomy and Diseases of the Breast. Lea & Blanchard, Philadelphia 1845

CORNER, G. W.: The hormonal control of lactation: positive action of extracts of the hypophysis. Amer. J. Physiol. 95 (1930) 43

CUTLER, M.: Tumors of the Breast. Pitman, London 1961; Lippincott, Philadelphia 1961

CUTLER, S. J.: Clinical Evaluation of Breast Cancer. Hayward, Bulbrook, London 1966

DAHL-IVERSEN, E.: Intramammary angioma. Hospitalstidende 76 (1933) 653

DALICHO, W. A.: Wahrnehmun gund Darstellbarkeit von Details im Röntgenbild. Grenzen und Grundlagen dargestellt an Harnsteinen im Ausscheidungsurogramm. Edition, Leipzig 1967

DANIELS, W. B.: Superficial thrombophlebitis; a new cause of chest pain. Amer. J. med. Sci. 183 (1932) 398

DA SILVA NETO, J. B.: Results of 22 cases of breast sarcoma over five years after surgery. Tumori 56 (1970) 39;
Benign tumors of the breast. Arch. Surg. 38 (1939) 79;
Supermammary breast. Arch. Surg. 39 (1939) 926

DE CHOLNOKY, T.: Accessory breast tissue in the axilla. N. Y. St. J. Med. 51 (1951) 2245

DECOURT, J., M. F. JAYLE, J. P. MASSIN: Étude de 49 cas de gynécomastie apparemment isolées de l'adolescence. Sem. Hôp. Paris 38 (1962) 1266

DELAND, FRANK H.: Ultraschalldiagnostik von Brustgeschwülsten. Röntgen-Bl. 23 (1970) 6

DE LUCA, J. T., J. H. WENTWORTH: Mammography in clinical practice. N. Y. St. J. Med. 66 (1966) 2113

DOANE, W. A., R. G. WILLIAMS: Mammography in the diagnosis of cancer of the female breast. Amer. J. Surg. 106 (1963) 317

DOBRETSBERGER, W.: Mammadiagnostik mittels Isodens-Technik. Radiol. Austriaca 13 (1962) 239
Die Fluidographie der weiblichen Brust. Elektromedica 4 (1967) 12;
Die isodensische Weichteilaufnahme (Fluidogramm). Radiologe 5 (1965) 28

DOHRMANN, R., R. LABUSCH: Über den Wert der röntgenologischen Mammadiagnostik. Chirurg 29 (1958) 3

DOMINGUEZ, C. M.: Estudio sistenatizado del cancer del seno. Dol. Liga. urug. Cancer 4 (1929) 145;
Estudio radiólogico de los descalcificadores. Bol. Anat. Patol. 1 (1930) 175

DONOVAN, R. J.: A new contour casette for mammographic roentgenography. Amer. J. Roentgenol. 91 (1964) 917

DOWDY, A. H., L. D. LAGASSE, P. ROACH, D. WILSON: Lay screeners in mammographic survey programs. Radiology 95 (1970) 619

DOWDY, A. H., L. D. LAGASSE, L. SPERLING, W. F. BARKER, L. J. ZELDIS, W. P. LONGMIRE, PH. H. COOPER: A combined screening program for the detection of carcinoma of the cervix and carcinoma of the breast. Surg. Gynec. Obstet. 131 (1970) 93

DUBREUILH, W.: De la mélanose circonscrite précancérense. Ann. Derm. Syph. (Paris) 3 (1912) 129

DUNN, J. E.: Epidemiology and possible identification of high-risk groups that could develop cancer of the breast. Cancer (Philad.) 23 (1969) 775

EGAN, R. L.: Mammography: Report on 2,000 studies. Surgery 53 (1963) 291
Mammography. Amer. J. Surg. 106 (1963) 421;
Reproducibility of Mammography. A preliminary report. Amer. J. Roentgenol. 40 (1963) 356;
Mammography. Thomas, Springfield 1964;
Fundamentals of mammographic diagnoses of benign and malignant diseases. Oncology 23 (1969) 126

ELLIS, R. E.: The distribution of active bone marrow in the adult. Phys. in Med. Biol. 5 (1961) 255

ESPAILLAT, A.: Contribution à l'étude radiographique du sein normal et pathologique. Thèse de Paris (1933)

FARROW, J. H.: Bilateral mammary cancer. Cancer (Philad.) 9 (1956) 1182
Clinical considerations and treatment of in situ lobular breast cancer. Amer. J. Roentgenol. 102 (1968) 652;
Current concepts in the detection and treatment of the earliest of the early breast cancers. Cancer (Philad.) 25 (1970) 468

FELDMANN, F.: Angiography of cancer of the breast. Cancer (Philad.) 23 (1969) 803

FELDMANN, S., M. MAHL, D. FRIEDMANN, A. L. DUNEWITZ: Mondor's disease. N. Y. St. J. Med. 54 (1954) 387

FELDMANN, F., D. V. HABIF, R. J. FLEMING, I. E. KANTER, W. B. SEAMAN: Arteriography of the breast. Radiology 89 (1967) 1053

FERGASON, J. L.: Liquid Crystals. Scientific American 211 (1964) 77

FIESSINGER, N., P. MATHIEU: Thrombo-phlebitis des veines de la paroi thoraco-abdominale. Bull. Soc. Méd. Paris 46 (1922) 352

FINSTERBUSCH, R., F. GROSS: Kalkablagerungen in den Milch- und Ausführungsgängen beider Brustdrüsen. Röntgenpraxis 6 (1934) 172

FISCHEDICK, O., R. EVERS: Möglichkeiten und Grenzen der Xeroradiographie der Brust. Fortschr. Röntgenstr. 119 (1973) 389

FISCHERMANN, K., I. BECH, P. FOGED, J. HOSTRUP PEDERSEN, J. B. LAURITZEN: Relation between cystic fibroadenomatosis and cancer of the breast. Acta chir. scand. 135 (1969) 671

FOCHEM, K., G. NARIK: Die Röntgenaufnahme der weiblichen Brust (Mammogramm) als Schwangerschaftsnachweis. Geburtsh. u. Frauenheilk. 17 (1957) 957

FOOTE, F. W., F. W. STEWART: Lobular carcinoma in situ; a rare form of mammary cancer. Amer. J. Path. 17 (1941) 491;
Comparative studies of cancerous versus non-cancerous breasts. II Role of so-called chronic cystic mastitis in mammary carcinogenesis, influence of certain hormones on human breast structure. Ann. Surg. 121 (1945) 197

FRANTZ, V. K., J. W. PICKREN, G. W. MELCHER, H. AUCHINCLOSS, jr.: Incidence of chronic cystic disease in so-called normal breast. Cancer (Philad.) 4 (1951) 762

FRANZÉN, S., J. ZAJICEK: Aspiration biopsy in diagnosis of palpable lesions of the breast. Acta radiol. (Stockh.) 7 (1968) 241

FRAY, W. W., S. L. WARREN: Stereoscopic roentgenography of the breasts. An aid in establishing the diagnosis of mastitis and carcinoma. Ann. Surg. 95 (1932) 425

FREILINGER, G., L. HOWANIETZ, F. RATH, W. WALDHÄUSL: Pubertätsgynäkomastie. Dtsch. med. Wschr. 96 (1971) 1744

FRIEDMANN, A. K., S. I. ASKOVITZ, S. M. BERGER, G. D. DODD, M. S. FISCHER, M. S. LAPAYOWKER, J. P. MOORE, D. E. PARLEE, G. N. STEIN, E. P. PENDERGRASS: A co-operative evaluation of mammography in seven teaching hospitals. Radiology 86 (1966) 886

GAJEWSKI, H., H.-P. HEILMANN: Experimentelle Untersuchungen zur optimalen Aufnahmetechnik bei der Mammographie. Fortschr. Röntgenstr. 115 (1971) 248

GALLAGER, H. S., J. E. MARTIN: The study of mammary carcinoma by mammography and whole organ sectioning. Cancer (Philad.) 23 (1969) 855;
Early phases in the development of breast cancer. Cancer (Philad.) 24 (1969) 1170

GATCHELL, F. G., M. B. DOCKERTY, O. T. CLAGETT: Intracystic carcinoma of the breast. Surg. Gynec. Obstet. 106 (1958) 347

GELBKE, H.: Wiederherstellende und plastische Chirurgie. Bd. II. Thieme, Stuttgart 1963

GERLACH, M., H. THIEMANN: Elektronenmikroskopische Untersuchung der metastatischen Kalzifizierung. Klin. Wschr. 43 (1965) 1262

GEROTA, D.: Zur Technik der Lymphgefäßinjektion. Anat. Anz. 12 (1896) 216

GERSHON-COHEN, J.: Breast Roentgenology, Historical Review. Amer. J. Roentgenol. 86 (1961) 879;
Detection of unsuspected breast cancer by mammography. Surg. Gynec. Obstet. 121 (1965) 97;
Medical and legal implications of mammography. Surg. Gynec. Obstet. 130 (1970) 347;
Atlas of Mammography. Springer, Berlin 1970

GERSHON-COHEN, J., M. B. HERMEL: Modalities in breast cancer detection: Xeroradiography, mammography, thermography, and mammometry. Cancer 24 (Philad.) (1969) 1226

GERSHON-COHEN, J., H. INGLEBY: Secretory disease and plasma cell mastitis in the female breast. Surg. Gynec. Obstet. 95 (1952) 497;

Roentgenography of cysts of the breast. Surg. Gynec. Obstet. 97 (1953) 483;
Roentgenography of abscess and mamillary fistula. Amer. J. Roentgenol. 79 (1958) 122

GERSHON-COHEN, J., L. MOORE: Roentgenography of giant fibroadenoma of breast/cystosarcoma phylloides. Radiology 74 (1960) 619

GERSHON-COHEN, J., S. SCHORR: The diagnostic problems of isolated, circumscribed breast tumors. Amer. J. Roentgenol. 106 (1969) 863

GERSHON-COHEN, J., S. M. BERGER, B. M. CURCIO: Breast cancer with microcalcifications: diagnostic difficulties. Radiology 87 (1966) 613

GERSHON-COHEN, J., M. B. HERMEL, S. M. BERGER: Detection of breast cancer by periodic X-ray examinations (A five-year survey). J. Amer. med. Ass. 176 (1961) 1114;

GERSHON-COHEN, J., H. INGLEBY, M. B. HERMEL: Calcification in secretory disease of the breast. Amer. J. Roentgenol. 76 (1956) 132

GERSHON-COHEN, J., H. INGLEBY, L. MOORE: Can mass X-ray surveys be used in detection of early cancer of the breast? J. Amer. med. Ass. 161 (1956) 1069;
Analysis of 2,514 examinations during early phases of an X-ray survey of the breast. Surg. Gynec. Obstet. 106 (1958) 478

GERSHON-COHEN, J., L. S. YIU, S. M. BERGER: The diagnostic importance of calcareous patterns in roentgenography of breast cancer. Amer. J. Roentgenol. 88 (1962) 1117

GERSHON-COHEN, J., H. INGLEBY, M. B. HERMEL, S. M. BERGER: Accuracy of preoperative X-ray diagnoses of breast tumors. Surgery 35 (1954) 766

GERSHON-COHEN, J., H. INGLEBY, S. M. BERGER, M. FORMAN, B. M. CURCIO: Mammographic screening for breast cancer (Results of a ten-year survey). Radiology 88 (1967) 663

GESCHICKTER, C. F.: Diseases of the Breast, 2nd edn. Lippincott, Philadelphia 1945

GIBSON, A., G. SMITH: Aspiration biopsy of breast tumours. Brit. J. Surg. 45 (1957) 236

GILBERTSEN, V. A.: Survival of asymptomatic breast cancer patients. Surg. Gynec. Obstet. 122 (1966) 81;
Detection of breast cancer in a specialized cancer detection center. Cancer (Philad.) 24 (1969) 1192

GILBERTSON, J. D., G. R. MITCHELL, A. G. FINGERHUT: Evaluation of roentgen exposure in mammography. Part 1: Six Views. Radiology 95 (1970) 383

GILBERTSON, J. D., M. G. RANDALL, A. G. FINGERHUT: Evaluation of roentgen exposure in mammography. Part 2: Four Views. Radiology 97 (1970) 641

GILBRIDE, J. J.: Lymphatic injection with radiopaque substance for roentgen examination in carcinoma of mammary gland. Amer. J. Surg. 79 (1938) 617

GODWIN, J. T.: Chronology of lobular carcinoma of the breast. Cancer (Philad.) 5 (1952) 259

GOULD, H. R., F. F. RUZICKA Jr., R. SANCHEZ-UBEDA, J. PEREZ: Xeroradiography of the Breast. Am. J. Roentgenol. 84 (1960) 220

GOYANES, J., F. GENTIL, B. GUEDES: Radiography of mammary gland and its diagnostic value. Arch. esp. Oncol. 11 (1931) 111

GRALL, Y., J. TRICOIRE: La thermographie cutanée par cristaux liquides d'esters de cholesterol. C. R. Soc. Biol. (Paris) 161 (1967) 1309

GRAVELLE, I. H.: Schirmbildphotographie bei Brustkrankheiten. Odelca Mirror 8 (1969) 10

GREGL, A., H. POPPE: Klinische und röntgenologische Symptomatik der sezernierenden Brust. J. Radiol. Électrol. 48 (1967) 723

GRIESBACH, W. A.: Mammography as a possible screening examination using conventional techniques. Cancer (Philad.) 23 (1969) 874;
Screening for breast carcinoma. Oncology 23 (1969) 167

GRIESBACH, W. A., W. S. EADS: Experience with screening for breast carcinoma. Cancer (Philad.) 19 (1966) 1548

GROS, CH. M.: Radiographie des cancers intrakystiques du sein. J. int. Coll. Surg. 30 (1958) 674;
Radio-klinische Diagnose des Mammakarzinoms. Röntgen-Bl. 13 (1960) 373;
Les maladies du sein. Masson, Paris 1963;
Méthodologie. J. Radiol. Électrol. 48 (1967) 638. Berichtsheft: Proceeding Symposium Européen de Radiologie Mammaire, Strasbourg, July 1966

GROS, CH. M., S. BURG: Découverte radiologique d'un cancer occulte cliniquement. J. Radiol. Électrol. 38 (1957) 1084;
Radiographie des mastites carcinomatenses. J. Radiol. Électrol. 38 (1957) 769

GROS, CH. M., M. SIGRIST: La radiographie de la mamelle. Annuel Congrès des Médecins Électro-Radiologique de Culture latine, Brüssel 1951 (p. 11);
La radiographie et la transillumination de la mamelle. Strasbourg méd. (1951) 451

GROS, CH. M., P. BOURJAT, M. GAUTHERIE: Die Diagnose von Brustkarzinomen durch Infrarot-Thermographie. Fortschr. Röntgenstr. 116 (1972) 669

GROS, CH. M., Y. QUENNEVILLE, Y. HUMMEL: Diaphanologie mammaire. J. Radiol. Électrol. 53 (1972) 297

GROS, C. M., R. SIGRIST, S. BURG: La pneumomastographie. (Technique du radiodiagnostic des kystes du sein). J. Radiol. Électrol. 35 (1954) 882

GROS, CH. M., M. GAUTHERIE, P. BOURJAT, F. ARCHER: Les cristaux liquides en thermographie. Ann. Radiol. 13 (1970) 333

GROSSMANN, F.: Über die axillären Lymphdrüsen. Inaug. Diss. C. Vogt, Berlin 1896

GROW, J. L., E. F. LEWISON: Superficial thrombophlebitis of the breast. Surg. Gynec. Obstet. 116 (1963) 180

HAAGE, H., O. FISCHEDICK: Die Solitärzyste der weiblichen Brust im Röntgenbild. Fortschr. Röntgenstr. 100 (1964) 639

HAAGENSEN, C. D.: Lobular carcinoma of the breast. Clin. Obstet. Gynec. 5 (1962) 1093;
Diseases of the Breast, 2nd edn. Saunders, Philadelphia 1971

HABERMAN, J. D.: The present status of mammary thermography. Cancer (Philad.) 18 (1968) 315;
La thermographie dépiste les lésions des seins. Trib. med. 2/8 (1968);
The importance of thermal patterns in infrared thermogram evaluation of diseases of the breast. Paper presented at the 54th Ann. meeting of the Radiological Soc. of North America, Chicago 1968

HALSTED, W. S.: A clinical and histological study of certain adenocarcinomata of the breast. Ann. Surg. 28 (1898) 557

HAMPERL, H.: Über die Myothelien (myo-epithelialen Elemente) der Brustdrüse. Virchows Arch. path. Anat. 305 (1939) 171;
Zur Frage der pathologisch-anatomischen Grundlagen der Mammographie. Geburtsh. u. Frauenheilk. 28 (1968) 901;
Personal communication 1969;
Das lobuläre Carcinoma in situ der Mamma. Dtsch. med. Wschr. 96 (1971) 1585

HARDY, J. D.: Radiation of heat from the human body. The human skin as a blackbody radiator. J. clin. Invest. 13 (1934) 615

HAYASHI, S., T. WAGAI, G. MIYAZAWA, K. ITO, S. ISHIKAWA, K. UEMATSU, Y. KIKUCHI, Y. UCHIDA: Ultrasonic diagnosis of breast tumor and cholelithiasis. West. J Obstet. Gynec. 70 (1962) 34

HAYDEN, CH. W.: Use of mammography in the follow-up examination for the detection of localised or unsuspected carcinoma. Cancer (Philad.) 23 (1969) 818

HENNY, G. C.: Effect of Roentgen Ray Quality on Response in Xeroradiography. Am. J. Roentgenol. 79 (1958) 158

HERMANUTZ, D., R. MÜLLER: Mammakarzinom und verkalkte Fettgewebstransplantate nach beidseitiger Mammavergrößerungsplastik. Fortschr. Röntgenstr. 113 (1970) 530

HESSLER, CH., J. GERSHON-COHEN: Mastography-evaluation in 215 proven lesions. Acta radiol. (Stockh.) New Series Diagn. 3 (1965) 249

HEUSS, K., W. HOEFFKEN: Messungen der Oberflächendosis bei Aufnahmen mit Spezial-Mammographiegeräten. Fortschr. Röntgenstr. 117 (1972) 669

HILLS, T. H., R. W. STANFORD, R. D. MOORE: Xeroradiography: II. The Present Medical Applications. Brit. J. Radiol. 28 (1955) 545

HITCHCOCK, C. R., D. F. HICKOK, J. SOUCHERAY, T. MOULTON, R. C. BAKER: Thermography in mass screening for occult breast cancer. J. Amer. med. Ass. 204 (1968) 419

HOEFFKEN, W., H. GAJEWSKI: Vergleichsuntersuchungen zur Mammographie mit Weichstrahltechnik und Isodensmethode. Radiologe 6 (1966) 407

HOEFFKEN, W., C. HINTZEN: Die Diagnostik der Mammazysten durch Mammographie und Pneumozystographie. Fortschr. Röntgenstr. 112 (1970) 9

HOEFFKEN, W., K. MOCK: Die „weite Vene" als indirektes mammographisches Zeichen für Malignität von pathologischen Mammaveränderungen. Radiologe 10 (1970) 136

HOEFFKEN, W., K. HEUSS, E. RÖDEL: Die Notwendigkeit einer Belichtungsautomatik für die Mammographie. Radiologe 10 (1970) 154

HOFFMAN, R. L.: Thermography in the detection of breast malignancy. Amer. J. Obstet. Gynec. 98 (1967) 681

HOFMANN, W.-D., F. W. BOSCHBACH: Die fibrosierende Adenose der weiblichen Brustdrüse. Geburtsh. u. Frauenheilk. 30 (1970) 40

HONIG, C., R. RADO: Mondor's disease — superficial phlebitis of the chest wall. Ann. Surg. 153 (1961) 589

HÜPPE, J. R.: Optimierung der Mammographie aus klinisch-radiologischer Sicht. Radiologe 10 (1970) 128

HUTTER, R. V. P., F. W. FOOTE: Lobular carcinoma in situ. Long term follow-up. Cancer (Philad.) 24 (1969) 1081

HUTTER, R. V. P., R. E. SNYDER, J. C. LUCAS, F. W. FOOTE, jr., H. H. FARROW: Clinical and pathologic correlation with mammographic findings in lobular carcinoma in situ. Cancer (Philad.) 23 (1969) 826

ICHIKAWA, N., T. WAGAI, S. HAYASHI: The relation between ultrasonotomographic patterns and histological findings in mastopathy. Med. Ultrasonics 4 (1966) 13

INGLEBY, H., J. GERSHON-COHEN: Mammary abscess and mamillary fistula (pathology and roentgenology). J. A. Einstein med. Cent. (1957) 20;
Comparative Anatomy Pathology and Roentgenology of the Breast. Univ. of Pennsylvania Press, Philadelphia 1960

INGLEBY, H., L. MOORE, J. GERSHON-COHEN: Gestational breast changes; X-ray studies of human breast. Obstet. and Gynec. 10 (1957) 149

INGLIS, K.: Paget's disease of the nipple. Amer. J. Path. 22 (1946) 1

IRVINE, R. W., W. B. JAMES: Clinical and radiographic examination of the breast in well women. Scott. med. J. 14 (1969) 405

JACOBS, H.: Fortschr. Röntgenstr. 116 (1972)

JOHNSON, W. C., R. WALLRICH, E. B. HELWIG: Superficial thrombophlebitis of the chest wall. J. Amer. med. Ass. 180 (1962) 103

JONES, G. H.: Interpretation Problems in Thermography of the Female Breast. Medical Thermography. Karger, Basel 1969

KAPLAN, M., D. W. TRAPHAGEN: Superficial phlebitis of the breast. Amer. J. Surg. 94 (1957) 981

KAUFMANN, C.: Die Bedeutung der Mammographie für den untersuchenden und behandelnden Arzt. Geburtsh. u. Frauenheilk. 28 (1968) 927

KAUFMANN, C., H. HAMPERL, F. BALDUS, B. D. KI: Das lobuläre Carcinoma in situ der Mamma. Dtsch. med. Wschr. 96 (1971) 1581

KEATS, TH. E., G. F. KOENIG, K. L. RALL, D. D. WOOD: Soft tissue roentgenography of the breast. An analysis of the factors which influence roentgenographic quality and description of a new technique. Amer. J. Roentgenol. 90 (1963) 359

KENNEDY, B. J., R. BORNSTEIN, R. D. BRUNNING, D. OINES: Breast involvement in acute lymphatic leukemia. Cancer (Philad.) 25 (1970) 693

KETT, K., L. LUKACS: Direct lymphography of the breast. Lymphology 3 (1970) 3

KETT, K., L. LUKACS, G. VARGA: Über den Wert der indirekten Lymphographie beim Mammacarcinom. Bruns Beitr. klin. Chir. 218 (1970) 27

KETT, K., G. VARGA, L. LUKACS: Direct lymphography of the breast. Lymphology 3 (1970) 2

KIAER, W.: Relation of Fibroadenomatosis ("Chronic Mastitis") to Cancer of the Breast. Munksgaard, Copenhagen 1954

KISTER, S. J., C. D. HAAGENSEN: Paget's disease of the breast. Amer. J. Surg. 119 (1970) 606

KLEINSCHMIDT, O.: in ZWEIFEL-PAYR: Klinik der bösartigen Geschwülste, Bd. IV. Hirzel, Leipzig 1927

KÖNIG, F.: Mastitis chronica cystica. Zbl. Chir. 20 (1893) 49

KRAUS, F. T., R. D. NEUBECKER: The differential diagnosis of papillary tumors of the breast. Cancer (Philad.) 15 (1962) 444

KREMENS, V.: Roentgenography of the breast. Amer. J. Roentgenol. 80 (1958) 1005

KRUEGER, P.: Hilfsgerät für die Mammographie. Röntgenpraxis 25 (1972) 19

KÜBLER, E.: Über die Differentialdiagnose des pathologischen Mamma-Bildes. Fortschr. Röntgenstr. 82 (1955) 789

KÜCKENS, H.: Ein lokales Lymphogranulom der Brust in Form eines Mammatumors. Beitr. path. Anat. 80 (1928) 135

KUHN, H., H. GAJEWSKI: Die extrafokale Strahlung von Röntgendrehanodenröhren und ihr Einfluß auf die Bildqualität. Electromedica 4 (1971) 125

KUSHNER, L. N.: Hodgkin's disease simulating inflammatory breast carcinoma on mammography. Radiology 92 (1969) 350

KUZMA, J. F., W. A. D. ANDERSON: The Breast in "Pathology" vol. 2, 5th edn. Mosby, St. Louis 1966

KVASNICKA, I., J. DVORAK, B. STARA: Indirekte Mammalymphographie mit Verographin. Erste Ergebnisse. Fortschr. Röntgenstr. 115 (1971) 619

KYSER, K.: Ein Beitrag zur Diskussion über die Wahl der Strahlenqualität bei Weichstrahlaufnahmen. Vortrag auf dem Deutschen Röntgenkongreß in Düsseldorf, 1971

LAMBIRD, P. A., W. M. SHELLEY: The spatial distribution of lobular in situ mammary carcinoma. J. Amer. med. Ass. 210 (1969) 689

LANYI, M.: Quelques problemes du radiodiagnostic des tumeurs du sein non palpables. J. Radiol. Électrol. 48 (1967) 695;
Alkalmas-e a mammographia szürövizsgalatra? Magy. Rad. 19 (1967) 233;
Ist die Odelca-Kamera zur Mammographie geeignet? Röntgen-Bl. 23 (1970) 372

LANYI, M., I. LITTMAN: Die Entdeckung des klinisch okkulten Brustdrüsenkarzinoms mit der Mammographie. Chirurg 41 (1970) 169

LANYI, M., P. CITOLER, H. H. ZIPPEL: Das lobuläre Carcinoma in situ der Mamma. Symposium International Therapeutiques non mutilantes des cancéreuses du sein. Strasbourg, 27.—30. June 1972

LANYI, M., T. HERCZEG, L. TAPOLCSANYI: A mammographia jelentösége az emlödaganatok diagnosztikajaban. Orv. Hetil. 37 (1966) 1739

LANYI, M., GY. LASZLO, M. FARKAS: Kombinierte klinische und mammographische Reihenuntersuchung beim Mammakarzinom. Fortschr. Röntgenstr. 112 (1970) 18

LANYI, M., I. LITTMAN, P. RUTKAI: A klinikailag occult emlöcarcinomák diagnosztikája Mammographiaval. Orv. Hetil. 13 (1968) 697

LAPAYOWKER, M. S. u. Mitarb.: Thermographic patterns of the female breast and their relationship to carcinoma. Cancer (Philad.) 27 (1971) 819

LAVAL-JEANTET, M., M. L. AUBIN, J. VIGNAUD, R. LICHTENBERG, G. KORACH: Le rayonnement diffusé dans la formation de l'image des parties molles. Ann. Radiol. 12 (1969) 711

LAWSON, R. N.: Implications of surface temperature in the diagnosis of breast cancer. Canad. med. Ass. J. 75 (1956) 309

LEBORGNE, R.: Diagnostico de los procesos patológicos de la mamma por la radiograffia con la inyección de medios de contraste. Obstet. Ginec. lat.-amer. 2 (1944) 551;
Diagnosis of tumors of the breast by simple roentgenography. Calcifications in carcinomas. Amer. J. Roentgenol. 65 (1951) 1;
The Breast in Roentgendiagnosis. Impressora Uruguaya, Montevideo 1953;
Esteatonecrosis quistica calcificada de la mama. Tórax 16 (1967) 172

LEBORGNE, R., F. LEBORGNE, J. H. LEBORGNE: Soft tissue of the axilla in cancer of the breast. Brit. J. Radiol. 36 (1963) 494

LEDOUX-LEBARD, R., J. GARCIA-CALDERON, G. A. ESPAILLAT: Étude radiographique de la glande mammaire. Bull. Soc. Radiol. med. France 21 (1933) 418

LEE, R. M., G. M. STEVENS, R. D. CRESSMAN: A surgical appraisal of mammography-experiences with over 2000 mammograms. Surg. Clin. N. Amer. 43 (1963) 1331

LEIBER, B., G. OLBRICH: Wörterbuch der klinischen Syndrome, 3. Aufl. Urban & Schwarzenberg, München 1963

LEIS, H. P.: Presymptomatic diagnosis of breast cancer. Progr. Clin. Cancer 4 (1970) 133

LEONHARDT, T.: A case of Weber-Christian disease with roentgenographically demonstrable mammary calcifications. Amer. J. Med. 44 (1968) 140

LEVY, D. M., J. B. ERICH, A. B. HAYLES: Gynaecomastia. Postgrad. Med. 36 (1964) 234

Lewison, E. .F: Lobular carcinoma in situ of the breast. Amer. Surg. 31 (1965) 787;
The follow-up examination of the contralateral breast: From the viewpoint of the surgeon. Cancer (Philad.) 23 (1969) 809
Lewison, E. F., J. G. Lyons jr.: Relationship between breast disease and cancer. Arch. Surg. 66 (1953) 94
Lindell, M. M., J. J. Boyle: An improved method in diagnostic roentgenography of the breast. Amer. J. Roentgenol. 86 (1961) 178
Liszka, G., A. Kallo, I. Decker: Vergleichende radiologische und morphologische Untersuchung der Adiposomastie, Fibrosomastie und Gynäkomastie. Fortschr. Röntgenstr. 108 (1968) 233
Lockwood, I. H., W. Stewart: Roentgen study of physiologic and pathologic changes in mammary gland. J. Amer. med. Ass. 99 (1932) 1461
Lohbeck, H. U., H. J. Frischbier: Zur diagnostischen Treffsicherheit bei der Mammographie. Fortschr. Röntgenstr. Suppl. 172 (1969)
Lunn, G. M., J. M. Potter: Mondor's disease (subcutaneous phlebitis of the breast region). Brit. med. J. 1954/I, 1074

McDonald, I.: The natural history of mammary carcinoma. Amer. J. Surg. 111 (1966) 435
McMaster, R. C.: New developments in xeroradiography. Non-Destr. Testing 10 (1951) 8
Madding, G. F., L. R. Hershberger: Haemangioma of the breast, report of a case. Surgery 26 (1949) 685
Maier, W. P., G. P. Rosemond, P. Wittenberg, E. M. Tassoni: Cystosarcoma Phyllodes Mammae. Oncologia (Basel) 22 (1968) 145
Mannherz, K. H., P. Kuhwald: Röntgendiagnostik bei Brustdrüsenerkrankungen im Rahmen der Vorsorgeuntersuchungen. Mitteilungsdienst GBK 4 (1966) 409
Mari, Y., M. Matsuda, H. Kono, J. Moröki, N. Morishita, H. Omo: Ultrasonic diagnosis of breast diseases. Med. Ultrasonic 4 (1966) 12
Martinelli, A., U. Herrmann: Beitrag zur Mammographie, Gynecologia 167 (1969) 391
Massopust, L. C., W. D. Gardner: Infrared photographic studies of the superficial thoracic veins in the female. Surg. Gynec. Obstet. 91 (1950) 717
McDivitt, R. W., R. V. P. Hutter, F. W. Foote jr., F. W. Stewart: In situ lobular carcinoma. J. Amer. med. Ass. 201 (1967) 82
McDivitt, R. W., F. W. Stewart, J. W. Berg: Tumors of the Breast. Atlas of Tumor Pathology, 2. Serie, Fasc. 2. Armed Forces Institute of Pathology, Washington 1968
McGregor, J. K.: Hodgkin's disease of the breast. Amer. J. Surg. 99 (1960) 348
McNair, T. J., H. A. I. Dudley: Axillary lymphnodes in patients without breast carcinoma. Lancet 1960/I, 713
McWhirter, R.: Should more radical treatment be attempted in breast cancer? Amer. J. Roentgenol. 92 (1964) 3
McWilliams, C. A., F. M. Hanes: Leukemic tumors of the breast mistaken for lymphosarcoma. Amer. J. med. Sci. 14 (1912) 518—525
Menville, J. G., J. C. Bloodgood: Subcutaneous angiomas of the breast. Ann. Surg. 97 (1933) 401
Mestwerdt, W.: Die Tuberkulose der weiblichen Brustdrüse. Zbl. Gynäk. 91 (1969) 541
Mika, N., K. H. Reiss: Optimierung der Röntgenbelichtungstechnik mit Hilfe der Halbleiterspektrometrie. Röntgenpraxis 21 (1968) 164
Miller, H. W. jr., S. Kay: Infiltrating lobular carcinoma of the female mammary gland. Surg. Gynec. Obstet. 102 (1956) 661
Minagi, H., J. E. Youker: Roentgenography of breast specimens. An aid in the management of nonpalpable breast carcinoma. Amer. J. Surg. 115 (1968) 435
Misgeld, V., A. Albrecht, W. Höfer: Mammäre Leiomyomatose unter dem Bild einer Lymphangiosis carcinomatosa. Fortschr. Röntgenstr. 112 (1970) 649
Mondor, H.: Tronculite sous-cutanée subaigue de la paroi thoracique antére-latérale. Mém. Acad. Chir, 65 (1939) 1271
Muir, R.: Pathogenesis of Paget's disease of the nipple and associated lesions. Brit. J. Surg. 22 (1935) 728
Müller, J.: Über den feineren Bau und die Formen der krankhaften Geschwülste. Reimer, Berlin 1838
Muntean, E.: Ist die Röntgenuntersuchung der Mamma eine zuverlässige diagnostische Methode? Fortschr. Röntgenstr. 94 (1961) 509

Murad, T. M.: A proposed histochemical and electromicroscopic classification of human breast cancer according to cell of origin. Cancer (Philad.) 27 (1971) 288
Ultrastructure of ductular carcinoma of the breast (in situ and infiltrating lobular carcinoma). Cancer (Philad.) 27 (1971) 18
Musgrove, J. E.: Subcutaneous phlebitis of the breast. (Mondor's disease). Canad. med. Ass. J. 85 (1961) 36

Nagami, H.: Discussion of the x-ray characteristic of xeroradiographic plates. Electrophotography 4 (1962) 3
Nappi, R., A. Nibbio, G. Vita: Value of mammography and photofluorography in mass screening for breast cancer. Radiol. Electrol. 48 (1967)
Nathan, B. E., J. Jan, Burn D. P. Mac Erlean: Value of mammary thermography in differential diagnosis. Brit. med. J. 1972/II, 316
Newman, W.: Lobular carcinoma of the female breast. Ann. Surg. 164 (1966) 305
Nievelstein, J. Th. K. G.: De Isodens-Techniek of Fluidogrfie bij het Röntgen-Onderzoek van de Mamma. Diss. Schricks, Asten 1968
Notter, G., O. Melander: Klinische Diagnostik mit Thermovision. Röntgen-Bl. 21 (1968) 49

Oldfield, M. C.: Mondor's disease. A superficial phlebitis of the breast. Lancet 1962/I, 994
Oliphant, W. D.: Xeroradiography: I. Apparatus and Method of Use. Brit. J. Radiol. 28 (1955) 543
O'Mara, R. E., F. F. Ruzicka jr., A. Osborne, J. Connell jr.: Xeromammography and film mammography. Completion of a comparative study. Radiology 88 (1967) 1121
Ott, G., J. Ruef: Sarkome der Brustdrüse. Langenbecks Arch. klin. Chir. 297 (1961) 557

Paget, J.: On disease of the mammary areola preceding cancer of the mammary gland. St. Barth Hosp. Reports 10 (1874) 86
Lectures, Surgical, Pathology, Tumours, vol. II. Longman, Brown, Green & Longmans, London 1853
Palmer, R. C., R. L. Egan, B. K. Tanner, P. A. Barnette: Absorbed dose in mammography using three tungsten and three molybdenum target tubes. Radiology 101 (1971) 697
Pape, C., H.-E. Stegner: Vortrag Dtsch. Ges. für Elektronenmikroskopie. Karlsruhe 1971
Pascoe, H. R.: Tumors composed of immature granulocytes occuring in the breast in chronic granulocytic leukemia. Cancer (Philad.) 25 (1970) 697
Patil, K. F.: The influence of physical and biological factors on thermal patterns produced by breast tumors. Annual Scientific Meeting of American Thermographic Society. San Francisco, June 1972
Paulsen, C. A.: Gynaecomastia. In: Textbook of Endocrinology, 4th edn., ed by. R. H. Williams, Saunders, Philadelphia 1968
Petracic, B., F. K. Mörl, R. Bähr, R. Wenzel: Mammasarkome. Langenbecks Arch. klin. Chir. 326 (1970) 239
Philipp, R., B. Heymer, H. J. Maurer: Zur diagnostischen Leistungsbreite der Mammographie. Chirurg 35 (1964) 398
Picard, J. D., J. P. Desprez-Curely: Place de la mammographie parmi les éléments du diagnostic des lesions mammaires. Rev. Prat. (Paris) 24 (1968) 2755
van der Plaats, G. J., J. Th. K. G. Nievelstein: Die Mammographie nach Dobretsberger. J. Radiol. Électrol. 48 (1967) 656
Prager, W., V. Hasert: Zur Differentialdiagnose von Rundherden im Mammogramm. Radiol. Diagn. (Berlin) 10 (1969) 369
Price, J. L., P. D. Butter: The reduction of radiation and exposure time in mammography. Brit. J. Radiol. 43 (1970) 251
Prives, M. G.: Rentgenografia limfaticeskoj sistemy. Zit. nach: I. Kvasnicka, J. Dvorak, B. Stara: Indirekte Mamma-Lymphographie mit Verografin. Fortschr. Röntgenstr. 115 (1971) 619
Puente Duany, M.: Lipofibroadenosis de aspecto tumoral de las mamas. Arch. cuba. Cancer. 10 (1951) 326;
Hiperplasia adenofibrolipomatosa o fibrolipomatosis periglandular de aspecto tumoral de la mama. Arch. cuba. Cancer. 18 (1961) 361
Randall, K. J., J. E. Spalding: Primary Hodgkin's disease of breast. Guy's Hosp. Rep. 94 (1947) 137
Rasmussen, Th.: Centralsygehuset. Hjorring, Dänemark, Persönliche Mitteilung, 1967

RECLUS, P.: La maladie kystique des mamelles. Rev. Chir. (Paris) 3 (1883); Bull. Soc. anat. Paris 8 (1883) 428

REHM, A., M. AMIRFALLAH, O. FISCHEDICK: Rundherde der Mamma. Radiologe 10 (1970) 149

REIMANN, ST., P. S. SEABOLD: Correlation of x-ray picture with histology in certain breast lesions. Amer. J. Cancer 17 (1933) 34

REINARTZ, G., K. H. KÄRCHER, H. MISRI: Veränderungen im Röntgenbild der weiblichen Brust aufgrund hormoneller Einflüsse. Fortschr. Röntgenstr. 113 (1970) 443

REINHARDT, K.: Die Bedeutung der Mamma-Aufnahme für Diagnose und Verlaufsbeobachtung des Brustkrebses. Fortschr. Röntgenstr. 78 (1953) 714

RIES, E.: Diagnostic lipiodol injection into milk ducts followed by abscess formation. Amer. J. Obstet. Gynec. 20 (1930) 414

ROACH, J. F., H. E. HILLEBOE: Xeroradiography. Am. J. Roentgenol. 73 (1955) 5

ROACH, J. F., H. E. HILLEBOE: Xeroradiography. J. Amer. med. Ass. 157 (1955) 899

ROBBINS, G. F., J. H. BROTHERS, W. F. EBERHARD, S. QUAR: Is aspiration biopsy of breast cancer dangerous to the patient? Cancer (Philad.) 7 (1954) 774

ROGERS, J. V., R. W. POWELL, R. L. EGAN: Comparative mammography study. Amer. J. Roentgenol. 97 (1966) 748

ROMANO, S. A. E. M. MCFETRIDGE: Limitations and dangers of mammography by contrast mediums. J. Amer. med. Ass. 110 (1938) 1905

RONNEN, J. F. V.: Het Roentgenonderzoek van der Mamma zonder Toepassing van Contrastmiddeln. Mouton, Utrecht, Med. Fak., Diss. v. 1956

ROTTER, J.: Zur Topographie des Mammakarzinoms. Arch. J. Klin. Chir. 58 (1899) 346

RUMMEL, W., G. KINDERMANN, J. WEISHAAR: Thermographie — Galaktographie. Diagnostik 4 (1971) 523

RUZICKA, F. F. jr., L. KAUFMANN, G. SHAPIRO, J. V. PEREZ, E. E. GROSSI: Xeromammography and film mammography. A comparative study. Radiology 85 (1965) 260

SALOMON, A.: Beiträge zur Pathologie und Klinik der Mammacarcinome. Arch. klin. Chir. 103 (1913) 573

SAMUEL, E., G. B. YOUNG: Screening for breast cancer. Lancet 1968/II, 215

SCHERER, E., J. SEIFERT: Die Bedeutung der Mammographie als Reihenuntersuchung in der Tumorvorsorge. Fortschr. Röntgenstr. 109 (1968) 766

SCHIMMELBUSCH, C.: Das Cystadenom der Mamma. Arch. klin. Chir. 44 (1892) 117

SEABOLD, P. S.: Roentgenograpic diagnosis of disesaes of the breast Surg. Gynec. Obstet. 53 (1931) 461

SEEMANN, H. E.: Physikalische Betrachtungen zur Weichteil-Radiographie. Med. Radiogr. u. Photogr. (Kodak) March 1967 (p. 22)

SEIDEL, K.: Zur Technik der Mammographie, Fortschr. Röntgenstr. 101 (1964) 656

SELAWRY, O. S., J. F. HOLLAND: Cholesteric thermography for direct visualization of temperatures over tumors. Proc. Amer. Ass. Cancer Res. 7 (1966) 63

SEMB, C.: Pathologic-anatomical and clinical investigations of fibroadenomatosis cystica mammae and its relation to other pathological conditions in the mamma, especially cancer. Acta chir. scand. Suppl. 10, 64 (1928) 1

SHAPIRO, S., PH. STRAX, L. VENET: Evaluation of periodic breast cancer screening with mammography. Methodology and early observations. J. Amer. med. Ass. 195 (1966) 731
Periodic breast cancer screening in reducing mortality from breast cancer. J. Amer. med. Ass. 215 (1971) 1777

SHIMKIN, M. B.: End results in cancer of the breast. Cancer (Philad.) 20 (1967) 1039

SIMPSON, T. E., R. L. VAN DERVOORT, H. B. LYNN: Giant fibroadenoma (benign cystosarcoma phylloides). Report of case in 13-year-old-girl. Surgery 65 (1969) 341

SINNER, W.: Zur Frage der männlichen Mammasarkome. Strahlentherapie 114 (1961) 595

SMITH, B. H., H. B. TAYLOR: The occurrence of bone and cartilage in mammary tumors. Amer. J. Clin. Path. 59 (1969) 610

SNYDER, R. E.: Mammography and lobular carcinoma in situ. Surg. Gynec. Obstet. 122 (1966) 255

SPALDING, J. E.: Adeno-lipoma and lipoma of the breast. Guy's Hosp. Rep. 94 (1945) 80

SPRATT, J. S., S. T. DONEGAN: Cancer of the Breast. Saunders, Philadelphia 1967

STAPLEY, L. A., M. B. DOCKERTY, S. W. HARRINGTON: Comedocarcinoma of the breast. Surg. Gynec. Obstet. 100 (1955) 707

STEGNER, H.-E.: Erkrankungen der Brustdrüse. Histopathologie der Mammatumoren. In: Gynäkologie und Geburtshilfe, Bd. III, hrsg. von O. KÖSER, V. FRIEDBERG, K. G. OBER, K. THOMSEN, J. ZANDER. Thieme, Stuttgart 1972

STEIN, J. J.: The follow-up examination in the detection of localized cancer in the contralateral breast: From the standpoint of the radiation therapist. Cancer (Philad.) 23 (1969) 811

STEINTHAL, C. F.: Zur Dauerheilung des Brustkrebses. Beitr. z. klin. Chir. 47 (1905) 226

STEVENS, G. M.: Prospects of survey mammography. Sixth Annual Mammography Seminar, San Juan. Puerto Rico 1967 (lecture)

STEVENS, G. M., J. F. WEIGEN: Mammography survey for breast cancer detection. A 2-year study of 1,223 clinically negative asymptomatic women over 40. Cancer (Philad.) 19 (1966) 51;
Survey mammography as a case finding method for routine and postmastectomized patients. Cancer (Philad.) 24 (1969) 1201

STEWART, F. W.: Tumors of the Breast. Atlas of Pathology Sect. IX, Fasc. 34. Armed Forces Institute of Pathology, Washington 1950

STEWART, F. W., N. TREVES: Lymphangiosarcoma in postmastectomy lymphedema; a report of six cases in elephantiasis chirurgica. Cancer (N. Y.) 1 (1968) 64

STIEVE, F. E., L. WIDENMANN: Die Beurteilung der Güte eines Röntgenbildes. Röntgen-Bl. 20 (1967) 199

STRAX, PH., A. OPPENHEIM: New apparatus for mass screening in mammography. Amer. J. Roentgenol. 102 (1968) 941
Breast types in mammography, N. Y. St. J. Med. 66 (1966) 724

STRAX, PH., M. M. POMERANZ: Nonmalignant variations in mammography. Amer. J. Roentgenol. 92 (1964) 21

STRAX, PH., L. VENET, S. SHAPIRO, S. GROSS: Mammography and clinical examination in mass screening for cancer of the breast. Cancer 20 (1967) 2184

SUSTERIC, Z.: Über eine spontane beiderseitige Nekrose der Mamma. Chirurg 33 (1962) 485

SWEARINGEN, A. G.: Thermography: Report of the radiographic and thermographic examinations of the breast of 100 patients. Radiology 85 (1965) 818

TAYLOR, G. M., G. H. TENNEY: Field evaluation of industrial xeroradiography. Non-Destr. Testing 13 (1955) 12

TORTORA, M., A. TOTI, R. NAPPI: Our experience on mass breast screening with mammography. J. Radiol. Électrol. 48 (1967) 662

TOTI, A.: Die technischen Möglichkeiten der Schirmbildphotographie für die Mammographie. Odelca Mirror 8 (1969) 14

TRICOIRE, J., L. MARIEL, J. P. AMIEL, G. POIROT, J. LACOUR, S. FAJBISOWICZ: Thermographie en plaque. Presse méd. 78 (1970) 2483

URBAN, J. A.: The treatment of early cancer of the breast. Postgrad Med. 27 (1960) 389

URBAN, J. A., F. E. ADAIR: Sclerosing adenosis. Cancer (N. Y.) 2 (1969) 625

VAILLANT, W. K. TH.: Versuche zur Früherkennung des Mammacarcinoms durch Thermographie. Diss. München 1970

VELPEAU, A.: The diseases of the breast and mammary region. Zit. nach C. D. HAAGENSEN: Diseases of the breast. Saunders, Philadelphia 1956

VERHAGEN, H.: Local haemorrhage and necrosis of the skin and underlying tissues during anti-coagulant therapy with Dicumarol or Dicumacyl. Acta med. Scand. 148 (1954) 453

VOGEL, W.: Die Röntgendarstellung von Mammatumoren. Arch. klin. Chir. 171 (1932) 618

WACHSMANN, F., A. DIMOTSIS: Kurven und Tabellen für die Strahlentherapie. Hirzel, Stuttgart 1957

WAGAI, T., R. MIYAZAWA, K. ITO: Ultrasonic diagnosis of intracranial disease, breast tumors, and abdominal disease. In: Ultrasonic Energy-

Biological Investigations and Medical Applications; ed. by E. KELLY. University of Illinois Press, Urbana 1965 (pp. 346—364)

WARNER, N. E.: Lobular carcinoma of the breast .Cancer (Philad.) 23 (1969) 840

WARREN, ST. L.: A roentgenologic study of the breast. Amer. J. Roentgenol. 24 (1930) 113

WEBB, A. J.: The diagnostic cytology of breast carcinoma. Brit. J. Surg. 57 (1970) 259

WEINSTEIN, E. C., H. L. ENDLICH: Mammography. J. Amer. Geriat. Soc. 14 (1966) 394

WEISHAAR, J., W. D. RUMMEL, G. KINDERMANN: Die Milchgangsdarstellung mit wasserlöslichem Kontrastmittel (Galaktographie) bei sezernierender Mamma. Erste Ergebnisse. Fortschr. Röntgenstr. 112 (1970) 1

WILLIAMS, G. A.: Thoraco-epigastric phlebitis producing dyspnea. J. Amer. med. Ass. 96 (1931) 2196

WINSBERG, F., M. ELKIN, J. MACY: Detection of radiographic abnormalities in mammograms by means of optical scanning and computer analysis. Radiology 89 (1967) 211

WITTEN, D. M.: (Mayo Clinic, Rochester, Minnesota). Personal communications 1967 and 1968;
The Breast. Year Book Medical Publishers, Chicago 1969

WITTEN, D. M., D. L. THURBER: Mammography as a routine screening examination for detecting breast cancer. Amer. J. Roentgenol. 92 (1964) 14

WOLFE, J. N.: Mammography: Report on its use in women with breasts abnormal and normal on physical examination. Radiology 83 (1964) 244; 262;
Mammography as a screening examination in breast cancer. Radiology 84 (1965) 703;
Mammography: errors in diagnosis. Radiology 87 (1966) 214;
Mammography. Thomas, Springfield 1967;

A study of breast parenchyma by mammography in the normal woman and those with benign and malignant disease. Radiology 89 (1967) 201;
Mammography: ducts as a sole indicator of breast carcinoma. Radiology 89 (1967) 206;
Xerography of the breast. Radiology 91 (1968) 231;
Xeroradiography of the breast. Oncology 23 (1969) 113;
Xeroradiography of the breast. Cancer (Philad.) 23 (1969) 791;
Breast Xeroradiography. Cancer 24 (1969) 1222;
The prominent duct pattern as an indicator of cancer risk. Oncology 23 (1969) 149;
Xeroradiography of the Breast. Thomas, Springfield 1972-75

WOLFE, J. N., R. P. DOOLEY, L. E. HERKINS: Xeroradiography of the breast. Cancer 28 (1971) 1569

WRIGHT, D. J., F. M. NICHINI, H. M. STAUFFER: Beryllium window tubes for mammographic examinations. Brit. J. Radiol. 44 (1971) 480

WYNDER, E. L.: Identification of woman at high risk for breast cancer. Cancer 24 (1969) 1235

ZAJICEK, J.: Zytologische Untersuchung von Punktaten in der Diagnostik der Brustdrüse. Schweiz. med. Wschr. 99 (1969) 1271

ZINSER, H.-K.: Mammakarzinom. Diagnose und Differentialdiagnose. Thieme, Stuttgart 1972

ZOLTOWSKA, A., H. KOZLOWSKI: Investigations on the transformation of fibroadenoma of the breast into malignant cystosarcoma phylloides. Neoplasma (Bratisl.) 16 (1969) 549

ZUPPINGER, A.: In: Lehrbuch der Röntgendiagnostik, Bd. II, hrsg. von H. R. SCHINZ, W. E. BAENSCH, E. FRIEDEL, E. UEHLINGER. Thieme, Stuttgart 1952

ZWICKER, H., M. THELEN: Lymphogranulom in der Mamma. Fortschr. Röntgenstr. 116 (1972) 124

Index

Note: page numbers in italics refer to illustrations.